CLASSICS IN
CLINICAL
DERMATOLOGY

With Biographical Sketches

50TH ANNIVERSARY SECOND EDITION

50

50TH ANNIVERSARY · SECOND EDITION ·

WALTER BROWN SHELLEY, MD, PhD, MACP

and

JOHN THORNE CRISSEY, MD

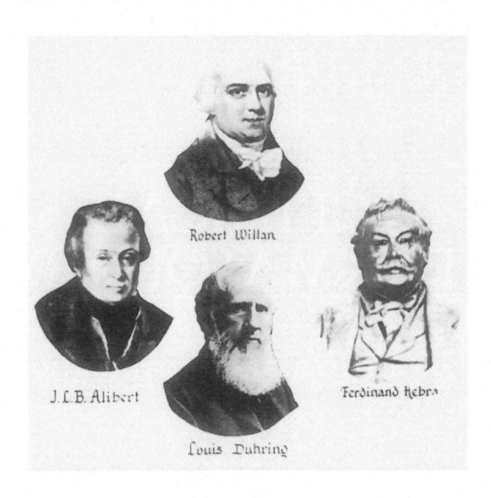

Robert Willan

J.L.B. Alibert

Louis Duhring

Ferdinand Hebra

CLASSICS IN CLINICAL DERMATOLOGY

With Biographical Sketches
50TH ANNIVERSARY SECOND EDITION

CLASSICS IN CLINICAL DERMATOLOGY

With Biographical Sketches

50TH ANNIVERSARY SECOND EDITION

WALTER BROWN SHELLEY, MD, PhD, MACP
Department of Dermatology, Medical College of Ohio, Toledo, Ohio

and

JOHN THORNE CRISSEY, MD
Department of Dermatology, Keck School of Medicine, University of Southern California, Los Angeles, California

The Parthenon Publishing Group

International Publishers in Medicine, Science & Technology

A CRC PRESS COMPANY

BOCA RATON LONDON NEW YORK WASHINGTON, D.C.

To
Our wives, Dorinda and Alice
For the joy and happiness they have brought into our lives

Library of Congress Cataloging-in-Publication Data
Classics in clinical dermatology with biographical
sketches/[edited by] Walter B.Shelley and
John Thorne Crissey. —2nd ed.
p. cm.
'50th anniversary.'
Previous ed. cataloged under: Shelley, Walter B.
Previous ed. published with title: Classics in
clinical dermatology.
Includes bibliographical references and index.
ISBN 1-84214-207-0 (alk. paper)
1. Dermatology. 2. Dermatology—History—
Sources. 3. Dermatologists. I. Shelley, Walter B.
(Walter Brown), 1917– Classics in clinical
dermatology. II. Shelley, Walter B. (Walter
Brown), 1917– III. Crissey, John Thorne, 1924–
R136.C56 2003
616.5'009–dc21
2003056381

British Library Cataloguing in Publication Data
Classics in clinical dermatology with biographical
sketches. —50th anniversary 2nd ed.
1. Dermatology 2. Dermatologists—Biography
I. Shelley, Walter B. (Walter Brown), 1917–
II. Crissey, John Thorne
616.5

ISBN 0-203-49383-4 Master e-book ISBN

ISBN 0-203-59642-0 (Adobe eReader Format)
ISBN 1-84214-207-0 (Print Edition)

Published in the USA by
The Parthenon Publishing Group
345 Park Avenue South
10th Floor
New York, NY 10010
USA

This edition published in the Taylor & Francis e-Library, 2005.

"To purchase your own copy of this or any of Taylor & Francis or Routledge's collection of thousands of eBooks please go to
www.eBookstore.tandf.co.uk."

Published in the UK and Europe by
The Parthenon Publishing Group
23–25 Blades Court, Deodar Road
London SW15 2NU
UK

Contents

Preface to Second Edition   xviii

Preface to First Edition   xx

Introduction to First Edition   xxii

Acknowledgements for First Edition   xxiv

Acknowledgements for Second Edition   xxvi

List of Illustrations   xxviii

PART I   **THE EARLY WORKERS**

    Robert Willan   2

1.   Purpose of a Treatise on Cutaneous Diseases;

2.   Definitions of Technical Terms;

3.   Psoriasis;

4.   Ichthyosis;

5.   Erythema Nodosum;

6.   Pemphigus

    Thomas Bateman   14

1.   Molluscum Contagiosum;

2.   Papular Urticaria;

3.   Eczema;

4.   Sycosis Barbae

    Michael Underwood   21

    Sclerema Neonatorum

    Jean Louis Alibert   24

1.   Lupus Vulgaris;

2.   Keloid;

3.   Mycosis Fungoides;

4.   Dermatolysis

     Armand Trousseau   35

     Cutaneous Diphtheria

     Luca Stulli   38

     Mal de Meleda

     Pierre François Rayer   41

1.   Ecthyma;

2.   Cheilitis Exfoliativa;

3.   Lingua Nigra

     Samuel Plumbe   45

1.   Acne Vulgaris;

2.   Tinea Capitis

     Alphée Cazenave   49

1.   Pemphigus Foliaceus;

2.   Lupus Erythematosus

     Julius Otto Ludwig Moeller   55

     Atrophic Glossitis

     Auguste Nélaton   56

     Malum Perforans Pedis

     Alphonse Devergie   59

1.   Nummular Eczema;

2.   Pityriasis Rubra Pilaris

     Max Burchardt   63

     Erythrasma

     Ernest Bazin   65

1.   Erythema Induratum;

2.   Hydroa Vacciniforme

     Thomas Addison   69

1.   Xanthoma;

2.   Morphea

      Camille Gibert   75

      Pityriasis Rosea

      Samuel Wilks   77

      Verruca Necrogenica

PART II   THE DISCIPLES

      Ferdinand von Hebra   80

1.   Erythema Multiforme;

2.   Lichen Scrofulosorum;

3.   Prurigo;

4.   Pityriasis Rubra (Exfoliative Dermatitis of Hebra);

5.   Rhinoscleroma;

6.   Impetigo Herpetiformis

      Jules Parrot   92

      Edema Neonatorum

      Erasmus Wilson   94

1.   Lichen Planus;

2.   Nevus Araneus;

3.   Exfoliative Dermatitis;

4.   Neurotic Excoriations

      Edward Nettleship   103

      Urticaria Pigmentosa

      Richard von Volkmann   105

      Cheilitis Glandularis

      Tilbury Fox   107

1.   Impetigo Contagiosa;

2.   Dysidrosis

      James Paget   112

      Paget's Disease

PART III   THE GOLDEN AGE

Louis Duhring — 116

1. Prurigo Hiemalis;

2. Dermatitis Herpetiformis

Isidor Neumann — 126

Pemphigus Vegetans

Walter G.Smith — 129

Monilethrix

Moritz Kaposi — 131

1. Dermatitis Papillaris Capillitii (Acne Keloidalis Nuchae);

2. Multiple Idiopathic Hemorrhagic Sarcoma;

3. Xeroderma Pigmentosum;

4. Kaposi's Varicelliform Eruption

William Augustus Hardaway — 137

Prurigo Nodularis

Alfred Goldscheider — 140

Epidermolysis Bullosa

Heinrich Irenaeus Quincke — 142

Angioneurotic Edema

Jonathan Hutchinson — 144

1. Hydroa Aestivale;

2. Solid Edema;

3. Arsenical Keratosis;

4. Angioma Serpiginosum

August Breisky — 151

Kraurosis Vulvae

Julius Friedrich Rosenbach — 153

Erysipeloid

Ernst Lebericht Wagner — 155

1. Colloid Milium;

2. Dermatomyositis

Henry Radcliffe-Crocker   158

1.   Dermatitis Gangrenosa Infantum;

2.   Dermatitis Repens (Acrodermatitis Continua);

3.   Erythema Elevatum Diutinum;

4.   Granuloma Annulare

Paul Gerson Unna   168

Seborrheic Dermatitis

Charles Quinquaud   174

Folliculitis Decalvans

James C.White   176

Keratosis Follicularis

J.J.Pringle   180

Adenoma Sebaceum

Thomas Colcott Fox   184

Erythema Gyratum Perstans

Ernst Schweninger   188

Multiple Benign Tumor-like New Growths of the Skin (Schweninger-Buzzi Anetoderma)

Sigmund Pollitzer   191

Acanthosis Nigricans

Ernest Besnier   196

Atopic Dermatitis

H.G.Brooke   199

Epithelioma Adenoides Cysticum (Trichoepithelioma)

William F.Milroy   202

Hereditary Edema of the Legs (Milroy's Disease)

Émile Vidal   204

Keratosis Blennorrhagica

Vittorio Mibelli   208

1.   Angiokeratoma;

2.   Porokeratosis

Andrew Rose Robinson   214

Hidrocystoma

John Addison Fordyce   217

1.   Angiokeratoma of the Scrotum;

2.   Pseudo-colloid of the Lips

Henri Rendu   222

Hereditary Hemorrhagic Telangiectasia (Rendu-Osler-Weber Syndrome)

Antonin Poncet   225

Pyogenic Granuloma

Domenico Majocchi   227

Purpura Annularis Telangiectodes (Majocchi's Disease)

Henri Hallopeau   231

1.   Lichen Sclerosus et Atrophicus;

2.   Acrodermatitis Continua

Benjamin Robinson Schenck   237

Sporotrichosis

Caesar Boeck   239

Sarcoidosis

PART IV   THE EXPANDING UNIVERSE

Jean-Louis Brocq   245

1.   Pseudopelade;

2.   Keratosis Pilaris;

3.   Neurodermatitis Circumscripta;

4.   Congenital Ichthyosiform Erythroderma;

5.   Parapsoriasis

Edvard Ehlers   256

The Ehlers-Danlos Syndrome

George Henry Fox   259

Fox-Fordyce Disease

Abraham Buschke   262

Scleredema Adultorum

Martin Feeney Engman   265

Infectious Eczematoid Dermatitis

Theodor Escherich   268

Erythema Infectiosum

Josef Jadassohn   270

1.   Macular Atrophy;

2.   Granulosis Rubra Nasi;

3.   Cutis Verticis Gyrata;

4.   Pachyonychia Congenita

Eduard Jacobi   278

Poikilodermia Vascularis Atrophicans

Felix Pinkus   282

Lichen Nitidus

Carl Leiner   286

Leiner's Disease

Grover Wende   288

Erythema Figurata Perstans

Jay Frank Schamberg   291

1.   Schamberg's Disease;

2.   Grain Itch

Louis Queyrat   298

Erythroplasia

J.E.McDonagh   301

Nevoxantho-Endothelioma

John T.Bowen   305

Chronic Atypical Epithelial Proliferation (Bowen's Disease)

Benjamin Lipschuetz   310

Ulcus Vulvae Acutum

Richard L.Sutton   312

1. Periadenitis Mucosa Necrotica Recurrens;

2. Leucoderma Acquisitum Centrifugum (Sutton's Nevus)

C.Guy Lane   317

Chromoblastomycosis

Max Winkler   320

Chondrodermatitis Nodularis Chronica Helicis

Jean Darier   323

1. Darier's Disease;

2. Pseudo-xanthoma Elasticum;

3. Erythema Annulare Centrifugum

Gustav Riehl   331

1. Tuberculosis Verrucosa Cutis;

2. Riehl's Melanosis

F.Parkes-Weber   335

Relapsing Non-suppurative Nodular Panniculitis

Aldo Castellani   338

Dermatosis Papulosa Nigra

Henri Gougerot and Paul Blum   340

Pigmented Purpuric Lichenoid Dermatitis

George Pernet   344

Symmetric Erythema of the Soles

Bruno Bloch   347

Incontinentia Pigmenti

Francis E.Senear and Barney Usher   350

Pemphigus Erythematodes

Erich Urbach   356

Necrobiosis Lipoidica Diabeticorum

G.A.Grant Peterkin   360

Orf

Marion B.Sulzberger and William Garbe   362

Exudative Discoid and Lichenoid Chronic Dermatosis (Sulzberger-Garbe Syndrome)

Hulusi Behçet 369

Triple Symptom Complex (Behçet's Disease)

Howard Hailey and Hugh Hailey 371

Familial Benign Chronic Pemphigus

João Paulo Vieira 375

Fogo Salvagem

Stuart D.Allen and John P.O'Brien 378

1. Tropical Anidrosis;

2. Actinic Granuloma (O'Brien's Granuloma)

Johannes Fabry 384

Angiokeratoma Corporis Diffusum (Fabry's Disease)

Agostino Pasini and Luis E.Pierini 387

Atrophoderma of Pasini and Pierini

Louis A.Brunsting 393

Pyoderma Gangrenosum

Friederich Wegener 396

Wegener's Granulomatosis

Albert Sézary 399

Sézary's Syndrome (T-cell Erythroderma)

Masao Ota 402

Nevus Fusco-coeruleus Ophthalmomaxillaris, Oculodermal Melanocytosis (Nevus of Ota)

S.William Becker 405

1. Necrolytic Migratory Erythema (Glucagonoma Syndrome);

2. Becker's Nevus (Melanosis and Hypertrichosis)

Clarence S.Livingood 410

Dhobie Dermatitis

Eugene M.Farber 414

Hypertensive Ulcer

Sophie Spitz — 418

Spitz Nevus (Benign Juvenile Melanoma)

PART V   **THE LAST 50 YEARS**

Walter F.Lever — 423

Bullous Pemphigoid

Max Jessner — 426

Jessner's Lymphocytic Infiltrate

Ferdinando Gianotti and Agostino Crosti — 429

Gianotti-Crosti Syndrome (Papular Acrodermatitis of Childhood)

Ian Bruce Sneddon — 433

1. Sneddon's Syndrome;

2. Sneddon-Wilkinson Disease

Darrell Sheldon Wilkinson — 436

Subcorneal Pustular Dermatosis (Sneddon-Wilkinson Disease)

Alan Lyell — 440

Toxic Epidermal Necrolysis (Lyell's Syndrome)

Walter B.Shelley — 443

1. Larva Currens;

2. Cold Erythema;

3. Aquagenic Urticaria;

4. Autoimmune Progesterone Sensitivity Dermatitis;

5. Piezogenic Pedal Papules;

6. Pincer Nails;

7. Mid-dermal Elastolysis Wrinkles;

8. Adrenergic Urticaria;

9. Non-pigmenting Fixed Drug Eruption;

10. Autoimmune Estrogen Dermatitis;

11. Abacus Nodule;

12. IgE Bullous Disease;

13. Aquadynia

William Bennett Bean   459

Blue Rubber-Bleb Nevus Syndrome (Bean's Syndrome)

Earl W.Netherton   462

Netherton's Syndrome

Harold O.Perry   466

Reticular Erythematous Mucinosis (REM Syndrome)

Albert M.Kligman   469

Telogen Effluvium

John Thorne Crissey   474

Calcaneal Petechiae (Black Heel, Talon Noir)

Robert W.Goltz   476

Focal Dermal Hypoplasia Syndrome (Goltz Syndrome)

Peter Samman   479

Yellow Nail Syndrome

R.D.Sweet   482

Acute Febrile Neutrophilic Dermatosis (Sweet's Syndrome)

André Bazex   485

1.   Acrokeratosis Paraneoplastica (Bazex Syndrome);

2.   Follicular Atrophoderma and Basal Cell Carcinoma Syndrome (Bazex Atrophoderma)

Ervin Epstein   489

Acanthoma Fissuratum

Marvin Chernosky   491

Disseminated Superficial Actinic Porokeratosis (DSAP)

Amir H.Mehregan   494

Reactive Perforating Collagenosis

Tomisaku Kawasaki   497

Kawasaki Disease (Muco-cutaneous Lymph Node Syndrome)

Thomas B.Fitzpatrick   500

The Ash Leaf Macule of Tuberous Sclerosis

Lawrence M.Solomon   503

Epidermal Nevus Syndrome (Solomon's Syndrome)

Ralph Grover   506

Transient Acantholytic Dermatosis (Grover's Disease)

Shigeo Ofuji   509

1. Eosinophilic Pustular Folliculitis (Ofuji's Disease);

2. Papuloerythroderma of Ofuji

George C.Wells   513

Eosinophilic Cellulitis (Wells' Syndrome)

Peyton E.Weary   517

1. Weary's Syndrome;

2. Cowden's Syndrome

Rona M.MacKie   521

Juvenile Plantar Dermatosis

Thomas J.Lawley   524

Pruritic Urticarial Papules and Plaques of Pregnancy (PUPPP)

Steven Kossard and Richard K.Winkelmann   527

Necrobiotic Xanthogranuloma

Grant J.Anhalt   531

Paraneoplastic Pemphigus

Index   534

Preface to Second Edition

This book began in 1946 as a dream of the senior author, who was then a resident in dermatology at the University of Pennsylvania. Like most beginners, he felt lost in the sophisticated disease discussions of the experts at clinico-pathologic conferences. He discovered, at last, that a marvelous key to enlightenment lay in the original articles in which would-be sponsors of 'new diseases' were forced, by the nature of the subject, to lay out the facts well enough to convince a knowledgeable and skeptical readership.

The book came to fruition when the senior was joined, in 1950, by the junior author, a new resident in dermatology at Penn, who shared his enthusiasm and insights. The two of us worked together happily and harmoniously for the next 3 years, collecting original disease descriptions and biographic material. We badgered the staff of the Philadelphia College of Physicians' Library and accosted relentlessly, by mail and telephone, the dermatologic cognoscenti and elite in all parts of the Western World.

The result, the *Classics in Clinical Dermatology,* appeared in 1953, 50 years ago. The present reincarnation of the work represents, to the best of our knowledge, the only time the second edition of a medical publication has appeared half a century after the first, brought up to date by the original authors.

Many of the diseases included in our pages had been described in one form or another by others in earlier times. Indeed, it is likely that an inspection of the thousands of case reports and disease vignettes buried in the published archives and society transactions of the past 150 years would raise the level from 'many' to 'most'. To explain, with scientific rigor, how certain of the new disease descriptions in this grand dermatologic database came to merit a place in the dermatologic textbooks of today is almost impossible. It would require the application of modern chaos theory by highly motivated individuals endowed with the morphologic skills of a Ferdinand Hebra and the mathematical genius of a Jules Poincaré.

It is, however, both possible and of interest to identify by historical study several paths that have led to the acceptance of many of our skin diseases as *sui generis*. A few of the entities are so striking or unusual that they were accepted on the spot as new by the dermatologists of the time who felt instinctively and correctly that they could not have been overlooked before. Others owe their success to clinicians with a special talent attached to what might be called the Jonathan Hutchinson genre—the ability, so prominently displayed by the English master, to store cases in the memory and identify similarities in subsequent cases, even when months or years pass between examples. Numerous instances of the exercise of this talent grace the pages of this book.

Still others owe their acceptance to clinicians endowed with an even more uncommon skill, the ability to synthesize, to determine by cogent observation that large numbers of disease entities cluttering up the literature under many different names are actually variants of a single entity. Erythema multiforme and dermatitis herpetiformis were created by the application of this skill. Finally, certain of the disease descriptions included in our pages triumphed over earlier versions of equal validity simply because they were published in more prestigious or widely read journals, or in languages spoken or understood by the influential in the medico-scientific world. Such are the facts of life.

Many of the entities included in this book are grave and of great importance. Others are trivial. Some readers may find this diversity disturbing, but we point out that this is exactly the mix that appears every day before dermatologists in their offices and clinics. It is the central strength of the specialty that its practitioners, familiar with both, can tell them apart.

Over the years both of us have received many requests for copies of the 'Classics', which has long been out of print. We believe the time has come to expand the work and make it available once again, both for the beginner who can use it as 'a marvelous key to enlightenment', and for the experienced who can appreciate and take pride in the talents and efforts of colleagues and predecessors.

Walter B.Shelley
John T.Crissey

Preface to First Edition

No previous attempt has been made to gather together, in English, the most significant of the clinical dermatologic writings. The task is one of selection. For some diseases there is no really definitive account; they have been a part of man's common store of knowledge since he began to record it. For others, such accounts exist, and it is with these that we have been concerned. The establishment of a disease picture requires of the observer the power to perceive the new as new, and although the 95 men whose 143 descriptions are presented here differed in every conceivable way—race, age, time, background, education, temperament, and ability—they had that one faculty in common.

The diseases depicted vary from daily clinic fare to the rarest of the rare. Some are case reports, lucky finds for individuals whose names are perpetrated because of a fortunate afternoon in the ambulatorium. Others are the fruit of countless hours in the meticulous study of many patients, the application of the mature mind to diversities and similarities in clinical material, masterpieces of conceptual and correlative thinking.

We have begun our work with Robert Willan's *On Cutaneous Diseases*. If there be any date in history to which one can point and say, 'Here is the beginning of modern dermatology', it is 1796, the year in which he began his treatise. With few exceptions, cutaneous disease descriptions prior to this time are difficult to identify, with any real assurance, with the entities we accept today. Willan's own indictment of his predecessors and contemporaries seems justified:

> 'They employ the same terms in very different significations. They also make artificial, and often inconsistent arrangements, some reducing all the diseases under two or three genera, while others, too studious of amplification, apply new names to different stages of appearances of the same complaint. Those who attempt to theorize on the subject are seldom clear and satisfactory.'

In the editing of the articles we have been very careful to preserve continuity. Histologic and purely laboratory particulars have been omitted. The important clinical material has been presented in its entirety, except in those few cases in which needless repetition was encountered. These accounts are not synopses. Every sentence appears exactly as its author wrote it. The length of the descriptions is not always proportional to the frequency of the disease, nor to its importance. It is, rather, a reflection of the enthusiasm and temperament of the author, or of the color inherent in the material he had at hand. Descriptions of the manifestations of syphilis have not been included. We feel that they merit a separate volume.

Unless otherwise stated, the translations given are our own. In this matter we have attempted, like all translators, to find that middle road between a rendering so stiff and literal as to be unreadable, and one so free that it can no longer be considered the work of the original author. Footnotes to the articles indicate the publication in which they appeared, and those to the biographies indicate the chief sources from which the biographical material was drawn.

That many of the greatest names in dermatology are missing from these pages is not to be construed as an indication of incompleteness. There are those whose talents have been directed always toward the elaboration, the detailing, the polishing of these disease entities, and toward the ultimate purpose of it all, the treatment of the patient. Others have devoted their lives to the advancement of our knowledge in the laboratory. The tremendous progress the specialty has made in the past 150 years has been due to this happy combination of careful clinical study and inspired laboratory activity.

Walter B.Shelley
John T.Crissey

Introduction to First Edition

The genealogy of medical disciplines, like that of individual human beings and racial stocks, too often seems to be a hobby of the declining years rather than a preoccupation of the young investigator. In this book one sees the comparative novelty of an effort on the part of the young investigators to re-discover for themselves and for us, the genealogy of the dermatological discipline. This is a bibliocretic research, a hunting out from the literature of the foundation stones of clinical descriptive medicine on which has been built the edifice of a modern specialty. Let us concede, before some caviller reminds us of it, that pre-occupation with the past may become an obsessive neurosis, obscuring the intentness of the forward gaze which carries us into the new, the unexplored reaches of yet-to-be-understood things. The backward look in this book is anything but an obsessive worship of history as such. Its purpose would seem rather, first to memorialize human achievement and to remind us that the growing world is seen through human eyes and felt through human touch. Secondly, this study pays tribute to mastery, the distinction of standing head and shoulders above, which in this heyday of the average, is still an inspiring picture. Thirdly, the study brings out the process of building a medical specialty; the formation of a language, the acceptance of words representing concepts in which to clothe descriptive thought; the vital significance of fitness and precision, the importance of detail that omits nothing, and is as conscious of the negative as of the positive. While it sometimes seems as if language, translated as 'lingo', is an almost intentionally erected fence to keep the Ignorami off the lot because they have not mastered the jargon, there can be no question that terminology and accurate description move hand in hand to define significant thought, and to make both synthesis and analysis of concepts possible. If this book can do something to lay the curse of fuzzy description which has fallen upon some dermatologists, or better some training and practice in medicine, general and special, it will be a beneficence in itself. The authors of the classic descriptions here presented saw describable entities and differentiated them by logic and reasoning. They created for dermatology the basic art of physical diagnosis. They did not take to diagnostic hallucinationism, go into a fugue or fog and come out of it with an 'impression' of the disease, which can be vulgarly translated by the American phrase 'street car diagnosis'. In today's understandable but a bit too eager scramble for the laboratory, it will do us good to be reminded that clinical medicine has advanced and still does advance, by the meticulous study of the patient. Each of us, like each of these, the masters, can bring in light through a window that does not have a laboratory pane in it. Or if it does, as when pathologic anatomy is utilized, it is in observation of describable differences that sharpen and define the picture.

The authors of this work have well brought out their desire to stress the vital contribution of constructive-mindedness to the progress which these classic descriptions of disease represent. It is easy to see the analytical mastery of detail; but to see the arc of synthesis flash across from analysis to concept—this is to be privileged to witness the lightning stroke of genius. Analysis may become picayune, lost in minuscule variations without it. And yet this seeming flash of synthesis has its hard-won mastery of detail built into it too. Fact linked to hard-won fact forms the cable over which the current of constructive thought is carried to the arcing terminal.

One sees in the material of this book and in the way the authors have developed it, great encouragement for the individual, the lone student of cutaneous disease, isolated by, or buried under the routine of his work. The gods still live and move among men visible to those whose eyes are open. A seeing eye can read in droplets of perspiration, in flush and color play, in gooseflesh; in distribution and configuration, in the glance of the eye and the movements of the respiratory cage, clues to new physiologic concepts, and to that vast *terra incognita* of functional entities and linkages which is the future.

There is always a lingering disposition to say that it was all very easy to be a Willan when dermatology was chaos, or a Benjamin Franklin when physics was young and one could snare immortality with a kite. Today, we sigh that there are no new clinical worlds to conquer; all the diseases are described, their histopathology known for better, or indeed sometimes for worse, if confusion from inadequate method be at work. It does seem true that descriptive dermatology has in some directions, published its last catalogue and should have published its last sterile case report. But a moment's thought in application of the spirit of the founding fathers, as their work leads us to conceive it, reopens the outlook in the direction of correlations, leading to etiologic syntheses, among what appear to be structurally or morphologically different entities. Seborrheic dermatitis is still seborrheic dermatitis, but its concentration in the flush area of the center face brings in that fascinating play of psychosomatic factors that has been coming to light in recent years as the rosacea complex. It is possible to construct spectra of so-called disease entities which have morphologic being, but represent, so to speak, differing wave lengths of a yet to be discovered common element or agency. Such a spectrum is an idea to toy with in the range between lichen planus, through lichen sclerosus et atrophicus, to morphoea and the sclerodermas. The staphylodermias constitute another field ripe for morphologic integrations.

With the stage set for clinical progress, assisted but not replaced by the laboratory, an inspiration to thoroughness in analysis, rigor in differential logic and constructive vision such as these vignettes of the master in action in the past, is more than timely. It is a spur to an even more distinguished future.

John H.Stokes, MD
Professor of Dermatology and Syphilology
Graduate School of Medicine
University of Pennsylvania

Acknowledgements for First Edition

Our first acknowlededgment is to the men from whose writings this chrestomathy has been prepared. It is made with the great admiration and respect their work commands.

It would never have been possible to make the literary acquaintance of many of these authors without the magnificent facilities afforded us by the library of the College of Physicians of Philadelphia. Here, with the kindly and efficient assistance of Mrs M.G.Maines, reference librarian, the many tomes, texts, and journals pertinent to the work were consulted. We are grateful to W.B.McDaniel, II, PhD, chief librarian, to Elliott Morse, assistant librarian, and to the entire staff for their continued interest and assistance in this undertaking. It was their realization, as well as our own, that this volume would give the reader some small idea of the College of Physicians' dermatologic treasure trove.

Dr Donald M.Pillsbury, Professor and Director of the Department of Dermatology and Syphilology of the University of Pennsylvania, School of Medicine, has aided us at every turn. Our special appreciation is due him for the ways he found to remove the administrative difficulties which always beset a work of this kind.

Professor John H.Stokes has earned our gratitude by his gracious consent to prepare the foreword to this volume.

Miss Edna Brand has been our right hand. To her we are deeply indebted for a technically superb manuscript. Her enthusiasm, expertness, and exquisite attention to detail have been a delight to us.

Robert Morris of the Deats Photographic Agency, Philadelphia, has been our constant friend and adviser. Through his cameras has passed all of the pictorial material, and we thank him for the meticulous attention he gave to it.

Many people of many lands have given us biographic and bibliographic aid. For direct assistance we are grateful to the following:

Harry L.Arnold, Jr., MD	Honolulu
William Bennett Bean, MD	Iowa City
Herman Beerman, MD	Philadelphia
Nils Danbolt, MD	Oslo
Oscar Gans, MD	Frankfurt
Sven Hellerstrom, MD	Stockholm
Sir Archibald Gray	London
Erich Hoffman, MD	Bonn
Herman M.Jahr, MD	Omaha
Pierre Mallet-Guy, MD	Lyon
Lowry Miller, MD	New York

Samuel X.Radbill, MD	Philadelphia
R.V.Rajam, MD	Madras
Herbert Rattner, MD	Chicago
Gustav Riehl, Jr., MD	Vienna
G.A.Rost, MD	Berlin
Ali Paris Sümen, MD	Istanbul
Fred D.Weidman, MD	Philadelphia
Samuel J.Zakon, MD	Chicago

The funds for this project were derived from a grant made in 1948 by the Rockefeller Foundation to the Department of Dermatology and Syphilology of the University of Pennsylvania.

Charles C.Thomas and Payne Thomas have won our special gratitude for their realization of the need for such an anthology as this, and for their abiding interest in the history of medicine.

W.B.S.
J.T.C.

Acknowledgements for Second Edition

No longer can we sit and write at the foot of the great portrait of Duhring, surrounded by the limitless treasures of the College of Physicians in Philadelphia. Now our debt of gratitude goes to Liz Fabian and Barbara McNamee, librarians at the Medical College of Ohio, who did computer searches and secured photocopies of the references we needed. The following sources in our personal library were of real help:

- Dyall-Smith D, ed. *Dermatological Discoveries of the 20th Century.* Parthenon Publishing, 1999

  - This is a color atlas which brilliantly illustrates the conditions described in the book you now hold.

- Braun-Falco O, *et al. Dermatology,* 2nd edn. Springer, 2000

  - A source book of 'firsts' in clinical dermatology

- Crissey JT, *et al. Historical Atlas of Dermatology and Dermatologists.* Parthenon Publishing, 2002
- Wallach D.Vintage descriptions. In Wallach D, Tilles G, eds. *Dermatology in France.* Pierre Fabre Publication, 2002:77–107
- Teraki Y, Nishikawa T.Skin diseases first described in Japan. *J Dermatol (Japan)* 1994; 21:139–51
- Gold S. *A Biographical History of British Dermatology.* British Association of Dermatologists, 1996

Georgiann Monhollen has been our valued associate in preparing a meticulous print and disc copy of the manuscript for publication.

Angela Campbell, the Medical College of Ohio Dermatology Division Secretary, has given us the power of e-mail, totally unimaginable a half century ago. Indeed, months of intercontinental correspondence for the First Edition have been reduced to but moments.

Jack Meade, our Medical College of Ohio Photographer, transferred our motley collection of portraits onto a CD using the modern magic of digital computerized imagery.

Pamela Lancaster, Medical Editor at Parthenon Publishing, has given us genius in design, layout and typography, as well as accouchement for this baby, our book.

Again, many people from many lands have given us biographies and bibliographic aid. For direct assistance we are grateful to the following:

François Abboud   Iowa City, Iowa
A.Bernard Ackerman   New York
Margaret Aguiar   Detroit, Michigan

Jacques Bazex	France
Martin M.Black	UK
Margaret Blackburn	Toledo, Ohio
Bess Brennan	Higland, Indiana
Ruggero Caputo	Italy
Enrico Ceccolini	Italy
J.Stanley Comaish	UK
Suzanne Connolly	Scottsdale, Arizona
Selma Epstein	Piedmont, California
Ruth Farber	Portola Valley, California
Malcolm W.Greaves	Malaysia
David Grinspan	Argentina
David Harris	Campbell, California
Karl Holubar	Austria
Atsushi Kukita	Japan
Darius R.Mehregan	Monroe, Michigan
Leo Montes	Argentina
Jean Paul Ortonne	France
Bill Radl	Iowa City, Iowa
Terence Ryan	UK
John S.Strauss	Iowa City, Iowa
Nickolai Talanin	Washington, DC
James S.Taylor	Cleveland, Ohio
Ronnie Wacker	Cutchogue, NY
Wolfgang Weyers	Germany
Darrell S.Wilkinson	UK
Victor Witten	Miami, Florida

Special thanks go to E.Dorinda Shelley for her continuing advice, research, encouragement and proofreading.

Finally, we express our deep gratitude to our publisher, David Bloomer, a man of exceptional charm and action. Achieving this unique 2003 imprimature is in no small part due to him.

List of Illustrations

Frontispiece The four greatest dermatologists   i

Figure 1.	Robert Willan	3
Figure 2.	Title page to Willan's *On Cutaneous Diseases*	5
Figure 3.	Psoriasis	8
Figure 4.	Ichthyosis	11
Figure 5.	Pemphigus	13
Figure 6.	Molluscum contagiosum	16
Figure 7.	Eczema	18
Figure 8.	Sycosis barbae	20
Figure 9.	Jean Louis Alibert	25
Figure 10.	Lupus vulgaris	27
Figure 11.	Keloid	29
Figure 12.	Mycosis fungoides	31
Figure 13.	Dermatolysis	33
Figure 14.	Armand Trousseau	36
Figure 15.	The island, Meleda (Mljet)	39
Figure 16.	Pierre François Rayer	42
Figure 17.	Ecthyma	44
Figure 18.	Alphée Cazenave	50
Figure 19.	Title page to Cazenave's *Annales des Maladies de la Peau*	50
Figure 20.	Auguste Nélaton	57
Figure 21.	Alphonse Devergie	60
Figure 22.	Ernest Bazin	66
Figure 23.	Thomas Addison	70
Figure 24.	L'Hôpital Saint Louis	76
Figure 25.	Ferdinand von Hebra	81
Figure 26.	Erythema multiforme (circinatum)	82
Figure 27.	Pityriasis rubra	88
Figure 28.	Rhinoscleroma	90
Figure 29.	Erasmus Wilson	95
Figure 30.	Title page to Wilson's *Journal of Cutaneous Medicine*	97
Figure 31.	Tilbury Fox	108
Figure 32.	James Paget	113
Figure 33.	Louis Duhring	117
Figure 34.	Isidor Neumann	127
Figure 35.	Moritz Kaposi	132

Figure 36.	Dermatitis papillaris capillitii	133
Figure 37.	Jonathan Hutchinson	145
Figure 38.	Arsenical keratosis (the hands of the American physician)	149
Figure 39.	Angioma serpiginosum	149
Figure 40.	Henry Radcliffe-Crocker	159
Figure 41.	Dermatitis gangrenosa infantum	161
Figure 42.	Erythema elevatum diutinum	163
Figure 43.	Granuloma annulare	166
Figure 44.	Paul Gerson Unna	169
Figure 45.	Seborrheic dermatitis	170
Figure 46.	James C.White	177
Figure 47.	J.J.Pringle	181
Figure 48.	Adenoma sebaceum	183
Figure 49.	Thomas Colcott Fox	185
Figure 50.	Erythema gyratum perstans	186
Figure 51.	Multiple benign tumor-like new growths of the skin	189
Figure 52.	Sigmund Pollitzer	192
Figure 53.	Acanthosis nigricans	194
Figure 54.	Ernest Besnier	197
Figure 55.	H.G.Brooke	200
Figure 56.	Epithelioma adenoides cysticum	200
Figure 57.	Émile Vidal	205
Figure 58.	Angiokeratoma	210
Figure 59.	Porokeratosis	212
Figure 60.	Hidrocystoma	216
Figure 61.	John Addison Fordyce	218
Figure 62.	Angiokeratoma of the scrotum	220
Figure 63.	Fordyce's disease	220
Figure 64.	Domenico Majocchi	228
Figure 65.	Henri Hallopeau	232
Figure 66.	Caesar Boeck	240
Figure 67.	Boeck's sarcoid	242
Figure 68.	Jean-Louis Brocq	246
Figure 69.	L'Hôpital Saint Louis	246
Figure 70.	Edvard Ehlers	257
Figure 71.	George Henry Fox	260
Figure 72.	Abraham Buschke	263
Figure 73.	Josef Jadassohn	271
Figure 74.	Cutis verticis gyrata	275
Figure 75.	Pachyonychia congenita	276
Figure 76.	Eduard Jacobi	279
Figure 77.	Poikilodermia vascularis atrophicans (Jacobi's case)	279
Figure 78.	Felix Pinkus	283
Figure 79.	Grover Wende	289
Figure 80.	Jay Frank Schamberg	292

Figure 81.	Grain itch	295
Figure 82.	Erythroplasia	299
Figure 83.	J.E.R.McDonagh	302
Figure 84.	Nevoxantho-endothelioma	302
Figure 85.	John T.Bowen	306
Figure 86.	Richard L.Sutton	313
Figure 87.	Periadenitis mucosa necrotica recurrens	315
Figure 88.	C.Guy Lane	318
Figure 89.	Max Winkler	321
Figure 90.	Jean Darier	324
Figure 91.	Keratosis follicularis (one of Darier's original cases)	326
Figure 92.	Erythema annulare centrifugum	329
Figure 93.	F.Parkes-Weber	336
Figure 94.	Henri Gougerot	341
Figure 95.	Paul Blum	341
Figure 96.	Symmetrical lividities of the soles of the feet	345
Figure 97.	Bruno Bloch	348
Figure 98.	Francis E.Senear	351
Figure 99.	Barney Usher	351
Figure 100.	Pemphigus erythematodes	351
Figure 101.	Erich Urbach	357
Figure 102.	Necrobiosis lipoidica diabeticorum	359
Figure 103.	G.A.Grant Peterkin	361
Figure 104.	Marion B.Sulzberger	363
Figure 105.	William Garbe	363
Figure 106.	Typical discoid and lichenoid elevated plaques on posterior axillary fold; and typical diffuse lichenification	366
Figure 107.	(a) Howard Hailey; (b) Hugh Hailey	372
Figure 108.	João Paulo Vieira	376
Figure 109.	Stuart D.Allen	379
Figure 110.	John P.O'Brien	379
Figure 111.	Johannes Fabry	385
Figure 112.	Agostino Pasini	388
Figure 113.	Luis E.Pierini	388
Figure 114.	Louis A.Brunsting	394
Figure 115.	Friederich Wegener	397
Figure 116.	Albert Sézary	400
Figure 117.	Masao Ota	403
Figure 118.	Ota's original illustration	404
Figure 119.	S.William Becker	406
Figure 120.	Clarence S.Livingood	411
Figure 121.	Eugene M.Farber	415
Figure 122.	Sophie Spitz	419
Figure 123.	Walter F.Lever	424
Figure 124.	Max Jessner	427

Figure 125.   Ferdinando Gianotti   430
Figure 126.   Agostino Crosti   430
Figure 127.   Ian Bruce Sneddon   434
Figure 128.   Darrell S.Wilkinson   437
Figure 129.   Alan Lyell   441
Figure 130.   Walter B.Shelley   444
Figure 131.   William Bennett Bean   460
Figure 132.   Earl W.Netherton   463
Figure 133.   Harold O.Perry   467
Figure 134.   Albert M.Kligman   470
Figure 135.   John Thorne Crissey   475
Figure 136.   Robert W.Goltz   477
Figure 137.   Peter Samman   480
Figure 138.   R.D.Sweet   483
Figure 139.   André Bazex   486
Figure 140.   Ervin Epstein   490
Figure 141.   Marvin Chernosky   492
Figure 142.   Amir H.Mehregan   495
Figure 143.   Tomisaku Kawasaki   498
Figure 144.   Thomas B.Fitzpatrick   501
Figure 145.   Lawrence M.Solomon   504
Figure 146.   Ralph Grover   507
Figure 147.   Shigeo Ofuji   510
Figure 148.   George C.Wells   514
Figure 149.   Peyton E.Weary   518
Figure 150.   Rona M.MacKie   522
Figure 151.   Thomas J.Lawley   525
Figure 152.   Steven Kossard   528
Figure 153.   Richard K.Winkelmann   528
Figure 154.   Grant J.Anhalt   532

PART I

THE EARLY WORKERS

Robert Willan

1. *Purpose of a Treatise on Cutaneous Diseases*

2. *Definitions of Technical Terms*

3. *Psoriasis*

4. *Ichthyosis*

5. *Erythema Nodosum*

6. *Pemphigus*

ROBERT WILLAN was born November 12, 1757, near Sedburg in Yorkshire. He was the son of a practicing physician and a Quaker. Little is known of his younger days. He was an assiduous scholar and acquired great facility in Latin and Greek, which stood him in good stead in his later historical researches. His medical education was begun in 1777 at Edinburgh, and was completed there in 1780 with the publication of his thesis, *On Inflammation of the Liver*.

After an unsuccessful year of practice at Darlington he moved to London in 1782, and in 1783 was appointed physician to the newly established Public Dispensary in Gary Street. This dispensary became, then, the birthplace of modern dermatology, for Willan was the first modern dermatologist. It served the poor in the vicinity of Clare Market, Drury Lane, Chancery Lane, Templebar, Strand, Holborn, Fleet Street and Market, Ludgate and Black and White Friars. Willan remained associated with it almost to the end of his life. It was here that he conceived and perfected a classification of cutaneous disease based on the morphology of the essential lesion, an approach which, expounded in his *On Cutaneous Diseases* (1798–1808), established order where little but chaos had existed. It is difficult to overestimate the effect this work has had on the specialty. Leaders in other dermatologic centers— Rayer and Biett in France, Hebra in Germany—were greatly influenced by it, and through these great men, as well as Willan's own pupils, many of the Willan concepts have been perpetuated. Rayer said: "The greatest characteristics of Willan's writings are the impress they bear of the scientific spirit that guided him in his researches: the great precision and the purity of his descriptions; the particular pains he takes to select well and to use judiciously his technical expressions; lastly, the sound judgment he displays in his interpretation of the ancients."

In about 1801 Willan met Thomas Bateman, and being impressed by this fellow Yorkshireman he invited the young man to become his pupil at the Dispensary. Bateman did so, grasped quickly Willan's approach to dermatologic problems, and soon became his most trusted assistant, friend, and finally biographer and successor. It was Bateman who brought Willan's great work, interrupted by his death, to its logical

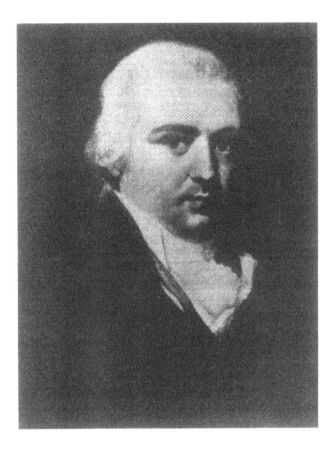

Figure 1 Robert Willan

conclusion in his own *Synopsis of Cutaneous Diseases* (1813) and *Delineations of Cutaneous Diseases* (1814–1817), the latter being the first dermatologic atlas.

As a clinician, Willan's keenness and skill were remarkable. He was, however, skeptical of the therapeutics of his day.

Bateman stated: "As a practitioner, he was a close and faithful observer of diseases, and by the peculiar quickness with which he detected their characteristic appearance, however obscured by complication, he had obtained a copious store of sound experience. Yet, it has been remarked that he did not always prescribe with that vigour and decision, which so much discriminative talent would have authorized."

Willan was, in addition to his other recommendations, an extremely tolerant and likeable man, though somewhat reserved in manner. From Bateman's biography of his teacher: "In his intercourse with his professional brethren he was liberal and independent and extremely tender of giving offense. His early education, his studious mode of life and retiring disposition prevented that display of his various and extensive knowledge in mixed society, which delighted the privacy of a small circle of friends, and which was dispensed with much playfulness and simplicity of manner. In all the relations of domestic life, indeed, he was an object of general esteem and attachment. The gentleness and humanity of his disposition were equally conspicuous in the exercise of his professional duties, in the patient attention with which he listened to the complaints of the sick whom, in his fullest occupation, he never dismissed from his presence dissatisfied with the brevity of his inquiries and in the liberty with which he imparted his assistance, yet refused the remuneration to which he was entitled, when the circumstances of the patient appeared to render it oppressive."

Willan was stricken at the height of his fame and skill with a cardiac disease which increased gradually in severity over the last two years of his life. He died April 7, 1812, at the age of 55.*

It is difficult to limit oneself in the selection of material from Willan's masterful work. We have reproduced his objectives, as he stated them, and his definitions of the terms which he used in his work, which first made exact dermatologic description possible. The pieces chosen are representative of his accurate, comprehensive, yet concise, descriptions.

Accounts suggestive of psoriasis, pemphigus, and ichthyosis have been known since antiquity, but due to the carelessness of the ancients in their use of terms they are of limited value.

PURPOSE OF A TREATISE ON CUTANEOUS DISEASES*

In a systematical treatise on cutaneous disease, we should endeavour:

1. To fix the sense of the terms employed by proper definitions.
2. To constitute general division or orders of the diseases, from leading and peculiar circumstances in their appearance, to arrange them into distinct genera, and to describe at large their specific forms, or varieties.
3. To class and give names to such as have not been hitherto sufficiently distinguished.
4. To specify the mode of treatment for each disease.

To complete adequately a plan so extensive must be considered an undertaking of much difficulty, and perhaps exceeding the powers of any individual. My own observations are principally founded on the cutaneous diseases occurring in London, and its vicinity. I intend, however, to compare them with the accounts of similar complaints in ancient and modern writers.

DEFINITIONS OF TECHNICAL TERMS*

Consistently with the principles above laid down, I proceed in the first place to define the sense of several technical terms employed in the following pages.

Definitions

1. **Scurf (Furfura).** Small exfoliations of the cuticle, which take place after slight inflammation or irritation of the skin, a new cuticle being formed underneath during exfoliation.
2. **Scale (Squama).** A lamina of morbid cuticle, hard, thickened, whitish and opaque. Scales have at first the figure and extent of the cuticular lozenges, but they afterwards often increase into irregular layers, denominated crusts. Both scales and crusts repeatedly fall off and are reproduced in a short time.

---

* Lane, J.E.: *Arch. Dermat. and Syph., 13:737,* 1926.

* On Cutaneous Diseases. London, 1808, p. VII.

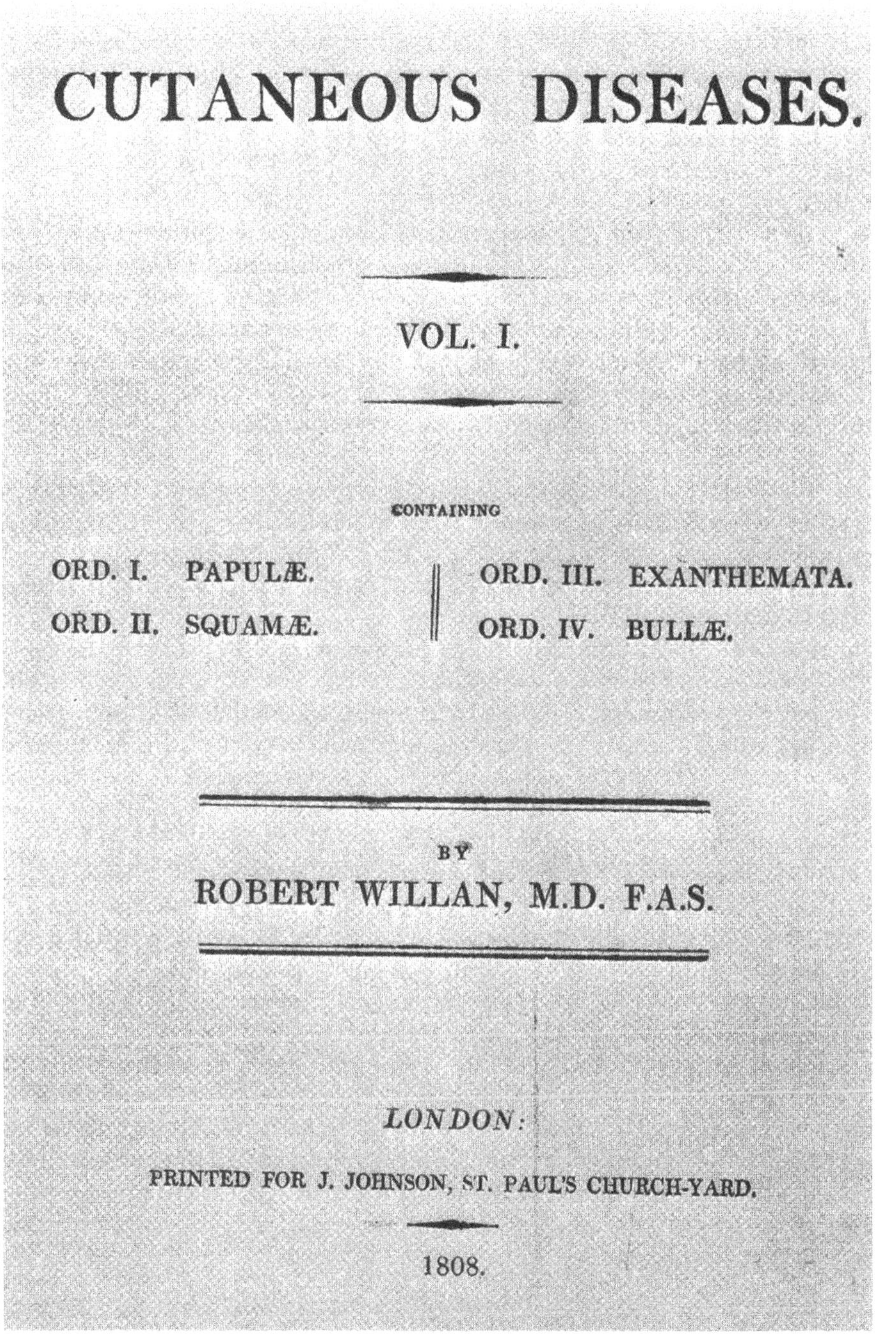

CUTANEOUS DISEASES.

VOL. I.

CONTAINING

ORD. I. PAPULÆ.	ORD. III. EXANTHEMATA.
ORD. II. SQUAMÆ.	ORD. IV. BULLÆ.

BY

ROBERT WILLAN, M.D. F.A.S.

LONDON:

PRINTED FOR J. JOHNSON, ST. PAUL'S CHURCH-YARD.

1808.

Figure 2 Title page to Willan's *On Cutaneous Diseases*. Courtesy, College of Physicians, Philadelphia

3. **Scab.** A hard substance covering superficial ulcerations, and formed by a concretion of the fluid

discharged from them.

4. **Stigma.** A small bright red speck in the skin, without any elevation of the cuticle. Stigmata are generally distinct or apart from each other. When they coalesce, and assume a dark red, or livid colour, they are termed *Petechiae.*

5. **Papula.** A very small and acuminated elevation of the cuticle, with an inflamed base, not containing fluid, nor tending to suppuration. The duration of papulae is uncertain, but they terminate for the most part in scurf.

6. **Rash (Exanthema).** Consists of red patches on the skin, variously figured, in general confluent, and diffused irregularly over the body, leaving interstices of a natural colour. Portions of the cuticle are often elevated in a rash, so as to give the sensation of an uneven surface. The eruption is usually accompanied with disorder of the constitution, and terminates in a few days by cuticular exfoliations.

7. **Macula.** A permanent discolouration of some portion of the skin, often with a change of its texture, but not connected with any disorder of the constitution.

8. **Tubercle.** A small, hard, superficial tumour, circumscribed, and permanent or proceeding very slowly to suppuration.

9. **Wheal.** A rounded or longitudinal elevation of the cuticle, with a white summit, hard but not permanent, not containing a fluid, nor tending to suppuration.

10. **Vesicle (Vesicula).** Small, orbicular elevation of the cuticle, containing lymph which is sometimes clear and colourless, but often opaque and whitish, or pearl coloured. Vesicles are succeeded either by scurf or laminated scabs.

11. **Bleb (Bulla).** A large portion of the cuticle detached from the skin by the interposition of a transparent watery fluid. Soon after the water is discharged, the excoriated surface is covered with a flat, yellow, or blackish scab, which remains 'till a new cuticle is formed underneath. Both vesicles and blebs, when they have a dark-red or livid base, are by medical and chirurgical writers, denominated Phlyctenae.

12. **Pustule.** An elevation of the cuticle, with an inflamed base containing pus. Pustules are various in their size, but the diameter of the largest seldom exceeds two lines.

Some forms of pustules have been distinguished by specific appellations, as:

1. **Phlyzacium.** A pustule of the size represented in Pl. I, Figure 13, raised on a hard circular base, of a vivid red colour. It is succeeded by a thick, hard, dark-coloured scab.

2. **Psydracium.** A minute pustule, irregularly circumscribed, producing but a slight elevation of the cuticle, and terminating in a laminating scab. Many of these pustules usually appear together, and become confluent. After the discharge of pus, a thin watery humour exudes, which often forms an irregular incrustation.

3. **Achor.** An acuminated pustule of intermediate size between the two foregoing, which contains a straw-coloured matter, having the appearance and nearly the consistency of strained honey. It appears most frequently about the head, and is succeeded by a thin brown or yellowish scab.

4. **Cerion or Favus.** This pustule is somewhat larger than achor, and contains a more viscid matter. Its base is but slightly inflamed, and it is succeeded by a yellow, semi-transparent and sometimes cellular scab, like a honeycomb.

---

* On Cutaneous Diseases. London, 1808, p. IX.

I propose to arrange cutaneous diseases in eight orders, to be characterized by the different appearance of papulae, scales, rashes, bullae, vesicles, pustules, tubercles and maculae. By comparing together the 2nd, 5th, 6th, 7th, 8th, 10th, 11th and 12th definitions, the distinguishing characters of each order may be readily understood. They will also be further illustrated in treating of the orders respectively.

PSORIASIS

Scaly Diseases of the Skin*

The second Order of Cutaneous Diseases includes those affections, which are characterized by an appearance of scales, arising from a morbid state of the cuticle, as specified in the second definition. The cuticle is not, however, the only seat of these complaints. They often originate from indurated papulae, or larger elevations of the true skin which by pressure or distension injure the texture of the cuticle, and produce thickened irregular layers of it. The scales or crusts, thus formed, have not always been distinguished from scabs succeeding confluent pustules, or superficial ulcerations, whence we find in medical writers several dissimilar diseases connected together. I shall endeavor to avoid such inaccuracies by strictly observing the second, and third definitions.

I. The *Lepra vulgaris* at first exhibits small, distinct elevations of the cuticle which are reddish and shining, but never contain any fluid. Their surface, when examined through a magnifying glass, appears tense and smooth. Within 24 hours, however, thin white scales form on their tops. After three or four days the small elevations are flattened, and at the same time dilated by an extension of their bases to the size of a silver penny. These patches continue to enlarge gradually, till they become nearly the size of a crown piece. They always retain a circular or oval form, are covered with dry scales, and surrounded by a red border. The scales accumulate on them, so as to form a thick prominent crust (Def. I), which is quickly reproduced, whether it falls off spontaneously or has been forcibly detached. On its removal, the surface appears, through a magnifier, to be porous, and irregular or wrinkled, but the furrows do not coincide with the lines of the contiguous found cuticle. The eruption is not attended with any pain or uneasiness, excepting a slight degree of itching, felt when the person affected becomes warm in bed, and a sensation of tingling upon any sudden change in temperature of the atmosphere.

This species of Lepra sometimes appears first at the elbow, or on the forearm, but more generally about the knee. In the latter case the primary patch forms immediately below the patella. Within a few weeks several other scaly circles appear along the fore parts of the leg and thigh, increasing by degrees 'till they come nearly into contact. The disease is then often stationary for a considerable length of time. If it does advance further, its progress is towards the hip and loins, afterwards to the sides, back and shoulders and about the same time to the arms and hands. In a great number of cases, the hairy scalp is the part last affected, although the circles formed on it remain for sometime distinct, yet they finally unite and cover the whole surface on which the hair grows with a white, scaly incrustation. This appearance is attended, more especially in hot weather, with a troublesome itching, and when any part of the crust is detached a watery discharge takes place and continues for several hours. The pubis in adults is sometimes affected in the same manner as the head, and if the subject be a female, there is usually an internal pruritus pudendi, as has been already observed. In some cases of the disorder, the nails, both of the fingers and toes, are thickened, and deeply indented longitudinally. Either the whole or some part of each nail is harder and more prominent

---

* On Cutaneous Diseases. London, 1808, p. 105.

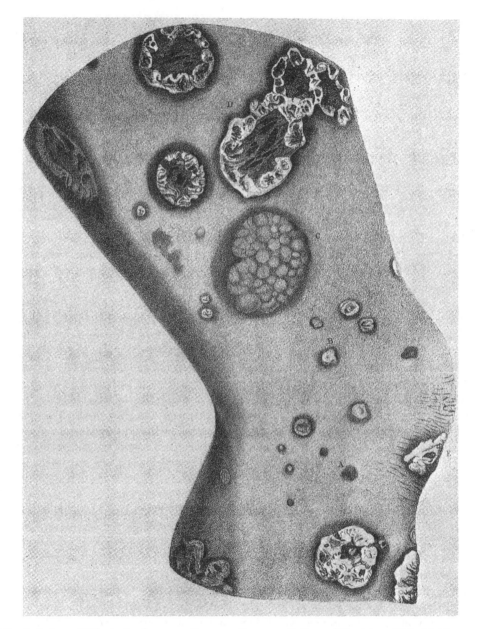

Figure 3 Psoriasis. From Willan's *On Cutaneous Diseases*. Courtesy, College of Physicians, Philadelphia

than usual. Under several of them also may be observed one, two or three round yellowish specks, which on advancing to the end of the nail will be found to have originated from a deposition of curdly, sebaceous matter, having an extremely fetid smell.

When the Lepra extends to all the parts above mentioned, it becomes highly disgusting in its appearance and inconvenient from the stiffness and torpor occasioned by it in the limbs. The disease, however, is seldom disposed to terminate spontaneously. It continues nearly in the same state for several years, or sometimes during the whole life of the person affected, not being apparently connected with any disorder of the constitution.

A regular diet with an appropriate course of medicine acts very slowly on the Lepra, yet will at length accomplish its cure. The steps by which it proceeds to a termination are as follows. First, the incrustation separates from about the centres of the patches, and is no longer reproduced. The scales being farther and farther removed, a circle of red shining cuticle deeply indented appears within the original patch, which still retains a broad, hard, scaly ring or border. This border continues 'till the cuticle within it assumes the usual colour and texture. It then gradually softens, and the cuticular lines being extended over it; every vestige of the disease is erased.

There are some other circumstances in this form of Lepra which merit attention:

1. The scaly patches are generally situated where the bone is nearest the surface, as along the shin, about the elbow, and upon the ulna in the forearm, on the scalp and along the spine, os ilium, and shoulder blades. They rarely appear on the calf of the leg, on the fleshy part of the arm and thigh or within the flexures of the joints.
2. The Lepra almost constantly affects both sides, appearing at each elbow or at each knee about the same time and extending from thence along the limbs in a similar manner.
3. Though fresh patches arise from time to time in different situations, there is no alteration in the state of the parts first affected, as happens in some other cutaneous diseases, but when the complaint is about to terminate, all the patches assume a favourable appearance at the same time, those nearest the extremities going off somewhat later than the rest.
4. The incrustation of the scalp encroaches a little on the forehead and temples, but I have never yet observed any of the scaly patches on the cheeks or chin, on the nose or near the eyebrows.
5. When the extremities, back, loins and head are all at the same time covered with dry crusts, it might be expected that the obstruction of the perspiration on so large a surface would produce disagreeable consequences which, however, is not found to be the case.

II. *Lepra alphoides.* In this form of Lepra, the scaly patches are smaller than in the Lepra vulgaris. They also differ by having their central parts a little depressed. The eruption usually begins about the elbow, with distinct hard protuberances not much larger than papulae, and of a dull red colour. These in a short time dilate to nearly the size of a silver penny. Two or three days afterwards the central part of them suffers a depression, within which minute white scales may be observed. The surrounding border, however, still continues to be raised, but it retains the same size and the same red colour as at first. All the forearm, and in many cases the back of the hand, is spotted with similar patches which seldom become confluent, but there is sometimes a white incrustation round the point of the elbow. This eruption appears in the same manner upon the joint of the knee, but without spreading far along the thigh or leg. I do not remember to have seen it on the trunk of the body, nor on the face. It is a disease of long duration and not less difficult to cure than the foregoing species of Lepra. Even when the scaly patches have been removed by a perseverance in the use of suitable applications, the cuticle remains for a long time red, tender and brittle, but the small hairs of the skin are not destroyed nor altered in their colour, and texture as some authors have stated.

III. The *Lepra nigricans* does not much differ from the Lepra vulgaris with respect to its form or distribution. The most striking difference is in the colour of the patches, which are dark and livid. They appear first on the legs and forearms, extending afterwards to the thighs, loins, neck, back and hands. Their central part is not depressed as in alphos. They are somewhat smaller than the patches of the Lepra vulgaris, and have a livid or purplish border. The skin likewise appears of a livid colour through the scaly incrustations, which are seldom very thick. It is further to be observed that the scales are more easily detached than in the other forms of Lepra, and that the surface remains longer excoriated, discharging lymph, often with an intermixture of blood, 'till a new incrustation forms, which is hard, brittle, and irregular. This complaint is particularly troublesome when it covers the scalp.

ICHTHYOSIS

Ichthyosis*

Ichthyosis is characterized by a permanently harsh, dry, scaly, and, in some cases, almost horny texture of the integuments of the body, unconnected with internal disorder. Psoriasis and Lepra differ from Ichthyosis in being but partially diffused, and in having deciduous scales.

There is a peculiar arrangement, and distribution, of the scales in this disease. Round the olecranon, on the arm, and near the patella on the thigh and leg, they are small, rounded, prominent or papillary, and of a black colour. Some of the scaly papillae have a short, narrow neck, and broad, irregular tops. On some parts of the extremities, and on the trunk of the body, the scales are flat, and large, often placed like tiling, or like the scales on the back of a fish; but in a few cases they have appeared separate, being intersected by whitish furrows. There is usually in this complaint a dryness, and roughness of the soles of the feet, sometimes a thickened, and brittle state of the skin in the palms of the hands, with large painful fissures, and on the face an appearance of scurf rather than of scales. The inner part of the wrists, the hams, the inside of the elbow, the furrow along the spine, and the inner and upper part of the thighs are perhaps the only parts of the skin always exempt from scaliness. Patients affected with the ichthyosis are occasionally much harassed with inflamed pustules (Phlyzacia, Def. X.I.) or with large, painful boils on different parts of the body: it is also remarkable that they never seem to have the least perspiration or moisture on the skin.

This disease did not, in any case presented to me, appear to have been transmitted hereditarily, but I have seen two or three children of the same parents affected with it. In several instances the disease was said to have appeared immediately after birth, but in others to have occurred at the age of two or three months: in one case it appeared soon after the smallpox, at the age of two years, and had continued six or seven years without alteration.

When a portion of the hard scaly coating is removed, it is not soon produced again. The easiest mode of removing the scales is to pick them off carefully with the nails, from any part of the body while it is immersed in hot water. The layer of cuticle which remains after this operation is harsh and dry; and the skin did not, in the cases I have noted, recover its usual texture and softness; but the formation of the scales was prevented by a frequent use of the warm bath, with moderate friction.

---

* On Cutaneous Diseases. London, 1808, p. 199.

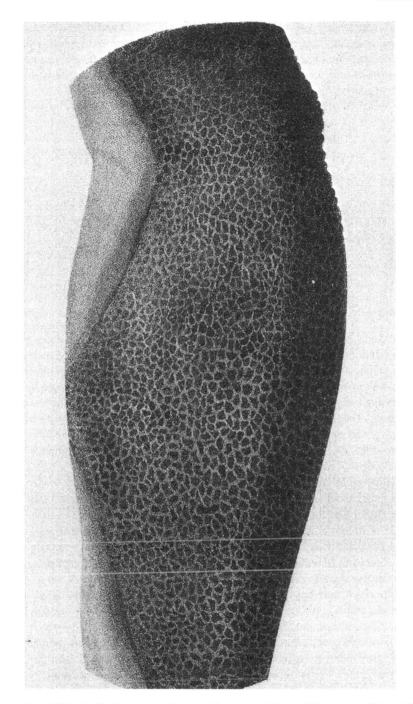

Figure 4 Ichthyosis. From Willan's *On Cutaneous Diseases*. Courtesy, College of Physicians, Philadelphia

ERYTHEMA NODOSUM

Erythema nodosum*

In the *Erythema nodosum,* many of the red patches are large and rounded. The central parts of them are very gradually elevated, and on the sixth or seventh day, form hard and painful protuberances, which are often taken for imposthumes, but from the seventh to the tenth, they constantly soften and subside, without ulceration. On the eighth or ninth day, the red colour changes to bluish or livid, and the affected limb appears as if it had been severely bruised. This appearance remains for a week or 10 days, when the cuticle begins to separate in scurf.

The Erythema nodosum usually affects the fore part of the legs. I have only seen it in females, most of whom were servants. It is preceded by irregular shiverings, nausea, headache, and fretfulness, with a quick unequal pulse, and a whitish fur on the tongue. These symptoms continue for a week, or more, but they usually abate on the appearance of the Erythema, so that in the latter stages of the disease, the only sensations of uneasiness are, languor, thirst, and disrelish for food.

The remedies prescribed by me in this complaint were calomel, or sometimes a milder purgative at first, and afterwards Peruvian bark, in considerable doses, either alone, or combined with vitriolic acid, wine, etc. These medicines were effectual in every case of the Erythema nodosum, but they proved fruitless in the Erythema tuberculatum.

PEMPHIGUS

Pompholyx diutinus[†]

The Pompholyx is an eruption of Bullae, without any inflammation round them, and without fever.

The *Pompholyx diutinus,* is a tedious and painful disorder chiefly affecting persons of a debilitated constitution, and particularly severe in those who are of an advanced age. It commences with numerous bullae or vesications on the face and arms, and is diffused, by a gradual progression, to the neck and breasts, and round the body, to the groins, thighs, and legs, and sometimes to the tongue, fauces, and the inside of the cheeks. The vesications seem to arise from red tingling elevations of the cuticle, nearly resembling the larger sort of papulae: within 24 hours they are the size of a pea, and perfectly transparent, but if permitted to dilate, they afterwards become as large as a walnut, sometimes assuming a yellowish hue. If the fluid be discharged from any of them from a small orifice, they are again filled with lymph during the succeeding night. When the vesications are rubbed off, or otherwise removed prematurely, the excoriated surface is extremely sore and inflamed, and does not heal for a considerable time. Ulcerations of this kind being multiplied as the disease advances, a slight paroxysm occurs every night, and the patient suffers much from pain, loss of sleep, and confinement. Since the bullae or vesications arise in succession upon different parts of the body, and often re-appear on the parts first affected, we are not able, at the beginning of the complaint, to judge, with any degree of certainty, what will be the extent or duration of it. In some cases under my own observation, it continued two months, in others, three or four, or even five months, so that the whole number of bullae, amounted to several thousands. After a cessation of some weeks, or months, the eruption frequently returned again, and proceeded in the same manner as before.

In a man, aged 46, the vesications first appeared on the scrotum and about the groins, during the month of October, 1789: the eruption afterwards extended to other parts of the body, and to the tongue: it was removed in about two months. He continued free from the complaint till February 1790, when a few vesications appeared on his wrists; others arose on his arms, neck, sides, scrotum, and lower extremities.

---

* On Cutaneous Diseases. London, 1808, p. 483.

[†] On Cutaneous Diseases. London, 1808, p. 544.

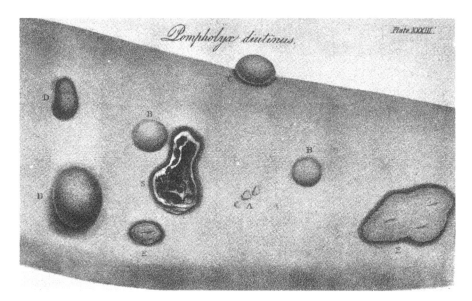

Figure 5 Pemphigus. From Willan's *On Cutaneous Diseases*. Courtesy, College of Physicians, Philadelphia

Those on the legs were slightly inflamed, and their contents became turbid from an admixture of pus: the rest were pellucid, and without any redness or inflammation around them. The disorder continued nearly three months: after it had disappeared; the patient enjoyed good health but he was again affected with the eruption, at the latter end of June, in the year 1790.

In a widow, aged 38, the vesications began to appear on the cheeks and round the eyes, at the latter end of December 1786. About the middle of January 1787, the eruption took place on her neck and breasts, and afterwards affected successively the shoulders, arms, back, and lower extremities. The vesications then arose from time to time, on different parts, without any regular order; some of them, which were nearly an inch in diameter, were succeeded by painful ulcerations. The complaint wholly disappeared in April, but returned again on the 12th of May, and continued for about a month.

The Pompholyx diutinus is usually preceded, for several weeks, by sickness, headache, and pains of the limbs, with a sensation of languor and lassitude. These symptoms do not always abate, on the appearance of the vesications. The causes of this disease, or the circumstances under which it appears, are not uniform. In some of the cases presented to my own observation, it was imputed to fatigue, anxiety, watching, and low diet: in others, it seemed referable to intemperance in eating, and excess in drinking spirituous liquors.

Thomas Bateman

1.   *Molluscum Contagiosum*

2.   *Papular Urticaria*

3.   *Eczema*

4.   *Sycosis Barbae*

THOMAS BATEMAN was born at Whitby in Yorkshire on April 29, 1778. His early childhood gave no indications of the ability which afterwards distinguished him. He was remarkably silent and reserved, and never opened a book for his own amusement.

At the age of 19, having become a fine scholar as he grew older, he went to London, studied at St. George's for a year, transferred to Edinburgh, and finished his medical training there in 1801, entitling his thesis *Haemorrhea Petechialis*. He returned to London to practice in 1801, and shortly after became associated with Robert Willan at the Public Dispensary, an association which was to become far more than one of teacher and pupil, for Bateman became Willan's most trusted assistant, and the tremendous work of the latter interrupted by death (1811) was brought to its logical conclusion by Bateman in his masterful and most influential *Synopsis of Cutaneous Diseases* (1813). As with Socrates and Plato, it is difficult to determine where the work of the one ends and the other begins. Building also on Willan's concept of illustrating skin diseases, and completing the engravings of that man, he published the first atlas of dermatology (1814–1817).

Personally, Bateman was an unassuming man. His language was simple and direct and his whole deportment plain and without pre-tension. He was very religious, fond of music and a competent organist. A friend said of him: "It would be hardly too much to say that he never wasted a minute. His pen was always in his hand the moment he came downstairs in the morning. His papers and books were on the table during the short interval which elapsed before he breakfasted. In his daily rounds at the Dispensary he was equally careful not to waste time, taking every short-cut, and not disdaining to contrive how to save even a few steps, since all these savings in the aggregate procured him a little more time."

He was stricken at the height of his career with an undiagnosed disease of the digestive organs, and died in April, 1821, after months of suffering.*

The original accounts given here are from Bateman's synopsis. They demonstrate well the terse style of that important work, and the keen perception of its author.

MOLLUSCUM CONTAGIOSUM

Molluscum[†]

Since the second edition was printed, a patient was sent to me by a distinguished physician, affected with a singular species of molluscum, which appears to be communicable by contact. The face and neck of this young woman were thickly studded with round prominent tubercles of various sizes, from that of a large pinhead to that of a small bean, which were hard, smooth, and shining on their surface, with a slight degree of transparency, and nearly the color of the skin. The tubercles were all sessile, upon a contracted base, without any peduncle. From the larger ones a small quantity of a milk-like fluid issued, on pressure, from a minute aperture, such as might be made by a needle-point, and which only became visible on the exit of the fluid. The progress of their growth was very slow; the first tubercle had appeared on the chin 12 months ago, and only a few of them had attained large size.

She ascribed the origin of this disease to contact with the face of a child, whom she nursed, on which a large tubercle of the same sort existed; on a subsequent visit, she informed me that two other children of the same family were disfigured by similar tubercles. The parents believed that the first child had received the eruption from a servant, on whose face it was observed.

PAPULAR URTICARIA

Lichen urticatus*

There is scarcely any limit to the varieties of these papular affections, but I have observed one form, which is so uniform in its character as to be entitled to notice here. It may be called lichen urticatus; as its first appearance is in irregular inflamed wheals, so closely resembling the spots excited by the bites of bugs or gnats, as almost to deceive the observer. The inflammation, however, subsides in a day or two, leaving small elevated, itching papules. While the first wheals are terminating, new ones continue to appear in succession, until the whole body and limbs are spotted with papulae, which become here and there confluent in small patches. This eruption is peculiar to children. It commences, in some cases, soon after birth, and sometimes later, and continues with great obstinacy for many months. Both the wheals and the papulae are accompanied with intense itching, which is exceedingly severe in the night, occasioning an almost total interruption of sleep, and considerable loss of flesh.

ECZEMA

Eczema[†]

The eczema is characterized by an eruption of small vesicles, on various parts of the skin, usually set close or crowded together, with little or no inflammation round their bases, and unattended by fever. It is not contagious.

---

* Rumsey, J.: Some Account of the Life and Character of the Late Thomas Bateman. London, 1826.

[†] A Practical Synopsis of Cutaneous Diseases, 3rd Edition. London, 1814, p. 271.

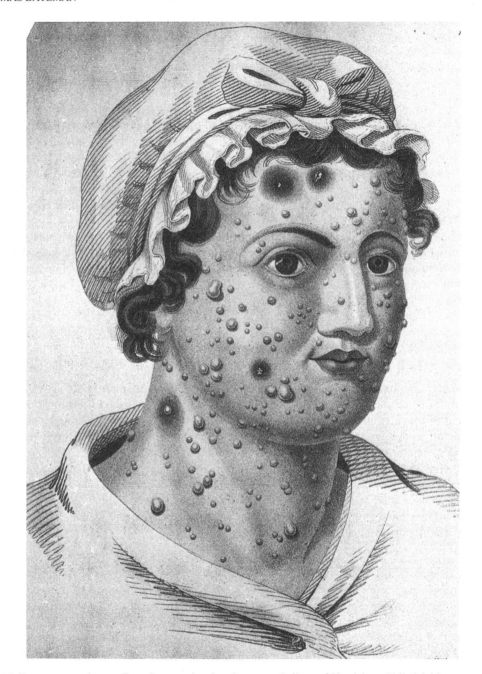

Figure 6 Molluscum contagiosum. From Bateman's atlas. Courtesy, College of Physicians, Philadelphia

Eczema Impetigenodes. A local eczema is produced by the irritation of various substances, and, when these are habitually applied, it is constantly kept up in a chronic form, differing from the Impetigo only in the absence of pustules. Small separate vesicles, containing a transparent fluid, and, like the psydracious pustules, imbedded in the skin, or but slightly elevated, arise, and slowly increase: they are attended with pain, heat, smarting, and often intense itching. When they break, the acrid lymph, that is discharged, irritates and inflames the surrounding cuticle, which becomes thickened, rough, reddish, and cracked, as in the impetiginous state. The alliance, indeed, of this affection with Impetigo is further proved by the circumstance, that, in some cases, vesicles and pustules are intermixed with each other; and, in different individuals, the same irritant will excite a pustular or a vesicular eruption respectively; the vesicular disease being always the most painful and obstinate. Of this we have an example in the affection of the hands and fingers, produced by the irritation of sugar, which is commonly called the *grocer's itch;* and which is in some persons vesicular, in others pustular. The acrid stimulus of lime occasions similar eruptions on the hands of *bricklayers:* and one of the most severe cases I have ever witnessed, occurred on the hands of a *filemaker,* being occasioned perhaps by the united irritation of the heat of the forge and the impalpable powder of steel with which they were constantly covered during his work. In like manner, both vesicular and pustular affections are excited by the local irritation of blisters, stimulating plasters, and cataplasms of mercury, tartarized antimony, the oil of the cashew nut, the Indian varnish, arsenic, valerian root, etc. These often extend to a considerable distance beyond the part to which the irritants were immediately applied, and continue for some time, in a successive series, after the stimulus has been withdrawn, especially in irritable and cachectic habits. Thus, when a blister is applied to the pit of the stomach, an eruption of vesicles, intermixed often with ecthymatous pustules, and inflamed tubercles and boils, extends, in some cases, over nearly the whole abdomen, or to the top of the sternum; or if the blister be applied between the shoulders, the whole of the back and loins becomes covered with a similar eruption. These tubercles and boils suppurate very slowly and deeply in some habits, and are ultimately filled with dark dry scabs, which do not soon fall off; and when the sores are numerous, they produce some degree of feverishness, and much pain on motion. In other respects, the constitution suffers no injury from this tedious eruption; although from its duration, which is sometimes extended to two or three weeks, it occasions more inconvenience than the original applications.

Eczema rubrum. The most remarkable variety of the Eczema rubrum, is that which arises from the irritation of mercury. But the disease is not exclusively occasioned by this mineral, either in its general or more partial attacks: it has been observed to follow exposure to cold, and to recur in the same individual, at irregular intervals, sometimes without any obvious or adequate cause.

The Eczema rubrum is preceded by a sense of stiffness, burning heat, and itching, in the part where it commences, which is most frequently the upper and inner surface of the thighs, and about the scrotum in men: but sometimes it appears first in the groins, axillae, or in the bend of the arms, or about the wrists and hands, or in the neck. These sensations are soon followed by an appearance of redness, and the surface is somewhat rough to the touch. This, however, is not a simple Erythema: for on examining it minutely between the light and the eye, or with a convex glass, the roughness is found to be occasioned by innumerable minute, and pellucid vesicles, which have been mistaken for papulae. In two or three days, these vesicles, if they are not ruptured, attain the size of a pin's head; and, the included serum then becoming somewhat opake and milky, the character of the eruption is obvious. It soon extends itself over the body and limbs in successive large patches, and is accompanied by a considerable swelling of the integuments, such as is seen in smallpox and other eruptive fevers, and by great tenderness of the skin, and

---

* A Practical Synopsis of Cutaneous Diseases, 3rd Edition. London, 1814, p. 13.

† A Practical Synopsis of Cutaneous Diseases, 3rd Edition. London, 1814, p. 250.

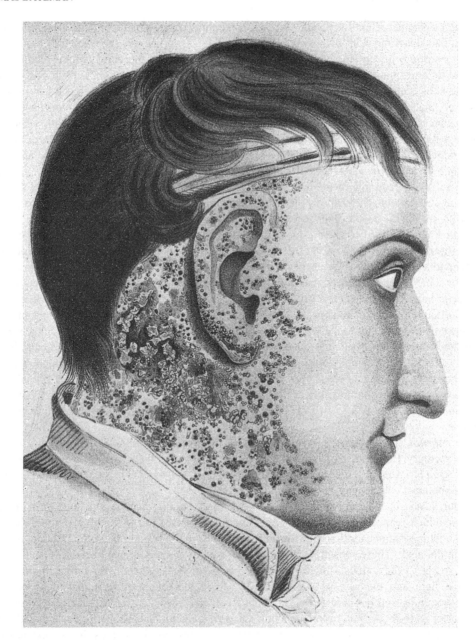

Figure 7 Eczema. From Bateman's atlas. Courtesy, College of Physicians, Philadelphia

much itching. When the vesicles begin to lose their transparency, they generally burst, and discharge from numerous points, a thin acrid fluid, which seems to irritate the surface over which it passes, and leaves it in a painful, inflamed, and excoriated condition. The quantity of this ichorous discharge is very considerable, and it gradually becomes thicker and more adherent, stiffening the linen which absorbs it, and which thus becomes a new source of irritation: it emits also a very fetid odour. This process takes place in the successive patches of the eruption, until the whole surface of the body, from head to foot, is sometimes in a state of painful excoriation, with deep fissures in the bends of the joints, and in the folds of the skin of the trunk, and with partial scaly incrustations, of a yellowish hue, produced by the drying of the humour, by which also the irritation is augmented. The extreme pain arising from the pressure of the weight of the body upon an extensive portion of such a raw surface, is sufficient to give rise to an acceleration of the pulse, and white tongue; but the functions of the stomach and of the sensorium commune are not evidently disturbed by this disease.

The duration of this excoriation and discharge is uncertain and irregular: when only a small part of the body is affected, it may terminate in 10 days; but when the disorder has been universal, the patient seldom completely recovers in less than six weeks, and is often afflicted to the end of eight or 10 weeks.

SYCOSIS BARBAE

Sycosis menti*

In the Sycosis *menti,* the tubercles arise first on the under lip, or on the prominent part of the chin, in an irregularly circular cluster; but this is speedily followed by other clusters, and by distinct tubercles, which appear in succession, along the lower part of the cheeks up to the ears, and under the jaw towards the neck, as the beard grows. The tubercles are red and smooth and of a conoidal form, and nearly equal to a pea in magnitude. Many of them continue in this condition for three or four weeks, or even longer, having attained their full size in seven or eight days; but others separate very slowly and partially, discharging a small quantity of thick matter, by which the hairs of the beard are matted together, so that shaving becomes impracticable, from the tender and irregular surface of the skin. This condition of the face, rendered rugged by tubercles from both ears round to the point of the chin, together with the partial ulceration, and scabbing, and the matting together of the unshaven beard, occasions a considerable degree of deformity; and it is accompanied also with a very troublesome itching.

This form of the Sycosis occurs, of course, chiefly in men; but women are not altogether exempt from it, though it is commonly slight, when it appears in them. Its duration is very uncertain: it is commonly removed in about a fortnight; but sometimes the slow suppuration goes on for many weeks; and sometimes the suppurating tubercles heal, and again begin to discharge. Occasionally the disease disappears for a season, and breaks out again.

* A Practical Synopsis of Cutaneous Diseases, 3rd Edition, London, 1814, p. 292.

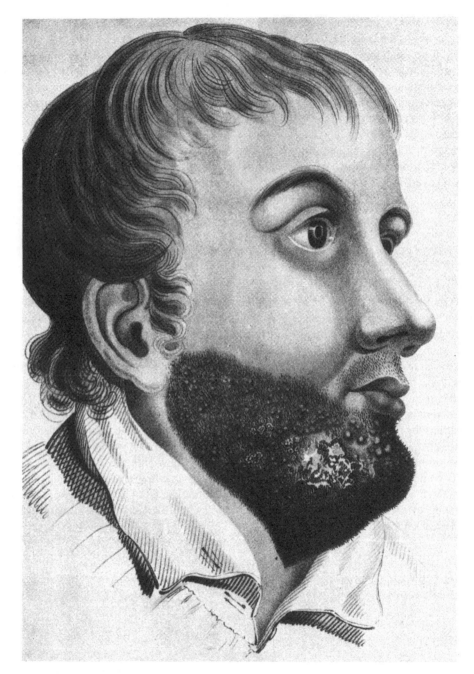

Figure 8 Sycosis barbae. From Bateman's atlas. Courtesy, College of Physicians, Philadelphia

Michael Underwood

Sclerema Neonatorum

MICHAEL UNDERWOOD was born September 29, 1737, in Surrey. After preliminary education at West Moulsey and Kensington he was placed with Mr. Caesar Hawkins (1711–1786), a skillful operator and sergeant-surgeon to King George II, and he eventually became a house-pupil at St. George's Hospital. At the conclusion of a sojourn in Paris he became a member of the Surgeon's Company, and started out in Margaret Street, Cavendish Square, combining the practice of obstetrics with his operative work.

Underwood was an able accoucheur; persons of rank and consequence were among his clientele. He attended the Princess of Wales at the birth of the Princess Charlotte. But it was in pediatrics that Underwood really excelled, and it is for his writings in this field that he is chiefly remembered. In 1784 he published his *Treatise on the Diseases of Children*. This remarkable book was the first English pediatric text, and remained the accepted authority for over 60 years, during which time 10 editions were published. Its direct style and delightful simplicity make it worthwhile reading even today. In addition to the original description of sclerema neonatorum presented here, it contained the first clear account of poliomyelitis.

Underwood was well on the way to wealth and position when the pressure of domestic afflictions forced him to retire in 1801. Melancholy and despondent for a number of years, during which time friends were forced to come to his rescue financially, he recovered somewhat and resumed his practice to a limited extent for the last few years before his death in 1820.*

SCLEREMA NEONATORUM

Skin-bound[†]

In the preceding edition, this disorder was considered only in a transient way, under the article of *Purging;* both from its being conceived to appear chiefly in the form of a morbid symptom attending certain bowel complaints, and because I had then neither seen, nor heard enough of the disease to enable me to offer to the public any very distinct account of it. I could indeed wish that this disorder were yet better understood, and that I were able to lay down a more successful method of treatment than has yet been made known: it is however in every view worthy of the most distinct consideration, as well as from the observations made in this country, as from the late researches by several physicians in *Paris,* as I shall have occasion to notice very soon.

That the present account of the disease may therefore be clearly stated, I shall first consider it as it has appeared in this country, and in the manner I had long ago intended, and had actually drawn up before I was favoured by some farther description of it by Dr. Audrey of Paris.

It has indeed, been much less common in this kingdom than on the continent, but is equally an hospital disease, and is seldom met with but accompanied with some bowel complaint, and still more rarely appearing at birth. It was first spoken of in public, I believe, by my friend Dr. Denman (when physician to the Middlesex hospital, and a teacher in midwifery); as I remarked in the former edition; and it is to him I was indebted for some account of it before I had at all noticed the disorder myself.

The *British Lying-in* hospital has been very little infested with it, and, possibly, by being solely appropriated to the reception of pregnant women, which the Middlesex hospital is not. I shall therefore first of all lay down the symptoms exactly as they were noticed in that infirmary, by Dr. Denman whose unwearied attention to it, though not with all the desired effect, does him more honour, than could have been derived from the most successful treatment of a disease less fatal than has proved wherever it has appeared.

The following symptoms may be considered as pathognomonic, or characteristic of the disease:

1. The skin is always of a yellowish white colour, giving the idea of soft wax.
2. The feel of the skin and flesh is hard and resisting, but not edematose.
3. The cellular membrane is fixed in such a manner, that the skin will not slide over the subjacent muscles; not even on the back of the hands, where it is usually very loose and pliable.
4. This structure often extends over the whole body; but the skin is peculiarly rigid in the parts about the face; and on the extremities.
5. The child is always cold.
6. The infant makes a peculiar kind of moaning noise, which is often very feeble; and never cries like other children.
7. Whatever number of days such children may survive, they always have the appearance of being dying.

This disease appears at no regular periods; but whenever it takes place it attacks several infants within a short time; and chiefly those, as I have just noticed who may be in the last stage of obstinate bowel complaints, in which the stools are of a waxey or clayey consistence. It has also been remarked, that it sometimes makes its appearance as an *original* disease, and even at the birth; in which case, the infant has never survived many days.

I have seen the rigidity extending beyond the cellular membrane, so as to affect the muscles, but only those of the lower jaw, which became perfectly rigid; but this *spasm* or *tetanus* is, by no means, a frequent symptom, and does not seize the extremities, as it is found to do in France; nor has the disease, in any instance that I have heard of, been attended with the *erysipelatous* afflictions constantly noticed in that country.

The Cause of this dreadful complaint, when congenite, or evidently supervenient to disorders of the first passages, seems to me to be a spasm depending very much upon a certain morbid state of those parts, and with which the skin is well known to have a peculiar sympathy. But when, though an original disease, it does not take place till some days after birth, which, I believe, is rarely, if ever the case except in large hospitals, and other crowded apartments; wherever the irritating cause, in such instances, may be seated, the disease seems

---

* Ruhräh, J.: Pediatrics of the Past. Hoeber, New York, 1925, p. 447.

† A Treatise on Diseases of Children, 2nd Edition. Philadelphia, 1793, p. 110.

to be an *endemic* of certain seasons, arising from that unwholesome air to which such places are peculiarly liable.

Jean Louis Alibert

1. *Lupus Vulgaris*

2. *Keloid*

3. *Mycosis Fungoides*

4. *Dermatolysis*

JEAN LOUIS MARC ALIBERT was born in Villefranche-de-Rouergue on May 2, 1768. He began his studies at a local school conducted by the Fathers of the Christian Doctrine, and later entered this order, passing his novitiate at Toulouse. He returned to his home to teach when the law of August 17, 1792 abolished all religious orders in France, and forced him to change his profession. After spending further time at a Paris normal school he was introduced by friends into the well known salon of Mme. Helvetius at Auteuil where he met the influential physicians, Roussel and Cabanis, who persuaded him to go into medicine. He matriculated in the Paris Medical School in 1796, and in 1799 submitted his thesis, *A Dissertation on the Pernicious or Ataxic Intermittent Fever*. The thesis was widely acclaimed, and the young Alibert began to come into prominence.

He now began to move in the circle of the most influential medical men in Paris and, in 1801, was appointed adjunct physician to l'Hôpital Saint Louis; within a year he was a full staff member. It was in 1801 that Saint Louis was set aside by law for the care of the more chronic disorders, under which category came most skin diseases at that time. The charge of these patients fell to Alibert, and it was his brilliant work there during the next few years that entitled him to his undisputed place as the founder of French dermatology; he was in no small measure responsible for establishing firmly the preeminence of Saint Louis in French dermatology—almost to the exclusion of other institutions, as a review of the work of French dermatologists included in this volume will bear out.

Alibert's Linnean classification of skin diseases, a *nosologie naturelle,* was impractical compared to Willian's which was based on the morphology of the essential lesion, and it was abandoned, even by his own pupils. Nevertheless, he was responsible for many fine clinical descriptions, couched always in a beautiful and flowery French difficult to render adequately into English. Many of his terms have persisted—dermatosis, syphilid, dermatolysis, and others. He fancied himself as an explorer in the vast unknown land of skin diseases, and never tired of bringing it to the attention of pupils and colleagues. He was a pioneer, with Willan, in dermatologic illustration, and the huge beautifully colored copper engravings which illustrate the work from which the selections given here are taken are superb from both the medical and artistic standpoints.

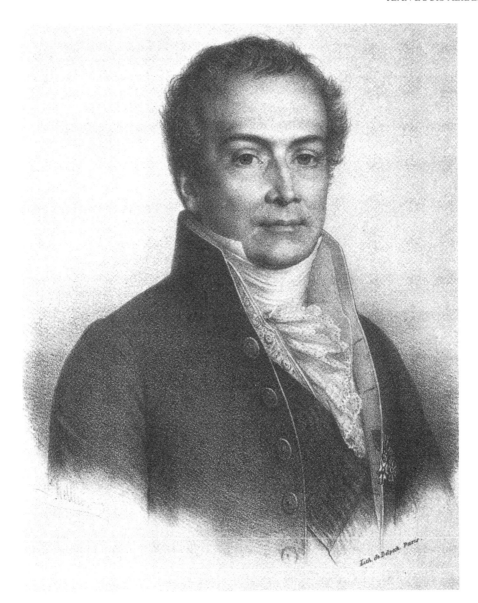

Figure 9 Jean Louis Alibert. Courtesy, College of Physicians, Philadelphia

Alibert was more than a well known dermatologist; he was the most renowned physician in all France. In addition to his tremendous private practice and his teaching at Saint Louis, he was the personal physician of Louis XVIII, a job which was no sinecure, for this was a sickly king.

Alibert's clinics were theatrical productions; he held forth in the garden of Saint Louis, *sous les tilleuls*. He was a magnificent speaker, bubbling with metaphor and simile, the more pungent for his strong southern accent. A syphilitic prostitute became "a priestess of Venus wounded by a perfidious dart of love." Patients were displayed on a platform and each bore the name of his disorder in one inch letters across his chest; tableaux of interesting cases were hung between the trees. Here was Alibert at his grandest.

He was made a baron by Charles X in 1827. This was at the height of his fame and power. He gave elaborate dinners, staged amateur theatricals, and counted among his guests the finest poets, musicians, writers, and artists in France.

Alibert died November 9, 1837, after a few months illness, only the last few days being spent in bed. The autopsy by Cruveilhier revealed an extensive gastric carcinoma.*

LUPUS VULGARIS

Tableau de la Dartre rongeante[†]

How many different features, indeed, are presented by the course of this disastrous affection when compared to the other species of Dartre! These latter commonly attack only the skin and the reticular body, but the Dartre we are dealing with here spares none of the different tissues of which the dermal system is composed. It is the seat of a deep ulceration whence escapes continually a purulent matter, fetid and corrosive, which leads to destruction of the muscles, vessels, membranes, cartilage, and even bone. It sometimes makes such progress on the face that it provokes a shedding of all the hairs, tearing up the face in some way. For a long time we saw a man at l'Hôpital Saint Louis who had lost his beard completely, due to the unhappy effect of this desperate affection.

The patients, to be sure, experience none of that pruritus which is so annoying, and which occurs particularly in the squamous and crustaceous Dartres, but they are victims of a torment devouring in intensity, almost insupportable, especially when, from the intensity of the causes, the Dartre is converted into an ulcerated cancer. However, it must also be said that the flesh is sometimes so slowly corroded that the patients complain of little but dull pains.

The Dartre rongeante shows several stages, from the point of view of the observer. Before this sort of phagadenic decomposition manifests itself on the living body, everything seems to proclaim the approaching malignity of those symptoms which are bound to announce themselves. The tissu muqueux of the skin reddens intensely, becomes hard, embossed, and uneven. A dull pain appears in the place in which the Dartre is beginning to develop. The cutaneous surface is attacked by an extremely annoying pruritus which the patient seeks vainly to assuage by a continual and most noxious rubbing. All of the nervous papillae are inflamed to such a degree that the more they are scratched, the more they dispose the dermal system to experience pruritus anew. At this time it might be possible to avert the formation of this horrible disease, or at least curb it at its outset, but the patients could scarcely know what this first point of irritation must become; very often no importance is attached to it, and no measure is taken to avert such a scourge.

Similar to those baneful germs of putrefaction that destroy with promptitude the interior substance of the finest fruits, this morbific germ of corruption soon spreads, unless one is able to arrest its course and its frightful development. The dreadful decomposition progresses at the pleasure of the forces that favor it; the epidermis elevates, opens, and falls away; the reticular body is broached; the entire skin becomes irritated, tumefied; from the heart of an ulcerated pustule springs an ichorous matter so acrid in quality that it inflames and reddens the surrounding parts, and becomes thereby one of the most active causes in the extension of

---

* Beeson, B., Arch. of Dermat. and Syph., 26:1086, 1932.

[†] Description des Maladies de la Peau. Paris, 1806, p. 65.

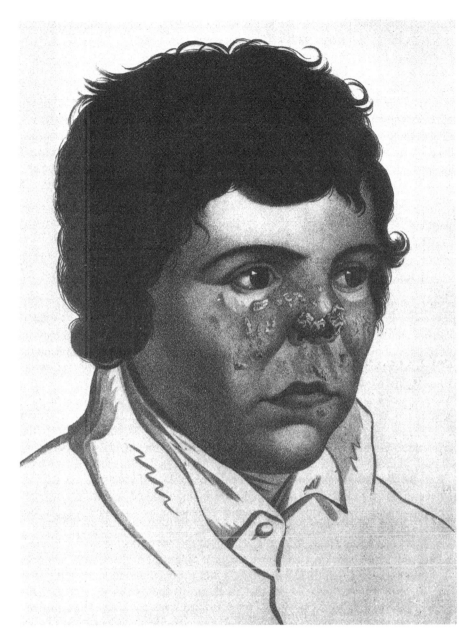

Figure 10 Lupus vulgaris. From Alibert's *Description des Maladies de la Peau*. Courtesy, College of Physicians, Philadelphia

the disease. For, the more abundant this matter is, the more phagadenic Dartre extends its ravages; in the opposite case, when the source of this humor dries up, the Dartre does not advance at all; it remains stationary. Almost always the pus concretes in the form of a large crust, forming a sort of cover on the corroded part of the Dartre; if this crust falls off, a second one forms, etc.

There is a third stage to this affection, in which it gains considerably in depth. It traverses, by corroding them, the adjacent parts of the dermal system. The bones are attacked and rotted, and it is then that the purulent matter becomes thicker, more fetid, and more corrosive. The patient's sleep begins to be interrupted; a low fever wastes him; the internal functions become troubled and deranged; a diarrhea appears which is certainly inauspicious inasmuch as it daily saps the strength.

Finally all the organic systems participate in the local infection. The lymphatic system takes it up, and all the abdominal viscera begin to engorge; the greenish color of the patient announces that the spleen is obstructed; the liver suffers the same alteration before long; an infiltration soon reaches the lower parts. The flux then becomes perpetual, instead of intermittent; it is, strictly speaking, a colliquative flux, to which death is the sequel.

KELOID

Tableau des principaux phénomènes que présentent' les Cancroïdes*

The Cancroïdes (Cancroides) are carniform excrescences, sometimes oval, sometimes oblong, situated horizontally on one or several parts of the integument, pale rose in color, covered by whitish lines and separated one from another, deeply adherent to the skin, the color of which is altered only in the elevated area, imitating quite well the cicatricial forms that follow severe scalds, extending out from their borders at times small bifurcated prolongations which bear some resemblance to the claws of a crab, which fact clearly justifies the name we have given to these extraordinary tumors.

The Cancroïdes which I have observed formed flat and compact tumors which were elevated at the edges and a bit depressed toward the center, especially when they were oval in configuration, protuberant, one or two lines above the level of the skin. They were shiny, a little wrinkled, hard and renitent to the touch. They were of a very reddish color, and on their surfaces were seen a multitude of small veins injected with a sanguineous liquid. Their circumferences were, however, much less dark in color. If they were compressed beneath the finger they blanched momentarily. The epidermis of the affected part was daily converted into fine scales, I have at times seen Cancroïdes which were cylindrical and set into the skin. They have the appearance of those oblong worms which the naturalists designate by the name dragonneaux, and which crawl about in cellular tissues.

There is ordinarily considerable increase in the warmth of the parts affected by Cancroïdes. The patients experience itching, intolerable pricking, and sharp and smarting pain in them, as if lances or hot needles were being shot into the skin. Often these pains extend into the neighboring parts, and sometimes there is even an internal sensation of twitching. One felt that his chest was about to burst. It is especially at night that the itching becomes fiery and most annoying. There are also cases in which these oval or longitudinal indurations are, so to speak, indolent. The individuals thus affected experience scarcely anything but a slight stiffness of the skin.

Most commonly there is but a single Cancroide on the skin, but at times one may see two or three on the same individual, sometimes even a greater number. This affection appears almost always in the area between the breasts, the posterior part of the arm or shoulder, on the lateral part of the thighs, etc.; it is   so

---

* Description des Maladies de la Peau. Paris, 1806, p. 113.

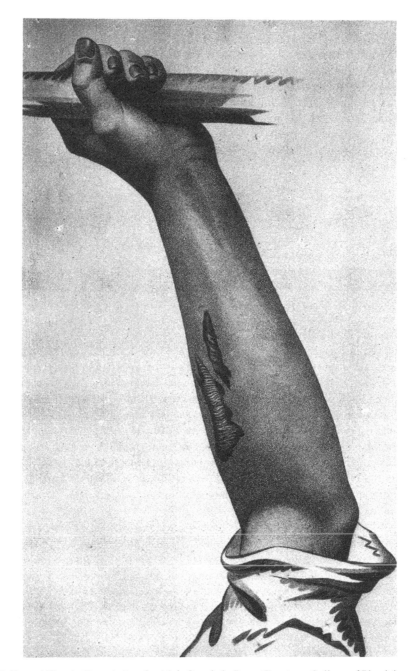

Figure 11 Keloid. From Alibert's *Description des Maladies de la Peau*. Courtesy, College of Physicians, Philadelphia

metimes seen along the back. When Cancroïdes multiply they become extremely painful. I have seen a patient so greatly affected that he could do no work whatsoever, and felt a general weakness in all his extremities.

Cancroïdes rarely disappear; they are as lasting as cancers. Ordinarily they remain on the skin for many years without progressing; this is a characteristic that merits emphasis. Nevertheless it may happen that they disappear spontaneously. The skin then sinks back and looks as though it were the site of a well healed cicatrix; that is, in that area the integument is whiter, thinner, and more wrinkled, indicating that there is a void in the tissue muqueux. It is known that a similar phenomenon occurs in cancer, in certain dartres, in the scrophules, etc., and that wherever these diseases heal, the skin remains depressed.

In general, women are much more subject to the Cancroïdes than men, which proves that in this affection the lymphatic system is radically impaired. In Paris several women are to be seen who, affected with this sort of tumor on the anterior superior part of the chest, seek to hide it beneath lockets or other jewelry which they hang about the neck.

MYCOSIS FUNGOIDES

Tableau du Pian fongoïde*

Bontius has mentioned this type of Pian; it manifests itself, according to him, by tubercles which have, as it were, the consistency and hardness of squirres. These nodules generally affect the face, and successively the arms, the lower extremities, etc. In time one sees them soften, open, and produce a thick gummy pus with a greenish color. This results in virulent ulcers; the liquid which flows from them is so acrimonious that it produces eschars on the skin.

Two periods can be distinguished, therefore, in the course and development of Pian fongöide. In the first period of its existence the growths are so hard and renitent that one would hardly suspect an approaching suppuration. But in the second period the skin which covers them opens, and each tubercle becomes a fetid ulcer; as decomposition progresses, these tubercles take on a greenish black color or a very dark violaceous tint. One can picture them as fruits rotting on the stem that bears them.

The pustules of Pian fongoïde resemble warts, for the most part, when they begin to develop; later they enlarge, taking the form of mushrooms, and spread out in great numbers over the surface of the body. There eventually comes a time when almost the whole cutaneous surface is covered.

This malady has definitely the mask of venereal disease; however, it causes scarcely any sharp pain. It is rather rare to see manifest exostosis, caries, or, finally, all those ravages syphilis produces about the mouth. But the external disorders are almost always more horrible.

The excrescences of Plan fongoïde are not all the same size; there are those of them which stay small for a long time, and are not much larger than a raisin seed or lentil; others are quite as large as morels on the ground, or those reddish fruits of the *solanun lycopersicon* ordinarily designated in the domestic economy by the name *tomatoes* or *love apples*.

After some months the tumors collapse and shrink; the withered and dried skin is so insensible that it may sometimes be cut with the scissors without the patient feeling the least painful sensation. The latter fall little by little into a state of emaciation that weakens them to the extreme; they end up succumbing, or leading a miserable life for many years.

---

* Description des Maladies de la Peau. Paris, 1806, p. 157.

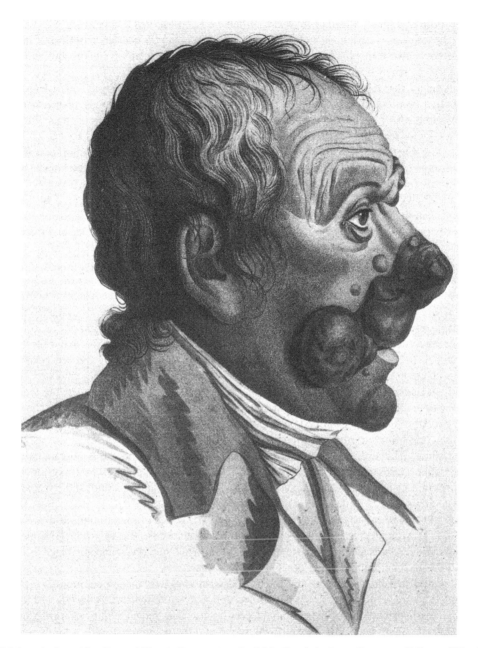

Figure 12 Mycosis fungoides. From Alibert's *Description des Maladies de la Peau*. Courtesy, College of Physicians, Philadelphia

DERMATOLYSIS

Histoire d'un berger des environs de Gisors (Dermatose hétéromorphe)*

Never, perhaps, has the skin offered so extraordinary an example of development as in the person of

J.B.Lemoine, born in a small village near Gisors. When we first observed this individual he was 45 years of age. His height was four feet four inches; his head made up almost a quarter or a fifth of his height; the trunk made up only two fifths: his legs and thighs were much longer than his height should have required; the sum total was a man of small stature, but quite well constituted.

The extraordinary development of his head was due to the folds formed by the skin which covered it. These folds were seen on the forehead, the left temple, and the entire right side of the head; they were enormous in extent. The first, occupying the forehead, took the form of a square, elongated at the superior and posterior angle on the right, and at the anterior and inferior angle on the left, almost reaching the frontal bossa on this side. The skin which formed these folds was thick, the cellular tissue a little swollen, but more in some places than in others. This skin was whitish pink and not at all adherent to the bone. The square that it formed was three inches in its greatest diameter, which was the transverse, by two inches six lines in its smallest diameter, which was vertical. After this first development the skin appeared to thin out, being always thicker than in the normal state, however, and continued in extent to the articulation of the occipital bone with the parietal; it extended over two thirds of the frontal bone on the right side and over the superior half of the parietal on the same side, over the superior part of the occipital, over all the left parietal, over the temporal and the cheek bone on the same side, and ended at the nasal apophysis of the frontal bone; from the nasal apophysis of the frontal it continued in its extent, forming new folds over the entire right side of the nose, over the whole of the upper lip, from the mental foramen of the lower jaw to its angle on the right side; it then reascended to the mastoid apophysis on the same side, to behind the ear, reached the temple on the same side, carrying over in front to the parietal bossa, which we took as its point of departure.

Over the entire vertex the skin showed no folds, but there were irregularities here and there which were due to a peculiar engorgement of the cellular tissue. All of that part covering the left parietal bone was increased in thickness, and flattened out on the temple on the same side, forming four or five large folds which joined with other such folds coming from the right frontal bossa, passing over the left superciliary arch to unite with the first over the temporal apophysis of the frontal bone.

The combination of these folds formed an uneven mass of pendant skin which by its own weight pulled down everything covering that surface of the head. It carried the eyebrow down two inches and caused it to fall upon the cheek. This eyebrow extended from the base of the nose to the zygomatic apophysis. The border of the upper lid extended like the snout of a carp, more tumefied in its external portion, and covering an eye starting from its orbit, so to speak; this eye was smaller than in the natural state; it was whitish and embossed at certain points.

The entire right side of the head and face was occupied by a series of longitudinal folds, five in number. The middle one was divided at its lower part into three other folds, one of which, the most posterior, terminated on the helix, reascending to become fixed there. The other two branches joined with the second longitudinal fold, and continuing with it, descended to the chest.

The first longitudinal fold, which was also the most anterior, began at the left commissure of the upper lip and was formed completely by this lip; it descended obliquely covering three quarters of the mouth, and came to an end on the lateral part of the chin; the lower lip also contributed a bit to its formation. The upper lid on the same side was found to be drawn down by the middle longitudinal fold. It too was a little loose, and covered an atrophied eye which had not left its orbit at all, but which, being very small, rested on the lower edge of the orbit, and left the upper part free, giving the appearance of an ugly recess in this area. The orbit was wider than in the normal state. The eyebrow was also found to be drawn down in the lateral part

---

* Monographie des Dermatoses. Paris, 1835, p. 796.

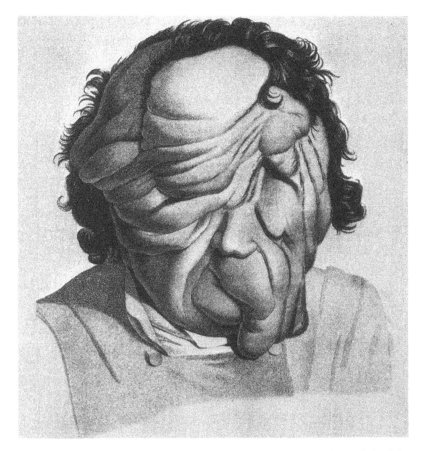

Figure 13 Dermatolysis. From Alibert's *Monographic des Dermatoses*. Courtesy, College of Physicians, Philadelphia

by this same middle fold; its medial part was adherent to the superciliary arch. The fourth longitudinal fold ended in the posterior division of the third, passing in front of the ear. The fifth, finally, after having passed between the ear and the fourth, was turned up like a drapery, and was fixed to the posterior part of the helix. These last three folds, united, dragged the ear down with them. Moreover, none of these folds appeared to be formed from diseased skin; on the contrary, the envelope was of a natural color; those parts destined to be covered with hair were so, but with hairs which were stronger and more thinly sowed than ordinary. It was not only the skin forming all these folds which contributed to the extraordinary volume of the head; the bones there also accounted for much of it. The frontal and parietal bones were a quarter larger than in the normal state; they were covered over with eminences which appeared to be due to the development of the pericranium. All these eminences, made up of bone, huge in dimension, gave him the most hideous appearance it is possible to imagine; one would not know to what to compare the form of the face; it was most monstrous.

This unfortunate had lost an eye at the age of six months; at twenty years he lost the remaining one, after having experienced most violent headaches. He despaired of ever being able to work again. When he went walking, directing himself with a cane, he was seized with boredom. He betook himself to a woods not far from his village and, wishing to make his walk fruitful, began to cut birches to make brooms. His first successes encouraged him so much that he felt himself able to look after cows; one could scarcely entrust him with more than one, however. Moreover, Lemoine recognized each place to which his steps led him. He knew how to distinguish between the meadows and grounds which were not too far from the woods he frequented. During the nearly 20 years in which he followed this profession he never lost his way; if he stepped from the path for a moment he soon recovered, directing himself by the sun, some glimmer of which he was still able to perceive through his eyelids.

We may add that he possessed all his intellectual faculties. One of the greatest sorrows his deformity caused him was that he had not been able to marry. He dearly loved his parents. He was sometimes seen to laugh, when one addressed some pleasantry to him; the mass of skin on the right side of his face, as well as the folds on the left side and his upper lip were then lifted and shaken with a convulsive movement. Lemoine did not let his beard grow; he shaved with extreme expertness those ribbons of skin that masked his hideous visage. He slept in a hovel to which everything necessary was brought, for this unfortunate had been excluded from his father's house following a vow made by his sister, when she married, never again to look upon his face, fearing lest one of her progeny bear one day the impress of his deformity.

Armand Trousseau

Cutaneous Diphtheria

ARMAND TROUSSEAU was born in Tours, October 14, 1801. After early schooling at the lyceums of Orleans and Lyons he became, at twenty, professor of rhetoric at the college of Chateau-roux. At an evening reception he met the great Bretonneau, who first clarified the pathology of diphtheria and typhoid fever, and at the older man's invitation began his medical training at the hospital in Tours. So assiduous was he at the post mortem table that his classmates dubbed him "Vultur-papa." During all this time he was almost a son to the childless Bretonneau. He took his Paris degree in 1825, and in 1828 was sent by the government to investigate a diphtheria epidemic in Sologne. After a period in Gibraltar studying yellow fever, and several preparatory hospital appointments, he came into his own at l'Hôtel Dieu de Paris where he remained the rest of his life.

Trousseau was a brilliant teacher. A pupil, Dieulafoy, left a vivid impression of his clinic:

"It was at the clinic of the old Hotel Dieu that I saw Trousseau for the first time…. I was astonished, I was dazzled. A great crowd of physicians of all nationalities, avid of instruction, were following the clinic. One of the most assiduous was Duchenne of Boulogne. Trousseau discussed the most disparate cases with equal competence. Whether it was general pathology, therapeutics, or internal medicine, he was equally on his own ground everywhere."

In addition to his great interest in diphtheria which was manifested early in his career, as evidenced by his account of cutaneous diphtheria which we have included here, Trousseau did important work on laryngeal phthisis and gastric vertigo, and made many important contributions to therapeutics. His name is connected with a diagnostic sign in infantile tetany, and a test for bile pigments. He performed the first tracheotomy in Paris, and more than anyone else was responsible for popularization of this procedure.

He made his last diagnosis in 1867, his own, and waited for the end with stoicism and fortitude.*

CUTANEOUS DIPHTHERIA

De la Diphthérite Cutanée[†]

The daughter of Josephine Pressoir, eight years of age, had had, the mother told us, several contacts with a family infected in the town, *les Rois,* and a short time later was seized with pharyngeal diphtheria.

When we saw her, the 13th of September, she was in the eighth day of her disease. M.Leménager had applied leeches to the neck, had touched the posterior pharynx three times with a silver nitrate solution, and had performed several alum insufflations. Besides this, the fear of a gangrenous affection had induced this

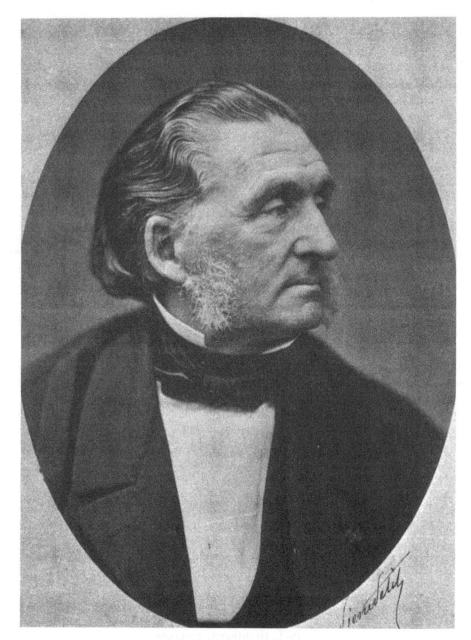

Figure 14 Armand Trousseau. Courtesy, College of Physicians, Philadelphia

physician to introduce injections of a decoction of camphorated cinchona into the throat, and to prescribe gargles of cinchona and alum. On the fifth day of the disease a vesicatory was applied to the nucha; abundant suppuration followed and the excoriated surface became covered with false membranes as was the case with an ulceration that the girl had had for a long time on the foot.

I will describe the condition in which we found the back of the child, the 13th day of September, the ninth day of the illness.

The vesication, which was in the beginning only three inches in diameter, is now more than six. It is horribly painful, and produces excessive suppuration. It spreads out over the back forming irregular projections resembling trick-track marks, and it is surrounded by a large erysipelatous aureola, much more marked at the lower portion than at the upper and on the sides. The part denuded of epidermis at this time appears depressed, and it actually is, with respect to the neighboring tumefaction. It is covered with superposed yellowish white fibrinous layers which, thickest in the center, thin out toward the circumference. In the center their thickness is two, three, up to four lines, and they look exactly like the dry pleuritic concretions that one finds in the chest cavity when resolution has already begun, and the secreted serous part is almost entirely resorbed. We lifted some of these concretions with a very thin metal plate, and we noted that they were very firmly adherent to the skin, and could be gotten off only with a certain amount of difficulty.

The surrounding erysipelas had a singular appearance. The redness was brighter toward the excoriated parts. The epidermis at many points was elevated by small quantities of a lactescent serosity in such a way that the skin was covered with vesicles, confluent in the neighborhood of the wound, less and less numerous toward the normal skin. Among the vesicles were those which appeared to have formed from the confluence of several; others, discrete or confluent, were ruptured, and at their sites the skin was seen to be covered with a white membrane; these ulcerations joined with other small ones, and then became confluent with the principal area; it was in this way that the disease spread from one area to another.

We should add, as a notable peculiarity, that the erysipelas had spread scarcely at all to the sides of the head or shoulders, and that in these areas very few vesicles were to be seen.

---

* Garrison, F.H.: Internal. Clin., *3:*384, 1916.

† Arch. Gén. de Méd, *23:*383, 1830.

Luca Stulli

Mal de Meleda

LUCA STULLI was born in Ragusa, September 22, 1772. He was educated at the Collegium in Piaristen, and at the age of 20 began at the University in Bologna, where he devoted himself to the medical sciences under Uttini, Mondini, and Galvani. He was graduated in 1795, and soon afterwards found it necessary to leave Bologna for political reasons. In Florence he came under the influence of the eminent naturalist, Felix Fontana, and maintained an active interest in this field for the rest of his life. After practice in Rome and Naples he returned to his fatherland, Dalmatia, where he died suddenly from a stroke in September, 1828.

Stulli's work was divided among three fields. As a physician he is best known for the observation given here, and for his pioneer work in mass vaccination, particularly in Dalmatia. As a naturalist he wrote much of the Mediterranean lands, including a series of papers on the Meleda geological detonation phenomenon he mentions below. In addition, he was an accomplished classical scholar, a poet, and successful playwright.*

MAL DE MELEDA

Lettre du Dr. Stulli, sur une espèce de maladie cutanée[†]

In a village on the island of Meleda, known for those faint detonations that are heard there, a cutaneous disease is observed which affects the extremities of some of the inhabitants and which, although a far cry from the petites cornes of Anna Jakson and the scales of the Lambert brothers, merits a place among all those anomalies observed in the organic tissues of animals.

Eleven individuals belonging to three families present the same alteration in the cutaneous envelope of the palms of the hands, of the palmar surfaces of the fingers, the soles of the feet and the heels, parts of the body in which the epidermis is thickest.

The first time this tissue alteration was observed was not more than half a century ago; there are no previous traditions from which it is possible to conjecture when and how it appeared on this island, and who the individual was, first affected with it. It is certain that in the course of 50 years it has always shown the same characteristics; it is therefore likely that it was no different in its nature in more remote times.

---

* Wurzbach, C.: Biograph. Lex. des Kaiserthums Oester. Vienna, 1879, Part 40, p. 192.

† Bull, des Sciences Méd., *21:*96, 1830.

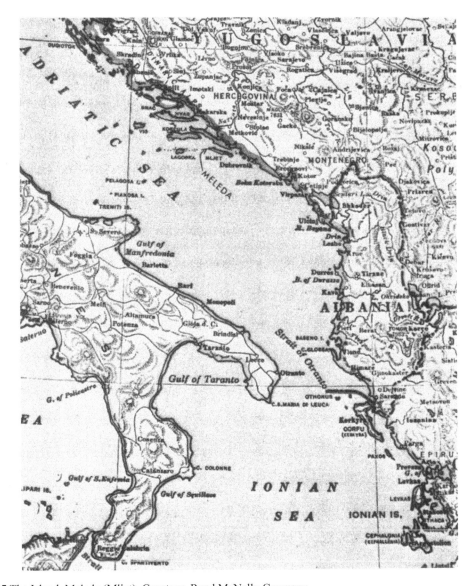

Figure 15 The Island, Meleda (Mljet). Courtesy, Rand McNally Company

Newborns show unquestionable signs on the palms of the hands of this alteration of the integument which progresses with age. The alteration in the tissue becomes little by little thicker and more compact, and extends in such a manner that it occupies the entire internal surface of the parts indicated above; it then spreads to the sides of the fingers and toes, and extends to the skin between them, and to the metacarpal and metatarsal articulations, and finally the skin takes on the appearance of a thick layer of yellowish tallow as resistant to pressure as leather; it is rough and uneven because of fissures which render it similar in appearance to the bark of the cork tree. Thus, the most superficial and external layer of the skin is transformed into an almost totally inorganic membrane, and indeed, in the parts indicated there is no sweating, no transpiration, and no sensibility, manifest indications that the vessels and nerves are destroyed. Because of this structure, there is no more of that albuminous transudation by which the epidermis renews itself as it is destroyed. A thickening of the epidermis of the elbows also takes place. Except in the case of those in whom the alteration has become most marked, the dermis and the corps muqueux form a single layer without including the superior portion of the skin, the reason why the integument of the carpus and tarsus appears wrinkled and dirty; that of the knees is also often covered with scales and excrescences similar to warts; moreover, the hands and feet are crippled.

The affected parts are devoid of any sensation whatsoever; the most violent contact is insufficient to render them sensible. There is no tumefaction at all, and it does not appear that the elevation of the skin is produced by a purulent, puriform, or viscous humor, nor by dirty and suppurating ulcers.

The principal cause of the stench given off by these villagers in the summer lies in the fissures that they have on the plantar surfaces of the feet; they are so deep that they traverse the entire thickness of the skin, and lay bare the muscular fibers which are visible, bloody to behold.

Children presenting these alterations of the skin are sometimes born of parents who are free of them, but who were themselves born of affected individuals; they are common to both sexes. Some siblings indict the stock from which they spring, others bear no mark; any suspicion of contagious propagation is inadmissible.

Pierre François Rayer

1.   *Ecthyma*

2.   *Cheilitis Exfoliativa*

3.   *Lingua Nigra*

PIERRE FRANÇOIS RAYER was born at Saint Sylvain, March 7, 1793. He studied medicine in Paris and received his doctorate in 1818 with a thesis entitled *Summary of a Brief History of Pathological Anatomy.* Named a Physician to the Hospitals of Paris in 1824, he spent seven years at Saint Antoine, and then transferred to the Charité where he spent the remainder of his hospital career. In addition to his many scholastic honors Rayer became the personal physician to Louis Philippe and Louis Napoléon. By imperial edict, in 1862, he was appointed dean of the Paris Medical School, but bitter opposition by the student body and a number of the faculty to what they felt was arbitrary use of imperial prerogative forced him to resign in 1864, a humiliation from which he never recovered. His death was in 1867.

Like Biett, Rayer was more or less a Willanist, but did not hesitate to alter the older man's work to suit his own experience. He was more appreciated abroad than at home, particularly in England, where several independent translations were made of his great *Treatise on the Diseases of the Skin,* from which the three definitive disease descriptions here included are taken. The terse style of this popular work is well shown by these selections.

Rayer was tall and rather stout, kindly, but forceful and authoritative. He was jealous of medicine's lofty position in France and defended it well. Beeson cites an anecdote in point:

One day a notorious financier asked him this question: "Is it true, Doctor, that the Roman physicians were all freed slaves?" "Yes," replied Rayer, "but that was the time when Mercury was the god of bankers and thieves."*

ECTHYMA

Chronic Ecthyma*

Chronic ecthyma, is a much more common disease than that which has just been described, and consists in several successive eruptions, which appear on the neck, extremities, and occasionally even on the face, at

---

* Beeson, B.: Arch. of Dermat. and Syph., *22:*893, 1930.

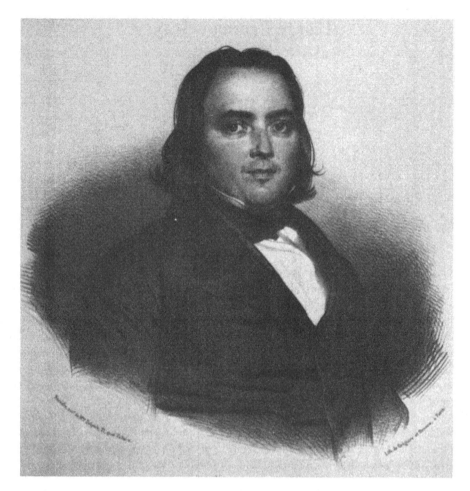

Figure 16 Pierre François Rayer. Courtesy, College of Physicians, Philadelphia

intervals more or less remote from each other. Each of these eruptions presents features in its course analogous to those which distinguish *acute* ecthyma. Whilst several of the pustules are appearing under the form of large red elevations, others are suppurating, and others are drying off and cicatrizing. It is not uncommon, for several eruptions of such phlyzacious pustules to take place over different regions of the body, within the space of a few months.

Besides this particular mode of making their appearance, the pustules of chronic ecthyma occasionally exhibit peculiar characters. In persons advanced in life, of indifferent constitution, affected with ulcers, etc., very large pustules are occasionally observed to be produced, with bases very similar in appearance to those of furuncles. The voluminous elevations which signalize their earliest stage, have a deep-red tint from their first appearance; the skin swells very slowly; the cuticle, distended with a blackish or sanguinolent serum, gives way at the end of six or eight days; the centres of the elevations soften, and become covered with a thick crust, which is prominent, black, very adherent, set, as it were, within a rim of the skin, and is not loosened before the lapse of several weeks.

When this crust is accidentally detached, or when it is removed by means of topical applications, it is found to conceal a small ulcer. Left to itself, this ulcer hardly becomes covered with a fresh scab; its surface discharges a sanguinous fluid.

These small ulcers may continue open for a very long time, and even spread, especially when they are situated on the lower extremities. When they are at length healed up, they leave cicatrices behind them which long continue of a livid or violet colour.

Ecthyma occasionally occurs during the exacerbations of lichen prurigo, scabies, and several other chronic inflammations of the skin; and the disease is a very frequent attendant upon convalescence from small-pox.

The continuance of chronic ecthyma, dependent on the number of successive eruptions that take place, and the state of the constitution, occasionally extends to a period of three or four months. The concomitant affections, if any exist, may get well before the pustules or continue after their disappearance.

Ecthyma attacks individuals of every age and of every variety of constitution; it occurs at all seasons, but is met with more particularly during the spring. A cold and damp habitation, filthy clothing, and indifferent food are causes common to this and a great number of other affections of the skin. Ecthyma is not a contagious disease, and its appearance may correspond with a disordered condition of the functions of the stomach and bowels.

CHEILITIS EXFOLIATIVA

Pityriasis labrum*

Pityriasis *labrum,* is a variety that has hitherto been confounded with psoriasis, a disease, however, from which it differs in being evolved on the lips and surrounding skin, not as papular elevations, followed by thick squamae, but under the semblance of minute red stains, to which succeed a general redness and a continual desquamation of the epithelium of the lips, and occasionally of the cuticle of the neighbouring skin. The desquamation goes on in the shape of little thin and transparent laminae, very similar to portions of the healthy epidermis dried, or of the epidermis whose inner surface has imbibed a little serum previous to desiccation. The lips, in this state, are affected with heat and tension; the epithelium gets yellow and thickened, it then cracks, and falls off in laminae of considerable size. It frequently happens that these continue to adhere for some time by their centre, when their edges are loose and already dry, so that a new epidermis is formed under the one about to be detached before it falls; this new cuticle then grows yellow, cracks, peels off, and falls in its turn, to be succeeded by another which undergoes the same changes and shares the same fate. This is always a long continuing and obstinate affection; every now and then it gets worse than usual, when the lips look swollen and of the brightest red. It is very different from that transient inflammation to which the lips are subject, attended with chapping and the detachment of the epithelium, which is induced by exposure to cold, or happens as a consequence of different acute diseases: this slight affection soon passes, whilst true pityriasis is always a lengthy and troublesome disease. The causes of pityriasis *labrum* are frequently obscure; I have observed it in two individuals, great talkers, who had a trick of always biting their lips.

---

* A Theoretical and Practical Treatise on the Diseases of the Skin (translation of Robert Willis). London, 1835, p. 531.

* A Theoretical and Practical Treatise on the Diseases of the Skin (Translation of R.Willis). London, 1835, p. 653.

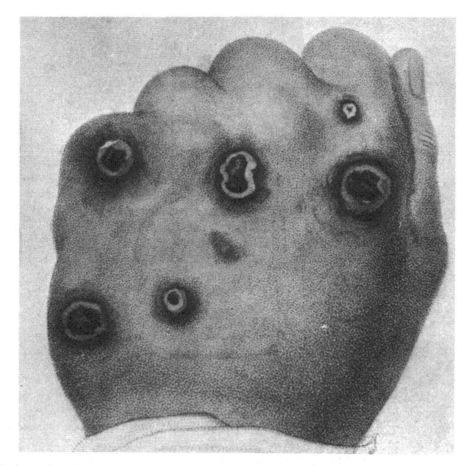

Figure 17 Ecthyma. From Rayer's atlas. Courtesy, College of Physicians, Philadelphia

LINGUA NIGRA

Nigrities*

I have seen several cases in which the tongue became black; the colouring matter, of a bluish black, is generally deposited on the edges of the organ, in small close spots, from whence it gradually extends over its upper surface. The tongue is otherwise perfectly healthy. It is necessary to distinguish these pigmentary discolorations from the artificial blackening, produced by food or medicine, and from those which the reaction of two substances, the one containing tannin, the other iron, might produce on being taken into the mouth at the same time, or shortly after each other.

---

* A Theoretical and Practical Treatise on the Diseases of the Skin (Translation of R.Willis). London, 1835, p. 938.

Samuel Plumbe

1. *Acne Vulgaris*

2. *Tinea Capitis*

SAMUEL PLUMBE (?–1837) flourished in that comparatively unproductive period in English dermatology between the death of Bateman (1821) and the maturation of the new and powerful schools of Erasmus Wilson, Tilbury Fox and Jonathan Hutchinson, in the latter half of the century. Although he suffers by comparison to these giants, he nevertheless made valuable contributions both to clinical dermatology and, more so than either Willan or Bateman, to the correlation of anatomy and physiology with skin disease.

Practically nothing is known of his early life, not even his birth date, nor of his training. He was active from 1821 to 1837. His most important work—from which the two important descriptions given below have been taken—was his *Diseases of the Skin*. It ran through four editions, the last (1837) being the most concise, practical and original.

Rosenthal said: "To judge from the quiet manner of his life and from the lack of notice taken of his death, it is safe to conclude that Samuel Plumbe was a simple, meek and unassuming man, imbued with an intense interest and zeal for his profession, who undoubtedly preferred labor at his studies in an unimportant dispensary service to publicity and who emerged into the public eye only at intervals with publications of genuine worth and the highest scientific merit."*

ACNE VULGARIS

Acne, or Obstruction and Simple Inflammation of the Cutaneous Follicles*

English authors have described four varieties of this affection, under the titles of acne, simplex, punctata, indurata, and rosacea; while Alibert, under the head of dartres, described the first and second of these as "dartre pustuleuse miliaire" and "dartre pustuleuse disseminée."

These varied designations create difficulties to the student, and are not necessary or useful. The circumstances on which they are founded are for the most part accidental and unimportant, and dependent merely on ordinary deviations from the regular progress of inflammation, or the degree of activity or its reverse which such inflammation may assume in the structure concerned.

---

* Rosenthal, F.: Arch. of Dermat. and Syph., *36:*348, 1937.

In its simple and most trifling form, the disease consists merely of obstruction of the sebaceous follicles, in consequence of their contents becoming too hard to pass readily to the surface. Inflammation of the follicle, and the production of what is called a pimple results, and is soon followed by the formation of matter; the follicle is destroyed by this process, the matter is discharged, a little redness remains for a day or two, and the part returns to the healthy state.

The situations in which the eruptions, designated as above, make their appearance, will generally be sufficient to enable us to determine their character. It has been observed in a preceding page, that the sebaceous follicles are chiefly distributed on the face, more particularly on the forehead, tip, and alae of the nose, and the adjoining cutis, and less copiously on the chin. Next to these the chest, below the clavicle, to about the fifth or sixth rib, and the back to an equal extent, are most liberally furnished with them; and as the disease consists in the derangement and inflammation of these structures, it is these parts solely in which it makes its appearance. Hence, it has been described as "an eruption of distinct hard inflamed tubercles which are sometimes permanent for a considerable length of time, and sometimes suppurate very slowly and partially; they usually appear on the face, especially on the forehead, temples, and chin, and sometimes also on the neck, shoulders, and upper part of the breast; but never descend to the lower parts of the trunk or to the extremities. As the progress of each tubercle is slow, and they appear in succession, they are generally seen at the same time in the various stages of growth and decline; and in the more violent cases are intermixed likewise with the marks or vestiges of those which have subsided.

In every case of this affection, a very considerable number of black points will be observed, imbedded in the cutis. These are nothing more than the blackened surfaces of the contents of the uninflamed follicles. The skins of different individuals differ greatly in the number, as well as size, of the sebaceous follicles; and hence, in a state of health, the complexions of some are said to be more clear than that of others; the copious distribution of the black spots which have been described, giving a dirty and less healthy appearance to the part, while their minuteness in size and numbers leaves the agreeableness of the red and white unimpaired. It is evident, however, that the simple appearance of such spots ought not to be considered as a disease, or as in any respect a deviation from a state of health. The most desirable change which can be effected, therefore, where they exist to an unpleasant extent, is that which frequent ablution and moderate friction only can produce.

There is great difference in the period elapsing between the commencement of the inflammation of different follicles, and its termination in suppuration; and consequently many of them are seen apparently only slightly inflamed, and presenting to the touch the resemblance of a small millet seed under the cuticle, while others have actually suppurated. It is not correct, however, as far as I have observed, that inflammation, as alleged by Willan and Bateman, when once begun, ever terminates in resolution; for each tubercle thus formed, if punctured with a lancet when assuming an appearance of subsiding, is found to contain matter: the orifice of the follicle is in such cases closed at the commencement of the inflammatory action, and if the latter has been less violent than usual, the quantity of pus produced does not lead to the rupture of the superincumbent structure, and absorption, more or less speedily, takes place.

In the case of an extensive affection of this kind, many tubercles are found in the state described, gradually subsiding without the appearance of matter on the apices. Where, however, matter makes its way to the surface, a few hours only elapse before it is discharged, and the only vestige remaining a day or two after, is merely a bluish red speck, which rapidly disappears. Minute scabs probably, for the first 48 hours, may be found covering this: these are intermixed with a considerable number of the reddened tubercles before

---

* A Practical Treatise on the Diseases of the Skin, 4th Edition. London, 1837, p. 15.

mentioned, and the blackened orifices of a larger portion of the uninflamed follicles. In most instances, when inflammation in the follicle begins its orifice is soon closed up by the attendant tumefaction, and the blackened speck disappears; but it sometimes happens, that the latter is observed in the centre of the pustule in which case, the sebaceous matter is surrounded by pus, and eventually discharged with it; still, however, it retains its solid form, though insulated in this manner, when it is easily detected by rubbing the contents of the pustule between the finger and thumb.

It has been constantly observed, that persons of a sanguine temperament and florid complexion have been most subject to follicular inflammation; and among these, that young men between the ages of 20 and 25 have been the greatest sufferers from it. Females, at the same age, are also subjects in whom its visitations are not infrequently manifested; but, in the latter, it rarely proceeds with such rapidity to suppuration, or produces such unpleasant appearances as to extent.

TINEA CAPITIS

Porrigo*

The forms I am about to describe, each occasionally occur spontaneously, but are also very frequently the results of infection. They have also the power of producing each other, as I have ascertained, beyond doubt, in a variety of instances; a fact which is, perhaps, by itself sufficient to establish their identity.

The first of these is that noticed by Turner, in which "the hair falls off not altogether from the root but by piecemeal." It is supposed by this author, and by Sennertus, to be produced by some insect, but they have not noticed the state of the skin of the affected parts. The attention is first attracted to it by the *falling off* of the hair of the part; there is little attendant itching, and no apparent fluid secretion on the spot. Sometimes, but not always, the patches are of a pretty regularly circular form, the margin being clearly defined, and exhibiting a line of scurf considerably thicker than that in the centre. In the centre of the spots the skin is scurfy, and the hair thinned, and easily extracted by the finger and thumb. What remains of it is unhealthy in appearance, some hairs being thin and delicate, others being the remains or stumps of those which have been broken or dropped off. There is a downy or towy looking substance just rising above, and mixing with the scurf, evidently formed by feeble attempts at the production of new hair. Two, three, or more of those spots, varying in dimensions are usually discovered on examining the head more particularly; and when the hair has been removed by shaving, they exhibit a red and slightly inflamed appearance. Several others in an incipient state will be discovered in different parts. The latter may be known before the hair begins to fall off, when they exhibit nothing beyond the appearance of a small discolouration about the size of a spangle; the hue is of a yellowish red, somewhat resembling the bran of the darker-coloured wheat. Others a little larger have decidedly assumed the ringed form.

With children of light complexion, with thin and delicate hair, with no constitutional disorder, or no great irritability of the skin, this will be the state in which the disease will always be found, provided no interference by stimulating or other applications has occurred; the margin of the spots not exhibiting any distinct appearance of pustulation. The diameter of these continue to enlarge rather slowly till they join each other, and a great part of the scalp is divested of its hair; but if stimuli in the shape of ointments be applied, a more active condition often takes place, and minute achores form, not only on the margins, but on other parts. Much irritation, heat, and itching arises; the disease spreads with greater rapidity, and changes its chronic inactive character for one directly the reverse. The pustules discharge their contents, and unless the head be washed frequently during the day, layers of lightish straw-coloured scabs are formed, under which the cutis is sometimes found to be abraded to a considerable extent.

At the commencement of the disease, and for some time after, spots evidently of the same nature as the affection of the scalp may be seen on different parts of the body; but the former being usually protracted for a considerable time, from causes hereafter to be more particularly mentioned, these spots generally disappear before much improvement is effected on the scalp.

The vesicles of the little patches, to which I allude as connected with ringworm of the scalp (if vesicles they may be termed) are, when unbroken, scarcely discernible to the naked eye, and are ruptured in a very few hours after their formation. They are, indeed, rarely seen unbroken; and when the attention is first directed to the spot, it exhibits the appearance of a small ring of scab, of a brownish colour; and in this state is well known under the name of ringworm, and quickly yields to the application of any mild escharotic application. The frequent occurrence of these spots simultaneously with the disease of the scalp first led me to the suspicion of connexion between them, and for the reasons I have detailed below, I now entertain no doubt of their identity, the apparent difference of character being solely the result of the *mischievous influence of the hair of the scalp.*

The other form of the disease to which I have alluded never assumes the circular figure just described: on the scalp it is pustular from the beginning, and marked during every stage of its progress by a much greater degree of irritation and itching. It is so generally diffused over a considerable space, even on its first appearance, as to warrant a designation founded on this feature, in contradistinction from the foregoing, which is so constantly circumscribed.

Like the latter, it appears to be readily identified with an affection of the skin of other parts, which is in part vesicular, but chiefly consisting of papulae of different sizes. These not being of much importance, are usually little noticed; but as soon as the disease appears on the scalp, alarm is immediately communicated to the parents, or others connected with the children who are subjects of it.

At this period much itching and irritation are found to exist. The pustules are very thickly dispersed over certain parts of the head, *every individual pustule having a hair growing through its centre,* and the scalp in the interstices being excessively red and inflamed. The child is feverish and irritable, the digestive organs evidently disordered, and a generally bad state of health will be found to have existed for a considerable length of time.

The absorbent glands at the back of the head, and those of the neck, are enlarged and tender, and in some neglected cases have proceeded on to suppuration; but this is by no means common. Small abscesses form here and there, from the inflammation of the cellular membrane under the scalp, which, in a few days, discharge their contents, and heal; the spots which they occupied remain in some cases ever after completely bald, the adipose structure secreting the hair having been destroyed.

As the pustules become ruptured, and their contents distributed over the adjacent parts of the scalp, these parts become inoculated, the disease spreads, and yellowish scabs are formed, of an unpleasant odour and aspect, which, unless frequent ablution be had recourse to, rapidly accumulate.

This diffused or pustular form of porrigo, is chiefly found among children of dark hair and unhealthy constitutions. It is not attended with immediate loss of hair, like the former; but this event takes place if the parts be frequently washed, in a short time.

---

* A Practical Treatise on the Diseases of the Skin, 4th Edition. London, 1837, p. 138.

Alphée Cazenave

1.   Pemphigus Foliaceus

2.   Lupus Erythematosus

PIERRE LOUIS ALPHÉE CAZENAVE was born in 1795, in Paris. His medical studies were concluded in that city, and an interest in dermatology was already manifest in his doctoral thesis, *Sur quelques propositions de médecine (maladies de la peau),* in 1827. He was a pupil of Biett, and therefore a Willanist, for it was his teacher who introduced the doctrines of Willan and Bateman into France. A year later he published, with Schedel, his *Pratique des Maladies de la Peau,* a very popular work in which he and the co-author gathered together Biett's clinical lectures. English translations soon appeared, especially in the United States, where it quickly became the most influential work in the field.

Cazenave founded the first journal devoted entirely to dermatology, the *Annales des Maladies de la Peau et de la Syphilis* (1843–52). In this journal appeared the first description of pemphigus foliaceus, and the definitive description of lupus erythematosus, both of which are given below. In addition to this, he was the author of important works on syphilis, describing in particularly great detail the secondary manifestations of this disease. He made notable contributions to syphilitic therapy, to the study of alopecia areata, linking it with vitiligo, and to the further understanding of eczema and diseases of the scalp.

His many active years in dermatology were spent at l'Hôpital Saint Louis. He died in 1877.*

PEMPHIGUS FOLIACEUS

Pemphigus Chronique, Général; Forme Rare de Pemphigus foliacé*

L..., 47 years of age, consulted me at l'Hôpital Saint Louis August 27, 1842 for an eruption of several years duration which occupied the entire surface of the   body, and which through its persistence had gravely compromised the health of the patient.

This woman, L..., had always been well until the age of 20 when she was attacked by an articular rheumatism which lasted for a very long time. Since then she has had two different attacks of *jaundice,* and still more recently, a gangrenous erysipelas of the leg.

---

* Goodman, H.: Urol. & Cutan. Rev., *51:*301, 1947.

* Annales des Maladies de la Peau, *1:*208, 1844.

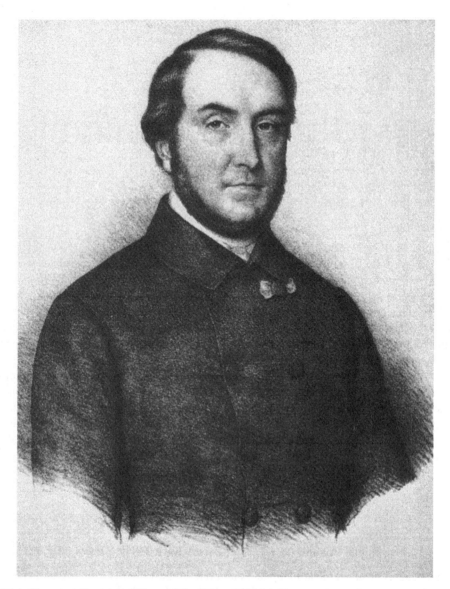

Figure 18 Alphée Cazenave. Courtesy, College of Physicians, Philadelphia

The present illness had already existed for 4 years. It was ushered in, according to the patient, by an erysipelas of the face which spread to the chest, and then involved successively the entire surface of the body. These erysipelatous plaques were, then, from the beginning the seat of the blisters of pemphigus. However that may be, for a long time the face, the abdomen, and the medial part of the thighs were continually the seat of large irregular elevations of the epidermis containing a serosity which was very limpid at first, but which soon became reddish. The eruption appeared usually without pain; the bullae, which were at first quite full and quite distended, ruptured or were lacerated by the least movement of the patient, and left more or less completely exposed a surface which became less and less red, and less and less

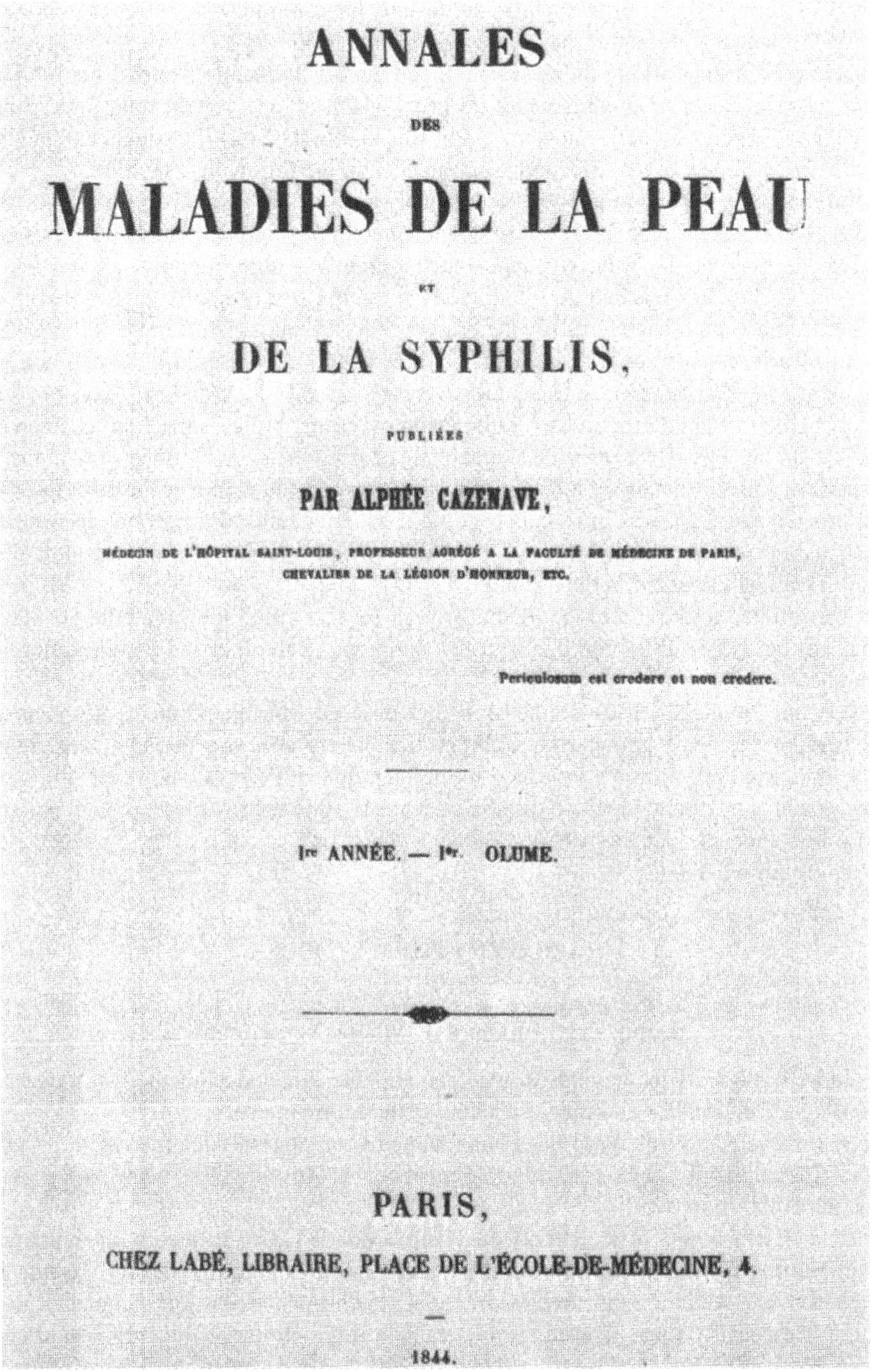

ANNALES

DES

MALADIES DE LA PEAU

ET

DE LA SYPHILIS,

PUBLIÉES

PAR ALPHÉE CAZENAVE,

MÉDECIN DE L'HÔPITAL SAINT-LOUIS, PROFESSEUR AGRÉGÉ A LA FACULTÉ DE MÉDECINE DE PARIS,
CHEVALIER DE LA LÉGION D'HONNEUR, ETC.

Periculosum est credere et non credere.

Iʳᵉ ANNÉE. — Iᵉʳ. OLUME.

PARIS,

CHEZ LABÉ, LIBRAIRE, PLACE DE L'ÉCOLE-DE-MÉDECINE, 4.

—

1844.

Figure 19 Title page to Cazenave's *Annales des Maladies de la Peau*. Courtesy, College of Physicians, Philadelphia

painful. New ones formed daily; little by little the lesions became more crowded, the bullae became less confluent; they formed less perfectly; they were less regular; still later, finally, they appeared as uneven, soft, scarcely elevated lesions lifting the epidermis in an almost insensible manner: the liquid flowed with difficulty and dried in place, producing a kind of crust which after a certain time formed into a general encasement with an entirely distinctive appearance. It was in this state that the patient entered the ward, four years, I repeat, after the onset of the affection. She was then in the following condition:

The face, the chest, and the abdomen were covered with a species of yellowish crusts, quite different from the thick and rugous crusts of impetigo; most of them, adherent only at one point and free around the rest of their circumference, presented a foliaceus appearance which was quite remarkable, and which one finds only in pemphigus which has reached this state. They formed a sort of continuous envelope in which one could, with a little attention, recognize easily the pre-existence of bullae. Thus most of them were extremely thin, and were clearly convex toward the center, while at the circumference, sometimes very strongly adherent, they lay one upon another; at times they were excessively thin, and showed wrinkling similar to that in the skin found puckered around each bulla. Moreover, true bullae, intact and characteristic, existed on the thighs and on the legs. They recurred several times during the patient's short stay in the hospital, and they established beyond the shadow of a doubt, if any had existed, the nature of the disease.

Moreover, this woman, L…, was in serious condition; with generalized infiltration from time to time she had a diarrhea that one could scarcely modify; she emitted a characteristic nauseating odor, and finally, she had a constant fever that increased in the evening.

Treatment was limited to the use of emollients at first, several mild tonics (café de gland), to the use of opiates, and a soft but quite substantial diet. But the symptoms increased, and 25 days after admission the patient succumbed.

Pemphigus is one of the diseases of the skin that deserves the attention of physicians; its history, however, is perhaps the least known. This observation offers an example of a rare form of chronic pemphigus, a form one finds scarcely indicated in the literature; it deserves, however, to be better known, since in every case it is confounded with a disease which is of little consequence, with impetigo. It is hardly necessary to dwell upon the dangers of such an error when one considers that for the bullous form the prognosis is almost always fatal.

LUPUS ERYTHEMATOSUS

Lupus érythémateux (Érythème centrifuge)*

Conference, June 4, 1851. After having shown four patients affected with the same disease (erythema centrifugum), M.Cazenave called attention especially to the following case.

In bed No. 68 of the Napoleon Ward lies a man named G.Prosper, a wine merchant, 38 years old, who first entered l'Hôpital Saint Louis the 3rd of September 1850, and after being out a few days, was readmitted on the 8th of May, 1851.

The eruption with which he is at present affected dates from 1841; it appeared without appreciable cause, and began with red spots, without elevation, without itching, the spots occupying at times the cheeks and at other times the ears, and which disappeared readily under the influence of a soft diet and tisanes. According to the patient, it is especially since he used a strong cantharides ointment that the disease has extended, and that the redness has spread more and more, and has reached the nose and all those parts of the face which it occupies today. The spots which are present on the hands date only from last year, and appeared a short time before his admission.

At the present time the following symptoms are observed: An erythematous reddening, light pink in color, disappearing on digital pressure and reappearing immediately on release, which occupies the superciliary arches, the two cheeks, the entire external surface of the nose, the eyelids (the edge alone on the right is unaffected), with an injection of their mucous surfaces which is quite marked, the free edge of the lips, the ears, and the hair line.

The face is the seat of a swelling which gives it a very particular appearance. Certain edematous *bourrelets* are present on the lower lids; this swelling does not yield to digital pressure.

The red areas are covered here and there by thin scales, very small, white, a little adherent, and later in their appearance than the erythematous spots.

Smooth pliant cicatrices of a bluish white are present on the root of the nose, and below the lids; they are the results of cauterizations already performed.

Somewhat similar spots are present on the neck, on the ears, especially on the lobes; they extend into the external auditory canal. At the hair line some of these spots are less pink colored, and the scales somewhat thicker, which makes them look somewhat like the plaques of psoriasis.

The lower extremities show nothing in particular. On both arms exactly demarcated spots are found which are quite dark red in color, and covered with a pronounced scale. They correspond to the scars of two vesicants which were applied some months before the entrance of the patient into l'Hôpital Saint Louis, after a suppuration lasting 18 months.

On the fingers and on the backs of the hands irregular spots of a wine red color are seen, in which the vessels ramify visibly, forming deep red trails.

The skin everywhere is soft, supple, and non-painful.

This case, interesting for several reasons, permits M.Cazenave to call to the attention of the practitioners a little known disease which exists usually in those with excellent general health, which, never presenting sores, ulcers nor crusts, proceeds by a thinning out, or sort of wearing out of the skin, and leaves indelible cicatrices.

This disease, which Biett indicated under the name *érythème centrifuge,* is a variety of lupus.

Without going into the general considerations of lupus, M.Cazenave felt it necessary to present several considerations on this curious variety which he calls *lupus erythematosus.*

Characterized by a redness which disappears on digital pressure, by a tendency to gradual and constant thinning out of the skin in the affected areas, and finally by cicatrices, lupus erythematosus presents, from the diagnostic standpoint, three important points: the redness, the thinning out of the skin without ulceration, and different appearances of lesions identical in nature.

Thus one may observe, but very rarely, an *urticarial* form. M.Cazenave has seen but very few examples of it. It appears almost always only in women. It sometimes localizes on the forehead, but most particularly on the cheeks; it appears in the form of somewhat raised plaques of true swellings which, instead of passing rapidly as simple urticaria, persist sometimes for quite a long time. This form is, in general, well demarcated, and when it passes always leaves behind a manifest thinning of the skin, or even cicatrices.

Lupus erythematosus appears in another form much more common than the preceding. Developing under the accidental influence of an external cause, it appears as a sort of chilblain. It consists of redness occupying the extremity of the nose. This redness may disappear, to return after longer or shorter intervals, and continue thus until it becomes permanent. With changes in temperature, for example, it is the seat of

---

* Annales des Maladies de la Peau, *3:*297, 1851.

pain, itching, and smarting. One, then, often mistakes lupus for a chilblain, and this diagnostic error is the more easy in some cases since the one sometimes succeeds the other, and the second may complicate the first.

When this form becomes permanent, it presents curious characteristics. It rarely involves all the nose; it is seated, on the contrary, only on the extremity of this organ, and is accompanied there by a mild swelling which may last a long time without progressing. However, if one examines it carefully, one sees that the skin is tense and shiny. Different places are dotted with depressions. Finally, the affected area becomes the seat of an exfoliation characterized by thin broad scales resembling the skin of an onion, and strongly adherent; without any apparent secretion to explain them, they constitute a true elimination product.

Lupus erythematosus has an almost exclusive predilection for the face; it localizes especially on the nose in women; in men, on the contrary, it is more frequent on the cheeks. It may, moreover, extend to the chin, the forehead, to the edges of the scalp, and sometimes to the scalp itself. One finds it rarely in other places, perhaps on the neck and hands. Samuel Plumbe attributes this erythema to dietary excess; this influence may be real, especially in the cases in which the congestive and inflammatory element dominates; but lupus erythematosus appears evidently under different conditions, and from different causes. Thus, it may be determined by the influence of cold, and also by the direct affect of a hot fire; it is also especially frequent in persons with a fine skin, women, and individuals exposed by occupation to great heat, as blacksmiths and cooks. One finds it also in messengers and coachmen, and it then appears to result from the direct action of the air.

In women, finally, this variety of lupus may accompany disorders of the uterus with menstrual troubles.

M.Cazenave feels it necessary, from the diagnostic point of view, to stress the very curious circumstance that lupus erythematosus co-exists in the majority of cases with excellent general health. He also brings out the fact that, contrary to what is observed in lupus in general, which appears especially in adolescence, lupus erythematosus develops only in the middle of life.

Julius Otto Ludwig Moeller

Atrophic Glossitis

JULIUS OTTO LUDWIG MOELLER was born in Koenigsberg, Prussia, on June 7, 1819. After studying in Koenigsberg, Berlin, Halle and Vienna, he began the practice of medicine in Koenigsberg in 1841, where he was made director of the polyclinic and later Professor of Medicine in the university. In 1863 he resigned these posts for political reasons. He wrote on numerous and diversified topics. His description of scurvy in rachitic infants is an early definitive account which led to the eponym, Moeller-Barlow disease. From the dermatologic standpoint he is remembered for his report, included here, of an unusual type of glossitis. Moeller died on August 28, 1887 in the city of his birth.[*]

ATROPHIC GLOSSITIS

Klinische Bemerkungen ueber eine weniger bekannte Krankheiten der Zunge[†]

Chronic excoriations appear not infrequently on the tongue, in the form of irregular bright red spots which are usually quite sharply circumscribed, and from which the epithelium has apparently been rubbed off, or is at least greatly thinned; the papillae appear hyperemic and swollen, projecting, then, above the level of the healthy surrounding area. A morbid secretion is never evident on them, nor does any deep inflammation ever develop; they show only a slight tendency to spread on the surface; indeed, once they attain a certain size and form, they usually maintain it very obstinately. They appear chiefly on the edges and tip of the tongue; identical spots are often found on the under surface of the tongue, and on the inner surfaces of the lips; I have never seen them in the posterior parts of the oral cavity. These excoriations produce a very unpleasant burning sensation which spoils the appetite and enjoyment of food in the patients affected, even when it is very mild, and stifles the taste completely. The articular motion of the tongue is sometimes somewhat painful as well.

I have seen this disease six times; all of the patients were middle aged women. In all these cases the excoriations had already been present for months when the patients came under my care, and they had shown themselves to be extremely resistant to the agents that had been used.

---

[*] Schönfeld, W.: Dermat. Wnschr., *123:*167, 1951.

[†] Deutsche Klinik, *3:*273, 1851.

Auguste Nélaton

Malum Perforans Pedis

AUGUSTE NÉLATON was born in Paris, June 17, 1807, son of a professional soldier who was later killed in Napoleon's Russian campaign. On completing his early education he entered the *College Bourbon* where he became associated with a tutor, Achille Requin, later to become famous in Parisian medical circles. Influenced by Requin, who was a medical student at the time, he too began the study of medicine, and pursued it with the same sober and uncompromising steadiness of purpose that characterized his every activity. It soon became clear that his talent was for surgery. After repeated applications for an internship with the great Dupuytren, the goal of all young surgical aspirants in that day, Nélaton finally succeeded in 1835, only to have the master's career terminate in death before his term had begun. A year later he submitted his doctoral thesis, *Sur l'affection tuberculeuse des os*.

Nélaton's rise to the peak of surgery in France was steady, and what with his great talent, inevitable. He was aided considerably, however, by the tremendous amount of international publicity he received for his part in the location of a musket ball which struck Garibaldi in the leg at the battle of Agramonte, in 1862. He acquired a huge private practice and became wealthy. Most of the surgical honors existent in France were bestowed upon him during his lifetime.

Nélaton was a perfecter, rather than an innovator. Besides the catheter, probe, and anatomical line which bear his name, he was responsible for a host of technical improvements in all aspects of surgery. As a teacher his direct and unhurried manner, his careful and explicit delivery, and complete command of the material won for him a great following of students. The description of malum perforans pedis given here was transcribed from one of his clinical lectures.

A breakdown in Nélaton's health occurred following excessive exertion in caring for the wounded of the 1870 revolution. He died September 21, 1873, of heart disease.*

MALUM PERFORANS PEDIS

Affection singulière des os du pied[†]

In bed 33 of the male ward, on the service of Prof. Nélaton, we have seen a man affected with one of the most singular conditions we have observed, and to which our readers will not judge it useless to turn their attention for a moment.

Here is, in a few words, a description of the disease.

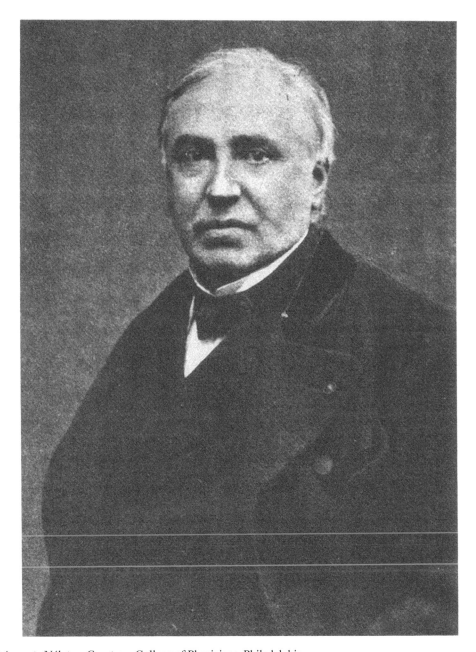

Figure 20 Auguste Nélaton. Courtesy, College of Physicians, Philadelphia

On the osseous prominences of the foot a blister appears. The epidermis elevates; under the epidermis there is a little purulent serosity. The epidermis perforates with or without the aid of surgery; the dermis becomes visible and has a pinkish color. It is more tender to touch than in the ordinary blister. For some time things remain in this state. Soon the dermis perforates in its turn, from the surface inwards, little by little. A small fistula is formed. This fistula reaches into the subcutaneous tissue; it persists, and produces a serosity which is somewhat purulent. Then, when one explores this fistula with a stylet after it has existed for four or five weeks, one finds a denuded and necrotic portion of bone. The sequestrum which is formed may be extracted, or it may separate itself.

Such are the phenomena reproduced many times in an unvarying fashion in this patient.

Twelve years ago a sequestrum formed at the head of the fifth metatarsal on the left. M.Ricord removed this sequestrum.

Two years later M.Blandin removed a sequestrum from the first phalanx of the second toe of the left foot. (Hôtel-Dieu)

Sometime after, at l'Hôpital Saint-Antoine, M.Nélaton removed a sequestrum from the first phalanx of the fifth toe of the right foot.

Eleven months later he performed the same operation on the fourth toe of the right foot.

Sometime later, the patient appeared at l'Hôtel-Dieu on the service of M.Boyer; a very deep greyish excavation was present on the head of the first metatarsal of the left foot. M.Boyer cleaned up all the exposed portion, extirpated all the soft parts, and cauterized the base of the wound with the hot iron.

Soon after, M.Michon removed the first toe of the left foot.

A little later M.Malgaigne performed a disarticulation of the first toe of the right foot.

Only a few months later the patient reappeared at l'Hôpital Saint-Louis with several fistulas at the heads of the metatarsals of the left foot. M.Malgaigne, to put an end to this, removed the heads of the five metatarsals in a single procedure. He performed the amputation at the middle of the metatarsals.

Thirty five days later, the patient left the hospital, only to re-enter a few months later.

The same process was reproduced on the end of the stump. Amputation was done by Lisfranc's method.

All these operations were necessitated by the same occurrences. One always met with the series of phenomena which we described in the beginning.

We should note in passing, without dwelling on it, that the patient underwent all these operations without chloroform.

The findings are the same at present. On the plantar surface of the left foot we find a large circular area devoid of its epidermis. There is a blister there which has opened, laying bare the dermis; in several days the dermis will perforate, a fistula will form, and one will find necrotic bone at the base of the fistula.

And that is not all. The second and third toes of the right foot are destined to the same finish. Beginning blisters are present on the osseous prominences; the patient has given these toes up for lost, and one may certainly agree with him, in view of what has previously been observed.

What name shall we give to this disease? M.Nélaton has not found one. He is satisfied to describe to his pupils the series of phenomena that occurred in this patient, without being able to attribute them to any known disease.

---

* Ashhurst, A.: U. of Penn. Med. Bull., *20:*246, 1908.

† Gaz. des Hôpitaux, 1852, p. 13.

Alphonse Devergie

1. *Nummular Eczema*

2. *Pityriasis Rubra Pilaris*

MARIE GUILLAUME ALPHONSE DEVERGIE was born February 15, 1798, in Paris, son of a humble hospital employee. He took an early interest in medicine, attended Dupuytren's Clinics, even at the age of 15, and received his degree in 1823, entitling his thesis, *An Essay on the Exploration of the Abdomen by the Aid of the Sight and Touch, Considered as to Its Connection with Diagnosis of the Diseases which Belong to Internal Pathology*. At the age of 29 he became physician to l'Hôpital Saint Louis, and in 1841 became Chief there, succeeding Biett.

Devergie led a sort of double medical life, being expert in two rather unconnected specialties. His work in legal medicine—the wounds of entrance and exit produced by firearms, where reason ends and insanity begins, asphyxia from coal gas, the Paris morgue, etc.—entitles him to recognition as one of the greatest authorities of his day in this field, and his *Treatise on Skin Diseases* (1857) and numerous lesser writings of a dermatologic nature make him one of the most important early workers in cutaneous medicine.

Though inflexibly honest, Devergie was an extremely stubborn man, one whose beliefs were well nigh impossible to alter. This and a certain stiffness of manner combined effectively to limit his popularity. He feuded constantly with his associates, notably Bazin, and was slow to accept the etiologic significance of ringworm fungi and the scabies acarus proposed by them.

For all this he was an excellent clinical observer, and this aspect of his work, as evidenced by the descriptions below, was certainly his forte. His long and active life came to a close in Paris in 1879.*

NUMMULAR ECZEMA

Eczema nummulaire*

Nummular eczema has nowhere been described. We observed it for the first time in a post office employee eight years ago, and since that time, having been impressed by its form, we have had occasion to see several examples of it a year. It is less remarkable for its nummular disposition than for its tenacity, and the difficulty experienced in treating it has led us to make it a particular species.

---

* Beeson, B.: Arch. of Dermat. and Syph., *21:*1030, 1930.

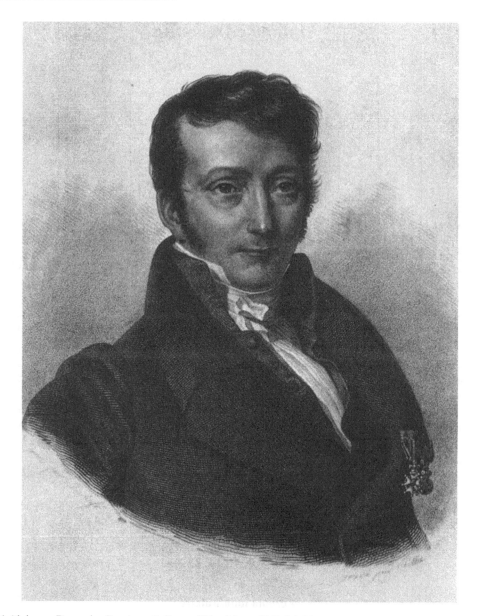

Figure 21 Alphonse Devergie. Courtesy, College of Physicians, Philadelphia

Nummular eczema has the special distinction of developing chiefly on the surface of the extremities, and notably the upper extremities, also on the surface of the trunk. It shows itself there as small plaques which attain immediately the size they are to have; they are rounded, the size of a five franc piece or a little more; they show no thickening, which distinguishes them from herpes; their periphery thins out and merges with the rest of the skin, as in ordinary eczema; they are accompanied, moreover, by redness, a punctate condition of the skin, itching, and serous secretions. They require, in general, several months for cure, and usually yield only to a combination of more or less energetic agents.

PITYRIASIS RUBRA PILARIS

Pityriasis pilaris[†]

The disease which I am about to describe, and which I observed for the first time at the end of the year 1854, has not yet drawn the attention of dermatologists.

It presents a new squamous form to add to those already known. I have assigned to it the name *Pityriasis pilaris,* although it possesses as well characteristics proper to psoriasis; but since it has constantly been preceded by pityriasis, since, moreover, the scales are very small, and are easily detached, I have inclined toward this name rather than toward that of *psoriasis pilaris.*

1. Its seat is essentially in the skin bearing the pilous bulbs, for it appears principally in those areas in which these are more prominent and developed. I say pilous bulbs and not hair bulbs, for I have never observed it on the head; it is, however, located on the external parts of the limbs, notably on the forearms and on the calves, and it attacks especially those groups of pilous bulbs disposed in ovoid plaques over the back of the first phalanges of the fingers. It can, however, appear over the whole surface of the body, the scalp excepted, though the parts may be very abundantly supplied with hair.
2. It leads to a thickening of the skin neighboring and covering the bulb of the hair, with chronic reddening of this tissue, in such a manner as to produce at the base of each hair a little conical pyramid from the summit of which the hair escapes. Each of these little pyramids is isolated from neighboring bulbs by an area of healthy skin in such a way that on the affected parts the skin presents an appearance that has been denoted by the term *chicken flesh.*
3. On the summit of these conoidal elevations which are traversed by the hair, there exists a small epidermal lamella, quite hard, partly free, partly adherent, and even strongly adherent to the touch, so that when one rubs the skin it conveys the sensation of a rough rasp.
4. A bath of short duration, or any aqueous lotion, suffices to detach all these epidermal lamellae, and to return to the skin the softness to the touch that it generally has, apart from the conoidal projections which persist to the same degree when the disease is established, but which disappear completely when it is recent, only to reappear several days later.
5. This affection is more often free of itching, and this circumstance tends to bring it closer to psoriasis; but one will notice that pityriasis produces this phenomenon only incidentally.

Such is the anatomico-pathologic picture of the disease. Let us now attempt to outline the general features which are characteristic of it.

In the four observations which I have been able to collect, the disease developed at about the age of 16 to 18 years. It has constantly been preceded by the following three affections: *psoriasis palmaria, pityriasis capitis* and *pityriasis rubra,* more or less generalized. These affections manifest themselves in the order of their enumeration.

---

* Traité Pratique des Maladies de la Peau. Paris, 1854, p. 237.
† Traité Pratique des Maladies de la Peau, 2nd Edition. Paris, 1857, p. 454.

Yet the form of palmar psoriasis which precedes it is entirely special, and in this respect one must remember that dermatologists have described palmar psoriasis as being very extensive. I have especially insisted in this work, more than any other author, on the differences that distinguish the two varieties of psoriasis palmaria. I have set up two forms, distinct both in course and in treatment. Indeed, in the variety of palmar psoriasis that precedes pityriasis pilaris, the entire palm of the hand is rapidly involved by the psoriasis; the palmar surface of the fingers is affected at the same time; the epidermal scales detach quite easily; the skin cracks, bleeds, and becomes pruritic, while in the pure or typical palmar psoriasis, the disease is very discrete; it progresses very slowly, and it occupies only the center of the palm of the hand.

Today that we know that this same variety of palmar psoriasis which progresses with rapidity, and which before long covers the entire palmar surface, constantly precedes *pityriasis capitis* and *rubra,* which themselves precede the development of *pityriasis pilaris,* we may ask whether this second variety of palmar psoriasis which dermatologists have described might not be a pityriasis rather than a psoriasis. I am inclined to believe so, for I recognize in that form the itching and rapid course of pityriasis, and I see there none of the characteristics of acute psoriasis, the rapidity of development of which might alone explain the so prompt invasion of the internal surface of the hands.

Until now Pityriasis pilaris has presented to our observation a chronic course and a very long duration.

Here, then, we have a new squamous form, even more refractory perhaps than any of those that have been described, ichthyosis excepted; but even more troublesome than this last, it attacks the exposed parts which ichthyosis respects, that is to say the face, the neck, the lower part of the forearms and the hands.

Max Burchardt

Erythrasma

MAX BURCHARDT was born January 15, 1831, in Naugard, in the old state of Pomerania. On completing his preliminary education, he began his medical studies at the Friedrich-Wilhelms-Institute in Berlin, a military medical school. He took his degree in 1855, submitting a thesis on abdominal ascites. During the next 20 years he served as a military physician at many different posts, and retained an active interest in army medicine for the rest of his life. In 1862 he journeyed to England and became one of Lister's first converts to the doctrine of antiseptic surgery. On his return to Germany, he became one of the leading proponents of the technique.

Burchardt was another example of the many sided physician of the 19th century, whom specialization has eliminated from the medical scene. In general medicine, he concerned himself particularly with the treatment of whooping cough, syphilis, and the diseases caused by intestinal worms, as well as with the problem of antisepsis. A polished dermatologist, he made important contributions to the study of scabies, especially from the military point of view, and fungous diseases, including erythrasma, his original description of which is given below. He is best known, however, as an ophthalmologist, and was one of the greatest pioneers in ophthalmoscopy, and in the development of visual tests.

Burchardt was gentle by nature, treated his patients with greatest kindness, and gave freely of his time in the care of the indigent. He worked tirelessly almost to his death in 1897.[*]

ERYTHRASMA

Über eine bei Chloasma vorkommende Pilzform[†]

The exanthem was first noted by the patient in the spring of 1857, and covered a part of the surface of the scrotum and the neighboring parts of the thighs at that time. It was located in the left axilla as well. The eruption spread peripherally in a centrifugal manner, but did not disappear in the center. At times it progressed more rapidly in one area, so that the simple arciform contour became irregular. At the time I first examined it, the exanthem extended from the scrotal folds downward onto both thighs, producing a sort of imprint of the scrotum there. The eruption was more extensive on the left than on the right. It occupied a continuous area which was sharply delineated from the normal skin. Outside the general border contour there were a number of small insular diseased areas of skin; the color of the diseased skin was reddish; the epidermis appeared thinned, a little wrinkled, smooth in places, and showed branny scaling. The reddish color was frequently more or less hidden by epidermal detritus, but could be made visible immediately by moistening.

On the larger diseased area, in the neighborhood of the border, and on a part of the insular areas of diseased skin, there were flat, yellowish brown scales, formed from thickened epidermis, which were easily removed, and under which the skin had the appearance described above. Identical manifestations were noted on the scrotum, except that the borders between healthy and diseased skin were not so sharp as on the thighs. The hair in the diseased areas of skin showed nothing abnormal. The eruption ordinarily itched mildly; severe itching appeared, however, following long walks, and especially as the result of chemical or mechanical stimuli.

---

* Hirschberg, J.: Charité-Annalen, *22*:356, 1897.

† Med. Zeitung, *2*:141, 1859.

Ernest Bazin

1. *Erythema Induratum*

2. *Hydroa Vacciniforme*

ANTOINE PIERRE ERNEST BAZIN was born near Paris, February 20, 1807, one of a large family of modest means. In both his preliminary and medical education he was a brilliant student. Although his early professional interest was not in dermatology, he was a most assiduous attendant at the clinics of Biett and the last lectures of Alibert. He submitted his thesis, *Researches on the Pulmonary Lesions to be Considered in the Morbid Affections Known as the Essential Fevers,* in 1834.

After a dozen years in general practice, he came to l'Hôpital Saint Louis where, following several years study with his characteristic driving energy, he became an associate of such distinguished men as Hardy, Devergie, Cazenave and Gibert.

Bazin was one of the first to popularize the acarus as the causative agent of scabies, although it had been proposed as such for many years. He was also a pioneer in applied mycology, recognizing ringworm and favus to be due to vegetable parasites, as maintained by Schoenlein, Gruby, and Remak. These two concepts were the subject of many bitter disputes in that day, and Bazin was frequently called upon to defend his beliefs against almost savage attacks, notably by Devergie and Cazenave.

Bazin also made important contributions to the study of syphilis, and particularly scrofula, the work from which the first description given below is taken, being perhaps his masterpiece.

He was a self-made man, and achieved his success, according to Besnier, through a combination of energy, unceasing toil, and confidence in the righteousness of his cause. Although kind to pupils and patients, he was in general an irritable and vindictive man, too free in his criticism of his colleagues.

Bazin in his etiologic thinking and insistence on consideration of the patient as a whole was ahead of his time. Brocq said of him, "Bazin arrived too soon in a medical world which was too much occupied with the sole anatomic lesion. That was his misfortune."

He died suddenly of acute pulmonary congestion in 1878, active almost to the end.*

ERYTHEMA INDURATUM

Scrofulides érythémateuses[†]

Erythema induratum, of a scrofulous nature, is not rare; it is characterized by red indurated plaques from which, with digital pressure, the redness disappears momentarily, soon to return. One feels an induration on the skin and in the skin which reaches more or less deeply into the subcutaneous cellular tissue. The redness,

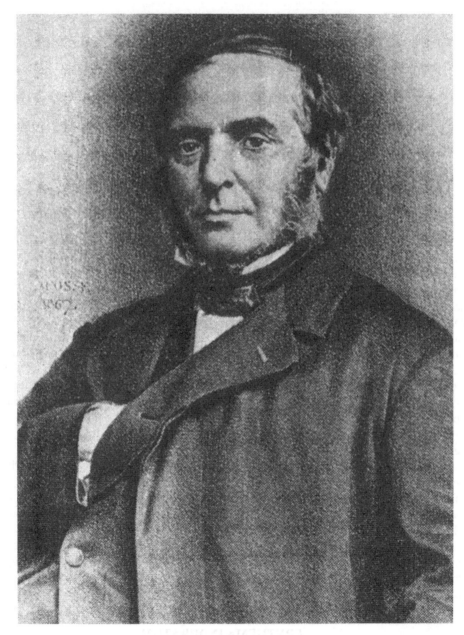

Figure 22 Ernest Bazin. Courtesy, *Annales de Dermatologie et de la Syphilographie*

which is more or less dark, quite often violaceous, and more marked in the center, blends insensibly at the periphery with the normal color of the skin. There is no itching in these plaques; digital pressure on them causes scarcely any pain.

This affection is observed commonly on the legs, more often perhaps in females than in males. I have often found it on the legs of young laundresses, young women with all the attributes of scrofulous corpulence and ruddiness. Its site of predilection is the lateral and lower part of the leg. At times one sees it located a little above the heel, along the Achilles tendon. Finally, one may also see it on the face, and I have seen it alternating with scrofulous ophthalmia in that region.

Observation. (Compiled and set down by M.Louis Fournier, interne du service.)

Van Koler (Aimée) 20 years of age,
    laundress, admitted 21 May, 1858

The present affection began six months previously with red plaques on the lower part of the right leg; these plaques were noticeably raised, and gave rise to itching which was quite severe. Two months later the lower part of the left leg was also attacked.

At present an irregular plaque is seen on the inferior internal surface of the left leg; it is five or six centimeters in size and has a red-violaceous color which disappears on pressure. To the touch it conveys the sensation of an indurated band situated under the plaque. There are several other small points presenting the same characteristics, and an elongated plaque which encroaches on the anterior tibial surface at its medial extremity, and which always shows the subcutaneous induration and red-violaceous color.

On the inner and lower part of the right leg there is another large irregular plaque, also red-violaceous with the induration band sensation to the touch. On the external part, there are disseminated points which show the same characteristics.

The induration of the plaques is regular, equal, superficial, and non painful to pressure, which distinguishes it from the painful, deep, tuberculous induration of erythema nodosum. Moreover, in the latter affection the color is not uniform; it often shows the various yellowish and yellow-greenish shades of ecchymosis which are never seen in the former.

HYDROA VACCINIFORME

L'Hydroa vacciniforme*

Hydroa vacciniforme has not been described by other authors; last year I had the opportunity to observe this singular eruption. I sent my patient to several hospital physicians for consultation; some felt that it was a syphilitic affection; others would not commit themselves as to the nature of this eruption. The affection was of a year's duration, and had been treated without success with a great variety of modalities. I induced the patient to take the waters at Bourbonne which had previously rid him of a rheumatic arthropathy; the eruption, rebellious to all treatments until then, was soon ameliorated; it finally disappeared completely. At present it has not recurred, and his health is excellent.

I do not believe that this affection has been described; it is, however, important to recognize it because of the grave errors it may otherwise occasion.

---

* Beeson, B.: Arch. of Dermat. and Syph., *20:*866, 1929.

† Leçons Théoriques et Cliniques sur la Scrofule, 2nd Edition. Paris, 1861, p. 146.

Symptoms. Hydroa vacciniforme appears following a walk in the open air, or after exposure to the hot sun. There is a little malaise and anorexia; the eruption appears first on the exposed surfaces, then on the other parts of the body. The buccal mucosa is also involved by the affection.

One sees, at first, red spots on which transparent vesicles which resemble those observed in herpes soon appear. On the second day these vesicles which are rounded show a very evident umbilication; in a short while a crust forms successively at the center, and at the circumference of the vesicle. When this crust comes off, it leaves a depressed cicatrix; in the case of the patient we spoke of above, the numerous cicatrices which covered the surface of the body would make one believe that he had formerly had variola.

The affection is prolonged for months by successive attacks; in the case we report the hydroa vacciniforme has lasted six months.

---

* Leçons Théoriques et Cliniques sur les Affections Génériques de la Peau. Paris, 1862, p. 132.

Thomas Addison

1.   *Xanthoma*

2.   *Morphea*

THOMAS ADDISON was born near Newcastle of humble parents in 1793, and although his early life is poorly documented; it is certain that he took his M.D. at Edinburgh in 1815, entitling his inaugural thesis, *De Syphilide*. Soon afterwards he repaired to London where he early studied with the eminent dermatologist, Thomas Bateman. In 1819 he became associated with Guy's Hospital as an internist, and his classic writings in this field, notably on diseases of the chest and suprarenals, are considered to be his greatest achievement; nevertheless, his early dermatologic training fitted him well for his accurate descriptions of morphea and the xanthomata, which we have included here. For years he personally supervised the preparation of the extremely effective wax models of dermatologic disease to be found at Guy's.

Addison was an acknowledged master of clinical observation in an age when this was the *sine qua non* of the physician. He had little time for anything not connected with medicine, and because of his superb lectures acquired a great student following. Because of a rather haughty and unapproachable manner, he was not personally attractive to his colleagues; he was nonetheless mightily respected by them.

In March 1860 he addressed the following letter to his beloved pupils:

"A considerable breakdown in my health has scared me from the anxieties, responsibilities, and excitement of the profession; whether temporarily or permanently cannot yet be determined, but, whatever may be the issue, be assured that nothing was better calculated to soothe me than the kind interest manifested by the pupils of Guy's Hospital during the many trying years devoted to that institution."

A short while later he was dead.[*]

XANTHOMA

On a Certain Affection of the Skin, Vitiligoidea[†]

The object of this communication is to call attention to a somewhat rare disease of the skin, which so far as our observations extend presents itself under two forms: namely, either as tubercles, varying from the size of a pinhead to that of a large pea, isolated or confluent, or secondly, as yellowish patches of irregular outline, slightly elevated, and with but little hardness. Either of these forms may occur separately, or the two

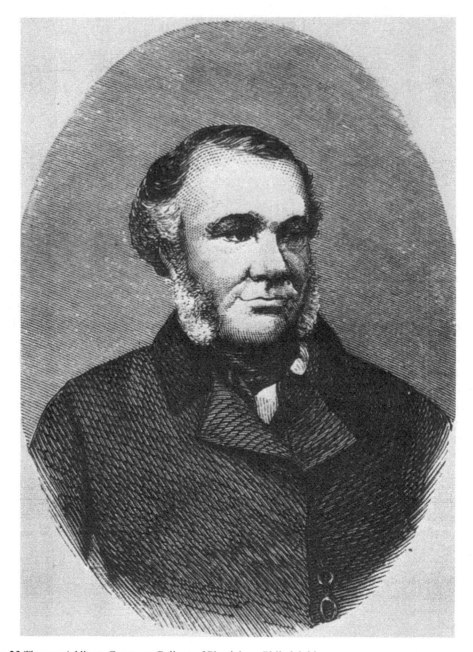

Figure 23 Thomas Addison. Courtesy, College of Physicians, Philadelphia

may be combined in the same individual. Under the latter circumstances we are able to trace the connection of the two through an intermediate series of gradations, which clearly demonstrate their essential relations.

It is doubtful whether this disease has been hitherto described.

The following is an outline of the history of the cases which we have observed:

Several years ago a young woman, aged 24, was admitted into the hospital with a peculiar eruption, extending across the nose and slightly affecting both cheeks. It consisted of shining tubercles, varying from the size of the smallest papule to that of ordinary acne. They were of a lightish colour with here and there superficial capillary veins meandering over them, giving them a faint rose tint. The changes they underwent were very slow; whilst some advanced others subsided. The further course of the case was not ascertained.

It was not until the winter of 1848 that our attention was again drawn to the subject, when the following case occurred: Mrs. B., aged 42, of fair complexion and blue eyes, married, mother of 11 children, had been the subject of jaundice for two years, with much pain about the right hypochondria. After the jaundice had lasted 14 months a change began in the integument, about the eyelids and in the palms of the hands and flexures of the fingers. The skin was at this time of a lemon tint. The affection of the eyelids consists of *patches of a light opaque colour, with the surface and edges slightly raised,* extending from the middle of the upper lid inwards around the inner canthus, and then outwards along the lower lid to nearly the same extent. There is a small isolated patch at the outer canthus. The disease affects both eyes equally and symmetrically, with the exception of two spots in the right lower lid, about the size of a hemp-seed, more elevated than the rest. The cuticle over the affected parts is healthy. There is no appreciable induration. The patches are more sensitive than surrounding parts. The capillaries of the cheeks are slightly tortuous. The palms of the hands are of an olive-brown. Along the ridges on either side of the flexures, both of the palms and fingers, there is the same opaque yellowish discoloration. The appearance is much as if the cuticle were thickened and the disease confined to it; but, on a complete investigation, it is evident that here, as on the face, it is healthy, and that the morbid change is seated on the cutis, which is rather thickened, altered in color, and has increased sensibility. The disease remained stationary until death, at the end of four years from the beginning of the jaundice. Towards the end the colour of the general surface deepened to a mahogany-brown. No affection of the skin, similar to that described on the face and hands, appeared elsewhere.

On the 18th of August, 1848, a patient was admitted into the hospital, under the care of Dr. Hughes, for diabetes. The following is an outline of his history at the time: John Sheriff, aged 27, of middle stature, by occupation a tailor, residing near Kingsbridge in Devonshire. About six months before he began to pass an unusual quantity of water, feeling at the same time weak and feverish, with a dry, harsh skin. On admission he presented the ordinary symptoms of diabetes. He voided four pints and a half of urine daily, sp. grav. 1050. The treatment pursued was various, but without any obvious improvement. On the 25th of January of the following year (1849), the quantity of urine was seven pints and a half, sp. grav. 1042. At this time an eruption somewhat suddenly appeared on the arms, at first apparently of a lichenous character. In the course of 10 days it had extended over the arms, legs and trunk, both anteriorly and posteriorly, also over the face and into the hair. It consisted of *scattered* tubercles of various sizes, some being as large as a small pea, together with shining, colourless papules. They were most numerous on the outside and back of the forearm, and especially about the elbows and knees where they were confluent. Along the inner side of the arms and thighs they were more sparingly present, and entirely absent from the flexures of the larger joints. Besides the compound character produced by the confluence of two or three tubercles, many of the single ones had also a compound character, or appeared to have such, as shown by the prominent whitish nodules

---

* A Collection of the Published Writings of the Late Thomas Addison. New Sydenham Society, London, 1868, Introduction.

† Thomas Addison and William Withey Gull, A Collection of the Published Writings of the Late Thomas Addison. New Sydenham Society, London, 1868, p. 157.

upon them. Some looked as if they were beginning to suppurate, and many were not unlike the ordinary molluscum, but when incised with a lancet they were found to consist of firm tissue, which on pressure, gave out no fluid save blood. They were of a yellowish colour, mottled with a deepish rosetint, and with small capillary veins here and there ramifying over them. They were accompanied with a moderate degree of irritation, hence, the apices of many were rubbed and inflamed. The nature of the eruption gave rise at the time to much discussion. On its first appearance some suspected it to have a secondary venereal affection, but there was nothing in the case, nor indeed in the character of the eruption, when carefully examined to support this view. The only cutaneous affection with which we could associate it, was that of a young woman, whose case we have given above, where the tubercles had occurred in the face only. The eruption continued almost stationary from the end of January to the beginning of March, when many of the tubercles began to subside, having no obvious change in the texture of the skin. At the end of March the patient left the hospital, and the further course of the case was not ascertained.

Up to this time we had, therefore, these three cases of anomalous affection of the skin, without our being able to do more than suspect a relation between the first and the third. Some further light was thrown upon the subject by the following case: Eliza Parachute, aged 33, of middle stature, moderately well nourished, mother of six children, catamenia regular. Her present illness began in 1848. She attributes it to fright, and to a blow received in the left groin whilst attempting to separate two men who were fighting. Two days after this she became jaundiced, and had from time to time severe paroxysmal pains about the hypochondria, lasting for a day or two, the liver being also enlarged and tender. Four months after the commencement of the jaundice (August 4, 1848) she was admitted into the hospital under the care of Dr. Hughes. She remained in until the 26th of September, and left much in the same state she was in when admitted. There was at this time nothing complained of beyond the itching and irritation of the skin common in jaundice. The present affection began after the jaundice had continued 14 months, when she again came under the care of Dr. Hughes. It first appeared in the hands, spreading across the flexures of the joints of the fingers and palms. Soon afterwards a yellowish patch of discoloration began near the inner canthus of the eyelid, and then a precisely symmetrical one at the same part on the opposite eyelid. These patches are very slightly raised, and not obviously indurated; they have extended very slowly. In the early part of the year 1850, two models were made of the case. At this time the patches on the face existed as above described. Along the ridges bounding the flexures in the palm and about the joints of the fingers, there were yellowish, opaque, irregular and somewhat raised lines. About the thumb, first joints of the fingers and inner and interior parts of the wrists, there is a gradual transition to a tubercular prominence of the affected parts, and some distinct tubercles exist on the elbow and knee. The diseased parts are tender, so as to give her pain in using a knife to cut bread. The whole surface of the body is of a dull lemon tint. Various means were employed without avail, the disease showing a tendency to progress slowly. Through the kindness of Mr. Startin, under whose care the patient now is, we have been able to observe it up to the present time. The jaundice still remains occasionally deepened by the exacerbation of the hepatic symptoms. The skin is of a dull lemon hue. During the last seven months the affection has become more tubercular, especially about the back of the joints of the fingers of the right hand. The patch of confluent tubercles on the right elbow has much increased since the model was taken. Both elbows are similarly affected. There are also tubercles on the right knee, on the superior surface of the great toe, and on both ears. On the hands the gradations from the plane to the tubercular variety are well marked, and the essential relations of the two forms demonstrable. The tubercles about the ears, elbows, joints of the fingers, etc., are of the same character they were in Sheriff's case. They are firm, rather irregular on the surface, have much the appearance at first sight of small compound follicles, but on closer inspection are proved to depend upon a change in the cutis. On the surface small venous capillaries may be here and there seen, producing a mottled appearance. In the hands we pass insensibly from the tubercles on the back of the joints to the state described in Mrs. B's case, namely, the slightly raised, opaque, yellowish lines about the flexures of the palms and fingers. The further identity of the disease in the two cases is shown by the presence of similar patches about the eyelids in both.

Mrs. J., aged 43, of spare frame, and below the middle stature, married, mother of two children, and in good health until about eight years ago when her catamenia ceased, probably from fright. After their cessation she was never well, had pains about the right side and through the shoulders, and for several years past, indeed, nearly ever since the commencement of her ailment, has been jaundiced. She was constitutionally of a dark complexion. This has now become a deep olive brown. During the last five years there has been a gradual change in the integument of the eyelids, giving her a strange expression. This affection of the skin began in the upper lid of the left eye, and extended round by the inner canthus to the lower lid. A similar affection then commenced in the right eyelid, and the appearances now presented by the two are remarkably symmetrical. The surface of the affected parts is slightly raised, and the edge defined. The colour is a light opaque yellow, "coloration feuille morte," with a mottling of the faintest rose tint, with a small meandering vessel or two especially on the patches, which are recent and extending. On passing the finger over the surface, there is a slight, yet but very slight, feeling of resistance. The older spots are the most raised. The cuticle is unaffected, and by slight tension of the skin, will be seen to pass unchanged from the normal to the diseased parts. The discoloured patches often smart, and to use the patient's expression, "seem as if gathering." They have also an increased sensibility.

It will be observed that as the disease extended it has run along the lids so as to avoid the Meibomian region, and that in the left eyelid are two sebaceous follicles, enlarged and filled with dark pigment cells. During the last two years a spot of black pigment has appeared on the mucous membrane of the lower lip. The whole course of the disease has been very slow, and its increase by degrees, almost insensible. There is no affection of the skin of any other part of the body, beyond the change in its colour above indicated.

The connection of this affection of the skin with hepatic derangement is obvious, and the exception which occurred in diabetes is of the more interest, in as much as modern pathology points to the liver as the faulty organ in this disease.

MORPHEA

On the Keloid of Alibert and on True Keloid*

What I have ventured to call "True Keloid" presents a very remarkable character, and leads to much more serious consequences than the keloid of Alibert. It is a disease, too, which so far as I know has not hitherto, with the exception of a slight allusion of Dr. Coley, been either noticed or described by any writer. Like the keloid of Alibert, it has its original seat in the subcutaneous areolar tissue, and is first indicated by a white patch or opacity of the integument, of a roundish or oval shape, and varying in size from that of a silver penny to that of a crown piece, very slightly or not at all elevated above the level of the surrounding skin, and probably unattended in the beginning with pain or any other local uneasiness or inconvenience, although a more or less vivid zone of redness surrounding the whole patch or a certain amount of venous congestion in its immediate vicinity sufficiently attests the vascular activity or inflammatory process going on in the parts beneath. Occasionally and especially when the original white patch is of considerable diameter, its surface presents here and there a faint yellowish or brownish tint communicating to the whole spot a somewhat mottled appearance. The slow and insidious change taking place in the areolar tissue either stops and the spot disappears, or it proceeds and at length begins to declare itself by a feeling of itching, pain, tightness or constriction in the affected part, and frequently by a certain amount of subcutaneous hardness and rigidity, extending beyond the site of the original superficial patch, although as yet without any necessary change in the appearance of the superincumbent skin. This hardness and rigidity can be distinctly felt and, especially when situated on the extremities, may sometimes be traced along the course of the neighboring tendons or fasciae, or stretching like a cord along the limb so as to bend or shorten it and even interfere with natural progression. At length the part originally affected becomes more or less hide-bound, and a similar change taking place around the more superficial fasciae and tendons, the latter becoming so tightened, fixed and rigid as to be no longer capable of performing their proper functions, and to such an extent that the whole of the limb, but especially the fingers, may be permanently contracted, bent, and rendered almost as hard and immovable as a piece of wood, thereby impeding progression, distorting the gait, and making the patient a poor miserable cripple for the remainder of his life.

As these changes proceed, the patient continues to experience itching, pain, or a sense of tightness or constriction of the parts, till at length the disease begins to tell upon both cutis and cuticle. The skin which may have previously presented only a slightly drawn or puckered look, imparting to a greater or less extent of it a ray-like appearance, now shrinks or shrivels. It assumes a dry, smooth or glistening aspect and undergoes a more decided change of colour, becoming reddish, pinkish, yellowish or of a dead leaf colour. The cuticle exfoliates, the cutis manifests a tendency to superficial ulceration or excoriation, with consequent scaliness or scabbing or, when not excoriated, is occasionally surmounted by obscure tubercular or nodular elevations—the whole appearance very closely resembling the remains of an extensive and imperfectly cicatrised burn. From some part of the boundary of the discoloured and shrivelled skin, there may now and then be seen reddish, elevated, claw-like processes of from half an inch to two inches in length, extending into the sounder integument, and bearing a very exact resemblance to those mentioned as being so characteristic of the keloid of Alibert. It must also be observed that, during the progress of the disease, it is by no means uncommon to find scattered over various parts of the apparently sound surface certain oval or roundish and flattened tubercular-looking elevations, which are somewhat hard to the touch, about the size of a split pea or horse bean, and without any other discoloration than what appears to be the result of accidental friction or irritation.

The above description of true keloid clearly points to some morbid change taking place in the subcutaneous areolar tissue, whilst the itching, pain and uneasiness experienced by the patient, the red zone surrounding the patch and the infection of the neighboring veins, as well as the subsequent appearances presented by the parts affected, would indicate that the morbid process going on in that tissue is one very nearly allied to inflammation, probably of a strumous kind. It would also appear that the inflammatory product, by its subsequent contraction, seriously interferes with the proper nutrition of the cutis, fixes it more or less firmly to the parts beneath and, when deposited in the immediate neighborhood of fasciae and tendons, may probably after the lapse of months or years lead to all those serious inconveniences which I have already described.

* A Collection of the Published Writings of the Late Thomas Addison. New Sydenham Society, London, 1868, p. 169.

Camille Gibert

Pityriasis Rosea

CAMILLE MELCHIOR GIBERT was born in Paris August 18, 1797. Little is known of his childhood. He served under Biett at Saint Louis as an interne in 1818 and 1819, received his M.D. in 1822, and entitled his thesis, *Some Reflections on Modern Medicine*. He became a Physician to the Hospitals of Paris about 1831, and often substituted for Biett, Lugol, and Manry at l'Hôpital Saint Louis. In 1840 he became permanently associated with Saint Louis.

Like Biett and Rayer, Gibert was a follower of Willan in his approach to dermatology; he did not hesitate, however, to alter the latter's system to fit the demands of progress.

Although best known for the description of pityriasis rosea given below, Gibert made many contributions to dermatology, notably in the diagnosis and treatment of syphilis. It was his successful inoculation of three subjects affected with lupus, with pus and blood taken from secondary syphilitic lesions that established the contagiousness of the disease in this stage, a fact which up to that time was vigorously denied by many, including such an authority as Ricord.

Gibert was a proud man, and prone to harbor enmity toward those who offended him. This was, however, more than compensated for by his professional skill, unusual intelligence, and great speaking ability.

He died during a cholera epidemic in Paris, July, 1866.*

PITYRIASIS ROSEA

Pityriasis*

The two most distinctive forms which we have observed in this eruption category are: 1. The one we have described above, the appearance of which recalls that of *lichen* sometimes, at other times psoriasis. 2. Another variety which one might designate by the name pityriasis *rosea,* and which presents the following characteristics: small furfuraceous spots which are very lightly colored, irregular, scarcely exceeding a fingernail in size, numerous and close set, although always separated by some interval of normal skin, pruritic, and which appear on the superior parts of the body, with a predilection for the neck, the upper part of the chest, and the upper part of the arms, but which may spread successively from above downwards as far as the thighs, in such a way that the total duration of the eruption, which disappears little by little from

---

* Beeson, B.: Arch. Dermat. and Syph., *30:*101, 1934.

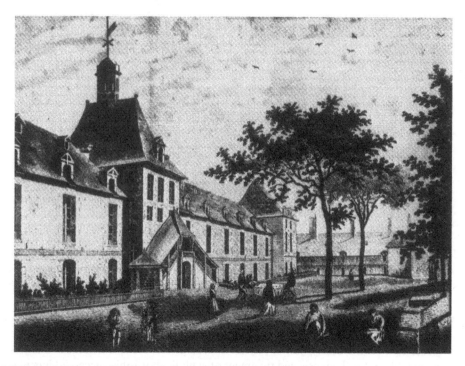

Figure 24 L'Hôpital Saint Louis. Courtesy, College of Physicians, Philadelphia

the parts first affected as it moves downward, is protracted quite commonly to six weeks or two months. This eruption, which is more common in the female than the male, is observed quite frequently in the warm season of the year. It is seen almost only in young people, and in individuals whose skin is fair, fine, and delicate.

---

* Traité Pratique des Maladies de la Peau, 5th Edition. Paris, 1860, p. 402.

Samuel Wilks

Verruca Necrogenica

SAMUEL WILKS was born June 2, 1824, in London. At the age of 11 he was tutored by the Reverend Dr. Spyers at Wallop, and when Dr. Spyers went to Alderham as head master, Wilks went along with him. In 1840 he was apprenticed to his family physician, but soon transferred to Guy's Hospital to continue his studies. In 1848 he took his bachelor's degree at the University of London, and in 1850 the degree, Doctor of Medicine, receiving the gold medal for scholarship at that time.

Wilks was an internist and a pathologist, and excelled at both. As much as any man in England, he pointed up the value of correlating clinical findings with pathological facts. In his double position as pathologist and curator of the museum at Guy's, it was only natural that he should wish to have models prepared of the lesion known as postmortem wart which he had noted in his autopsy work. It is from his notes on additions to the museum that we have taken his description of verruca necrogenica.

As a clinician Wilks made notable contributions to the study of diseases of the nervous system, particularly alcoholic paraplegia. He was one of the first to report on bacterial endocarditis, under the name "arterial pyaemia."

Wilks became one of the most noted citizens of his day, and was the recipient of many honors, both medical and otherwise. He was created a baronet in 1897, on the occasion of the Diamond Jubilee celebration of Queen Victoria. Ill health plagued him continually, following his retirement in 1901, but he lived another 10 years, death coming in 1911, in his 87th year.*

VERRUCA NECROGENICA

Disease of the Skin produced by post-mortem examinations, or Verruca necrogenica[†]

Those who have been engaged for any considerable time in post-mortem examinations, are aware that the constant contact of the hands with the morbid fluids of the diseased bodies produces a chronic thickening of the skin, which, in its general aspect, bears some resemblance to the early stages of epithelial cancer, and which we propose to call *verruca necrogenica*. As, however, the number of professional men thus occupied is very limited, it is not remarkable that the effect is not generally known, and for this reason we have requested our artist to produce some models of the disease. The first specimens are from the hands of a late assistant in the post-mortem room at Guy's, the others from a gentleman, who when a student, was occupied for some time in the same place. In his case he informs us the disease was so little recognized that, although he was aware that it originated in the inspection-room, yet its persistence made him at times fear that it was due to some malignant action of the skin; and he states also, that several medical men coincided in this view, whilst others considered it to be syphilitic.

In the case of another gentleman, who had not been engaged in pathological pursuits for some years, some remnant of the disease still existed, but no one in the company of several medical men could form a guess as to its nature.

In some cases the disease either begins as an active pustule, arising from a poison absorbed by the skin, or takes its origin in a wound; but, as a rule, the morbid change is a slow one, and commences without any evident breach of surface, the parts affected being not those liable to pustules, as the back of the hand or wrist, but the knuckles and joints of the fingers. If the disease should begin with a pustule, the latter bursts, but, instead of healing, a thickening of the cuticle takes place around it, and as, from time to time, a little fresh suppuration occurs, so the thickening and induration increase. Generally, however, the change of which we speak occurs slowly on the knuckles and on the first joints of the fingers, without any preliminary vesication. A warty thickening of the epithelium takes place, which, in course of time, becomes of a dark colour, and fissured until a kind of ichthyotic condition is produced.

In the case of the assistant in the post-mortem room, he left his duties about a year before the models were made, and yet the affection remained much the same as when he was actively engaged. It had existed on his hands for more than two years. The principal parts affected are the knuckles of the fore and middle f ingers of both hands, and also the ring finger of the left hand. These are covered with round patches of a brown colour, about the size of a shilling. They are raised about the surface, very rough and fissured. The most prominent parts are dry and brittle, so that pieces of the dry epithelium are constantly peeling off. If a portion be picked off, the part bleeds a little, but not otherwise.

In the other case—that of the former student—the disease had existed for three or four years, in spite of various remedies which he had used to cure it. He had applied caustics, and taken off portions of the epithelium, but the morbid process has still continued.

In the case of the other gentleman before alluded to, he had desisted from pathological pursuits for eight years, but there still remained on one of the knuckles a small, brown, thickened patch of epithelium.

A well known foreign professor, when in this country some years ago, was observed to have his fingers similarly affected, and his special occupation was recognized thereby.

In the case of the writer, the result was more fortunate, for a warty patch having existed for several months over one of the joints of the fingers, a desisting from irritating the part, and a frequent application of tinct. Iodin., caused it gradually to fade away until the merest trace now remains.

The entire want of knowledge as to knowledge of the affection expressed by those who have been subsequently informed of its character, is the reason for adding a representation of the disease to our collection. This fact, coupled with the counter one of its easy recognition by those who have any experience of it, is a sufficient proof of its peculiar and characteristic features. It appears to be produced by the constant irritation of the skin, from the acridity of the morbid fluids of the dead body, for we are not aware of any other irritant which is productive of the same effect, although it is possible that, should the skin be exposed to other exciting causes, a somewhat similar effect might be produced. We might add, that those who are subject to this affection still continue their avocation with impunity, as regards putrid absorption or inflammation of the lymphatics, for, as far as we have seen, neither these nor any constitutional symptoms result.

* Willius, F., and Keys, T.: Cardiac Classics. Mosby, St. Louis, 1941, p. 577.

† Guy's Hosp. Reports, 8:263, 1862.

PART II

THE DISCIPLES

Ferdinand von Hebra

1. *Erythema Multiforme*

2. *Lichen Scrofulosorum*

3. *Prurigo*

4. *Pityriasis Rubra (Exfoliative Dermatitis of Hebra)*

5. *Rhinoscleroma*

6. *Impetigo Herpetiformis*

FERDINAND VON HEBRA was born in Moravia, in 1816. He received his medical education at the University of Vienna and was graduated in 1841. As an assistant to the famed Skoda, he was placed at first in charge of patients afflicted with scabies. His interest in dermatology grew, and within four years he had proposed his classification of skin disease based upon the pathological anatomy, a classification which immediately superseded those that had gone before, including that of Willan, although Hebra had the greatest respect for the English master, and retained much of his nomenclature and descriptive methods.

Hebra's contributions to dermatology are so manifold that hardly any branch of the specialty was not altered and improved by his work. As a clinician he has never been excelled. Like Willan he wrought order from chaos in those disease groups to which he turned his special attention. He demonstrated experimentally the importance of external irritants in the production of inflammations of the skin. His therapeutic approach was refreshing—a sort of tempered application of the nihilism of Skoda. He weeded out hundreds of useless medications that had cluttered up the dermatologic armamentarium for years; he established the value of proper local therapy, and pointed up the value of doing nothing at all at times. Mercury was reinstituted in the treatment of syphilis largely through his efforts.

Hebra was a magnificent teacher. He gathered about him pupils destined to be among the most illustrious the specialty has known— Kaposi, Neumann, Heitzmann, Auspitz, Pick, Wertheim, and many others. His clinic became the mecca, and shifted the center of dermatology from England and France to Austria. He was a fascinating speaker—as Robinson put it—"in his speech blossomed that precious double flower—sympathy and satire."

The *Atlas der Hautkrankheiten* (1856–1876), and *On Diseases of the Skin* (completed by Kaposi in 1880) are his greatest achievements, truly monumental.

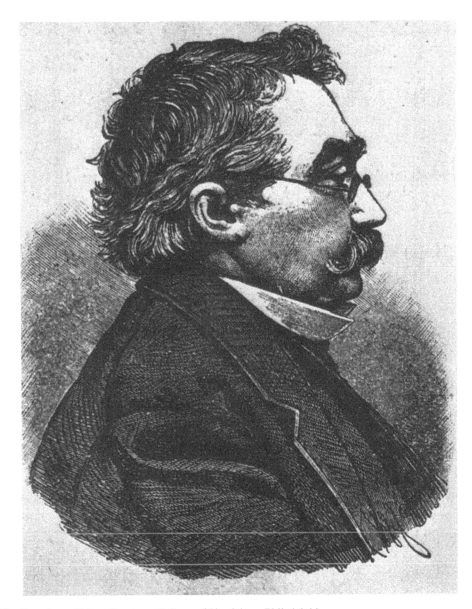

Figure 25 Ferdinand von Hebra. Courtesy, College of Physicians, Philadelphia

An observer described Hebra as a "short thick-set man with dirty fingers and a dress a good deal the worse for wear." Be that as it may, as Willan was the greatest dermatologist of the 18th century, so Hebra was by far the most important in the 19th.

Poor health prevailed in the last few years of his life, and he succumbed August 5, 1880, after 40 years as the "undisputed potentate of Hautkrankheiten."*

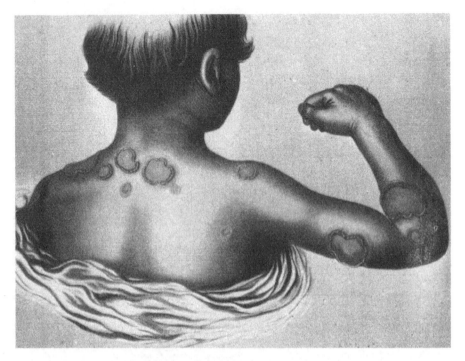

Figure 26 Erythema multiforme (circinatum). From Hebra's atlas

ERYTHEMA MULTIFORME

Erythema exudativum multiforme[†]

Willan speaks of six varieties of erythema, which is one of the diseases of the skin included in his third *order,* the *exanthemata* or rashes. Of these varieties the first, which he terms the E. fugax, is described by me among the hyperaemiae as belonging to that class of affections. The second, to which Willian gives the name of E. laeve, is not in my opinion a peculiar cutaneous affection, but is merely a simple erythema (E. fugax), presenting itself on the skin of parts which are oedematous. Hence it only remains for me to speak in this place of the *E. marginatum, E. papulatum, E. tuberculatum,* and *E. nodosum.* Certain authors, however, have mentioned other forms besides these. Thus, Rayer describes an *E. iris;* Biett, an *E. annulare, seu circinatum, seu centrifugum;* and Fuchs, an *E. gyratum,* an *E. urticans,* and an *E. diffusum.* But these various names by no means answer to as many distinct diseases, and therefore our first object must be to determine which of them apply merely to appearances developed in succession during the course of one and the same disease, and which of them are necessary to indicate cutaneous affections really different from one another.

Now, in reference to this point, experience has taught me that the *E. papulatum, E. tuberculatum, E. annulare, E. iris, E. gyratum* are merely forms of the same disease in different stages, the appearance

---

* Robinson, V.: Med. Rev. of Rev., *22:*719, 1916.

[†] On Diseases of the Skin. New Sydenham Society translation, London, 1866, Vol. I, p. 285.

varying according as the affection is undergoing development, or in a later period of its course or subsiding. To this malady I shall apply the name of *Erythema multiforme*.

The most striking character of this affection is its appearing on certain special parts of the body. Thus, in every instance, it is present on the dorsal surfaces of the hands or feet. In the more severe cases, but only in these, it may be observed on the forearms and legs, on the arms and thighs, and even on the trunk and face. It is, however, only in the very exceptional instances that it affects the regions last mentioned. When it is found on them, it invariably exists also on the backs of the patient's hands, where indeed this cutaneous disease first appears.

The efflorescence which I am now describing consists of flattened papules or tubercles of a dark blue or a brownish-red colour, and between lentils and beans in size. Their number varies in different cases. The skin immediately surrounding them is likewise reddened when they first make their appearance, but this is merely the effect of vascular injection, and lasts but a short time, subsiding at the latest within 24 hours. When it thus disappears this hyperaemic reddening leaves behind no pigment, and the dark red papules or tubercles then become still more plainly visible than they were before.

In the mildest cases the papules or tubercles which (corresponding to the *E. papulatum* and the *E. tuberculatum* respectively) constitute this affection persist only a few days. They are sometimes observed also on the fingers, where they closely resemble chilblains (Frostbeulen), and when they disappear are succeeded by a slight deposit of pigment.

When the disease is of longer duration, the tubercles become flattened, and their red colour spreads to the adjacent parts of the skin and fades from their centre. Hence, from each papule or tubercle is developed a red ring. This change constitutes the *Erythema annulare*.

Sometimes, however, the centre of such a circle is still indicated by a smaller papule, or again a second ring may develop itself round the first and at a slight distance from it, so that we find either a small ring with a papule in its centre or two concentric circles. These appearances characterize the *Erythema iris*.

In some cases the affection comes to an end when it has undergone these changes. Its whole duration is then very brief, the red colour of the circles soon subsides, and only a slight pigment deposit is left when they have disappeared. In other cases, however, the rings formed from the tubercles in the way above described do not so rapidly fade and disappear, but first spread at their margins. Hence the different circles, originally distinct, approach one another, touch, and at last coalesce. In this way are produced serpentine lines, arising from the union of the segments of several circles, and it is this appearance which constitutes the *Erythema* gyratum seu marginatum. After a shorter or longer interval these rings at length cease to spread, their red colour fades, and the affection terminates without giving rise to any further morbid changes, and is followed by slight desquamation and a scanty deposit of pigment.

It appears, then, from the description which I have given that the *Erythema papulatum* represents the lowest and the *Erythema gyratum* the highest grade in the development of this eruption. Hence, it will depend on the period at which the patient comes under medical observation, whether the case shall be diagnosed as an *Erythema papulatum* or as an *E. annulare,* or even as an *E. gyratum*. It is easy to understand how dermatologists who have seen such cases only at intervals (bei einer bloss ambulatorischen Betrachtung) have supposed that they belong to different species, whereas when these affections are made the subject of clinical observation, the view which I have taken cannot but be adopted, namely that they are all identical.

The *Erythema exudativum multiforme* gives rise to very trifling *subjective* symptoms. Some patients complain of a slight burning sensation, others of a slight itching. It is only when the papules on the backs of the hands are numerous and closely approximated, that the skin feels tense (Spannung) or thick and as if covered with a glove (Pelzigsein). The temperature of the surface is not, either subjectively or objectively, increased to any extent.

Concomitant and *febrile* symptoms are to be observed only in exceptional cases, in those cases, namely, in which the affection spreads over large tracts of the surface or even over the whole skin. No important complications, or sequellae, occur in the train of this eruption. Its whole duration varies between one and four weeks. I have seen the *Erythema papulatum* accompany a pneumonia of which the patient died. Each one of the papules was plainly visible on the dead body, and when they were cut through it became evident that they were caused by hemorrhagic exudation (durch hämorrhagisches Exudat).

The *Erythema papulatum* is peculiar in the time of its occurrence and in its liability to relapse. This affection presents itself only during those months, namely April, May, October and November, in which erysipelatous and herpetic eruptions are likewise most frequently observed. Moreover, its occurrence is connected with an annual type *(Typus annuus),* for there are persons in whom such an erythema breaks out, during many successive years in the course of the same month.

In some cases there appear simultaneously with these forms of erythema, eruptions which are of a similar kind, except that they are vesicular. These were, consequently, classed by Willan under the name of *Herpes.* It is, however, impossible to doubt that the *Herpes iris* and the *H. circinatus* arise from the same causes as the *Erythema iris* and the *E. annulare,* and differ only in the fact that in the first two affections vesicles running an acute course are developed, which are associated in groups and surround a common centre. All the other characters are the same in the two groups of the diseases, and the opinion long since expressed by Rayer that the *Erythema iris* and the *Herpes iris* are mere modifications of one affection is doubtless correct. There is, however, a practical advantage in retaining both these terms, because doing so enables us not only to adhere to the definitions of the two diseases (*Herpes* and *Erythema*), but also to indicate at once by the name which we employ which form is present in any particular case.

We are in a state of complete ignorance as to the cause of these erythemata. They are certainly never produced by local irritation, and no disease is known to us (with the exception, perhaps, of cholera) in the course of which they *regularly* present themselves.

I have seen these affections chiefly in young subjects who were in other respects perfectly healthy. They are more common in the male than in the female sex, but I have never been able to discover any predisposing cause for them in the patients themselves. These erythemata are often ascribed to catching cold or to errors of diet, or to mental emotions, but unless the real existence of these conditions can be proved, I regard such expressions as mere commonplaces and shibboleths (Gemein plätze and Schlagworte), and rather than avail myself of them, I shall confess that the cause of these diseases is altogether unknown to me. It is certain that they do not owe their origin either to the imbibition of alcoholic liquors or to eating any particular kind of food, whether sour, sweet or bitter, whether of animal or vegetable nature.

LICHEN SCROFULOSORUM

Lichen scroftilosorum*

The characteristic symptom of this disease is an eruption of miliary papules, which may be either pale yellow, brownish-red or of the same colour as the rest of the skin. They never contain any fluid. They are always placed in groups and sometimes form circles or segments of circles within which may occasionally be seen a few pigmented spots, indicating the seat of former papules and always covered with a very few minute scales. The papules of *Lichen scrofulosorum* produce but little itching and, being consequently not much scratched, present no excoriations and no little black crusts of dried blood. They remain long unaltered, and are subject to no metamorphosis beyond that of involution with shedding of the epidermis.

This affection is for the most part confined to the trunk, occupying the abdomen, chest, or back. It is very rarely seen on the limbs.

The course of the Lichen scrofulosorum is peculiarly slow. All the groups of papules, or at any rate a great many of them, generally appear simultaneously and quickly arrive at their full development; but, at this, they afterwards remain for a long time without change. As I have already stated, they give rise to no itching or other unpleasant sensation, and have no tendency to pass into vesicles or pustules. Hence their existence is commonly overlooked, escaping notice altogether until the groups of papules have developed themselves in large numbers, or until the affection has reached so high a pitch of intensity that the other morbid appearances present themselves. These consist in the formation of more or less numerous bluish-red tubercles as large as lentils, and quite distinct from one another. They appear in the intervals between the groups of papules and also on parts, such as the limbs and face, where there had been none of the lichenous papules. The tubercles resemble those of acne, and undergo exactly the same changes as in that affection. In some of them a purulent fluid develops itself, which afterwards dries up or is discharged, when the tubercles themselves disappear; others of them do not suppurate, but gradually subside. In either case they leave discoid, darkly pigmented maculae of the size of lentils, and they are followed by a fresh eruption at other spots. The cuticle of the surface between the tubercles is often cast off in small branny scales, having a fatty lustre, and this gives the skin generally a peculiar cachectic appearance.

The natural tendency of the disease is for the changes I have been describing to repeat themselves, so that it may go on interruptedly for many years if the conditions persists which originally gave rise to it.

It is, however, a fact worthy of notice, that a large majority (about 90 per cent) of the patients affected with this form of lichen are persons in whom the lymphatic glands (particularly those of the submaxillary and cervical regions and of the axillae) are greatly swollen, or who suffer from periostitis, caries or necrosis, with or without scrofulous sores, or who may be supposed to have disease of the mesenteric glands, being of cachectic aspect and generally badly nourished, and yet having the abdomen enlarged. Since all these conditions belong to the general state known under the name of scrofulosis, I am surely justified in applying the name of *Lichen scrofulosorum* to the cutaneous affection which I am now describing.

It may perhaps occur to some of my readers to ask what has been the state of the lungs in patients affected with this form of lichen. My answer to this question must be, that in no one of the cases (more than 50 in number) which have been under my observation has there been any symptom pointing to tubercular disease of these organs; and, as all the patients who have been under my care with the disease have recovered, I have had no opportunity of making an autopsy and examining the lungs.

PRURIGO

Prurigo*

In every case the earliest appearance is that of subepidermic papules as big as hemp-seeds and recognized rather by touch than by sight, since they rise but little above the level of the skin, and do not differ from it at all in colour. They are always isolated and, though they may appear in all sorts of places, constantly have some regions unaffected. They produce great irritation and thus, from being scratched, soon rise somewhat

---

* On Diseases of the Skin. New Sydenham Society translation, London, 1868, Vol. II, p. 52.

above the surface and also sometimes become red. Continued scratching destroys the epidermis at the summit of the papules, and by this means either their contents come into view—sometimes a transparent and colourless, sometimes a yellowish serosity—or else a papilla of the corium is at last wounded, and from its capillary vessel a drop of blood escapes which dries into a black crust at the top of the papule as big as a pinhead. There are always many papules developed, and this process repeated according to the extent of the eruption will produce the appearance presented by ordinary prurigo.

When, however, this disease has lasted for some time, fresh phenomena are added to those already mentioned. We notice a constantly increasing deposit of dark pigment in the epidermis which is proved to result from the patient's scratches by its always corresponding with the excoriations both in distribution and intensity. In all cases of long-standing prurigo we observe, moreover, that the slight depressions, lines and furrows which cover the surface of the skin in health, become gradually farther separated from one another and considerably deepened. This is particularly remarkable on the fingers, the back of the hand and the wrist. The numerous minute downy hairs which pierce the skin everywhere, as well as the thicker and longer ones, appear to be torn out by the sufferer's nails, and if not entirely absent, are much shorter and stiffer than they normally were. Lastly, the skin itself seems to be more hard and dense, and if a fold of it be pinched up, it feels much thicker than it does when in a healthy state.

Many cases of prurigo never show any other characters than these, more or less pronounced, even though the disease should last for a lifetime. But in other and more unusual cases, a further series of phenomena develop themselves, and these I will now describe. The first peculiarity of this more severe type of the disease which I will name *Prurigo agria s. ferox* is that all the characteristic symptoms of the ordinary form present themselves in an exaggerated degree. The papules are larger, the itching more intense, the excoriations more severe, and the blood crusts they cause more abundant. But, in addition to all this, we may observe upon the brown pigmented skin, between the black scabs of dried up blood, that the uppermost layers of epidermis are detached from the rest in the form of a white mealy dust which yet clings to the surface and thus simulates the appearance of Willan's *Pityriasis nigra,* or Alibert's *Ichthyosis nacrée.* In other cases of this severe form of prurigo, we may see all the phenomena of *Eczema rubrum* develop themselves, either over the entire surface or on many parts of the integument affected, until one might be tempted to look on the whole as a simple eczema, so completely does the secondary malady obscure the symptoms of the original one. Or, lastly, the fluid contained in the pruriginous papules may become purulent, each papule becomes a pustule, and either we find an eruption of these varying in size and number, but mingled with the primary efflorescence and afterwards turning to scabs or, if the papules are closely packed, the pustules into which they are transformed very easily come into contact, unite, and so form a continuous purulent layer beneath the cuticle which afterwards dries into crusts of large dimensions.

If we go over the different regions of the body in a patient affected with prurigo, we shall find the scalp quite free from any eruption, but the hair will appear dull, will feel dry to the touch, and often looks as if it were sprinkled over with dust. The face, especially in young patients, is usually clear and of a pale complexion, or a few scattered papules may be found on the cheeks, some intact, some wounded by scratching. Cases, however, occur in which a considerable number are observed in this region, or it may be the seat of an impetiginous eczema. It is rare to see any marked traces of prurigo on the throat or back of the neck, but the whole of the thorax, both in front and behind, is covered pretty uniformly with papules, some only to be recognized by the sense of touch, while others rise about the surface so as to become visible to the eye, and others again are tipt with a minute crust of dried-up blood. A similar aspect is presented by the

---

* On Diseases of the Skin. New Sydenham Society translation, London, 1868, Vol. II, p. 257.

skin of the abdomen, the sacral region and the buttocks, but the most intense form of the disease is displayed on the limbs, especially on their extensor surfaces. The skin is of darker hue than elsewhere and thickened in proportion to the duration of the malady. Its lines and furrows are more plainly marked on the extensor than the flexor surfaces, and most of all on the wrist, the back of the hand, the fingers, and the corresponding part of the ankle and instep, where may be seen deep and obvious lines more widely separated than in the normal condition. The eruption is less abundant above the elbow than on the forearm, on the thigh than on the leg, and on the upper than on the lower extremity. It is then below the knee that it is most intensely developed, and here one may with a little practice recognize every case of prurigo by the touch alone. The skin feels as rough as a file, and when *the closed hand* is passed over it, produces a sound like a short-haired nailbrush or rough paper, and causes a pricking sensation of the fingers. Not only do the lower extremities in ordinary prurigo present more papules and more roughness than other parts, but it is here also that we find the greater number of pustules, or the more severe eczema when these are super-added. It is, however, very remarkable that in all cases of prurigo the skin covering the bend of a joint either remains perfectly whole and appears smooth, soft and healthy or, in very rare and exceptional cases, offers a few papules or a slight degree of eczema. The armpits, elbows, flexor side of the wrists and palms, the groins, hams and soles are therefore almost always unaffected both to the sight and to the touch.

The prospects of an unfortunate patient afflicted with prurigo have been already depicted in no very cheerful colours. He may do whatever he pleases; his malady will follow him to his grave.

PITYRIASIS RUBRA (EXFOLIATIVE DERMATITIS OF HEBRA)

Pityriasis rubra*

As appears from its name, the affection which is termed pityriasis rubra consists in a reddening of the skin, which is also covered with scales. But as is well known, these characteristics are likewise found in other dermatoses such as psoriasis, lichen, eczema, and lupus erythematosus; and therefore, we have to give some additional symptoms belonging only to the disease in question, and absent in those which resemble it. In doing this, however, we must rely not so much on positive as on negative characters. In the above named affections, besides the redness and the scales, there are always other symptoms. Either there is infiltration of the cutis, with or without the presence of fissures; there is oozing of a fluid secretion; there is severe itching, which leads inevitably to scratching and consequently to the existence of excoriations; or lastly, the disease occupies some particular region, or presents certain peculiarities in its course. But in the pityriasis rubra all these are absent. In it there is nothing more than an intense redness, diffused over a large part of the skin, or even universal, disappearing beneath the pressure of the finger (when it gives place to a yellowish coloration) and accompanied by the presence of fine white loosely-adherent scales, which result from the constant shedding of the most superficial layer of the cuticle.

Now there can be no doubt that the recognition of an eczema squamosum (a species first described by Cazenave) has, so to speak, cut away the ground beneath the feet of pityriasis rubra, and that most of the cases which have been so termed would now, with more correctness, be considered to belong to the eczemata. Thus it happens that an eczema, either its commencement or while it is in course of involution, reaches a stage in which no vesicles or pustules are formed, in which there is no oozing, and in which the part affected is simply in a red scaly condition. To all such cases we may give the name eczema squamosum.

---

* On Diseases of the Skin. New Sydenham Society translation, London, 1868, Vol. II, p. 69.

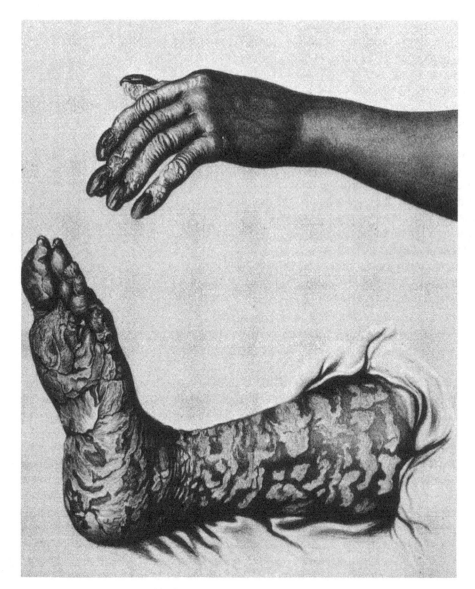

Figure 27 Pityriasis rubra. From Hebra's atlas

But there still remain others which may be fairly classed under the head of pityriasis rubra, in which reddening of the skin and gradual desquamation are the only characters, and in which there is no infiltration of the cutis, nor any other symptom. Such an affection cannot be termed eczema because the oozing and the vesicles which belong to that disease, are not present at any period of its duration.

Thus, then, I give the name pityriasis rubra to an affection in which, throughout its course, the only symptom is the persistent deep red coloration of the skin. In this disease there is no considerable infiltration of the cutis; no papules or vesicles are formed; no secretion is poured from the surface; the itching is slight, and does not lead to the formation of excoriations; no fissures make their appearance; and lastly, particular regions of the body are rarely affected, the whole surface of the skin being generally attacked.

Throughout the whole course of the disease, then, the only characters which it has presented have been those above described, except indeed that scales, consisting of dead epidermic plates, have accumulated in greater or less quantity. Towards the end of the patient's life, however (for, unhappily, diffused pityriasis rubra has always terminated fatally), the skin gradually becomes pale and turns at first of a yellowish, and ultimately of a dirty yellow tint. After death, even this is no longer to be discovered, and the appearance of the integument differs in no respect from that of a person who has died of some internal disease.

Before the occurrence of this melancholy termination, however, many years elapse. During the early part of this long period the patients have remained in good health, and have even been able to pursue their usual occupations; and if they had not been daily reminded of the existence of the disease by the change in the color of the skin, they would themselves have been ignorant of its presence since it gave rise to no unpleasant sensations. Little by little, however, they have begun to lose flesh and strength, so that they felt themselves no longer strong enough to carry on business; and it is this which has ultimately induced them to apply for medical relief. Such have been the circumstances under which cases of pityriasis rubra have come before me.

RHINOSCLEROMA

Über ein eigenthümliches Neugebilde an der Nase—Rhinosclerom*

Over a number of years I have had the opportunity to observe, in nine individuals (four men, five women), a skin affection which stands as a disease sui generis, both in its constant seat in the nose and immediate vicinity, and in the peculiarity of its manifestations.

To picture this disease, take a firm syphilitic sclerosis of the praeputium penis in its optimum form, and transplant it, in the mind's eye, partly to the outer structure of the nose, namely, in one case to the ala nasi, in another to the bridge of the nose, partly to the surface of the mucous membrane bordering the nostril, or, finally, to the skin of the regions about the nose, the upper lip, cheek, or forehead. In the nine cases observed, there were only two in which the disease was seen on the nose, cheek and forehead at the same time; in the others it was confined to the nose and upper lip alone. It was always sharply demarcated, appearing as a flat tumor sometimes projecting one and one-half inches above the level of the surrounding area, sloping off steeply at the edges. The color of this new growth varied from the color of normal skin to a dark brownish red. The surface of the diseased area was always smooth, and more or less shiny. The most striking objective symptom of the disease was the extraordinary hardness of the affected skin sites; they felt like ivory. The patients experienced very little pain in them, usually only when the growth localized on the inner surface of the nose, and pressure was applied to the raised areas.

Progress was very slow in all cases, and it took many years for the disease to reach a size sufficient to move the patient to seek the advice of a physician.

---

* Wiener Med. Wchnschr., *21:*1, 1870.

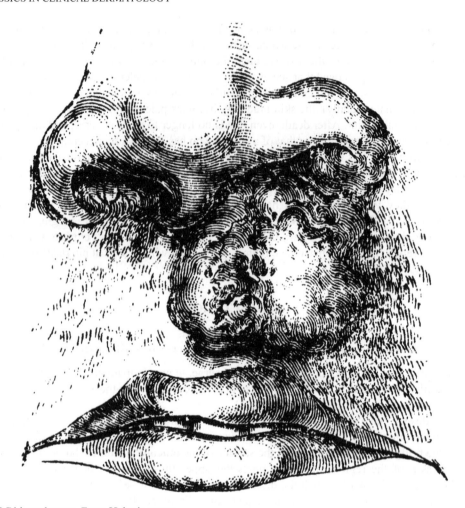

Figure 28 Rhinoscleroma. From Hebra's paper

IMPETIGO HERPETIFORMIS

Über einzelne während der Schwangerschaft, dem Wochenbette und bei Uterinalkrankheiten der Frauen zu beobachtende Hautkrankheiten.*

I will describe an eruption of the general surface of which I have only met with five examples occurring in pregnant and puerperal women, and of which, as far as I know, no account has ever been published. The eruption is characterized by pustules which are filled with pus at their first appearance, and by these effecting a peculiar mode of grouping and peripheric extension. In almost every case they have first appeared at the inner surface of the thigh, partly in groups the size of a kreutzer, and partly as separate pustules the size of a pin's head. Successive crops immediately follow, extending towards the periphery in a circular or iris form, so that in the course of a few days a gradual invasion takes place of the thighs, abdomen, legs, arms, hands, and feet, and afterwards of the neck, face, and hairy scalp. While at the center of each group the pustules become covered with flat dark-brown scabs, at the circumference new ones filled with yellow pus are being constantly produced. In this disposition they resemble the *herpes iris circinnatus;* but as from the very first it is a pustular disease, it must be regarded as a form of impetigo, and may, from its circular mode of grouping, be termed *impetigo herpetiformis.*

The affection throughout its whole course is attended by intense fever, a dry tongue, and great prostration. In three of these cases this reproduction of the pustules continued with more or less rapidity until the patient died, while in the other two after several weeks duration the pustules dried up, the thick scabs finally falling off and leaving the skin beneath healthy but strongly pigmented. Some of the pustules, instead of drying, especially at the bends of the joints, were converted into a grayish, stinking mass, which, lying on a red and moistened basis, assumed an eczematous appearance. No alterations occurred, and the discharges gradually dried into scabs, beneath which the epidermis was reproduced.

Only one out of the five cases finally survived. Each outbreak of pustules was preceded by shivering, which was followed by febrile action that lasted some days. Of the five women three had been delivered from two to five weeks before admission and two came in during the last month of pregnancy. The appearances of the skin were the same both before and after delivery. The autopsies of the four women who died revealed no certain cause of death; and neither the mode of life, employment or constitution of these patients threw any light upon the origin of this affection. In none of them was there any symptom of syphilis. In the absence of all other etiological data, and seeing that these cases all occurred in pregnant women, it may be stated, in connection with the cases already referred to in this paper, as most probable that these instances of herpetiformis impetigo were dependent upon a diseased change in the genital apparatus.

---

* Wiener Med. Wchnschr., *22:*1198, 1872 (translation from Am. J.Syph. and Dermat., *4:*158, 1873).

Jules Parrot

Edema Neonatorum

MARIE-JULES PARROT was born in Excideuil, Dordogne, November 1, 1829. He was the son of a physician. His initial studies were at the Paris Polytechnical School, and only later did he turn to medicine. While still a student he wrote a prize paper on herpes zoster. Following his graduation in 1857, he began practice in Paris. In 1876 he was appointed Professor of the History of Medicine on the Paris faculty, and in 1879, professor of pediatrics.

Parrot was an indefatigable worker. His publications touch on most phases of the pediatrics of his day. He was particularly interested in hereditary syphilis, and his work on the bony changes in this disease led to the eponym, the "pseudo-paralysis of Parrot." Parrot's most notable contribution to pediatrics lay in his work on the changes occurring in the nutrition of infants in various diseases, particularly in gastrointestinal affections. He presented his clinical and pathological observations in his *Clinique Nouveau-nés* (1867), under the name Athrepsia. It is from this work that we have taken the description of edema neonatorum given below.

Parrot was a meticulous clinician and a master of auscultation. Although charming personally, he was inclined to be temperamental; he habitually overworked, and was always in poor health. He died August 5, 1883.*

EDEMA NEONATORUM

L'Athrepsie*

But the most striking thing is the external appearance of athrepsia. The stamp of the disease, impressed upon the face and the entire body, is so profound and so characteristic that it is impossible to mistake it. The wasting is considerable, and presents something entirely special, for the destruction is manifest more in the fluids than in the solids. The entire organism suffers from aridity, and it could be said that the tissues have dried up. From this, a group of symptoms arise which are readily demonstrable to the hand and to the eye. The flesh has a special consistency. To compression it feels like congealed tallow, or wood. A marked rigidity of the extremities results; they remain completely rigid, as in tetany.

---

* Cornil, A.: Bull, de la Soc. Anat. de Paris, *59:*35, 1884.

In other subjects, where the soft parts have retained more suppleness, the skin is formed into numerous wrinkles. This is especially apparent in the face, where nothing remains but bony structure covered by a shriveled integument. Thus, the enlargement of the mouth, the prominence of the maxillae, and the hollow orbits lend something simian to the physiognomy of these tiny moribund individuals. At other times their wrinkled faces remind one of certain old men, the disease having done in a few days the work of many years. The cranium itself suffers notable modifications; the fontanelle becomes depressed, and elevations appear along the sutures, due to the overlapping of the osseous pieces which meet there. Around the buccal orifice and the eyes, the skin takes on a bluish color. The lids, imperfectly closed, expose an ocular globe decreased in size, and the cornea dry and lusterless, and the conjunctiva injected.

The infant utters cries less frequently than in the preceding period, but one can always recognize them by the anxiety they express. In calling them *cris de détress* I believe I have characterized them correctly.

When things have gone this far, life may cease at one moment or the next. The cry grows more feeble, and is finally extinguished; the heart sounds become more and more retarded, and the important functions are seen successively to be depressed before death becomes general.

---

* Clinique des Nouveau-nés: L'Athrepsie. Paris, 1867, p. 59.

Erasmus Wilson

1.   *Lichen Planus*

2.   *Nevus Araneus*

3.   *Exfoliative Dermatitis*

4.   *Neurotic Excoriations*

WILLIAM JAMES ERASMUS WILSON was born in London in 1809, of Scottish parents. He was educated at Dartford and Swanscombe, and in 1825 began his medical studies at St. Bartholomew's Hospital as a pupil of Mr. Abernethy, with whom he soon became a great favorite. In 1831 he was admitted to the Royal College of Surgeons of England, and soon afterwards became an assistant at University College.

During his early years Wilson devoted himself exclusively to anatomy and pathology, and acquired a nation wide reputation for his skill in this field. One of his earliest publications, the *Anatomist's Vade Mecum* became a standard student's text.

In his early thirties Wilson became interested in skin diseases, particularly in the as yet but little studied relationship between clinical disease and anatomical site, and turned his attention entirely to dermatology. The impress he made on dermatology in England can hardly be over-estimated. He revived interest in the specialty, which had flagged considerably following the death of Bateman; he published the first journal in England devoted exclusively to dermatology, the *Journal of Cutaneous Medicine* (1867), in which appeared the masterly and definitive description of lichen planus given here. He is best known for his account of exfoliative dermatitis, often called Wilson's disease, and for his *Lectures on Dermatology,* delivered before the Royal College of Surgeons, from which we have taken the first account of neurotic excoriations. The number of his publications is remarkable; they include a fine atlas, *Portraits of Diseases of the Skin* (1847), and the most widely used English text of the day, *On Diseases of the Skin* (1847).

By nature kindly and gentle, Wilson was one of the great medical philanthropists. He endowed chairs in dermatology and pathology, and made large bequests to various hospitals and to the Royal College of Surgeons, as well as to many non-medical institutions. He acquired national fame by bringing the obelisk known as Cleopatra's needle to England from Alexandria. For his many acts of bounty he was knighted in 1881 by Queen Victoria.

He fell ill in 1883 and, totally blind for more than a year, died in 1884, in his residence, The Bungalow, Westgate-on-Sea.*

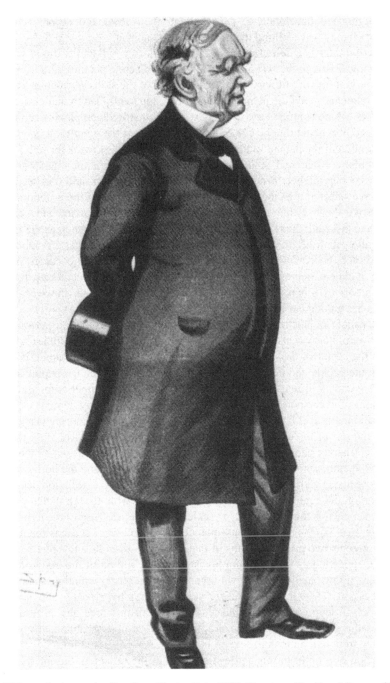

Figure 29 Erasmus Wilson. Caricature by Spy from *Vanity Fair,* 1880. Courtesy, The Free Library of Philadelphia

LICHEN PLANUS

Leichen planus[†]

Leichen planus is an eruption of pimples remarkable for their colour, their figure, their structure, their habits of isolated and aggregated development, their habitat, their local and chronic character, and for the melasmic stains which they leave behind them when they disappear.

The colour of the pimples is a dull crimson-red, more or less vivid, and suffused with a purplish or lilac tinge. It is most characteristic in the recently developed and discrete papules, and in the aggregated form is apt to assume the duskier hue of ordinary chronic affections of the skin. We incline to the belief that it is to this eruption that Hebra has given the name, leichen ruber, apparently led to that designation by the striking colour of the pimples, which contrast very strongly with the unattired complexion of the skin on which they are developed. Indeed, it is generally the colour and appearance of the pimples, without other symptom, that first attracts the attention of the patient to the disorder, and urges him to seek for relief.

In figure, the papulae are flattened, smooth and depressed on the summit, angular in outline, only slightly elevated, and of a size ranging between one and three lines in diameter, and this peculiarity of figure is so striking, that we have selected it as the pathognomonic characteristic of the eruption. The redness may be the first sign to strike the eye, but redness is a phenomenon common to many eruptions of the skin. Although, as we have just said, the redness of leichen planus is peculiar, whereas the flatness of the summit of the papulae is   altogether different from anything that is met with in other affections of the skin, and the flatness is rendered more conspicuous by the summit of the papulae being occupied by a thin, horny semi-transparent lamina of cuticle, depressed on the surface, and marked in the center by the aperture of a follicle which represents a sort of hilum. It is to this peculiarity of figure that the word planus is especially applicable, and this has guided our use of the term.

In structure the papule of leichen planus is a hyperaemia with exudation surrounding a follicle, and covered by a thin layer of horny transparent cuticle, while the aperture of the follicle and its conical epidermic plug are visible in the center of the horny plate. The horny covering of the papule is in no wise a scale; it rises and falls with the papule and neither separates nor exfoliates. When the papule subsides in the course of cure, its horny covering still remains, and disappears by degrees without exfoliation. In one form of the affection, the summit of every pore has its little horny plate, without any papular elevation whatever, and the surface of the skin looks as if it were inlaid with minute spangles or glittering particles of mica, perfectly homogenous with the rest of the epidermis. This applies, we need hardly say, only to the discrete form of the affection, to the separate papules. In the aggregated form of the disease, a new element is introduced, namely, diffused exudation, exfoliation, and desquamation take place, and the horny covering of the papule already described exfoliates with the rest of the cuticle. Whenever this exfoliation occurs, it is interesting to note the continuity of the under surface of the horny plate with the epithelial lining of the follicle. Nevertheless, not even then is the horny plate a "scale" in the proper sense of the term, but merely a portion of exuviated cuticle, cast like the rest as a consequence of the temporary suspension of nutrition.

Leichen planus presents two principal forms of manifestation, discrete and aggregate. It usually begins as a discrete eruption, appearing as isolated pimples in some one region of the body or dispersed on various parts. Here and there, a few papules are thrown up near to each other, sometimes simultaneously, but more frequently in succession. Then the intermediate skin becomes hyperaemic and infiltrated, and a patch results, consisting of an aggregation of papulae united by an inflamed and infiltrated base. With these aggregated patches the discrete form of the eruption is more or less abundantly commingled, and the patches range in size from half an inch to several inches in diameter, sometimes covering the greater part of the internodial portion of a limb. In this aggregated form of the affection, the interpapular congestion and

---

* Editor: Brit. Med. J., *2:*347, 1884.

† J.Cutan. Med., *3:*117, 1869.

JOURNAL OF

CUTANEOUS MEDICINE

AND

DISEASES OF THE SKIN.

A QUARTERLY RECORD OF

DERMATOLOGICAL SCIENCE.

EDITED BY

ERASMUS WILSON, F.R.S.

VOL. I.

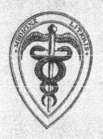

LONDON :
JOHN CHURCHILL AND SONS, NEW BURLINGTON STREET.
MDCCCLXVIII.

Figure 30 Title page to Wilson's *Journal of Cutaneous Medicine*. Courtesy, College of Physicians, Philadelphia

infiltration assume the most important place in our consideration, the infiltrated skin often rises up to a level with the summit of the papulae, the papulae are as it were submerged, and blended in the general exfoliation and desquamation which ensue, and we are driven to seek, in the circumference of the patch or in other regions of the body, isolated papulae in order to confirm our diagnosis. Nevertheless, with close inspection the figure of the separate papulae may still be detected in the midst of the patches, and especially that peculiarity of structure already noted, namely, the continuity of the desquamating cuticle with the epithelium of the follicle. Not infrequently, the aggregated patches are circular in figure and of a small size, and might very easily be mistaken for lepra vulgaris, the more especially as patches of this kind are apt to grow by the circumference and become depressed in the center. But in this case, the scale of lepra is always absent, and the history of the case, the seat of the eruption, and the presence of isolated papules confirm the diagnosis. At other times, the broader patches of the aggregated form of the affection so closely resemble those of any chronic eczema, that a mistake on the part of those unfamiliar with cutaneous disease would be perfectly pardonable. We lately saw a patient suffering under this disease, in whom it was named by an experienced dermatologist, "lichen agrius pruriginosus."

The habitat of the eruption is also characteristic of the identity of leichen planus; it is pretty constantly met with on the front of the forearm, just above the wrist, in the hollow of the loins, on the lower half of the abdomen, on the hips, around the knees, particularly over the mass of the vastus internus muscle, on the forearms and calves of the legs, and in women around the waist and in the grooves occasioned by garters. We have seen it also, but less frequently, on the palm of the hands and sole of the feet, and in two instances on the tongue, the buccal membrane, and the mucous lining of the fauces.

Leichen planus is essentially chronic and local in its habits. In 27 out of 50 cases examined, the eruption at the time of application for treatment, had lasted between six months and one year; and in six, between one year and seven. In distribution it is generally symmetrical, but occasionally is limited to one side of the body, sometimes occurring on one side in the upper extremity, and on the other in the lower. It has no constitutional symptoms of its own, and frequently prevails with very little constitutional disturbance of any kind.

The melasmic discolouration of those parts of the skin where the eruption has existed, and where it has disappeared, is a characteristic feature which leichen planus possesses, in common with lepra vulgaris, but it is not commonly met with in other affections. These stains are often very remarkable, they give rise to a strange mottling of the skin, and may be accepted as a pathognomonic character when taken in association with the signs already considered.

The separate papules of leichen planus sometimes enlarge sufficiently to produce a raised border, with a depressed center, and so to constitute a distinct ring, while at other times the ring results from the peripheral elevation of the border of a small patch, or the ring may itself be composed of a chain of papules. In either case a configuration results, which we have termed leichen planus annulatus. Sometimes these annuli are small and round or oval in figure; at other times they are extensive, one while encircling the axilla, as in case 39; and another while [encircling] the perineum, as in case 17. Occasionally the circles are broken, and only an irregular curved line remains to indicate the border of the vanished patch, in which case the term leichen planus marginatus is appropriate. Leichen planus scarcely deserves to be classed among the pruritic affections. The itching is generally very trifling, but in some instances, as in cases 18, 28, 33 is intolerable. Such cases as the latter have suggested the term leichen planus pruriginosus, which is then strikingly applicable.

This eruption is most commonly met with in the adult of middle age, the greatest number falling within the decade between 40 and 50 years.

NEVUS ARANEUS

Eruptive Angeiomata*

A publican, aged 30 years, had for some time yielded to the temptation of his calling, and had thereby injured his health, when he was suddenly attacked with epistaxis and to the epistaxis succeeded copious bleeding from the gums. At the same time, and subsequently, there appeared on the face, the neck, the hands, and the arms, an eruption of red papulae with a diffuse areola. On presenting himself for consultation there were six of these papular spots on the face, chiefly on one cheek, two on the neck, and three or four on the hands and forearms. It was evident, on careful examination, they were angeiomata; the central prominence was vascular, and around this was a plexus of venules spreading out to the breadth of a quarter or half an inch. In one or two of the spots the central prominence was absent and a plexus alone existed, resulting from angeiektasia, or multiplication and hypertrophy of the venous capillaries of the skin. The case is very rare, a sudden eruption of angeiomata, and its association with haemorrhage from the mucous membrane of the nose and mouth is very instructive. We are unaware of the conditions of the economy which may tend to the sudden hypertrophy of blood vessels, but we can easily understand how such an occurrence, taking place upon the mucous membranes, might lead to serious haemorrhage; and there is no reason to suppose that the cause of the epistaxis in the instance before us, and the bleeding of the gums may not have been a sudden hypertrophy of blood-vessels such as we have just described as appearing on the skin. And it appears to us that as a result, to the well-known haemorrhagic diathesis as a cause of hemorrhage, there must also be added a sudden hypertrophy of blood-vessels and rupture of their coat as exemplified in the case before us.

EXFOLIATIVE DERMATITIS

On Dermatitis Exfoliativa[†]

General dermatitis is sufficiently rare to excite some attention and interest whenever a case of the kind comes under notice. I have already published in my work, *On Diseases of the Skin,* two instances of this disease and one of a local form, and I now present to the profession the details of another example of the same affection. Heretofore, I have followed the nomenclature of Devergie and Hebra, and have called it "pityriasis rubra," but on the present occasion, I have ventured to employ a term which, I believe, will convey to the mind a better idea of the nature of the complaint than the name given to it by my colleagues, and which at the same time is calculated to escape controversy. There may be some doubt as to the true meaning of pityriasis and as to the appropriateness of the application of the name to the disease in question, but there can be none as to the term "dermatitis exfoliativa"; that is to say, inflammation of the skin accompanied with exfoliation of the epidermis, the inflammation being of an unusually intense kind, and the exfoliation of cuticle profuse, amounting in fact to a state of positive flux.

The case which I am about to describe may be briefly stated as follows: A punctated exanthema, following a shock to the nervous system occasioned by chill, nausea, perspiration and checked perspiration; the exanthema developed in a few hours and rapidly diffused, until the whole body presents a bright red color; excessive heat with soreness and stiffness of surface; well marked infiltration and condensation of the

---

* J.Cutan. Med., *3:*198, 1869.

[†] Med. Times and Gaz., *1:*118, 1870.

skin; tendency to crack into fissures on motion; in six or seven days incipient exfoliation of the epidermis in thin laminae with elongated base; the line of fracture of the cuticle corresponding with the grooves of motion of the skin and, when the laminae are only partially separated, projecting from the skin in narrow frills sometimes several inches in length. Incessant exfoliation of cuticle so as to fill the patient's bed with thin laminae; no pruritus; no general perspiration, and but slight partial perspiration from the forehead and back of the hands; tendency to oedema about the ankles; scanty urine loaded with urates; no albumen; pulse quick and excitable; tongue clean; appetite and digestive organs undisturbed, and strength but little affected.

The patient, a young man, aged 28, enjoying average health, and engaged in a brewery, was attacked with eczema erythematosum, which was developed in small circumscribed patches on his limbs, chiefly those of the lower extremity. This occurred in the month of May, 1869, the eruption desquamating and continuing without other change until October. At the latter date he left home with his wife for an afternoon's holiday. The day proved to be wet, and his clothes were saturated with moisture. He stood under an archway waiting for a cab for nearly an hour, and on reaching his house was seized with nausea. He then went into his garden to relieve himself by vomiting, but was unable to do so, and became suffused with perspiration. While in the garden he experienced a chill, which he was unable to shake off the whole evening, and he has remained abnormally sensitive to cold ever since. On the following morning it was perceived that his skin was covered with a bright red and punctated exanthema, which in the course of the two following days spread over the whole surface of his body. Nevertheless, the rash was unattended, and did not therefore confine him to the house. The inflammation of the skin, with great redness and excessive heat, lasted without breach of surface for about a week, but after this time the epidermis began to crack and exfoliate, and has continued to do so up to the present time—namely, about six weeks from the beginning of the attack.

On November 201 saw the patient with Dr. Locke. His face presented the usual remarkable character of this foliaceous form of dermatitis—a deep red hue, with tightening and contraction of the skin, and an unusual expansion of the eyelids, which gave to the countenance a staring expression, and, added to this, the white edges of numerous partially separated stripes of epidermis, which marked the forehead and face all over as if it had been tatooed. The ears also were deeply red, and looked parched, and there were dark scabs at the root of the pinna and at several points on the helix, produced by the oozing of blood occasioned by his habit of picking at the scales.

From the head down to the feet the same characters prevailed, although in a heightened degree. The skin everywhere exhibited the appearance of tightening and contraction; it was vividly red, covered with loose frills and shreds of epidermis, was hot and parched, and exhaled an unpleasant valerianic smell, while the lower sheet was covered with similar shreds and flakes. The exfoliation of the epidermis was, however, most remarkable on the back, which was covered with small gauze-like shreds ranged for the most part transversely, the rows being situated at short distances apart. The derma had the appearance of being thinner than ordinary, and the grooves of flexion were strongly marked. The only parts of the skin which had escaped the general dermatitis, but those only partially, were the soles of the feet and palms of the hands, the latter being moistened with perspiration. But, at a later period, the cuticle of the palm was raised by numerous pimples, was hard, stiff, and subsequently exfoliated, as did that of the soles of the feet.

The symptoms accompanying this state were a feeling of burning heat with occasional transient chills, of soreness and stiffness; he had difficulty in opening his mouth when told to put out his tongue, and he dreaded movement from the fear of cracking his skin. There was no itching, and he had had none from the first.

NEUROTIC EXCORIATIONS

Neurotic Excoriations*

I may better illustrate the kind of affection to which I am referring by the narration of a case.

Case I. A maiden lady, aged 47, has the face spotted over with small abrasions from which the epidermis has been recently removed. The excoriations are oval or polyhedral in figure, for the most part square or oblong, and sometimes pointed towards the inferior margin; they are about a quarter of an inch in diameter. There are from 15 to 20 spots of this kind scattered over the forehead and face, but of this number only three or four are perfectly fresh, the rest represent advancing but more particularly declining stages of the affection. The patient's attention is first directed to their existence by a sensation of fulness, burning, and tingling, and this sensation will continue for some hours, indeed, until she is driven to seek relief from the irritation by rubbing or scratching. The effect of a very slight rub is to detach the cuticle, which seems to slide off the spot and thus bring into view the excoriated patch which I have just been describing, and the excoriation is accompanied with bleeding to a greater or less degree.

The pathological history of the affection is that of a hyperaemia, which gives rise to a flat, circumscribed induration, accompanied with slight redness, and with the sensation of fulness, burning, and tingling already noticed; and then a slight serous exudation beneath the horny epidermis sufficient to loosen the cuticle but rarely sufficient to develop a blister; these several processes occupying only a few hours in their progress. Moreover, the morbid process is chronic, having existed in this lady for nearly two years, and the development of the spots being successive, they present, at the same time, a series of stages of growth. In one place a slight redness, occupying an indurated base without prominence and consequently neither a papule nor a tubercle; in another, a bleeding excoriation; in a third an excoriation encrusted with blood, sometimes a dry spot of a reddish-brown colour; and after healing, a pigmentary stain of various depths of hue.

The appearance of the patient whose case I am now narrating is that of a decidedly nervous person; she is shy, silent, dejected, seemingly occupied with her inward self, and desirous of shunning observation. The face is darkened by pigmentation, as well as being spotted by abrasions and their consequences. She complains of pains in her head, occipital and frontal, and also of much exhaustion and debility. The pulse is weak; her nutritive functions are defective; but those of digestion and excretion are fairly regular. Amenorrhea has prevailed for about three years, and she has some ovarian pain on the right side.

Her previous life had been one of average health; but at the age of 20 she was subject to occasional attacks of fainting, and of recent years has had considerable strain thrown upon her nervous system. For a few weeks previously to the affection of the skin she was engaged in reading to a deaf person, five hours a day, in a close, hot room. This gave rise to considerable exhaustion, which was increased by her anxiety to perform her duty satisfactorily; and the nervous excitement and debility consequent on her exertions became a predisponent of the cutaneous disorder. In this state, a trivial cause—namely, the eating of ice— became the first motive impulse of the affection of the skin, which at once broke out around her mouth. She then by accident bruised her nose, and a second attack of the disorder showed itself on and around the injured organ, while a third attack became developed on the forehead, as the consequence of a draught of cold air. The swarthiness and deep pigmentation of her skin became manifest about six weeks after the commencement of the cutaneous affection; and in reference to the spots, she observed that they were

---

* Lectures on Dermatology, 1874–75. London, 1875, p. 192.

introduced by a feeling of fulness, burning, tingling, pricking, and itching; if left to themselves, they frequently gave rise to a small blister, but that in general she had no chance of peace until she had rubbed them or scratched them and produced a flow of blood, and in that case the uneasiness ceased.

The form of disease which I am now describing is local, but it appears occasionally as a general affection. In the present instance it was limited to the face—a region more liable to its occurrence than any other part of the body. I have likewise seen a well-marked example restricted to the forearm, and especially to the district supplied by the ulnar nerve. When it occurs as a general affection, it is apt to be mistaken for ordinary prurigo; and although more common in the female than in the male, I have also met with the general form in an adult man.

This curious affection brings to our mind cases which some of us may have seen, and others have found reported, under the denomination of spontaneous haemorrhage from the skin, haemitidrosis, and vicarious menstruation, and notably those more extraordinary cases of religious neuropathia which are manifested by haemorrhage from the hands and feet and from the left hypochondriac region—the so-called *stigmata* of the crucifixion of our Lord. By the pathology of neuropathic excoriations of the skin, we are supplied with two out of three factors necessary to the production of such *stigmata,* namely, general neuropathia and local cutaneous haemorrhage; the third factor only is wanting, and that it is evident must stand in the relation of a predisposing cause to the rest of the phenomena. Thus it is not difficult to conceive, that, in one case, the predisposing cause may be a perverted religious enthusiasm, while in another case it may be a sexual irritation.

Edward Nettleship

Urticaria Pigmentosa

EDWARD NETTLESHIP was born at Kettering in Northamptonshire, March 3, 1845. He studied at Kings College Hospital in London, the London Hospital, and the London Veterinary College. In 1873 he became curator of the Moorfield Ophthalmologic Hospital, and later held important positions at St. Thomas's Hospital. The case of Urticaria pigmentosa given here was described by him early in his career, before his specialization in ophthalmology.

Nettleship wrote a widely used ophthalmologic text, *The Student's Guide to Diseases of the Eye* (1879), and was sufficiently interested in research in his field to quit private practice in 1902 to devote himself entirely to it. He died at Hindhead in Surrey, October 30, 1913.*

URTICARIA PIGMENTOSA

Rare Forms of Urticaria[†]

We group together today three examples of very unusual forms of urticaria. The first is peculiar in that the eruption has been persistent for nearly two years, and began at the early age of three months. A remarkable feature also is that the wheals have brown stains. The appearance produced is very singular and, the child being of beautifully fair skin, the brown patches are the more conspicuous. At first sight, the diagnosis of chloasma would occur to most, but the entire absence of branniness and the early age of the patient are fatal to this suspicion. It has also been set at rest by the microscope. The urticarious irritability of the child's skin is proved at once on scratching it.

Emile P., aged 2 years, living at Blackheath Hill, was admitted to the hospital for skin diseases on July 27th, 1869. She was the subject of chronic urticaria, and the eruption was peculiar in leaving stains of a light brown colour, their tint being very like that of chloasma, for which the disease might have been mistaken at first glance. She had light hair and a very fair complexion. The mother says that the child "has never suffered from any illness since her birth" and she is in excellent health. There was no history of urticaria in other members of the family. The present eruption began when she was three months old, and she has never been free from it since. The mother's account is that the spots began as "white lumps like the sting of a

---

* Fischer, I.: Biog. Lex. der Hervor Arzte. Berlin, Urban and Schwarzenberg, 1933, p. 1107.

† Brit. Med. J., *18*:323, 1869.

nettle"; these itch severely, and on subsiding, leave the curious brownish stains above noticed. The rash, on admission, thickly covered the neck and trunk, the extremities being more sparsely affected. There were no spots on the face, but a few brown stains of former wheals at the margin of the scalp on the forehead. There were no red wheals, but some slightly raised patches of light brown colour with slight congestion, and some stains of former wheals. The true nature of the raised patches was proved by their centres, turning nearly white when the skin was stretched. The wheals are of uniform size, and about as large as three-penny pieces. It was noticed that a scratch with the fingernail produced, in a few minutes, an ordinary urticaria wheal, with white center and red edges, and at a subsequent occasion a number of recent patches of elevated and erythematous skin were observed. These had not yet become brown. When the child first came, there was little or no evidence of scratching, but several weeks afterwards it is noted that "in addition to the urticaria, there are scratched papules, like those of prurigo; no lice can, however, be found." At her last attendance five weeks from admission, she was in much the same condition as at first, excepting the pruriginous spots.

We do not find any mention of a similar condition in our standard works. The patient is still attending, and can be seen by anyone interested in it.

Richard von Volkmann

Cheilitis Glandularis

RICHARD VON VOLKMANN was born August 17, 1830, in Leipzig, but spent the rest of his life in the university town, Halle, in Saxony where his father was Professor of Anatomy and Physiology. His student days, although poorly documented, must have been profitably spent, for at the age of 26 he was chosen to act as deputy to Professor Blasius, director of the Surgical Clinic of Halle. During this time his great talent in surgery came to be recognized, and he was appointed to the Chair of Surgery in 1867. In the Franco-Prussian War (1870), Volkmann had his first opportunity to put to the test the antiseptic doctrines Lister had begun to popularize some three years before. Although less than satisfied with his results in the field, he introduced the technique into the clinic, upon returning to Halle, with such great success that his clinic became the mecca for surgeons on the continent.

Volkmann's greatest contributions were made to the technique of surgery, particularly orthopedic surgery, his special province. His works on dislocations and on the ischemic contracture named for him are the pieces for which he is most remembered. In addition, he wrote much of subjects of dermatologic interest—of the treatment of lupus and chronic ulcers, as well as cheilitis glandularis, his account of which we have included here.

He was an elegant and bold operator. His appearance was aristocratic, though he was of but medium height and rather stoutly built. He was kindly in manner, and an excellent and deliberate speaker.

Volkmann also achieved considerable success in writing children's stories, poems, and fairy tales.

Afflicted for some years with a painful affection of the spinal cord, he died of pneumonia in 1889 in Jena, to which city he had taken a patient for consultation.*

CHEILITIS GLANDULARIS

Einige Fälle von Cheilitis glandularis apostematosa (Myxadenitis labialis)[†]

On five occasions thus far, I have seen a peculiar type of chronic inflammation of the lower lip, concerning which I have been able to find no account in the literature.

All the patients were adults. Three of them had had constitutional syphilis a short time before, and in one, some areas of palmar psoriasis were still demonstrable, whereas in the others, with the exception of some slightly enlarged lymph nodes, no further local syphilitic affections could be found. Two were perfectly healthy, and maintained never to have been ill with syphilis.

The course of the inflammation of the lips was in all five cases very similar, although differing in severity. The lower lip gradually became swollen without any particular pain, and became hard and firm, so that the face acquired an unpleasant puffy expression. The mobility of the lip was greatly reduced, indeed almost abolished in some cases. The swelling extended through the entire thickness and width of the lower lip, up to its transition into the chin. In one case it involved both angles of the mouth on the upper lip, so that in this patient the corners were diseased to the extent of a finger-breadth on both sides. The integument was slightly reddened in the diseased area. Precise examination showed that the mucous glands of the lip were swollen to the size of a hemp seed and larger, and were palpable through the mucous membrane as lumpy masses, unusual in number and extent. If the mucous membrane of the lip were everted, the excretory ducts could be seen, widely dilated, some to the extent that they could be penetrated with a fine eye probe. With pressure, which caused only moderate pain, a turbid mucous or mucopurulent secretion could be expressed from them, so that either the whole lip, previously carefully dried, appeared covered over by a thin film, or thick drops of almost pure pus appeared here and there.

True abscesses occurred only three times, and likewise arose, apparently, either from the glands, or at least from the surrounding periacinous connective tissue. With relatively slight pain, furunculoid inflammatory changes developed deep in the lip, and soon broke through a small opening in the outer skin, or more frequently in the mucous membrane; they showed a very great tendency to become fistulous, and drained a muco-purulent secretion for weeks or months. In one case there were 12 to 15 of these fine openings present simultaneously on the mucous membrane side of the lower lip, readily admitting a somewhat coarse eye probe, and leading to irregular fistulous tracts passing through the lip. These openings at the surface never progressed to true ulcers, nor could any syphilitic ulcers or plaques be discovered on the lip itself, or on other parts of the oral and pharyngeal mucous membrane. However, in all cases there was a rather marked oral and pharyngeal catarrh.

---

* Ross, J.: St. Bart. Hosp. J., *38:*47, 1930.

† Archiv für path. anat., *50:*142, 1870.

Tilbury Fox

1. *Impetigo Contagiosa*

2. *Dysidrosis*

WILLIAM TILBURY FOX was born in 1836, the son of a well known physician, in southern England. After preliminary studies at University College he began at the University of London, and in 1857 was graduated M.B., with honors in surgery and the gold medal for scholarship in medicine. At the beginning of his professional career he became house-surgeon at the General Lying-in Hospital, Lambeth, and gave much attention to obstetric subjects, writing an important paper on phlegmasia alba dolens, and another on puerperal fever. He soon became interested, however, in the mycologic aspects of certain diseases of the hair and skin, and thereafter devoted himself to the study of dermatology.

With Erasmus Wilson, Fox pioneered in dermatology as a specialty apart, and the specialty is in no small measure indebted to him for establishing it as a worthy division of medicine in England.

Besides his work on fungus diseases, which he elaborated in his monograph, *Skin Diseases of Parasitic Origin* (1863), Fox wrote one of the most popular and influential texts of the day, his *Treatise on Skin Diseases* (1864). He was a prolific contributor to the journals of the time, particularly to the *British Medical Journal,* in which appeared the two pieces we have included here, the two for which he is most remembered —impetigo contagiosa, and dysidrosis. The number and scope of his publications is remarkable when one considers that he was active only about 16 years.

In character Dr. Fox was bright, lively, and even effervescent, pleasant and kindly in manner. He saw to the education of his younger brother, Thomas Colcott Fox, who became a noted dermatologist in his own right.

Although Tilbury Fox died at the early age of 43 (1879), his death was not entirely unexpected. He had been known to have heart disease for some six years previously. It was believed to have resulted from a severe attack of acute rheumatism he had suffered while touring the East in the study of cholera and dermatologic disease early in his career.*

IMPETIGO CONTAGIOSA

On Impetigo Contagiosa or Porrigo[†]

At the outset, I had better state clearly that impetigo contagiosa must not be confounded with ordinary impetigo. They are absolutely distinct. Mr. Startin, if report be correct, fully recognizes the existence of a contagious form of impetigo, but I am not aware of any published account from that gentleman's pen. In the *British Medical Journal* for November 28, 1863, is a description by my colleague, Mr. R.W.Dunn, of

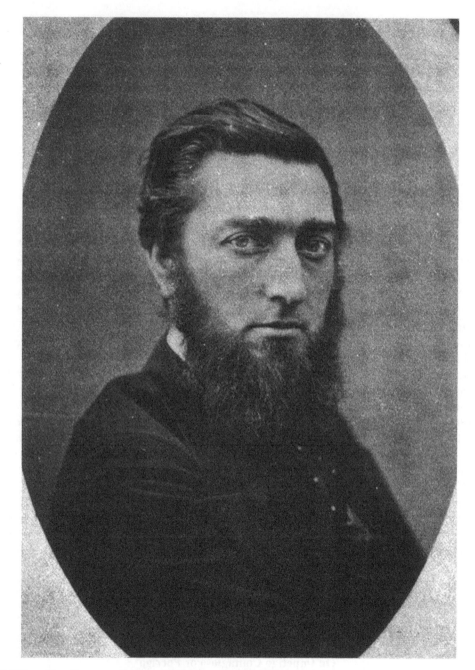

Figure 31 Tilbury Fox. Courtesy, College of Physicians, Philadelphia

porrigo. He says it consists of large dirty straw-coloured spots, flattened, of irregular shape, seeming as if they were stuck or glued on the part, without any inflammation at their bases, mostly seated on the scalp, but found also on all parts of the body. When the face is attacked, the spots are a little more regular. They discharge and commence originally as papules, which become pustular. Mr. Dunn thinks it is of parasitic nature; from this opinion, I entirely dissent.

Characters. The disease varies considerably in aspect, according to its seat, as I have narrowly observed. It occurs mostly on the face, where it is generally unilateral, and seated especially about the angle of the mouth and the side of the nose, also on the limbs, anteriorly and posteriorly, on the trunk especially about the shoulders, the neck, and the buttocks. The constitutional symptoms which usher in the complaint are generally sufficient to make the friends declare the child "poorly," unable to take its food properly, "mopish," and the like. The local characters of the disease show themselves as little white, apparently vesicular, or more truly pustular points, just tinged at their bases with slight redness, and generally possessed of little pain. These points, which are always isolated and distinct at the outset, speedily enlarge and umbilicate to a more or less perfect degree. Now and then, coalescence takes place between two or more pustules. This is seen especially on the face. The next change is the assumption of the characters of a perfect pustule, which may desiccate, leaving a dark dry scab, depressed in the centre generally, through or from beneath which oozes out a little thick pus or puriform discharge. Each spot increases in a perfectly centrifugal manner, until in about a week it attains the size of a shilling or so. A characteristic aspect is then presented. The disease looks like a flattened bleb, whose central part is depressed and shrunken, the contents giving an opacity. The margin of the bulla, as it now may be termed, is formed by a perfect ring of varying breadth, which has the look of wet soddened white leather, just as though the central part were circumscribed by a collar composed of upraised and blebbed epidermis, and this circumferential ring enlarges *pari passu* with the bleb.

It becomes an interesting question to determine the exact value to be attached to the umbilication in impetigo contagiosa. I hold it to be almost diagnostic. Of course, it is only seen perfectly in the early stages.

The so-called bleb or pustuloid may attain to a considerable size. The contents are peculiar. There is generally more or less pus, and always at the early stage, at the bottom a little pellet or *bouton* of mucous consistency (aplastic lymph), which can be removed, and then leaves to view a little conical pit of ulceration. The discharge dries into crusts, tolerably thick, which adhere for many days and then fall off leaving ulcerated surfaces. If the crusts be detached by the finger, a nasty sticky puriform fluid is seen to cover the surface of the ulcers. These latter give out a greater or less amount of discharge, which again concretes in crusts. Fresh pustulations occur, so as to prolong the disease for a period of from three to six or eight weeks. Each spot lasts a variable time—10 days or more—leaving in process of cure a dull red stain. The scabs may become quite black from the commingling of dirt with the discharge.

The disease is always characterized by the presence of *circular* umbilicated *quasi*-bullous spots, which increase centrifugally, and become covered by yellowish flat crusts, which cover over superficial ulcerations of an unhealthy kind, leaving in process of cure dull red stains.

Modifications. There are several modifications worth considering. There may be but one solitary spot. A short time since, I saw a most typical example in a patient of Dr. Frodsham. The crust was of about the size of a florin, or nearly so. This solitary spot may be seated on the face or head, rarely on the trunk, except as the consequence of direct contagion or inoculation. When seated on the head, the crusts are very perfect, inasmuch as the hairs help out the matting together of the mass. On the scalp, the disease possesses the characters ascribed to it by Mr. Dunn. The so-called porriginous spots always commence as small elevated

---

* Unsigned Obit., Brit. Med. J., *1*:915, 1879.

† Brit. Med. J., *1*:467, 1864.

isolated points. They are always a primary form of the disease. The crusts are circular, or nearly circular, isolated, yellowish, adherent, granular, and pretty dry.

I have seen this form of impetigo associated with strumous ophthalmia, and with otitis, both of an acutish kind. More than this, I have seen the mucous surfaces affected, all these states being dependent evidently upon the cause which gives rise to the impetigo.

On the face, it is not unusual to notice several separate foci of disease, running together into an irregular, oozy, cracked, scabbed patch. In this state, it is not unlike eczema impetiginoides, but almost invariably the peculiar umbilicated pustuloid or peculiar ulceration will be found. Again, on the surface (and head especially), there is usually little if any redness around the bases of the different spots, though they may be as large as a shilling. Occasionally, however, there is a marked exception to this rule, and there may be an intense inflammatory areola. I have seen a considerable degree of inflammation of the derma and subcutaneous cellular tissue, the erythema having a dull red hue.

DYSIDROSIS

On Dysidrosis, an Undescribed Eruption*

Gentlemen, I am desirous today of directing your attention to a disordered condition of the sweat follicles and the sweat function which you will not find described in books. In fact, I shall depict to you for the first time a disease of the skin which is, as a rule, diagnosed as eczema, but is a separate and distinct affair.

Its anatomical seat, as seen in the earliest stages of the disease, is clearly the sweat follicles. The vesicles result from distension of these follicles by sweat, which on examination is not found to bear any resemblance to the fluid exuded in inflammation, nor does it contain pus or give place to crusts. The bullae are formed by the coalescence of vesicles; the papulae, by the abortion of vesicles; the white patches of uplifted cuticle, by the maceration of the latter by sweat which becomes, from the access of air, acrid and sour.

Now, at first sight, this disease looks like an acute eczema, but it is not so, though the acrid sweat may so far irritate as to excite an eczema. Do not forget this. You will have observed that this disease does not begin as a serous catarrh of the papillary layer, as does eczema, but by distension of the sweat follicles. When there is no sero-purulent discharge about it, the fluid in the vesicles remains quite clear so long as it is confined, and during the whole course of the disease there is no crusting. It is altogether unlike eczema with its sero-purulent discharge, stiffening linen and drying into thin yellow crusts.

The disease may look like erythema papulatum, but only insofar as there are abortive vesicles present, and these clearly do not constitute the chief feature.

The disease varies greatly in extent and duration. It may happen that one or several successive outbursts of the eruption occur, and the disease may last a week or 10 days, or several weeks if there are successive outbursts. The case which I have described is a very marked one. In some cases we have a few little flattened itchy vesicles about the sides of the fingers, succeeded by a drying up of their contents and a mere peeling off of the cuticle. In some cases the feet are affected, and then we have between the toes, especially at the junction of the toes with the foot, small white patches produced by uplifting and maceration of the cuticle by acrid sweat. These cases are confounded with and always called eczema. There is often-times a great deal of very troublesome itching, especially at night, and patients complain of it bitterly, as it is

* Brit. Med. J., *2*:365, 1873.

excessively annoying and disturbs them from getting a fair night's rest. In other cases we have the whole foot affected, in others coincidently the hands and feet or the face and arms. I have noticed in gouty subjects that the disease is intensified in severity, I suppose on account of the irritable character of the blood.

The disease, gentlemen, is not described in books since it is always regarded as eczema, but I have explained to you that it is wholly unlike eczema. The resemblance is accounted for by the fact that in both diseases there are vesicles which are crowded together, but the character of the fluid uplifting the cuticle and its subsequent behavior, the source of this fluid, the anatomical seat of the disease, are wholly and entirely different.

James Paget

Paget's Disease

SIR JAMES PAGET was born at Yarmouth on January 11, 1814, son of a prosperous shipowner and merchant, and one of 17 children. As a boy he was intensely interested in botany and entomology, and after completing his preliminary education at a day-school in his native city, he was apprenticed to a local physician, Mr. Charles Costerton. Having completed his apprenticeship in 1834, he came up to London, and entered St. Bartholomew's Hospital. Paget was one of the most brilliant students St. Bart's has ever known. There is hardly a student honor he did not carry off easily. He made his well known discovery of the Trichina parasite in his first year of training. He was graduated in 1836.

After a short period of study in France, he returned to England, became curator of St. Bartholomew's Hospital Museum, and acquired such great facility in pathology that he was appointed a lecturer in the subject at the request of the students. He later became a lecturer in the expanding science of physiology. As an assistant surgeon to the Hospital (in 1847), he gave a series of lectures for the College of Surgeons. These were so successful in correlating the newer concepts of pathology and physiology with anatomy, that they firmly established Paget as the most promising young man in English medicine. From there on, his rise to the top of English surgery, indeed, to the position as "first surgeon of his day" was assured.

The energy Paget exhibited in his multitudinous activities was boundless. In addition to carrying on one of the heaviest, and most remunerative practices in the land, he found time for much teaching and organizational work, and opportunity to write many communications on all aspects of surgery, both technical and clinical. One may mention his works on osteitis deformans, tuberculosis in the aged, the sequellae of typhoid fever, peripheral nerve injuries, as the most outstanding, as well as his description of the disease which bears his name, given below.

Paget was warm hearted and sensitive, brief and direct in his manner. He had few enemies. He disliked sports, played whist well, knew a great deal about music, and enjoyed hiking. His last years were spent peaceably, death coming on December 30, 1899.*

PAGET'S DISEASE

On Diseases of the Mammary Areola Preceding Cancer of the Mammary Gland[†]

I believe it has not yet been published that certain chronic affections of the skin of the nipple and areola are very often succeeded by the formation of scirrhous cancer in the mammary gland. I have seen about 15

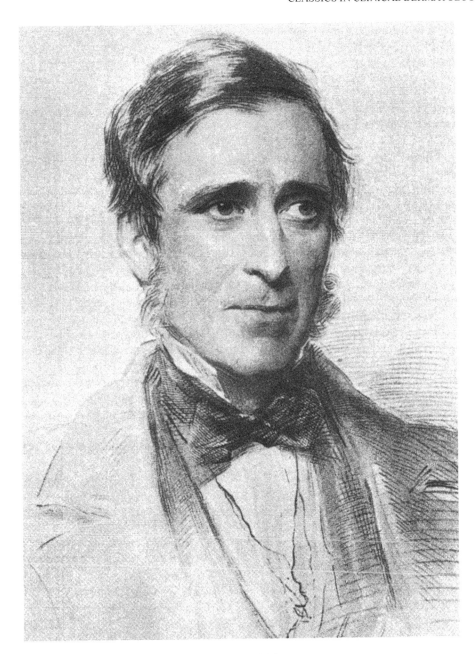

Figure 32 James Paget. Courtesy, College of Physicians, Philadelphia

cases in which this has happened, and the events were in all of them so similar that one description may suffice.

The patients were all women, various in age from 40 to 60 or more years, having in common nothing remarkable but their disease. In all of them the disease began as an eruption on the nipple and areola. In the majority it had the appearance of a florid intensely red, raw surface, very finely granular, as if nearly the whole thickness of the epidermis were removed; like the surface of very acute diffuse eczema, or like that of an acute balanitis. From such a surface, on the whole or greater part of the nipple and areola, there was always copious, clear, yellowish, viscid exudation. The sensations were commonly tingling, itching, and burning, but the malady was never attended by disturbance of the general health. I have not seen this form of eruption extend beyond the areola, and only once have seen it pass into a deeper ulceration of the skin after the manner of a rodent ulcer.

In some of the cases the eruption has presented the characters of an ordinary chronic eczema, with minute vesications, succeeded by soft, moist, yellowish scabs or scales, and constant viscid exudation. In some it has been like psoriasis, dry, with a few white scales slowly desquamating, and in both these forms, especially in the psoriasis, I have seen the eruption spreading far beyond the areola in widening circles, or, with scattered blotches of redness, covering nearly the whole breast.

I am not aware that in any of the cases which I have seen the eruption was different from what may be described as long persistent eczema, or psoriasis, or by some other name, in treatises on diseases of the skin; and I believe that such cases sometimes occur on the breast, and after many months' duration are cured, or pass by, and are not followed by any other disease. But it has happened that in every case which I have been able to watch cancer of the mammary gland has followed within at the most two years, and usually within one year. The eruption has resisted all the treatment, both local and general, that has been used, and has continued even after the affected part of the skin has been involved in the cancerous disease.

The formation of cancer has not in any case taken place first in the diseased part of the skin. It has always been in the substance of the mammary gland, beneath or not far from the diseased skin, and always with a clear interval of apparently healthy tissue.

In the cancers themselves, I have seen in these cases nothing peculiar. They have been various in form; some acute, some chronic, the majority following an average course, and all tending to the same end; recurring if removed, affecting lymph-glands and distant parts, showing nothing which might not be written in the ordinary history of cancer of the breast.

The single noteworthy fact found in all these cases is that which I have stated in the first sentence, and I think it deserves careful study.

* Marsh, H.: St. Bart. Hosp. Reports, *36:*1, 1900.
† St. Bart. Hosp. Reports, *10:*87, 1874.

PART III

THE GOLDEN AGE

Louis Duhring

1. *Prurigo Hiemalis*

2. *Dermatitis Herpetiformis*

LOUIS ADOLPHUS DUHRING was born in Philadelphia, December 23, 1845. His family was prominent and well-to-do. As a boy he was studious, an avid reader. After an elementary education in private Philadelphia schools, and undergraduate work at the University of Pennsylvania, he entered the medical school of this university and was graduated in 1867, submitting a thesis entitled *Nervous Gout*. During his residency at the Philadelphia Hospital (Blockley) his interest in cutaneous medicine first became manifest, aroused in the beginning by a case of painful neuroma of the skin occurring in an old man under his care. On completion of his residency he traveled to Europe for special training in dermatology in which there was then little interest in this country. He spent the next two years studying European methods with the enthusiasm and intense concentration that marked every undertaking of his life. Berlin, Paris, and London in their turn came under his scrutiny, but it was in Vienna that he spent his most profitable months. Even the master of masters, Hebra, was impressed with his brilliant work. He also studied oriental skin diseases in Constantinople and leprosy in Norway. In 1871 he was appointed Lecturer on diseases of the skin at the University of Pennsylvania, Clinical Professor of Dermatology in 1876, and full Professor in 1890. He remained directly associated with the school until his retirement in 1910.

Duhring's worth cannot be calculated in terms of any single contribution to cutaneous medicine. More than any other man he was responsible for the establishment of dermatology as a respected specialty in this country and maintaining in its formative years the highest of standards. Yet the acme of his work is clearly his famous series of papers on dermatitis herpetiformis, one of which is presented here. His *Atlas of Skin Diseases* (1876) and *Practical Treatise on Skin Diseases* (1877) were his two most extensive completed works, and the latter did much to spread his fame in Europe as well as at home. He began a tremendous encyclopedic work entitled *Cutaneous Medicine* and completed the first two parts in 1895 and 1898, but a fire destroyed all the accumulated material for the third part, so disheartening to the author that he was never able to complete the task.

Duhring's philanthropy, for he became rich, did much toward furthering the greatness of the University of Pennsylvania and expanding the magnificent library of the College of Physicians in Philadelphia.

Although fond of social functions, cheerful, and light-hearted early in life, he later became reserved and serious so that Arthur Van Harlingen, one of his very closest friends, said, "In after years I cannot recall any occasion when I have seen his smile or heard him laugh. His absorption in his work was absolute and complete." It has been suggested that the untimely death of a young lady precipitated this change.

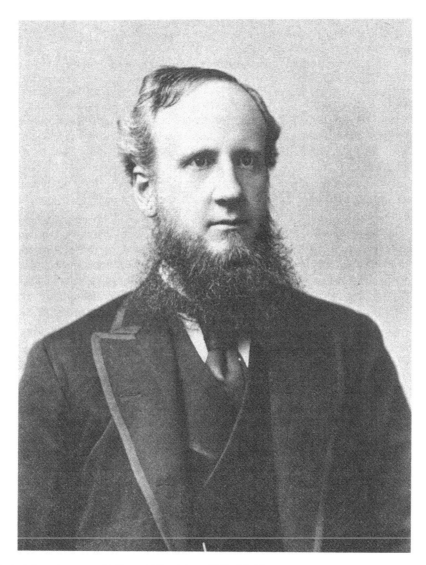

Figure 33 Louis Duhring. Courtesy, College of Physicians, Philadelphia

Duhring was plagued with illnesses vague in nature throughout his life. Symptoms of cardiac irritability and ill-defined abdominal uneasiness predominated. A nervous breakdown in 1885 nearly terminated his career. He died May 8, 1913 directly or indirectly from a constricting band over the ileum.*

PRURIGO HIEMALIS

Pruritus hiemalis—an Undescribed Form of Pruritus[†]

The affection consists in a peculiar state of irritability of the skin, which manifests itself in the autumn or even as late as the winter season. Generally it first makes its appearance with the advent of our cool October weather, or at about the time of frost. It may, however, not be noticed until later in the season— as late as December. In Philadelphia it commonly occurs towards the latter part of October, and continues usually until the cold weather has been thoroughly established, or even through the winter. Its duration is variable. In some cases it lasts but for a few days or weeks, and then disappears entirely. In other instances it remains present persistently for several months or longer; but it is never present after the cold weather has passed. With spring it always vanishes, to be absent at least until the succeeding autumn. It is rare, however, to observe it continuing in any marked degree through the entire winter. It is an affection of the cool weather only, and more particularly of the fall and winter season. It is never present in the summer months. It is found upon individuals of all ages, from childhood to old age. No particular period of life appears to be more susceptible than another. I have never met with it in young children, nor indeed much before the age of puberty. It occurs in both sexes in about the same proportion. It may exist upon any part of the body, though prone to attack certain regions in an almost invariable manner. It is confined, not entirely, but to a great extent, to the lower extremities, and it is here that it shows itself typically. It occasionally is found upon the arms, and more rarely upon the trunk, but never to the same extent and degree as upon the thighs, buttocks, and legs. The hands, feet, face, and scalp are never involved. Its common seat is upon the inner surface of the thighs, about the knees, in the popliteal space, upon the calves of the legs, and around the ankles. It affects the non-hairy portions of the limbs rather than the hairy parts. The outer surface of the thigh and the region of the tibia are more rarely involved than, for example, the calf of the leg. The calves of the legs are favorite localities for the trouble. It attacks both lower extremities symmetrically. Occasionally only the ankles and calves are affected, but in most cases it extends well up upon the thigh. It is not a localized affection, — that is, cannot be said to exist upon any given portion of the body exclusively. The sensation may be most intense here or there, as the case may be, or it may move from time to time from one locality to another. But the same regions are usually attacked day after day, and the symptoms remain there until they disappear entirely; and hence, although it cannot be said to be localized, yet, if present at all, it is almost invariably to be found upon the regions which I have particularized.

The affection may be said to be characterized by a certain itching of the skin, more especially of the lower extremities, which comes upon the individual rather suddenly, in the course of a few days, during the autumn or early winter, and which may be described as an itching, smarting, tingling, burning sensation, as though a person were clothed in new flannel or woolen-wear, and the same were rubbing and chafing the skin. The amount of irritation present varies with different cases, and may be either very slight, so as barely to attract attention, or it may be so severe and troublesome as to cause the sufferer very great annoyance and distress. It possesses one peculiarity which is striking, and generally present,—namely, the tendency to become aggravated towards night. It is always worse in the evening than at any other period in the 24 hours, and in many cases is present only at this time. In the mild form it is scarcely noticeable during the day, coming on with evening, and continuing through the night until sooner or later the patient retires and falls

---

* Parish, L.C.: Louis A.Duhring, M.D., Pathfinder for Dermatology. Charles C.Thomas, 1967.

[†] Phila. Med. Times, 4:225, 1874.

asleep. It is when taking off the clothes, at night especially, that the itching is most noticeable and severe. At this time the desire to scratch and rub the affected parts is almost irresistible, and the person usually gratifies this desire either until some relief is obtained or sleep terminates the suffering. A certain amount of relief follows severe scratching, and a marked burning sensation takes the place of itching, which is far more grateful to the feelings of the patient. According to the amount of disturbance and the irritability of the cutaneous nerves, will the sleep be more or less interfered with. At times the skin is so excited and disturbed that the person obtains but imperfect rest, and at least the earlier part of the night is passed in scratching and in making cooling applications of one kind or another to the parts. In other cases the itching is simply unpleasant and annoying upon retiring, but not sufficiently so to interfere with sleep.

Upon awaking in the morning, a little of the pruritus may still exist, but usually it has quite subsided, and no further thought is given the subject until the following evening, when the same symptoms reappear, and are exactly repeated. In this manner it continues day after day, with but slight intermission, until, at the end of an indefinite period, it gradually vanishes. The patient now remains free of it until the next autumn, when in all probability it will recur and run a similar course. It may relapse in this way year after year, or at the end of the first attack it may disappear, not to return. It is apt, however, to attack the same individual several seasons in succession, and then remain away permanently. It may also continue through a lifetime.

There is no *primary* eruption of any kind connected with the affection, either at its commencement or at any time during its course. This is an important point to be remembered in connection with the diagnosis. If the skin be minutely and carefully examined at the beginning of an attack, we see nothing indicative of a disease, or anything, indeed, which would enable one to account for the itching present. Inasmuch as the condition is always most marked and typical about the lower extremities, I shall describe the appearance of the skin as seen in a well-defined case the first day of its existence, for later the appearances are quite different, and call for a separate description. When the trouble is first noticed, then, the skin looks quite healthy, with the exception that it is apt to be somewhat dry. The epidermis seems normal, and there is no desquamation. The skin is neither hot nor hyperaemic. The hair-follicles are neither inflamed nor obstructed, and appear to be in order. There is no accumulation of epidermis or other matter about their openings. They are not prominent nor visibly altered. In fact, after close inspection, it is impossible to distinguish any sign of derangement in connection with the follicles, which parts, upon first thought, we might imagine to be the seat of the disorder. Here and there an inflamed follicle may exist, but this condition, however, occurs only occasionally at this stage of the trouble.

The condition of the sudoriferous glands it is difficult to determine, further than that they do not work very actively; but there is no reason for supposing that they are in any serious way deranged, or more so upon these localities than upon other portions of the body. There is no perceptible functional derangement of the skin. Neither is there any organic alteration observable. The subjective symptoms, which the patient communicates, alone convey any idea of the condition.

But if the case be seen several days or longer after the first symptoms, the skin looks different. Certain secondary changes now exist which, if error is to be avoided, must be viewed as such. For to regard these *secondary* lesions, which at this stage are present, as the *primary* lesions of the affection, would certainly be misleading as to the nature of the disorder. It must be remembered, too, that this stage is the one in which cases are usually seen, for advice from the physician is rarely sought before the trouble has existed for some time.

The skin now may be rough and harsh, resembling xeroderma or mild ichthyosis. Many of the hair-follicles are red and more or less inflamed and irritated, with an accumulation of epidermis and sebaceous matter about their openings. Many of the hairs are also torn and broken off short, close to their follicles. Here and there, or over a considerable surface, the whole skin looks red and irritated, as though it had been well rubbed and scratched. Upon close inspection, the epidermis bears unmistakable evidence of having been torn and wounded. The marks of the finger-nails are everywhere to be seen, often in the form of long streaks up and down the limbs. In fact, all the phenomena just detailed, which are so marked and prominent, are produced solely by the hands of the patient. They are all *secondary* lesions. They are the *results* of the pruritus. To view them as the primary lesions would give a very wrong idea concerning the nature of the trouble. The line of distinction between the primary lesions and the secondary symptoms must be clearly drawn. The primary symptoms are subjective alone. The secondary symptoms, those usually seen clinically, are both subjective and objective, the latter being an artificial product, caused by external irritants.

Such is a description of the disorder as I have encountered it through a number of seasons, and which it has been my pleasure to study and note as opportunity for observation upon new cases offered.

DERMATITIS HERPETIFORMIS

Dermatitis herpetiformis*

Under the name "Dermatitis Herpetiformis" I propose to place a number of cases of skin disease that I have encountered from time to time. These cases present are for the most part nameless, having been regarded and diagnosed either as peculiar manifestations of one or another of the commoner and well-known diseases, as eczema, herpes, or pemphigus, or in some cases as undescribed diseases.

That such a protean disease as I have intimated exists, and that these varied cutaneous manifestations are all but forms of one pathological process, there can be no doubt, and I shall elucidate this point by describing the several important varieties, which as in the case of eczema are based upon the predominance of certain lesions. Before doing this, however, I may refer to certain symptoms common to all forms of the disease, to which no particular allusion has as yet been made. In severe cases prodromata are usually present for several days preceding the cutaneous outbreak, consisting of malaise, constipation, febrile disturbance, chilliness, heat, or alternate hot and cold sensations. Itching is also generally present for several days before any sign of efflorescence. Even in mild cases slight systemic disorder may precede or exist with the outbreak. This latter may be gradual or sudden in its advent or development. Not infrequently it is sudden, one or another manifestation breaking out over the greater part of the general surface diffusely or in patches in the course of a few days, accompanied by severe itching or burning.

A single variety, as for example the erythematous or the vesicular, may appear, or several forms of lesions may exist simultaneously, constituting what may very properly be designated the multiform variety. The tendency is, in almost every instance, that I have observed, to multiformity. There is, moreover, in almost every case a distinct disposition for one variety, sooner or later, to pass into some other variety, thus for the vesicular or pustular to become bullous, or *vice versa*. This change of type may take place during the course of one attack or on the occasion of a relapse, or as is often the case, it may not show itself until months or years afterwards. I have notes of several cases where, during a period of from two to five years, the erythematous, vesicular and bullous varieties were all in turn manifested. Permit me, however, to state again that not only multiformity of lesion, but irregularity in the order of development, is the rule, whether during attack or later in the course of the disease.

---

* J.A.M.A., *3*:225, 1884.

Itching, burning or pricking sensations almost always exist. When the eruption is profuse they are intense, and cause the greatest suffering. As in the case of eczema, before and with each outbreak they become most violent, abating in a measure only with the laceration or rupture of the lesions.

The disease is rare, but is of more frequent occurrence than I formerly supposed. I have encountered 15 cases during a period of as many years, drawn from hospital, dispensary and private practice. All, with one exception, were adults, including both sexes in about equal proportion. The natural history is interesting. The process is in almost all instances chronic, and is characterized by more or less distinctly marked exacerbations or relapses, occurring at intervals of weeks or months. The disposition to appear in successive crops, sometimes slight, at other times severe, is peculiar. Relapses are the rule, the disease in most cases extending over years, pursuing an obstinate emphatically chronic course. All regions are liable to invasion, including both flexor and extensor surfaces, the face and scalp, elbows and knees, and palms and soles. Excoriations and pigmentation, diffuse and in localized areas, are in old cases always at hand in a marked degree. The pigmentation is usually of a mottled, dirty yellowish or brownish hue, and is persistent. I have seen it as pronounced as in chronic pediculosis corporis.

The more important forms of the disease may now be considered:

Dermatitis Herpetiformis (Erythematosa). The erythematous variety manifests itself in patches or as a diffuse efflorescence, as an erythema or superficial inflammation, usually of an urticarial or erythema multiforme-like type. The urticarial element may be marked, the skin showing a disposition to acute oedematous infiltration in a diffuse form. Urticarial complication, rather than urticaria, is suggested by the condition of the skin; in like manner, a resemblance to diffuse erythema multiforme may be noted. At times the patches, whether discrete or confluent, are circumscribed, and later by their coalition show irregularly shaped, marginate outlines, as in erythema multiforme. The colour varies with the shape, being at first bright red, but soon becoming deep red or violaceous, mottled, and tinged with yellowish hues. The variegation is usually pronounced in the later stages of the process, at which period more or less diffuse pigmentation is also present. Together with the erythematous inflammation there may form maculo-papules or circumscribed or diffuse flat infiltrations, variable as to size and shape; also vesico-papules, the process now bearing a resemblance to the first stage of herpes iris. It will thus be noted that the eruption, in its general aspect and course, is much like that of erythema multiforme. In severe cases the outbreak is preceded by and accompanied with malaise, chilliness, or slight febrile disturbance. The itching is generally violent, the disease differing in this respect from erythema multiforme.

Its course is variable. It may continue for days or weeks, or as is usually the case it may pass into the multiform variety, to be described later. It may be the first manifestation, or it may follow other varieties as a relapse.

As a variety it is not as clearly defined as the vesicular, bullous, or pustular, in some cases appearing to be but the first manifestation of one of the first-mentioned forms. But it is important that its features be described, for the reason that it is liable to be met with as a clinical picture, and may readily be confounded with other diseases, notably urticaria, erythema multiforme and eczema. I recall two cases where the diagnosis was at first difficult, and it was not until other manifestations appeared on the skin that the true nature of the process became evident.

Dermatitis Herpetiformis (Vesiculosa). The vesicular variety is that most frequently met with. It is characterized by variously sized, varying from a pinhead to a pea, flat or raised, irregularly shaped or stellate, glistening, pale yellowish or pearly, usually firm or tensely distended vesicles, as a rule unaccompanied by areolae. In their early stages they can be seen only with difficulty, and are liable to be overlooked in the examination. Sometimes they can only be detected or seen to advantage in an oblique light. This observation I have repeatedly noted, and it arises from the fact of the lesions being flat, translucent and without areolae. In size they vary extremely, large and small being formed side by side, and in this respect they differ from the vesicles of eczema. Here and there papules, papulo-vesicles, vesico-pustules, and small blebs will sometimes be encountered. Concerning their distribution, the eruption as a whole is disseminate, the lesions existing scattered more or less profusely over a given region, as for example the neck or the back, but they are for the most part aggregated in the form of small clusters or groups of two, three, or more, or there may be patches here and there as large as a silver dollar, upon which a number will be seated. When in close proximity they tend to coalesce, as in herpes zoster, forming multilocular vesicles or small blebs. When this occurs they are generally slightly raised, and are surrounded with a pale or distinctly reddish areola, which shows forth the irregular, angular, or stellate outline of the lesion. At this stage, moreover, the little cluster will generally present a "puckered" or "drawn up" appearance, indicative of its herpetic nature.

The eruption is usually profuse, sometimes to the extent of the upper extremities, and thighs, all being especially liable to invasion.

The most striking symptom is the itching. Not infrequently burning is also complained of. Itching, however, predominates and is in all cases violent or even intense. Patients state that it is altogether disproportionately in excess of the amount of eruption. It is, moreover, a persistent itching, causing the sufferer to scratch constantly. It generally precedes the outbreak, and does not abate until the lesions have been ruptured. Old sufferers familiar with the natural course of the process have informed me that they can obtain no relief until the lesions have been ruptured. From my observation I should say that the itching was both more severe and more lasting than in vesicular eczema. The vesicles made their appearance slowly, so that several days or a week may be required for their complete development. Notwithstanding that scratching is indulged in in the early stages of the disease, excoriations are not prominent, owing to the fact that the walls of the vesicles are tough and do not rupture, and that they incline to refill immediately on being evacuated.

The diagnosis in some cases is attended with difficulty on account of the resemblance to vesicular eczema. I recall the embarrassment experienced in the classification of the earlier cases encountered, and the provisional diagnoses of "vesicular eczema?" made at the time. But the irregularity in the size and form of the vesicles, their angular or stellate outline, their firm tense walls, with no disposition to rupture, and their herpetic character will all serve to aid in the diagnosis. In some cases the constitutional disturbance and the magnitude of the eruption, as regards profusion, distribution and multiformity, showing a more formidable disease than eczema, will also be striking. The itching and burning will usually be found to be more continuous and intenser than in eczema. The obstinacy of the disease to the ordinary treatment of eczema, moreover, must also soon become apparent, the usual milder remedies so frequently of service in acute vesicular eczema being of little or no benefit in this disease. Finally, the tendency to repeated relapses and the chronicity of the affection must strike the observer as peculiar. This variety cannot be confounded with herpes zoster, herpes iris, or pemphigus. Its relations to the "herpes gestations" of some authors will not be considered in this paper, further than to state that in my opinion they are probably one and the same disease. On a future occasion I shall deal more at length with this point.

Dermatitis Herpetiformis (Bullosa). In the bullous variety the lesions are more or less typical blebs, tense or flaccid, rounded or flat, usually the former, filled with a serious or cloudy fluid, seated upon a non-inflammatory or slightly inflamed base. In size they vary from a pea to a cherry or walnut, and are for the most part irregular or angular in outline. They incline to group in clusters of two or three, the skin between them in this event being reddish and puckered. Sometimes in immediate proximity—almost contiguous—will exist one, two, or three or a part of a circle of small pinhead sized, flat whitish pustules. Vesicles of all sizes, flat or raised, are also generally found nearby, or disseminated over the affected surface. As in the other varieties, all regions may be attacked, especially the trunk, upper extremities, and thighs. In several cases I have seen the greater part of the general surface invaded most profusely in which event the lesions are usually smaller than where comparatively few exist. They incline to appear in crops at irregular intervals, as in the other varieties. The lesions are generally ruptured in the course of a few days, and then crust over with a yellowish, greenish, or brownish crust. They are accompanied by burning and itching which may be very severe. They bear resemblance to those of pemphigus vulgaris, with which of course they may be readily confounded, but they are more herpetic in character. They differ in that they incline to group, and have a more inflammatory herpetic aspect, the type of which picture is seen in herpes zoster. Moreover around and near the bleb will usually be found vesicles and pustules, the latter often in close proximity, the whole manifestation being quite different from that of pemphigus.

Dermatitis Herpetiformis (Pustulosa). The pustular variety is generally less clearly defined than the vesicular, because the lesions are often intermingled with vesicles, vesico-pustules, and blebs. In typical cases the pustules are acuminate, rounded or flat, tense or flaccid, usually the former, and vary in size from a pinpoint to a pea or silver quarter-dollar. Vesicles and blebs in some cases precede the pustules. The smallest lesions are generally flat, or on a level with the surrounding skin, and as stated are frequently not larger than a pinpoint or pinhead. Larger pustules, the size of a pea, are generally rounded or acuminate, and are surrounded by a reddish inflammatory areola. Later they incline to flatten, and to increase in size by spreading peripherally, and drying in the centre.

Sometimes they are seated on a slightly raised base. When fully matured they generally present an "angry appearance," the skin immediately around them having a "puckered" look, from the fact that the pustule itself is irregular in outline, as sometimes is the case in herpes zoster.

They incline to form in groups of two, three, or more, and moreover often appear in patches of two or more groups. Such an arrangement is generally met with on the trunk. The grouping is further peculiar in that a central pustule will often be immediately surrounded by a variable number of smaller pustules, sometimes in a circinate form, as in herpes iris.

In other localities, however, no such peculiarity occurs, the lesions being discrete, and even disseminate. The pustules are usually opaque, and of a whitish colour; sometimes they are yellowish, though they are seldom so yellow as in pustular eczema. Not infrequently, slight hemorrhagic exudation occurs, as in the later stages of herpes zoster, giving them a reddish, bluish, or brownish hue. They are generally accompanied by sensations of heat, pricking or itching. In some cases, these symptoms precede for several days the eruption. They pursue a slow course, from one to two weeks being usually necessary for their full development. In other cases their maturation occurs more rapidly. In some cases, together with the pustules are found vesicles and blebs of various shapes and sizes, and these often form immediately by the side of, or in close proximity to, the pustule. Papules and papulovesicles may also be present. In a given area, say of a few square inches—as for example upon the abdomen—there may exist all of these lesions in various stages of evolution. This multiformity is striking, and presents a curious and peculiar mixture of lesions. The attacks last from two to four weeks, after which there generally follows a comparative respite of from one to six weeks. The disease may thus be kept up indefinitely, the outbreaks being at one time slight, at another time severe.

Sometimes it has preceded other varieties. In other cases it has followed the bullous variety, while in some instances that have been under observation for a long period it has at intervals of months alternated between the vesicular and bullous varieties. After what has previously been said, it need scarcely be stated that this variety is identical with the "impetigo herpetiformis" of Hebra, although in but few of the cases observed by me have the symptoms been so pronounced as in Hebra's experience, if I may judge from the portraits in his *Atlas of Skin Diseases*. The account given by me relates to the disease as I have encountered it. Hebra's account has already been given, and need not be repeated here. The difference of experience concerns chiefly the severity of the process. Thus in none of my cases has it proved fatal, while it will be remembered that four out of five of Hebra's cases died, and according to Kaposi (Hebra's successor) 10 out of 11 cases observed by him have perished. Finally I have observed it to occur about as often in men as in women, and also in the latter, apart from pregnancy. Hebra, on the other hand, met with it only in women, and moreover only in the parturient state.

Concerning the constitutional symptoms, they may be stated to vary with the gravity of the attack. Usually, however, they are more marked than in the other varieties, rigors and alternate paroxysms of heat and cold being especially noticeable. It is the most serious phase of the disease.

Dermatitis Herpetiformis (Papulosa). The papular variety is in my experience rarer than any other form. I have met with only two cases, one in an adult, the other in a boy, and in both of these the eruption was scanty. It is characterized by the formation of small or large pea-sized, irregularly-shaped, usually firm, reddish or violaceous papular lesions, occurring for the most part in groups of two or three, scattered here and there over the affected surface. They are of variable size, large and small ones not infrequently existing side by side, and are as a rule ill-defined, being neither acuminate nor flat, but resemble the papular infiltrations sometimes met with in abortive herpes zoster. They are of an acute or subacute inflammatory type, and as stated bear resemblance to abortive herpetic lesions, and also to certain phases of chronic relapsing papular eczema. Their surfaces are generally excoriated from scratching, and may be covered with blood crusts, or with slight, adherent, thin epidermis scales.

The itching is severe, so much that comparatively few lesions may so torment the patients as to interfere with the night's rest.

Ill-defined papulovesicles are also met with here and there, as in the case sometimes of papular eczema. The lesions pursue a slow, chronic course, lasting from one to two or four weeks, when they gradually disappear, leaving more or less pigmentation. Relapses are the rule at longer or shorter intervals.

As I have intimated, this variety bears a close resemblance to chronic papular eczema, and the earlier cases encountered by me were so diagnosed; but, the irregularity in the size and form of the lesions, the disposition to group, the usually slow evolution of the lesions, the tendency to appear in crops at irregular intervals, the chronicity of the process, and the extreme obstinacy to local and internal treatment are all peculiar. It is the mildest phase of the disease.

Dermatitis Herpetiformis (Multiformis). This may be regarded in the light of clinical variety, one that is eminently useful from a practical standpoint. It is a variety of the disease in the same sense that eczema rubrum is a variety of eczema. It is important to consider it for the reason that it is a picture which may at any time show itself in the course of the disease. It is a phase not infrequently met with, and on account of the great mixture of lesions, and the difficulties presented in diagnosis, is worthy of special description. The multiform variety consist of erythematous, sometimes slightly raised, urticarial patches of variable size and outline, often confluent, of a reddish or violaceous, yellowish, dusky, sometimes variegated colour, not unlike that of erythema multiforme. In addition there often exist more or less well-defined, irregularly-shaped or rounded maculo-papules and flat infiltrations, papules and vesico-papules, all in various stages of evolution. Small blebs and pustules, pinpoint sized or larger, may also be present, though with the vesicular element predominating it is not usual to meet blebs or pustules of large size nor in numbers. As the disease is in an early or late stage of its existence will pigmentation and excoriations be slight or marked. Briefly, then, to recapitulate, there exists a mixture of lesions, with no single type predominating, calling to mind in its behaviour eczema, although it is far more capricious and protean. It must also be remembered that the process may at any period change its type, such an occurrence usually taking place with an exacerbation or a relapse. Thus the vesicular variety may exist for a variable period, to be followed in a few weeks or months by an attack of blebs, or it may be pustules, or by a mixture of blebs and pustules. This mingling of several varieties is a marked and peculiar feature of the disease, giving a very striking, dermatological picture, different from that seen in any other disease of the skin.

In conclusion, permit me to summarize by saying that I have endeavored to show:

1. The existence of a distinct, well-defined, rare, serious, inflammatory disease of the skin, manifestly of an herpetic nature, characterized by systemic disturbance, a great variety of primary lesions, by severe itching and burning, and by a disposition to appear in repeated successive outbreaks.
2. That the disease is capable of exhibiting itself in many forms, all having a tendency to run into or to succeed one another irregularly in the natural course of the process.
3. The principal varieties are the erythematous, papular, vesicular, bullous, and pustular, which may occur singly or in various combinations.
4. That it is a remarkably protean disease.
5. That the pustular variety is the same manifestation as the disease described by Hebra under the name "impetigo herpetiformis," this being the only form hitherto described.
6. That the several other and equally important forms are worthy of special remark.
7. That the term "dermatitis herpetiformis" is sufficiently comprehensive and appropriate to include all varieties of the process.
8. That it may occur in both sexes, and in women independent of pregnancy.
9. That it usually pursues a chronic, variable course, often lasting years, and is exceedingly rebellious to treatment.

Isidor Neumann

Pemphigus Vegetans

ISIDOR VON NEUMANN was born March 2, 1832, in Moravia (Czechoslovakia), the country of Hebra and Auspitz. He took his M.D. in Vienna in 1858. After training under Dittel and Türck, he became an assistant to Hebra, and in 1862 a Privatdozent. His rise in the academic circles in Vienna was steady, and in 1881 he succeeded von Sigmund to the Vorstand of the University Syphilis clinic, which post he held until his death in 1906.

In the tradition of the Vienna school, Neumann's greatest achievements lay in the field of clinical medicine. Besides the description of pemphigus vegetans (Neumann's disease) which is given below, he made important contributions to the study of lichen planus, bromoderma, verruca senilis, and the idiopathic atrophies of the skin. An expert microscopist, he was one of the first to correlate clinical disease with histologic change, particularly in connection with senile degeneration of the skin, and argyria. He made notable investigations on the lymph vessels of the skin. Neumann had to his credit a successful dermatologic text and atlas, but his truly monumental work was his treatise on syphilis, which entitles him to his place with Fournier as the master syphilologist.

Neumann worked constantly for the acceptance of dermatology as a specialty apart, and the chair in the specialty was established in Vienna largely through his efforts.*

PEMPHIGUS VEGETANS

Beitrag zur Kenntnis des Pemphigus*

It is certainly the desire of every author to be able to cite a goodly number of cases as the basis for his observations. It is also his duty, however, to record rare occurrences, particularly when neither his own nor other's experience provides similar material. One should consider the following communication from this point of view; it presents both in the clinical picture and microscopic findings something new.

At the end of January, 1875, I was consulted by Kinderarzt Herrn Docenten und Director Dr. Pollitzer concerning the skin disease of a certain Frau B. who was under his care.

The history was that the patient had been hitherto well, had borne two children, the youngest of which was two years old at the time; menses were regular. The skin complaint had been present since the end of May,

---

* Rille, J.: Deutsch. Med. Wchnschr., *32:*2119, 1906.

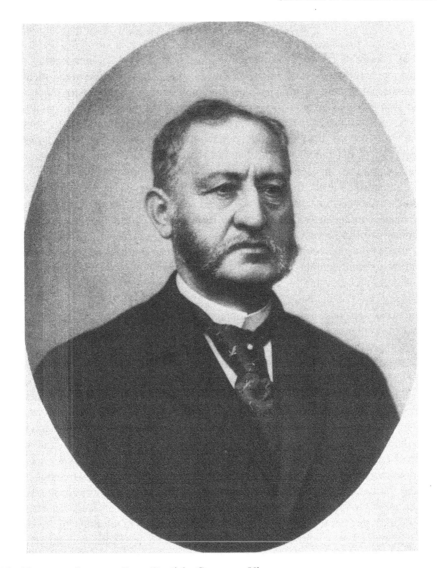

Figure 34 Isidor Neumann. Courtesy, Franz Deuticke Company, Vienna

1874; moreover, it had developed first as blisters which remained discrete on the skin of the right axillary fossa, and from which the epidermis was quickly lost. The bases of these did not heal over, despite the application of ointments and treatment with Lapis; the appearance of the eruption was preceded for a few days by mild anginal difficulties.

Present status. I found the patient well developed and well nourished. She complained only that the lesion kept her from going out, and that she experienced slight pain on swallowing.

On the skin of the right axilla there was an area larger than a thaler, dark red in color, denuded of epidermis, the eroded and uneven surface of which was somewhat raised above the level of the surrounding skin. It appeared traversed by furrows, and secreted a thin serous fluid.

Since outside of a slight swelling of the tonsils, on which discrete scattered points similar to aphthae were noted, no other symptoms presented themselves, the diagnosis was left in *suspenso,* and we prescribed only a mild solution of potash (0.2:150). However, even in the first week of observation the excrescences increased at such a rate that they extended almost 2 cm. Despite painting with Solutio Plenkii, and intensive treatment with caustic potash, the excrescences became more and more prominent. Soon the epithelium of the lower lip too was elevated in the form of flat bullae, the contents of which quickly dried up; after removal of the crust one could see a raw area covered over by a tough white layer. The number of lesions on the mucous membranes of the lips, the mouth, and throat increased to such an extent that taking of nourishment became difficult; almost nothing but fluids could be taken; the temperature of the skin was normal, the bowels regular, the menses somewhat scanty, the urine free of albumen.

On the 8th of February I noticed, for the first time, a walnut-sized, very tense blister filled with serous fluid on the right arm a short distance from the axilla, and around it four lentil-sized bullae of the same type. The bullae broke open spontaneously on the next day leaving on the site a flat, dark red colored excoriation which was circumscribed by the rest of the epidermal covering which was still adherent. After six days there appeared, almost in the center of the excoriated area, lentil-sized, raised, evenly epithelized excrescences, similar to condylomata lata, which increased continually in height and width, while at the periphery the epidermis was elevated by a serous exudate, forming a sinuous border. A week later equally large excrescences appeared on the belly wall, the inguinal folds, as well as the labia majora. The lesions on the mucous membranes kept pace in their development with those on the skin, but there the trouble was much greater, and even after the mildest treatment of these areas which were covered with a diphtheritic layer, marked swelling of the lips occurred, so that only simple greases could be used in these regions.

As it progressed only a few of the older diseased areas on the belly wall and forearm retained the characteristic appearance of central condylomatous excrescenes; the new lesions presented the purest picture of pemphigus vulgaris. On circumscribed erythematous areas bullae developed which through continuous multiplication gradually involved the greater part of the skin surface. These were hemispherical, pea to hazel-nut-sized, with gummy contents. Most of them were located on the chest and belly wall, on the back, discrete in the left axilla, confluent in many places; in the areas in which the epidermis had been lost large raw surfaces were exposed to the air, as in a second degree burn. There was a great deal of pain; the appetite failed completely, and even liquid nourishment caused great pain in the mucous membranes of the mouth when taken through a glass tube. Since the mucous membrane of the nose was also covered with bullae, the patient could breathe only through her mouth. The lips were dry and covered by a diphtheritic membrane, with deep fissures at the angles of the mouth; the mucous membranes of the cheeks, the tongue and the throat were covered over with dry crusts and whitish exudate. There were numerous bullae on the eyelids; the bulbar and palpebral conjunctivae were injected, and secreted a purulent material. Singultus and frequent vomiting began; the urinary output was small. The air in the sickroom took on a penetrating ammoniacal smell which persisted despite ventilation and greatest cleanliness.

With increasing marasmus the patient died on March 30, 1875, after four months of illness.

---

* Wiener Med. Jahrb., 1876, p. 409.

Walter G.Smith

Monilethrix

WALTER GEORGE SMITH was born in Dublin in 1844. He was educated in Trinity College, and took his M.B. degree in 1867. Like most Dublin physicians he did not limit himself to any special branch of medicine, but he took a special interest in dermatology, and was most sought after for his knowledge in this field. His powers of observation are well attested to in his original description of monilethrix which we have included here. He also devoted much time to Materia Medica, and as professor of this subject was one of the first to base his lectures on the newer concepts of physiology and biochemistry, which he followed zealously.

Smith was affectionately called "Wattie" by his students. He had an extreme dislike of pomposity and was sufficiently outspoken in the matter to reduce it to a minimum in meetings he attended. He worked ceaselessly at his many physiological and chemical projects, even commencing the study of the Russian language when past 80 years of age that he might consult the works of Pavlov in the original. In the last year of his life, 1932, works on relativity, and the books of Eddington and Jeans were frequently in his hands.*

MONILETHRIX

A Rare Nodose Condition of the Hair*

Dr. Smith exhibited and described specimens of a remarkable affection of the hair which had lately come under his notice. A healthy girl, aged 19, applied for advice concerning partial loss of hair, which began to fall out about four years ago without any apparent cause. Previously to that time, she had always possessed a good head of hair, reaching down to her shoulders. The hair was uniformly thinned over the whole scalp, and the longest hairs measured about five inches. Upon close inspection, a singular appearance was noted. Nearly all the shorter hairs presented a regular succession of swellings along the shaft, one nodosity corresponding on an average, to one millimetre of length of hair. The eyebrows were thin; but no beaded hairs could be detected either among them or in the eyelashes. The axillary hair was scanty, but normal; and on the pubes one hair was found with three of the characteristic fusiform swellings. The microscopical characters of the affected hairs were very remarkable, and were illustrated by drawings and specimens. There was scarcely a trace of scale-imbrication on the nodules; but it was tolerably well marked in the

* Irish J.Med. Sc., *6:*185, 1932.

contracted portions. Brown pigment was deposited outside the axis in streaks, much more abundantly in the nodes; and thus each hair, viewed by the naked eye, presented the appearance of being checked alternately brown and white. There was no trace of cells in the axis of the nodules. No account of this curious condition had hitherto been published; but Dr. R.Liveing had a similar case under his charge some years, the details of which were given in the paper. Dr. Walter Smith took occasion to point out that these nodose hairs exhibited no evidence of any fungoid elements, and that they could not be confounded either with piedra or with the tricosyphilis of Wilson. From trichorexis nodosa, with which it might be supposed they had affinity, they differed in several particulars. 1. There was little tendency to partial fracture of the cuticle, or brush-like splitting of the cortex. 2. The nodose hairs occurred in multitudes on the scalp. 3. When a hair was broken, the fracture was usually clean, not fibrous, and occurred through a constriction, never through a node. 4. The nodes were opaque, and constituted the darkest parts of the hair. 5. The nodules were very numerous, and succeeded each other in regular order like beads on a necklace.

---

* Brit. Med. J., *2*:291, 1879.

Moritz Kaposi

1. *Dermatitis Papillaris Capillitii (Acne Keloidalis Nuchae)*

2. *Multiple Idiopathic Hemorrhagic Sarcoma*

3. *Xeroderma Pigmentosum*

4. *Kaposi's Varicelliform Eruption*

MORITZ KAPOSI was born Moritz Kohn, October 23, 1837, in Kaposvar, Hungary. He completed his early education at Pressburg, and in 1861 took his M.D. at the University of Vienna. From 1866 to 1869 he served as an assistant to Hebra; he later married his teacher's daughter. After terms as Privatdozent and Associate Professor, he took over the chair at the University in 1881, following the death of Hebra, and remained at this post until his own death, March 6, 1902.

It is difficult to summarize in any way Kaposi's contributions to dermatology. As Hebra's successor, actually and spiritually, he had a hand in almost every clinical advance of the time. From the great number of his publications, we have chosen the four clinical descriptions for which he is most remembered, all of which have borne his name. Had he done nothing else but complete Hebra's *Diseases of the Skin* his fame would have been assured. In that work, and in his own *Pathologie und Therapie der Hautkrankheiten* (1881), he displays his complete mastery of dermatology not only from the clinical standpoint, but also with respect to pathology and therapy.

Kaposi's clinics were truly cosmopolitan. Physicians streamed into Vienna from all parts of the world to follow his teachings, and in many cases the patients they saw had traveled great distances to be there. His ability to seize upon the essentials of a case, and to communicate them clearly to his hearers won him a huge following of students. In keeping with this academic zeal, he took a leading part in the organization of dermatologic societies, local, national and international. Noted for the charm and originality of his speech, and the vivacity of his temperament, he became quite excited in debate, and no one defended his opinions and doctrines with more ardor and energy than he.*

DERMATITIS PAPILLARIS CAPILLITII (ACNE KELOIDALIS NUCHAE)

Dermatosis papillomatosa capillitii (Framboesia non syphilitica capillitii)†

In the fall of 1867, Herr E.G., a manufacturer from Rheinpreussen, came under the private care of Professor Hebra, and later under my care. Patient 30 years old, strongly built, completely healthy, glowing in appearance, in excellent condition. His affliction is of many years duration.

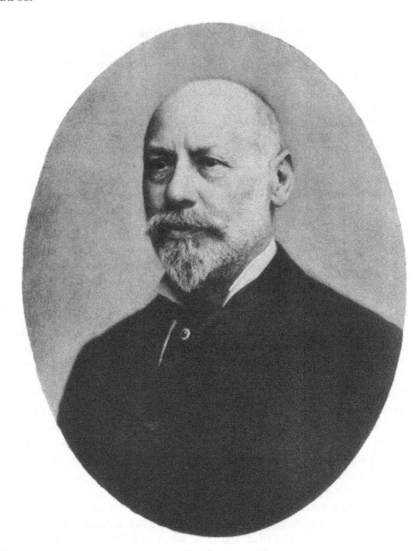

Figure 35 Moritz Kaposi. Courtesy, Wilhelm Braumueller Company, Vienna

On the neck, close below the hair line, in the region of the sparse hair at the nape, there was a tubercle the entire base of which was irregularly oval, about the size of a thaler, raised some two inches above the level of the skin, slopping off precipitously at the edges, of the same color as the normal skin, very firm, feeling like a hard scar or keloid. Its surface was broken by superficial and deep pits and furrows, and as the result of this, knobby or warty in appearance. The individual papules had the same red color and firm quality as the base of the elevation. A number of hairs, gathered in tufts, projected here and there from the pits and furrows, while the smooth parts of the swelling bore no hairs for the most part. If a single hair from a furrow in the tubercle were grasped with the cilia forceps it could only rarely be drawn out successfully; if so, it was noted that it must certainly have had a long and tortuous path to its follicle—so long was the hair shaft exposed. Furthermore, the hair was very thin, dry, and bore only rarely on its lower end the detached

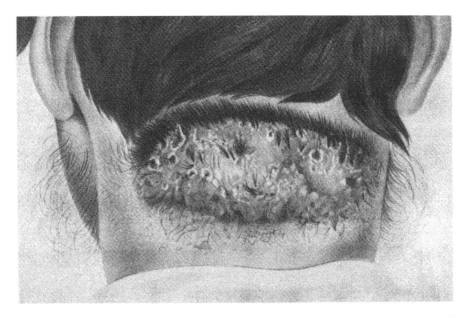

Figure 36 Dermatitis papillaris capillitii. From Kaposi's atlas. Courtesy, College of Physicians, Philadelphia

whitish scales which are the remainder of the inner root sheath—never moist adherent cells (from the external root sheath). Usually, however, it was not possible to pull the hair out at all, in that it broke off in the attempt.

In the immediate vicinity of this large tubercle, in the nuchal region, as well as partially within the hairy area on the occiput, there were papules scattered here and there which were discrete, pinhead sized, roundish, conical, flat or somewhat tabulated—knobby, and very firm, and which were either bald, or bore hairs which were single or gathered in tufts of two or more. These latter resisted attempts to pull them out as has already been described.

The tubercles were, however, painful either spontaneously or to pressure. They itched moderately at times. Each time the patient scratched open individual points on the papules with the fingernails or with the comb, yellowish gummy crusts were seen, adherent here and there.

The affliction was of many years duration. A great many things had been tried for it; in particular, the patient said, it had often been cauterized.

With regards to this, we considered whether the large tubercle might not have been a scar from cauterization. On the other hand, epidermal tissue was quite clearly recognizable there, which was certainly not compatible with the character of a scar. Moreover, the great number of other isolated smaller papules spoke against such a postulation, in that they themselves showed obviously genuine formations.

---

* Besnier, E., and Doyen, A.: Ann. de dermat. et syph., *3:*177, 1902.

† Archiv für dermat. und syph., *1:*390, 1869.

MULTIPLE IDIOPATHIC HEMORRHAGIC SARCOMA

Idiopathisches multiples Pigmentsarkom der Haut*

We can summarize, in the following, the characteristics of the disease as they appear from the observations reported here, and in supplementary case reports.

Brownish red to bluish red nodules, corn or pea to hazel nut size, arise in the skin, without any known local or systemic cause. Their surface is smooth, their consistency firmly elastic, sometimes erectile, as in a hemangioma. They remain isolated, and when they enlarge project as domes; they may also group together and remain more flat. In the latter case the central nodules of the plaque involute and leave behind a darkly pigmented scarred depression. They regularly arise first on the soles and on the dorsa of the feet, soon thereafter on the hands, and are also developed in the greatest number on these parts, associated there with a diffuse thickening of the skin and disfigurement of the hands and feet.

Later in the course, isolated and grouped nodules appear on the arms and legs, and the face and trunk as well, but always lesser in number and irregular in arrangement.

The nodules may involute partially, with atrophy. They ulcerate, it appears, sooner or later, with subsequent development of gangrene.

The lymph glands are not remarkably enlarged.

Finally, similar nodules form on the mucous membrane of the larynx, trachea, stomach, and intestines; they are especially profuse in the colon, up to the anus, and also in the liver.

The disease ends in death, and within the short space of time of two to three years.

XERODERMA PIGMENTOSUM

Xeroderma, Parchment Skin*

By this name, I shall indicate a characteristic disease coming under the designation of Atrophy of the Skin, of which I have seen two modifications. The first presented a remarkable abnormality of pigmentation, whilst, in the second form, the latter was absent.

I have only had the opportunity of observing the first kind of this undoubtedly rare affection in two cases.

A girl, 18 years of age, belonging to a well-to-do family in one of the northern German states, had suffered from the malady from early childhood. In the year 1863, she came under the care of Professor Hebra, and I had an opportunity of seeing her.

The skin of the face, ears, throat, neck, shoulders, arms, and of the breast, to the level of the third rib, exhibited a peculiar alteration. It was remarkable, in the first place, owing to its checkered appearance, for it appeared to be abundantly dotted over with pigmented spots of the size of pins' heads or of lentils, and of a yellowish-brown colour; it was also tightly stretched, as if contracted, was pinched up into a fold with difficulty, and felt very thin. Its surface was smooth in some places, whilst in others, fine epidermic lamellae peeled off; or, there were quite flat, linear furrows marked out on the epidermis, so that the surface appeared as dry as parchment, and wrinkled, whilst the skin itself was tightly stretched. In places, it was of a white colour and was without pigment, whilst there also existed, as has been mentioned, numerous scattered,

---

* Archiv für dermat. und syph., *4:*265, 1872.

* On Diseases of the Skin. New Sydenham Society translation, London, 1874, Vol. III, p. 252.

punctiform or lentil-shaped, yellowish or dark-brown, pigmented spots resembling those of frecldes. Here and there, could be seen a bright red telangiectasis of the size of a pin's head or of a lentil. The subcutaneous fatty tissue was not markedly diminished. The skin felt rather chilly. Fine, downy hairs could be distinctly recognized on the diseased skin. The sensibility was not diminished. Beyond a sensation of tightness, the patient had no pain and no sense of itching. At the level of the third rib, and at the upper third of the arm, the alteration in the condition of the skin ceased with an almost abrupt line of demarcation. From thence downwards, the skin of the mammae, of the whole trunk, and of the extremities was quite normal, smooth, pliant, fine. The general state of the health and of the menstruation was normal.

In addition to the parchment-like dryness, thinness, and wrinkling of the epidermis, the checkered pigmentation, and the small dilatations of the vessels, the most remarkable symptoms were the contraction and, at the same time, thinning of the skin. In consequence of the first, the lower eyelids were drawn downwards; on the left side, this was so considerable that the eye could not be closed. As a result the cornea was ulcerated, and rendered opaque in its lower half, which was always uncovered. The nose, towards its tip, appeared compressed, owing to the shrinking of its skin, and the external ears at their free extremities appeared indented here and there owing to the shrinking. The lips could only be slightly separated from one another.

I have been informed by two medical men who attended her, that she died of dropsy, resulting from cancer of the peritoneum, in September, 1872.

The second case which came under my observation was that of a girl ten years of age, who had also suffered from the disease from her earliest childhood. The child had attended Professor Hebra as a private patient, and thus came under my notice a year before, and now presented herself a second time for treatment. In this child, when first seen, the skin of the face, as far as the sub-maxillary region, and that of the extensor surfaces of the arms and hands, showed checkered pigmentation described. The epidermis, especially on the eyelids and on the cheeks was wrinkled and shrivelled, the upper eyelids being in consequence drawn somewhat downwards, and the lower ones drawn downwards and everted (ectropion), the eyes, therefore, seeming, from above, too small, and from below, incompletely covered. In the same way, the oral and nasal apertures were somewhat diminished. In addition, the skin was moderately tense, and was less readily than normally pinched up into a fold, but this could always be accomplished. The subcutaneous layer of fat was not altered.

In August of this year (1870) the child again came under care. The condition of the skin had not materially changed. The nose, however, was occupied by a pear-shaped, red, granulating, fissured tumour, secreting an offensive, sanious fluid. It began by a broad edge at the margin of the nares, and involved the alae and middle line of the nose symmetrically, and at a distance of about three-quarters of an inch, gradually dwindled away towards the root of the nose, reaching close to the two inner canthi. We recognized the growth to be an epithelioma, and destroyed it in great part. There remained, however, a perforation at the lower border of the right triangular cartilage. On the left cheek and on the left side of the upper lip there was a hyaline, fissured tubercle of the size of a pea.

KAPOSI'S VARICELLIFORM ERUPTION

Complication des Eczema larvale infantum*

As a very alarming complication of Eczema larvale infantum I have seen, in some cases, an acute eruption of vesicles which are numerous, partly disseminated, arranged in groups and clusters for the most part, lentil sized and somewhat larger, filled with clear serum, transparent, flat, and usually delled as well.

Because of the picture described they give the impression of varicella lesions, but they certainly are not. The skin of the face affected in this way, already swollen to various degrees by the eczema, now appears intensely turgid, even stretched taut, more edematous than solid. The little patients run a high fever, up to 40° and more, and are very restless. The eruption appears very acutely, as overnight, in the greater number, and frequently continues for three to four days or even a week with fresh outbreaks while the efflorescence of the first day involute, either dry up or, as is usual, break open and lay the corium bare, or become crusted and fall off. The greatest and most thickly clustered numbers of these varicella-like vesicles are located on the previously eczematous skin; separate and small groups of them appear on the previously intact skin in the neighborhood—on the forehead, the ears, the neck region, even on the shoulders and arms. I have never seen any appear anywhere else.

The course of this peculiar affection in the cases observed so far has been favorable, and has ended with the healing of the vesicles as described and the epithelization of the denuded surfaces in two to three weeks, in which time the fever has subsided in relation to the local affection. In many places pigmented spots persist, or even flat scars. The previously existing eczema is altered in character only as much as is influenced by the necessary local treatment used. I have seen a death from convulsive seizures in a six month old child on the sixth day of the illness when the eruption had healed almost entirely, and there was complete defervescence.

I am puzzled that I should be the one to describe this varicella-like exanthem which complicates the usual Eczema larvale infantum in such a dangerous way, which pediatricians of great experience here have never picked up, while I myself have seen it some ten times, and which would be regarded unhesitatingly by them, not as varicella, but as something of a special nature. Eczema herpetiforme would perhaps be most appropriate.

I am able to say even less about the cause of it. I cannot help thinking, however, that it has to do with the effect of a local contagion or, of course, fungus which finds suitably susceptible ground in the epidermis damaged by eczema, causing through its vegetation the eruption's characteristic lesion, great numbers of which constitute the dermatitis. Because the cases have all been so alarming we have as yet had no opportunity to carry out suitable microscopic investigations on these little patients.

The dangerous fever, however, is not to be regarded as the expression of a blood infection, rather, the effect of the local dermatitis determines its entire behaviour; it is proportional to this effect in intensity and progress.

---

* Pathologie und Therapie der Hautkrankheiten, 3rd Edition. Berlin, 1887, p. 483.

William Augustus Hardaway

Prurigo Nodularis

WILLIAM AUGUSTUS HARDAWAY was born June 8, 1850, in Mobile, Alabama. After a literary education at the University of Virginia, he began his medical studies at the St. Louis College of Physicians and Surgeons, and was graduated from Missouri Medical College in 1870, and remained with that institution, and with Washington University in St. Louis with which it merged, until his retirement in 1910. A founder of the *American Dermatological Association* (1876), he was in every sense a pioneer in American dermatology.

His most notable work was in the field of clinical dermatology. He is particularly remembered for his description of prurigo nodularis (the name was later given to it by Nevins Hyde) which we have included here, for his publications on papilloma cutis, and for his popularization of electrolysis for the removal of hair (1877).

He was courteous, kindly, well read, and noted for his sense of humor. He disliked exercise and abhorred mathematics.

On his death in 1923, a friend noted:

"It was a rare treat as well as a precious privilege, consultation hours over, to sit in his office, having accepted a cigarette tendered with an engaging smile and a brief eulogy of the brand, and to hear him set forth his thoroughly digested ideas and conclusions of his long and rich experience. His innermost thoughts, which he might have hesitated to set down in cold print, he would at times convey to his intimates in unstudied phrases between puffs of smoke, probably interlarded with bits of reminiscences on apt illustrations drawn from his retentive memory."*

PRURIGO NODULARIS

Case of Multiple Tumor of the Skin Accompanied by Intense Pruritus[†]

L.K., unmarried female, aged 51, residing in St. Charles, Missouri, was referred to me by Dr. F.N.Love, of St. Louis.

The disease commenced 22 years ago, and made its appearance upon the hands. She declares that the initial lesions were "blisters" which were accompanied by much itching, and that wherever any of the fluid from these "blisters" came into contact with the healthy integument, other similar places would form. Very soon after this, she does not recollect how long the tubercles, tumors, etc., from which she now suffers, made their appearance, and have continued without change up to the present time.

The disease with which she is affected involves the hands and the arms up to within a short distance of the shoulders, and then ceases rather abruptly. The feet are likewise implicated, and the legs up to the knees. The rest of the body is absolutely free from blemish of any sort, and has never been involved at any period since the commencement of her malady.

After a casual inspection of the parts affected, one is struck by the dark, pigmented and rough-looking appearance of the skin. Upon closer view, the integument between the lesions is found to be coarse and much thickened, particularly the extensor surfaces.

The principal lesions are made up of tubercles and tumors, varying in size from a large pea to almost the dimensions of a hickory nut and in about equal proportions as to numbers. The smallest of these growths is very perceptibly elevated above the skin, and the largest to the height of five or more millimeters.

In every instance they are covered by thick, scaly epidermis, except where it has been removed by scratching. Many of them have had their epidermal covering removed in that way, and present a roughened, frayed aspect, and bleeding excoriations. To the touch, they have a resistant, horny feel, which is quite characteristic.

In some places these tumors have run together, and appear in nodulated patches the size of a silver dollar. In other places, instead of a nutshaped tumor, are found plates of skin, apparently involving its entire thickness, and as large as a child's palm. Some of these plates are long and narrow, perhaps of the width and half the length of the adult finger. These plates, however, are few in number, not over eight altogether, the tumors largely preponderating.

Most of the lesions are situated on the outer aspects of the arms and legs, although this rule is not without exceptions. The palms and soles are not spared, and the lesions in these locations are particularly painful, as they crack open and leave painful, raw fissures. The sides of the fingers are likewise implicated, as also around the ankles, wrists, and elbows.

According to the patient's statements, when a lesion appears on one member, a corresponding one is sure to appear on the other. Upon inspection, I find this assertion borne out as regards the feet and hands, since the affection presents a remarkably symmetrical arrangement.

One of the most pronounced features of the case is the intense and intolerable pruritus. The itching is confined to the tumors and plates of thickened skin and to their immediate neighborhood; the healthy skin does not seem to give rise to it. The patient states that the formation of a new tumor is generally preceded by pruritus, and also that there is a great deal of swelling of the parts at times.

There are in all probability about 60 lesions, that is to say, tumors, tubercles and plates or patches. They are most closely aggregated in and about the hands and feet, and more widely scattered elsewhere. The pigmentation to which I have referred presents nothing peculiar as to color or form, and is identical with that deepening tint which follows pruritic conditions generally. Here and there this dark background is relieved by a very few white cicatricial-looking spots. This gives rise to the interesting question as to whether they are really the cicatrices of former lesions. It is very difficult to give a satisfactory reply to this query. The disease, during its years of existence, had become such a matter of course to the patient that she had long ceased to pay close attention to its manifestations, so that I am most unfortunately at a loss in reference to many interesting points and here, as elsewhere, can give only the patient's impressions previous to the time she came under my observation. The patient declares that these lesions have never disappeared since their first appearance, and that even when they had ulcerated, as she says they have formerly

---

* Unsigned Obit., Arch. of Dermat. and Syph., 7:640, 1923.

† Arch. of Dermat., 6:129, 1880.

or after they had been deeply bored into with caustic, they would invariably return. It must be remembered in this connection that the various lesions did not appear at once, but have been gradually evolved in the course of years. It is pertinent to remark here that, according to my own observation and the patient's belief, no new lesions have appeared in the last 16 months, nor have those already there undergone any change whatsoever. Another remarkable fact is that a large hickory nut sized tumor, situated near the elbow, which was thoroughly and completely excised (enucleated) for microscopical examination 16 months ago is now replaced by a tumor assuming its original dimensions and other external physical properties. Moreover, the cicatricial-looking spots are few and not much larger than a pea, therefore, out of proportion both as regards size and number to the lesions which now, at any rate, are mostly large and numerous.

The tumors, plates, etc., are not painful, except from the fissuring produced by scratching. The pruritus, which is the prominent feature of the case, and the only thing for which the patient seeks relief, when I first saw her was almost unbearable, and had been so for many years. It is the same in intensity at all times, both as to season and hour. She thinks it has diminished in the past few months, although when I saw her a few weeks ago the scratch-marks were painfully apparent. The mere touching of the lesions causes the most intense desire to scratch.

Alfred Goldscheider

Epidermolysis Bullosa

ALFRED GOLDSCHEIDER was born August 4, 1858, in Sommerfeld (near Frankfurt). The son of a physician, he was educated at the Friedrich-Wilhelms-Institute in Berlin, and graduating in 1881, embarked on a military medical career. After a preliminary period in provincial garrisons, during which time he described the case of epidermolysis bullosa we have included here, he returned to Berlin and worked at Leyden's Clinic. He later held posts at the Moabit and Virchow hospitals in Berlin, and in 1910 took over the Poly clinic University Institute; he remained connected with this institution until his death in 1935.

Goldscheider's most notable contributions to medicine were made early in his career. While still a student he began his famous investigations on the special sense organs of the skin, and on the nature of deep muscle and postural sense. At Leyden's clinic he became interested in physical medicine, and with his teacher may be considered to have laid the ground work for that specialty. Most of his publications deal with the use of physical modalities. Goldscheider was a fine clinician as well. He was interested particularly in physical diagnosis, and putting his neurophysiological training to practical use, he published a number of clinical neurological papers.

Goldscheider was an outstanding teacher. Stiff and unyielding, he applied Prussian military methods to the control of students. He said, "We must not train our students in geniality, but rather in correct and dependable work." He had no use for dilletantes, and engaged frequently in polemics with those whom he felt guilty of "diffuse thinking."*

EPIDERMOLYSIS BULLOSA

Hereditäre Neigung zur Blasenbildung[†]

The 22 year old musketeer, K., who enlisted in the troop last year, found that after each march his feet were dotted over with blisters; one could count 30 and some at one time. The affliction proved so obstinate that he had to be discharged as unfit for military service. He had already been discharged from the Guard-corps the year before because of the same illness. He gets these blisters on all parts of the body as soon as the skin undergoes friction, for example on the abdomen in the belt area, on the hands after hard work. He has never been able to take long walks. His father, who is 52 years old, has had the same affliction throughout his whole life, although it has become insignificant during the past few years. The father's mother, until her death at the age of 82, had suffered with it, likewise with slight improvement in old age; her brother was duly discharged from the military service in Potsdam because of the same disease. The genealogical tree cannot be traced any further. K. has a brother and sister, both of whom suffer from bullae formation. Of the four children of the sister, the affection has occurred in the first and third; the second is free from it; all three are girls; the fourth child, a boy, is only a year old, and has as yet, shown no bullae. K. himself has never been ill otherwise. He is a strongly built rather lean man, with perfectly healthy organs, an especially healthy circulatory system, and is intelligent. He shows no signs of sweaty feet; his skin is also not unusually dry, and presents nothing special in its appearance. The bullae brought on by marching look like ordinary pressure blisters; they contain a watery, clear, only slightly sticky fluid which secretes delicate gelatinous fibrin on standing.

If one rubs the skin on any part of the body moderately hard with the finger for some two or three minutes a bulla will form on the spot in a few hours. Mere pressure is not effective, nor chemical irritants, as tincture of iodine, acetic acid. After one has rubbed for a time one notices that the epidermis slides easily back and forth. On some parts of the body a small piece of epidermis is easily detached by strong rubbing and here, instead of bulla production, a more prolonged suppuration takes place. Bullae produced in this manner show faint reddening about them. The content is identical with that of the bullae not artificially produced. If left alone they will, like the others, continue to enlarge until about the third day, and then dry up. If they are opened, the base appears moist, not covered with fibrin; after drying up it appears whitish, faintly shiny, and covered with red dots. It becomes covered again very quickly with a moist film which reappears though wiped off repeatedly. If one leaves it to dry, the fluid accumulates in drops after five minutes. If one dresses a lesion, it becomes covered by the next day with a thick fibrin film and is deeply reddened beneath this; it then heals in eight to 10 days with an exceptionally copious secretion of watery pus.

To sum it up in a few words, the affection here described is characterized by an exquisitely hereditary tendency of the prickle cell layer to detachment, with consequent inflammatory exudation. I know of no analogous cases in the literature.

---

* Bergmann, G.: Deutsch. Med. Wchnschr., *61:*1053, 1935.

† Monatshfte. für Prakt. Dermat., *1:*163, 1882.

Heinrich Irenaeus Quincke

Angioneurotic Edema

HEINRICH IRENAEUS QUINCKE was born in August, 1842, in Frankfurt-am-Oder. He was the son of a physician and did his medical studies in Würzburg, Heidelberg, and Berlin, taking his degree in the latter city in 1863. After preliminary work in physiology in Vienna he became an assistant to Frerichs in Berlin, and in 1873 became a Professor of Internal Medicine in Bern. In 1878 he took a Professorship at Kiel and spent the next 30 years there, returning to Frankfurt in 1908 when he retired.

There is hardly any aspect of internal medicine to which Quincke did not make significant contributions—heart disease, visceral syphilis, gastric physiology, the icterus problem, skin diseases, and hemopoietic diseases in particular. The term poikilocytosis was coined by him. Besides the account given here, his best known works deal with the capillary pulse and the lumbar puncture. He introduced this last procedure as a therapeutic and diagnostic aid. He was gadget-minded and introduced many new pieces of apparatus into medicine.

Quincke was one of the ablest and most enthusiastic workers in the most active period of German medicine. He died May 19, 1922.*

ANGIONEUROTIC EDEMA

Ueber akutes umschriebenes Hautoedem*

This disease manifests itself by the appearance of an edematous swelling of the skin and subcutaneous tissue in circumscribed areas two-to 10 centimeters or more in diameter. These swellings are usually located on the extremities, especially in the neighborhood of the joints, but also on the trunk and on the face, here especially on the lips and the eyelids. The swollen parts of the skin are not sharply demarcated from the surrounding area; they are, moreover, the same color as the latter, or even pale and translucent, rarely somewhat reddened. Usually the afflicted experience in them only some feeling of tension, rarely itching. The mucous membranes may be affected simultaneously by similar swellings, specifically those of the lips, the soft palate, pharynx and laryngeal passages, even to such an extent that considerable respiratory difficulty results. Such circumscribed swellings venture also to appear on the mucous membrane of the

---

* Fischer, I.: Biog. Lex. der Hevor. Ärnte. Urban and Schwarzenberg, Berlin, 1932, p. 1260.

stomach and bowel, causing paroxysmally appearing gastric and intestinal symptoms in one case. In one case repeated serous effusions in the joints occurred.

These swellings appear, then, suddenly at multiple sites at the same time, reach their maximum in one to several hours and disappear quite as quickly after lasting several hours to a day. While the disappearance of one is taking place, more frequently new eruptions on other distant sites are beginning, so that in this manner the illness can be prolonged for several days or even weeks.

The general health is usually not disturbed; in some cases, besides subjective prodromal indisposition, a general feeling of illness, dizziness, thirst and diminution of urinary output occur during the eruption. Elevation in temperature is never observed.

Once the acute edema has been present in an individual it readily returns in new attacks and indeed usually at the earlier sites of predilection. The recurrence takes place sometimes at regular intervals, and sometimes in regular weekly attacks, repeated for years.

As the cause of appearance one can occasionally establish chilling of the skin, colds, bodily strain.

The malady affects men more frequently than women. The affected individuals were otherwise healthy, several nervous and irritable. The illness was transmitted to the son of one patient, whose attacks occurred at rather regular intervals, and appeared in the child as early as the first year of life.

---

* Monatshfte. für Prakt. Dermat., *1:*129, 1882.

Jonathan Hutchinson

1.   *Hydroa Aestivale*

2.   *Solid Edema*

3.   *Arsenical Keratosis*

4.   *Angioma Serpiginosum*

JONATHAN HUTCHINSON was born at Selby in 1828, of an old Quaker family. He began his medical career as an apprentice to Mr. Caleb Williams, a York surgeon, and in 1847 he entered St. Bartholomew's Hospital qualifying M.R.C.S., L.S.A. in 1850. Among his more important appointments were those in Blackfriars Hospital, Metropolitan Hospital, and London Hospital.

Hutchinson's accomplishments in medicine are astonishing. He was eminently skilled in dermatology, syphilology, surgery, ophthalmology, and neurology. He is most remembered for his work in syphilology, particularly for the "Hutchinson's triad" of the congenital form of the disease. In this field his only peer was Fournier. His contributions to dermatology were many, and chiefly clinical in nature. He was a most careful observer, kept detailed notes of his unusual cases and pioneered in the pictorial illustration of skin diseases. He was a zealous and fascinating teacher, an early advocate of postgraduate medical education in England.

Graham Little remembered Hutchinson as a "tall, stooping, spare figure, wearing a straggling unbeautiful beard to the end, when beards were mostly obsolete." He further noted that he "was totally devoid of any sense of humor and like most humorless men incredibly obstinate in clinging to his opinion (such as his fish theory of leprosy) long after they had been demonstrated to be untenable."

Today, Hutchinson's freckle (lentigo maligna) maintains his eponymic fame.

On his death in 1913 the British Journal of Dermatology remarked:

"We recognise that a great figure has passed from the scene, and that we shall not meet his like in the future. Modern research exacts such a development of specialism that we can never expect to see combined in one person the all-round excellencies of Jonathan Hutchinson."*

HYDROA AESTIVALE

Summer Prurigo[†]

Gentlemen—I have had much difficulty in finding a name which should be even tolerably appropriate to the disease which we are about to consider. I am not aware that it has been named or described by authors. Its prominent features consist in its tendency to relapse, or to continue without slight intermission over many

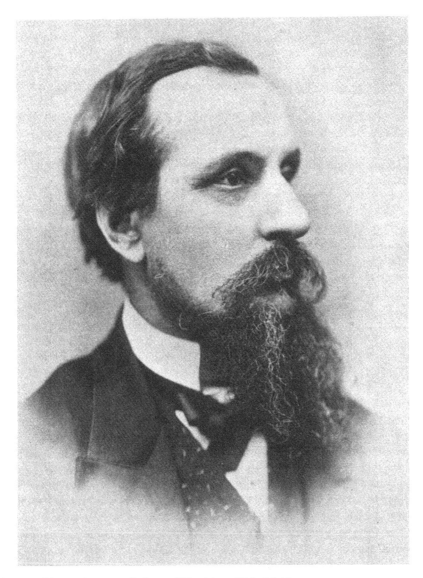

Figure 37 Jonathan Hutchinson. Courtesy, College of Physicians, Philadelphia

years and in spite of treatment, to affect by preference the face and the upper extremities, to be worse in summer weather, and to commence usually at or about the age of puberty. It is generally more or less pruriginous, but not by any means intensely so, and the eruption consists of small red papules which look as if they were about to form pustules, but which never do so (abortive pustules). Unless they are scratched no ulceration takes place and no crusts form. Although, however, there are no crusts, yet minute scars are constantly produced. On the cheeks there is usually a good deal of diffuse erythema, much more than is shown in the portrait which I now exhibit.

In the boy who was the subject of this portrait the disease affected the trunk as well as the upper limbs and face, but in most cases the eruption is limited to the face, neck, and upper extremities. The disease differs in some marked features from that known as "Hebra's Prurigo." First, the pruriginous element is very much less marked and the erythematous much more; secondly, the face is always affected, and the lower extremities less so than other parts; and lastly, whilst Hebra describes his form of prurigo as being always worse in winter, the reverse is the fact in this malady.

It would appear to have some alliance with, and on the face might easily be mistaken for, that disease, but none of the spots ever pass into acne pustules, nor does it restrict itself, on the *trunk,* to the acne positions. Probably it has supplied part of the material from which the descriptions of *Strophulus pruriginosus* were given by the old writers; and the *lichen urticatus* of Bateman may possibly have included some examples of this malady in its earliest stage.

The portrait which we have before us is that of a boy named Charles P., and was taken in August, 1867, when he was under my care in this hospital. At the conclusion of our lecture I shall produce the lad and show you that his skin disease has at length quite disappeared. He is now under my care for another malady. The portrait was taken when he was 13 years of age. He had been the subject of an eruption almost from infancy. It was believed to have begun at six months old. For a long time it always got well in winter and relapsed in summer. He was covered from head to foot with the spots, all his extremities being affected, the palms of the hands and soles of the feet alone being exempt. The spots were everywhere scattered, not arranged in patches. They presented conical elevations of a light red tint, and in the centre of some of them were minute accumulations of fluid. Most of them might be described as abortive pustules, for they looked in the early stages as if threatening to become definitively pustular, whilst but few really did so. The skin when he first came to me was marked all over with very shallow white cicatrices which the eruption had left. He had never had small-pox. The eruption showed but little preference as regards different regions. It was, however, especially copious on the cheeks, forehead, and back of the neck. He was thin, and his skin was somewhat harsh and brown, but he considered himself in good health. The eruption did not seem to occasion him any great annoyance; he said that it itched only at night, and gave him no trouble in the daytime. He asserted that usually it got quite well in the winter, only coming out in warm weather; but on the present occasion his attack had begun at Christmas, and had persisted during four months of cold weather. He did not notice any difference in his general health.

The following note records the state of the lad several years later:

He has grown well and appears to be in good health. The eruption is at present out only on the backs of his arms, slightly on the forehead and over the buttocks. His skin is everywhere spotted with small cicatrices, most of them very superficial, but so abundant that on his chest, back, and arms a marbled appearance is produced. His mother, who comes with him, states that the first outbreak in infancy occurred after measles, and was supposed to be "measles rash." She says also that it has at times covered the whole surface of the body with the exception of the flexures of the joints and the palms and soles. He has always had it less on the legs than elsewhere, and the parts most severely affected have been the face, backs of the hands, and arms. He has had repeated bad attacks since the portrait was taken, although on the whole the disease appears to be getting milder. For two months at midsummer of this year the eruption was very freely out, and his legs were so much swollen that he was obliged to stay at home. As a rule he continues regularly

---

* Brit. J.Dermat., *25:*225, 1913.

† Med. Times and Gaz., *1:*161, 1878.

at his work, and suffers but little inconvenience from his eruption. He complains somewhat of irritation when he is hot, and he habitually scratches, but he states that he is never kept awake at night by itching.

SOLID EDEMA

On Certain Diseases Allied to Erysipelas*

Let me next ask your attention to certain cases of recurring erysipelas of the face, leading to elephantoid hypertrophy of the eyelids and cheeks.

Of this malady I have seen many examples, and in both sexes. The history is always nearly the same. At some former period, perhaps years ago, an attack occurred which was called erysipelas, and which was attended by sharp illness, and all the usual conditions of the idiopathic form. The swelling on the first occasion probably showed a tendency to spread, and involved the scalp as well as the face. Subsequent attacks may have occurred once every few months, or oftener, and very probably have not been attended by any tendency to spread. In them there has been simple oedematous swelling of the eyelids and cheeks with slight feverishness. The eyes usually become closed for a day or two and the attacks last not longer than a week or 10 days. After each successive attack the oedema subsides only imperfectly and when the recurrences are frequent a condition of permanent swelling is produced. Mr. Waren Tay has kindly lent me a photograph which will illustrate this state (portrait shown). Between the permanent solid oedema with hypertrophy of the skin, which finally results, and a true elephantiasis, the differences are, I would submit, only those of degree. The question is, have we any right to call this disease by the name of erysipelas. I rely upon the history of the first attack, upon the nature of the exciting cause in the subsequent ones, and upon the constant phenomena of oedema and congestion, when I say that I think we have.

From cases such as these to true elephantiasis it is but a few steps, and I avow my conviction that we shall make a definite simplification in our nosology when we class the latter disease as in the main a result of chronic and recurring erysipelas. These results are rendered peculiar, and become in all respects exaggerated, by the peculiarities of the part affected in reference to their circulation. As is well known, elephantoid hypertrophy is seldom seen except in dependent parts—the feet and legs, the scrotum and penis, the labia, etc.—and it is obviously helped by difficulties in the return of blood. But these difficulties do not explain the whole. There is inflammation as well as passive or venous edema, and the lymphatic system is probably more especially concerned than the blood vessels. All observers agree that elephantoid parts are prone to attacks of erysipelas; that they swell up and inflame for a time, with general febrile disturbance, and that each successive attack leaves them worse than before. Let us change the mode of expression, and say, not that elephantiasis is liable to erysipelas, but that it is in large degree a result of it. It is, perhaps, not the fact that in all cases the disease dates its beginning from an attack of erysipelatous swelling, but I am sure that in many cases such a statement would come very near the truth. There is some slight wound of the foot or leg, some sore on the genitals, around which inflammatory oedema has occurred, and from that oedema the elephantoid process takes its origin. I have seen several cases in which this has certainly been the case; and whilst I would by no means assert that such first attacks are always, or even often, conspicuously "erysipelas," I feel no doubt they are closely allied to that process. In saying this I by no means overlook the influence of climate, race, and diathesis as predisposing factors.

---

* Med. Times and Gaz., *1*:4, 1883.

ARSENICAL KERATOSIS

Report of the Pathological Society of London*

Arsenic Cancer. Mr. Jonathan Hutchinson, F.R.S., desired to make the proposition that the internal administration of arsenic in large doses over long periods might produce a form of cancer which was of the epithelial variety, but presented certain peculiarities. He showed a drawing of the foot of a gentleman who had taken arsenic for psoriasis for many years; a corn on the sole of the foot ulcerated, and at first had the appearance of a perforating ulcer. Perfect immobility was not followed by any improvement. The palms of the hands also became affected, small corns developing. The growth in the foot was excised, and the patient recovered. The patient was now under the care of Professor Chiene; the microscopical examination was inconclusive. He also showed drawings of the hands of an American physician who had taken arsenic for long periods in considerable doses. A rough condition of the palms and soles developed though the psoriasis was cured. These early growths in these cases he observed parenthetically, were corns not warts, and the growths were never papillary. This patient then got on the front of the wrist of the left hand a growth in the subcutaneous tissue, the other hand also became affected; the growths perforated the skin and fungated; they had the appearance of a syphilitic lesion, but the patient had never had that disease. The growths were scraped away and also excised; microscopical examination was again at first inconclusive, but the opinion finally leaned to the view that the disease was cancer. The patient then came to Europe, and in deference to the opinion of several surgeons, anti-syphilitic remedies were fairly tried, but gave no result. Both hands were amputated; the patient died 18 months later. Nodules of epithelial cancer were found in the axillary glands on the left side, in both lungs, in the suprarenal capsules, in a rib and in other parts. He also showed drawings from another case of a lesion of the palms, exactly resembling the corns seen in the other cases. This patient had a cancerous growth in his neck, and took arsenic in large doses, for months together; the skin became muddy and thick, and patches like psoriasis developed upon the elbows and other parts, but in the palms and soles the corny masses formed but were not followed by cancer. About five years ago Dr. Clifford Albutt had given him the particulars of a case of a young lady who had taken arsenic for pemphigus for many years with occasional intermissions. An ulcer had developed on the crest of the ilium, the glands enlarged, a tumour formed in the thigh, and the patient died at the age of 25, owing to the enlargement of these growths. Mr. Hutchinson also mentioned a case which had been under the care of Mr. Waren Tay and himself. The patient was a clerk, aged 34, who had taken arsenic for a long time for psoriasis. The palms of his hands and soles of his feet were speckled over with corns when he applied at the skin hospital; finally, epithelial cancer of the scrotum appeared, and was excised; the patient was then lost sight of. He thought the facts he had brought forward warranted him in advancing the theory that the cancers in these cases were due to arsenic with the hope that attention might thus be more generally directed to the point.

---

* Brit. Med. J., *2:*1280, 1887.

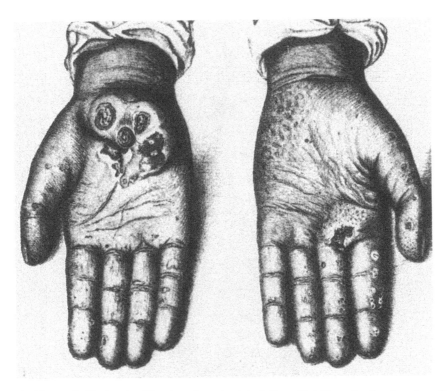

Figure 38 Arsenical keratosis (the hands of the American physician). From Hutchinson's atlas. Courtesy, College of Physicians, Philadelphia

ANGIOMA SERPIGINOSUM

A Peculiar Form of Serpiginous and Infective Naevoid Disease*

This portrait, which was taken from the arm of a young lady about 15 years of age, purposes to illustrate a very peculiar condition of serpiginous or infective naevus. Although naevi often increase in size and in number during the first few months of life, it is very rare indeed for the growth to continue to spread. Such, however, was the case in this instance, and with the addition of other peculiarities. A very slightly marked port-wine stain was observed at the back of the arm soon after the infant's birth. For some years it scarcely spread at all, and no notice was taken of it. It then began slowly to advance, and the condition shown in the portrait was gradually produced. A careful inspection of the plate will show that the mode of advance is somewhat peculiar, and that it has not been by a continuous edge. It would appear as if little satellite spots had been produced, which had spread into circles, and, by gradually advancing by infective edges, had coalesced, producing the irregular pattern which is here displayed. Some very good examples of these spreading circles are seen over the elbow, quite isolated from the rest of the disease. These conditions are no ordinary part of naevoid disease. They were extremely superficial, and it was even difficult to be sure whether or not they left any state of scar behind them. I have, however, no doubt that such was their

* Arch. Surg., *1:* Plate IX, 1890.

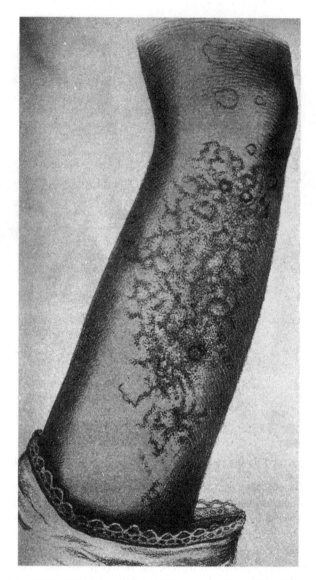

Figure 39 Angioma serpiginosum. From Hutchinson's atlas. Courtesy College of Physicians, Philadelphia

tendency, and that in some places a slightly-marked superficial scar could be demonstrated. The enlarged capillaries could be partially emptied by pressure, but not wholly, and in many places little tufts were distended with deep-purple venous blood, which could not be pressed out.

August Breisky

Kraurosis Vulvae

AUGUST BREISKY was born at Klattau, in Bohemia, March 25, 1832. He pursued his medical studies at Prague, and took his degree at the age of 23. After serving as an assistant in pathological anatomy for a time, he became associated with Professor Seyffert's obstetrical clinic where he qualified in that specialty. Breisky was called to the Chair of Obstetrics in Salzburg in 1866, and a year later to Berne where he remained seven years. He then returned to Prague, and on the death of Professor Spaeth took over at the University of Vienna, which post he occupied until his death in 1889.

Breisky made a great many contributions to the obstetrical literature, dealing particularly with myomectomy, Porro's operation, and pelvic measurement and deformity. His best known works are the description of kraurosis given here, and his extremely popular book *Diseases of the Vagina* (1887).

Breisky was genial and kindly, with a cordial smile and a warm handshake. He continued to work up to the end, although he had been in ill health for several years. He was seized with the symptoms of his fatal disease while performing a myomectomy.*

KRAUROSIS VULVAE

Ueber Kraurosis vulvae*

On the external genitalia of adult females I have observed, in a few cases—12 in all—peculiar alterations, an atrophic shriveling of the skin, localized to the vestibule, the labia minora with the frenulum and prepuce of the clitoris, the inner surfaces of the labia majora to the posterior commisure and on the neighboring skin of the perineum. These localizations were not always affected at the same time nor to the same degree; in three cases, however, they were, thereby producing a peculiar and striking picture of atrophy of and defect in the genital folds which to my knowledge has not been described in the literature. So far I have found nothing resembling it, at least in looking over the pathology, dermatology and gynecology handbooks.

In such exquisite cases one finds, on spreading the labia majora apart, that the labia minora are apparently missing, in that they are plastered to the mucous surface of the labia majora, so that the edges alone remain indicated by shallow furrows. From the mons veneris to the urethral orifice the integument is drawn tight over the clitoris, except for a trace of the preputial or frenular fold which may be found. Occasionally a

---

* Mundé, P.: Am. J.Obst., *22:*717, 1889.

white scarlike or raphe-like line may run down the middle of this area. The glans of the clitoris is either hidden completely behind the shriveled skin so that it cannot be exposed, or it lies within a small rounded aperture in the integument, the persisting remnant of the original space between the frenulum and prepuce. When the labia majora are drawn apart, the skin above the urethral orifice is stretched into tense transverse projecting folds. In a similar fashion, but with less striking alteration in form, this shriveling develops in the posterior part of the vulva. Here also, the generally contracted and unyielding skin resists dilatation attempts, and forms tense folds.

The general effect of this extensive shriveling is a striking smallness and inflexibility of the vestibular portion of the vulva, a definite though not extreme *Stenosis vestibularis* which may indeed, as we have observed, offer abnormal resistance to dilatation of the external genitalia in childbirth, and even in coitus, presenting thereby a distinct clinical picture. The skin in the areas of greatest shriveling appears whitish and dry, occasionally covered by a thick and somewhat roughened epidermis, as in the area of the glans clitoridis, on the skin between the clitoris and urethra, and in the area of the labial frenulum, while the adjacent skin parts involved are shiny and dry, pale reddish grey, covered also with faded whitish spots, and show ectatic vascular branchings here and there. The sebaceous glands of the pudendal folds are extremely scanty. The remaining portions of the external genitalia show no constant skin changes except for a moderate degree of relaxation and wasting.

---

* Zeitschr. für Heilk, *6*:69, 1885.

Julius Friedrich Rosenbach

Erysipeloid

JULIUS FRIEDRICH ROSENBACH was born December 16, 1842, at Grohnde. He studied at Heidelberg, Göttingen; Vienna, Paris, and Berlin, taking his degree in 1867. He became an assistant to Baum and Schweigger, qualified in surgery in 1872, and in 1877 began as a Professor of Surgery and Chief of the Surgical Polyclinic in Göttingen.

Rosenbach is best known for his fundamental work in wound infections and published much along that line. The description of erysipeloid given below, although of dermatologic importance, was a phase of this work. He died December 6, 1923.*

ERYSIPELOID

Ueber das Erysipeloid[†]

The disease which has long been known under the name Erysipelas chronicum, Erythema migrans, etc., and which I have named erysipeloid, plays no very prominent role in pathology. It is purely local and produces, except for some burning sensations, no symptoms at all. Nevertheless, gentlemen, I should like briefly to call your attention to this disease because it occupies a special place in the wound infection group because of its purely local course, and, more particularly, because of its etiology.

Erysipeloid presents a typical clinical picture. No one who has observed it frequently will doubt that it must be considered as a disease *sui generis*. Erysipeloid is a wound infection of no great virulence which is never transmitted directly, which, rather, is acquired only sporadically by inoculation of exogenous infectious material into wound sites. The infectious material is found in all sorts of dead and decomposing animal materials. Thus we see preponderately affected those people who have contact with dead animals, or wild animals, for example, cooks, restaurateurs, animal keepers, particularly butchers, tanners, fish mongers, oyster openers, etc., less often tradesmen who acquire erysipeloid through inoculation from cheese, herring, etc. Since such materials come into contact almost only with the fingers we have observed the affection for the most part only there. Of course infection at other sites on the integument is possible. A dark red, frequently livid swelling, with sharp borders, very similar to erysipelas, extends from the site of inoculation. This

* Fischer, I.: Biog. Lex. der Hervor. Ärzte, Urban and Schwarzenberg, Berlin, 1932, p. 1321.

† Verhandl. der Deutsch. Gesell. für Chir., *16:*75, 1887.

erythematous area itches and prickles in a painful way. The general status and temperature are unaffected. The affection advances slowly; when, for example, it begins on the tip of the finger, it reaches the metacarpus in about eight days; in the next eight days it advances further, well onto the back of the hand, and creeps then onto the neighboring finger. The peculiar appearance, the sharp borders, the livid redness, the steady progression, arrests the patient's attention and alarms him; the pain is never significant. The affection has no definite duration; it usually involutes spontaneously in one-two-three weeks. Long after the first affected areas have faded out, the progression at the periphery ceases, and the entire area returns to normal.

Ernst Lebericht Wagner

1. *Colloid Milium*

2. *Dermatomyositis*

ERNST LEBERICHT WAGNER was born in Dehlitz, March 12, 1829. He was raised in the home of his uncle, a Saxon country doctor. His medical studies were pursued in Leipzig, Prague, and Vienna, under Wunderlich, Oppolzer, Skoda, and Rokitanski. Finishing his studies, he set up practice in Leipzig, and here this man who was to become the most sought after and authoritative of the Saxon physicians failed miserably. After another try in a small Bohemian border town he returned to Leipzig, turned his interests to the rapidly developing field of histopathology, and gradually achieved greatest success in it. Most noted are his monograph on cancer of the uterus and his investigations on the pathology of fat embolism, phosphorus poisoning, the syphilomas, diphtheria, and lymphadenomata.

Great as were his contributions to pathology, it is as the master clinician that Wagner is most remembered. As the successor to Wunderlich at the medical clinic in Leipzig, he became one of the most renowned physicians in Germany. Pupils flocked to him; his diagnostic acumen never ceased to amaze. He added much to our knowledge of Bright's disease, the pneumonias, abdominal typhus, and perforative peritonitis. His approach to therapy was a bit nihilistic (Skoda rearing his head again). The original report of the disease we now know as dermatomyositis, which we have included here, was written shortly before his death in 1888, the description of colloid milium much earlier.*

COLLOID MILIUM

Das Colloid-Milium der Haut[†]

In May of this year a 54 year old woman sought help at the medical Polyclinic for a peculiar disease of the skin. She said that in the fall of last year she had had violent pains in the scalp six to eight weeks in duration, the nature of which cannot clearly be determined. The present illness then developed gradually and without pain.

This otherwise healthy woman exhibits the following cutaneous findings over the entire forehead, from the vicinity of the hairline down to the eyebrows, extending laterally from the orbits, over the upper parts of the cheeks, running together over the bridge of the nose, rather sharply demarcated: The skin over the whole is clearly thickened, and presents four or five marked longitudinal creases on the forehead which are intersected by numerous, shallower, diagonal, almost vertical creases. While the depths of these creases appear normal and white, the rest of the skin is yellowish brown, strikingly shiny, and shows projections which are set close together, mostly small, a few larger than millet seeds, for the most part round or roundish, not confluent. To the eye these look like vesicles, although they feel remarkably firm, and cannot be broken open either with the finger tip or with the nail. Insertion of a needle, which was as painful as usual and must therefore have been comparatively deep, produced no trace of fluid, occasionally a small drop of blood. Strong laterally applied pressure with the fingernail produced, along with slight bleeding, a whitish or pale yellowish translucent substance which reminded one of a firm colloid and which was in the form of round or sausage-shaped masses. The rest of the skin areas mentioned were in the same condition; the skin of the cheeks was less affected, the skin of the bridge of the nose more. The eyelids and the skin of the eyebrows were normal—moreover, all the skin sites were sparsely furnished with lanugo hair. Orifices of the sweat glands and sebaceous glands were not visible. The regional lymph glands were normal.

Macroscopic examination of the masses expressed showed the characteristics of ordinary colloids.

DERMATOMYOSITIS

Ein Fall von acuter Polymyositis*

A 34 year old female cook named Schellenberg. Father was addicted to drink, very fat; mother insane. Had typhus years ago. No puerperium. No menses past six years. For the past year, cough, expectoration, night sweats. Since the end of June, for no known reason, with no cold, in particular—pain in the back and lumbago. Stiff neck and stiff joints, severe pains in the nucha, in the shoulders, wrists and legs—one week's duration. Shortness of breath for same length of time.

Admitted July 19, 1886. A well nourished strongly built woman. No fever. Movement of the head difficult at upper neck articulations. Neck and nuchal muscles tender to pressure. Evidence of left sided apical tuberculosis, cough with bacilli present in the sputum. Heart normal. Liver somewhat enlarged. Spleen, kidneys, stomach, and bowel normal. Stiffness in both shoulder articulations, this latter painless. A little bilateral edema of the backs of the hands and the forearms, as well as the legs.

On July 24, the patient complained of itching and numbness in both forearms. The edema the same in degree. Nerves not tender to pressure.

On July 28, the arms became swollen, the forearms more so. The skin of both upper extremities was now so taut that the muscle contours could neither be seen nor felt through it; it was white, not shiny, and did not pit to moderate finger pressure. Movement was impaired, respiration extremely difficult, apparently as much from the edematous skin as from the muscles, which have a peculiar doughy feel. No tenderness to pressure, also none in the accessible nerves. No fibrillary twitching, touch and localization senses normal. Electrical investigation on the nerves and muscles of the arms produced no abnormal reactions. Faradocutaneous sensibility of the arms considerably diminished, on the skin of the pectoral areas and on the neck, on the other hand, normal. Treatment consisted of cautious massage and Faradization; it seemed to the physicians and to the patient to be successful.

On the 3rd of August the swelling was somewhat diminished and softer. With greater pressure one could penetrate more deeply; also the muscle contours could be felt somewhat. The evening temperature ran from 38° to 38.4°.

---

* Sudhoff, K.: Münch. Med. Wchnschr., *56:*1545, 1909.

† Arch. der. Heilk., *7:*463, 1866.

On August 7, the swelling was even softer. Pits made in the skin persisted for a long time. On the extensor surface of the left arm an erysipelas-like redness developed from the elbow down; it disappeared on pressure; its borders were on the whole similar to those of erysipelas, only strikingly scalloped. On the 12th of August this same redness appeared on the extensor surface of the right arm. By the 17th this redness had extended up and down, bilaterally. The swelling itself of the arm was much reduced; the normal folds in the skin were again visible. The back of the right hand alone was more swollen. The evening temperature reached 39° more frequently. The tuberculosis seemed to progress; increased cough and sputum.

On August 24, the redness on both arms disappeared completely. The swelling of the arms and forearms had, with daily massage, diminished even further; the arms themselves were movable. The patient complained of a deep seated pain in the right thigh for a few days; nothing objective was found. From that time on the patient had a very tormenting cough, and attacks of extreme shortness of breath. These last increased continually both in number and frequency, although no certain cause for them could be found, either in the lungs or heart. On the 29th, difficulty in swallowing began, as well as spontaneous attacks of asphyxia with loud tracheal rattles between times. Death came in the evening in one such attack.

---

* Deusch. Arch. für Klin. Med., *40*:241, 1887.

Henry Radcliffe-Crocker

1. *Dermatitis Gangrenosa Infantum*

2. *Dermatitis Repens (Acrodermatitis Continua)*

3. *Erythema Elevatum Diutinum*

4. *Granuloma Annulare*

HENRY RADCLIFFE-CROCKER was born in Brighton in 1845, and began his medical training in a northern English colliery district in the old fashioned manner of apprenticeship. Later entering the University College Hospital in London he was graduated in 1875 with many scholastic honors. His resident training was done at the Brompton Hospital, and the University College Hospital. It was Tilbury Fox who influenced Crocker to turn his attention exclusively to dermatology, and with the sudden death of the former in 1879, Crocker was elected to the post of Physician to the University College Hospital at the early age of 43, a post he held until his death.

Radcliffe-Crocker's contributions to dermatology were principally in the clinical and educational fields; they were many. His finest achievements were his textbook *Diseases of the Skin* (1888–1903), the leading text in English in its day, and his colored *Atlas of Skin Diseases*.

He was a man of untiring energy and powers of organization; a happy man with a devoted wife and a wide circle of friends. He died while vacationing in Switzerland August 22, 1909.*

DERMATITIS GANGRENOSA INFANTUM

Multiple Gangrene of the Skin of Infants and Its Causes[†]

There are thus a dozen cases of varying degrees of severity, some so mild and chronic that were it not for the intermediate links we should hesitate to class them with those gangrenous cases at the other end of the chain, which are fatal in a few days.

From a consideration of these and 21 other cases published by Mr. Hutchinson and other authors, we may draw up the following general account of the disease.

The place of onset, and mode of development varies according to whether it appears early or late in the course of the varicella, or is independent of that disease. If it begins while the varicella lesions are still present, it commences on the head or upper part of the body, and instead of scab being thrown off from the pock, ulceration takes place beneath it, and often a pustular border with a red areola is formed, the whole resembling a vaccination pustule, the process extending both in depth and peripherally. A black slough is

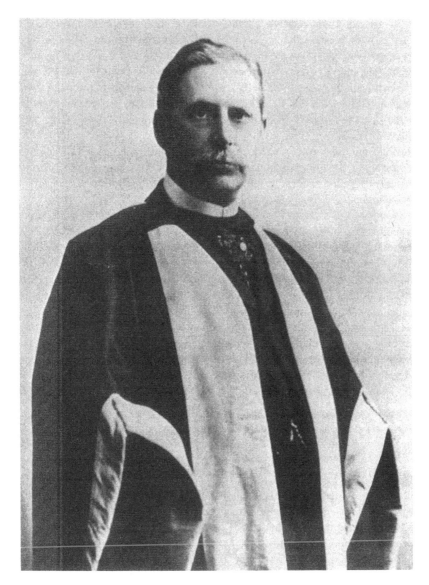

Figure 40 Henry Radcliffe-Crocker. Courtesy, *British Journal of Dermatology*

formed from a quarter to an inch or more in diameter, the smaller ones still with a pustular border and areola. After attaining a certain size, varying much, the process of separation sets in, and when completed a sharp edged roundish or oval conical ulcer is formed deep or shallow in proportion to the diameter of the slough, some of the largest being quite three quarters of an inch in the centre. Extension of the ulcer seldom takes place after the separation of the slough has commenced. When the lesions are closely aggregated coalescence will probably ensue and then very large ulcers, irregular both in contour and floor, are produced. If any fresh crops are formed, or when it commences after most if not all of the varicella lesions have cleared off, perhaps a fortnight or more from the onset, or in cases following vaccination or otherwise unconnected with varicella, the ulcerative lesions usually commence on the lower half of the body. They especially affect the buttocks and thighs as a pinhead sized papulopustule, which extends to the size of a pear or larger, ruptures, and except on the buttocks or wherever it is kept moist, dries in the centre to a scab with the pustular border and red areola like vaccinia, and from this point follows the same course as those which started in a varicella pustule. In some cases the buttocks and parts in contact with the napkin, and sometimes the legs and thighs, are fairly riddled with ulcers of all sizes, shapes and depths. On the trunk and rest of the body they   are not usually numerous, and though some may be very large and deep the majority are comparatively superficial.

Where the lesions are numerous and deep there is naturally much constitutional disturbance, the temperature ranging up to 104° or even higher. Lung complications, tubercular, pyaemic or inflammatory, are very frequent, and determine or hurry on the fatal issue. Should the child survive it is surprising how rapidly the lesions cicatrize, of course leaving deep and indelible scars.

There are all grades of the disease. In the mildest form ulceration may be quite superficial, the lesions reaching to the vaccinia-like stage and then drying up, often accompanied by pruritus and lasting by successive crops for a considerable period. There may also be simultaneously observed mere excoriation up to pretty deep ulceration, with or without a few lesions going on to gangrenous sloughs, while in the most extreme cases haemorrhage occurs into all the vesicles which become rapidly gangrenous and lead to the death of the child in a few days, either with a general tuberculosis or pyaemic lesions. When less severe than this, the contents of the vesicles are not haemorrhagic, but a large proportion of them become gangrenous and death is likely to ensue, but may be deferred for some time, and is usually due to a secondary complication.

As regards etiology, all the cases hitherto recorded have occurred in infants or young children. An analysis of my own and 11 of other authors, in which the age is stated, shows that by far the majority occur under one year, the figures being 14 not exceeding one year, six not exceeding two years, and three under three years of age. The youngest was three months old.

DERMATITIS REPENS (ACRODERMATITIS CONTINUA)

Dermatitis Repens*

This is a peculiar form of dermatitis, of which I have seen three instances, and as I have not found it described elsewhere, and it is most difficult to treat, I desire to call attention to it.

The first case was a young man who had a part of a finger amputated from injury. It healed up normally, but at the border of the wound, a dermatitis commenced, which extended gradually up to the palm, and then over half the hand and down the fingers. My colleague, Mr. Godler, then sent him to me. The general aspect suggested an eczema rubrum. The thin surface was denuded of epidermis, extremely red, with oozing points from which a clear fluid exuded in drops like sweat at the border of the inflammation, which was sharply defined. The epidermis was undermined by fluid and slightly raised. The disease extended steadily and uninterruptedly at the rate of about one-eighth or one-fourth of an inch per week, and was not arrested for some months, when it had involved the whole forearm up to the elbow, while the hand had got well,

---

* T.C.F.: Brit. J.Dermat., *21:*331, 1909.

† Med. Chir. Trans., *70:*397, 1887.

---

* Diseases of the Skin. London, 1888, p. 128.

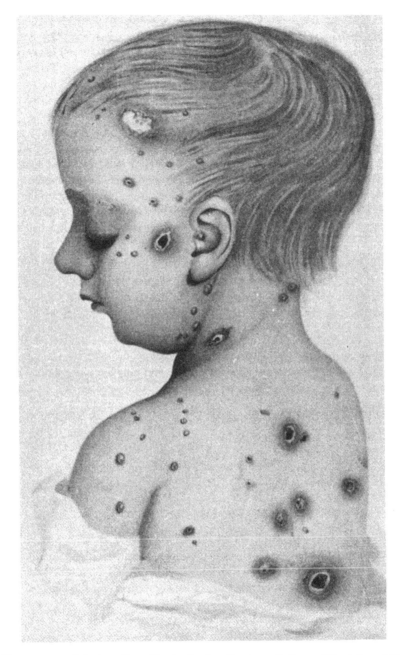

Figure 41 Dermatitis gangrenosa infantum. From Crocker's atlas. Courtesy, College of Physicians, Philadelphia

leaving the skin red and tender. There was no manifest departure from health, he was well fed, and there was no great amount of itching.

The treatment at first was that for eczema; this failing, snipping away the spreading edge, and afterwards sulphate of copper. The copper seemed to have some effect; it spread more slowly and not uniformly. It failed, however, to really stop the disease. Finally, after many trials, lactate of lead wrapped round it night and day seemed to be the curative agent. A continuous arm bath made it spread faster.

Case two was a lady, aged 28, whose general health was not satisfactory. She was weak, nervous, and suffered from irritative dyspepsia, but was better since the eruption, which began six months before I saw her, on the flexor surface of the wrist, with a crop of red papules, which coalesced and discharged. The eruption then spread down to the hand and up the arm, while the oldest part gradually got well, but was very red. The margin was well defined, and covered with thick, dirty-looking crusts, but there were very few elsewhere. At the upper border, the crusts were about an inch across, but at the lower, the skin was only undermined. The rest of the surface, though very red, was almost dry. In four months it spread from below the elbow up to the middle of the biceps. Four months later, it had traveled all up the right arm, across the back of the neck, and down the left arm to the elbow, the old parts healing. When last seen, it was almost well, owing apparently to the last treatment adopted. The general health was attended to and lactate of lead, which had succeeded with the other case, was tried here and failed. Tar, boracic acid, and many other treatments were tried in vain, but ultimately Beissel's permanganate of potash treatment after two months arrested the disease. A 10 per cent solution of permanganate of potash was painted on three times a day till it formed a crust, cutting away the undermined skin before it was applied.

The third was a much milder case, a man, aged 19. The eruption began as small blisters in the wrist a year previously, and spread up the arm and down the hand, so that the whole palm and fingers, except the terminal phalanges, was affected, but the back of the hands were free. He got well in about three months.

M.Nepvew read a case at the French Congress of Surgery in 1886 which probably belongs to this category. The patient was a woman, in whom a vesicular eruption commencing in a superficial wound of the thumb, spread over the whole body. Bacteria were found in the vesicles, and the disease was checked by an iodoform dressing.

Although the commencement in these cases was like an eczema, its subsequent course was very different, but the cases are too few to ground general statements upon, so I simply have them on record until more cases appear.

ERYTHEMA ELEVATUM DIUTINUM

Erythema Elevatum Diutinum*

The advantage of a pictorial record of rare cases in producing the recognition of similar instances when they are met with by other observers is universally acknowledged. It is in the hope, therefore, of eliciting fresh facts that the following case is described and figured, and comparison made between it and other recorded cases more or less resembling it.

Amy H., aged six years, was brought first to the Victoria Hospital for Sick Children in October, 1893, and on the 21 st was sent on from there for diagnosis, to University College Hospital. There was a very strong history of gout and rheumatism, on the mother's side. The mother's grandmother suffered badly from rheumatism; the mother's father and brother had gout badly, and her sister had rheumatism. The father's family history was unknown, but he himself was in good health.

The patient's general health had always been quite good, and she had never had any serious illness except measles in infancy.

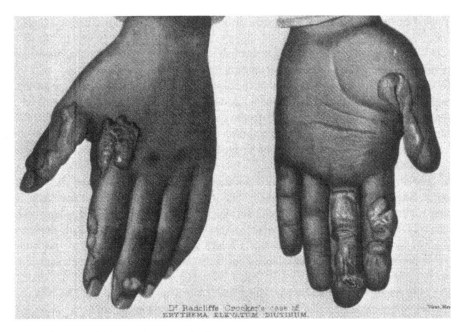

Figure 42 Erythema elevatum diutinum. From Crocker's paper

The disease of the skin began simultaneously on both knees five months before she came under notice; next, it developed on the buttocks, elbows, and finally on the hands, which have been affected for two months.

Positions. The lesions are situated on the left hand, on the knuckle, and on the first terminal phalanx at the border of the nail of the thumb, first and second fingers, on the palmar surface of the same fingers, over the whole of the second finger, and over all but the proximal phalanx of the index finger. On the thumb, it affects only the bend and the proximal phalanx.

On the right hand. The same fingers but not the thumb are affected, all up the palmar surface of the index finger, and the distal end of the second finger; the back is only slightly affected on the terminal phalanx of the index finger and the joint between the proximal and second phalanx of the first and second fingers.

The most highly developed lesions are over the first knuckle of the left hand and the inter-phalangeal joints of the right hand.

The one on the right index finger may be taken as a type; here the lesion was raised one-eighth of an inch, convex, sharply defined, pale purplish-red in colour, with a few dilated vessels over it, somewhat whiter on pressure, but diminishing very little in size; firm to the touch, very tender; but not painful except when pressed upon. It did not itch or burn.

Over the elbow-joints there were lesions evidently of a similar character, but retroceding. At the border the skin was wrinkled, and there was a brownish discoloration.

On the knees involution was still more complete; the left was almost well, except some slight discolorations and thickening in one part.

---

* Brit. J.Dermat., *6*:1, 1894.

On the right there were still three prominent lesions; the rest had involuting, leaving a dull, slightly reddened tint.

The buttocks were quite well, only a faint purplish stain remaining, and on the right side lower down, where the mother said there had been several tumours, even the stain had faded.

While the lesions on the back of the hands were conspicuously nodular, those on the palmar surface were more diffused from coalescence of the component nodules, which were only just discernible, and the whole infiltration was less raised and defined. The affected parts were hotter to the touch, very slightly scaly here and there, but most of the nodules were quite smooth.

The child was not subject to chilblains nor to factitious or other variety of urticaria, but was a well-nourished, apparently healthy girl.

The case clearly did not fit into any known category, and our patient was therefore shown at the Dermatological Society on November 11th to elicit opinions, but no one had met with any case corresponding to it. Subsequently Mr. Hutchinson suggested that it resembled a case published with a coloured plate by Dr. Judson Bury in the *Illustrated Medical News* of February 23rd, 1889, and republished in Mr. Hutchinson's *Archives of Surgery,* Vol. II No. 8, plate lxi. Although there are some differences, careful comparison shows that the resemblances outweigh them, and that the two cases are clearly of the same nature.

Bury refers to two cases described by Mr. Hutchinson as resembling his own. The first was described in the *Illustrations of Clinical Surgery,* plate VIII, page 42. The second in the *British Journal of Dermatology,* for November 1888, under the title of "Symmetrical purple congestion of the skin." But they do not appear quite to correspond with our case, and that of Bury.

Since the first portion of this paper was written, I have seen the drawing of another case like Bury's and my own, in a woman of about 22, in whom it had been present, I believe, about five years, but it will no doubt be published before long.

The cases of this form have the following features in common:

All of them were of the female sex, and the disease commenced in childhood or early youth. Of the two published cases, Bury's had acute rheumatism; and in mine there was a strong family history of gout and rheumatism. Bury's case had intermittent albuminuria. In both, the lesions developed over the articular prominences of the fingers, the elbows and knees, and also on the palms. In addition, in Bury's case, the toes were affected, in mine, the buttocks.

In both, there was a tendency to involution on the elbows and knees, but on the hands in Bury's case the tendency was to further development, while in mine involution occurred in the hands also, and there is some hope of complete recovery.

Nevertheless, the persistence of many of the lesions is a very striking feature in the disease, and on the whole greatly exceeds the tendency to involution.

While the primary tint of the lesions is pink, they soon acquire a purplish hue, which becomes more marked the longer the duration of the lesions; how very long that may be, is strikingly shown in Bury's and the unpublished case, well earning the title of "diutinum," or persistent. The older lesions become much firmer to the touch, almost cartilaginous, but at no time are they otherwise than firm and incompressible. The sharp line of demarcation between the diseased and healthy skin is to be noted.

There can be no question about the identity of the nature of these two published and the one unpublished cases, but with regard to Mr. Hutchinson's type, the differences between that and what in justice to the first recorder I may call the Bury type, are considerable, and we may compare them in parallel columns as on page 207.

The two types differ in the age and sex of the patient, in the position of the lesions, and in the older cases the nodular character was less developed, being oedematous, and lacking the firmness of the Bury type of the nodules and patches.

They resemble each other in the gouty diathesis of the patients, their being primarily nodular in character, becoming confluent and forming patches, and in the purple tint, the age of the patients perhaps accounting for the deeper hue of the Hutchinson type.

Bury type	*Hutchinson type*
All females.	All males.
All young.	All elderly.
Gouty or Rheumatic in Self or Family.	Very gouty personally.
Lesions situated over articulations and on the palmar surface.	Lesions not any special localization or over flat bony surfaces.
Erythematous at first, but becoming purplish.	Purplish from the first.
Began as nodules, but became confluent, still showing nodular character.	Began as flattish nodules, became confluent, and lost their nodular character.
Lesions, some very persistent, others involuting. Never spread over a large area.	All lesions persistent throughout life, and spreading widely.
Lesions paled but very firm, and otherwise unaffected by pressure.	Lesions paled only at the border. The elevation was chiefly due to oedema, and could be almost removed by continued pressure, and there was oedema in the neighborhood.

I think it is evident, therefore, that at present it is not safe either to affirm or deny that the two types may be phases only of one affection; but until, and perhaps even after, we have discovered connecting links, it will conduce to clearness of conception to regard them as distinct types, and not to endeavor to weld all the symptoms of the two varieties into one comprehensive description.

It may be safely assumed that the number of cases is too small to afford us a complete symptomatology of these forms of disease, which can so clearly be traced to what French writers would term "arthritism."

Practically, the microscope does not explain the real pathogeny of the process, and the name placed at the head of the paper is justified simply by the clinical features, which are those of an erythematous, raised, persistent lesion.

GRANULOMA ANNULARE

Granuloma annulare*

There are thus six cases which possess definite characters in common which show that they belong to one clinical group. Summing up these characters, they are as follows:

Nodules or papules of slow development which tend to form circles by aggregation or partial coalescence, leaving component nodules still visible. They tend to undergo slow involution, so that the circle is broken and often only a crescent is left, or a gyrate patch where two or more crescents join. The inner or involuted side of the ring slopes down gradually into the normal skin, leaving the part which has been affected slightly reddened for some time; the outer border is more abrupt, but crenate or distinctly nodular, and there may be

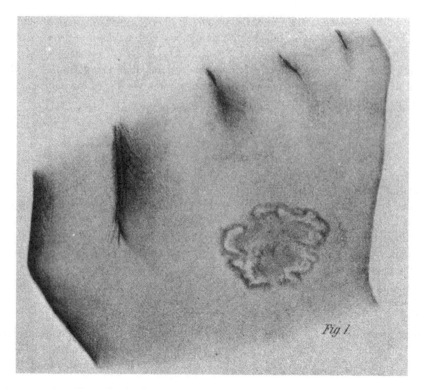

Figure 43 Granuloma annulare. From Crocker's paper

a very narrow areola. The colour of the lesion maybe violaceous red, or quite pale, as in Figure 1. The nodules are firm, and some of them may have a slightly warty character, whilst others are flat and rather suggestive of Lichen planus. The distribution is chiefly on the wrists and backs of the hands and fingers, but also on the neck, and it is curious that in no less than four cases there have been papules on the nape near the hair-line. They have also been seen on the head behind the ears and on the upper part of the face; only in the boy were they on the lower extremity over the knee. They seem to have a preference for bony prominences, such as the knuckles, radial and ulnar extremities, etc., but are not exclusively there. The characters in the case of the boy were not quite so definite as in the others.

In connection with their slightly warty appearance, it will be noted that in two cases there were common warts both as antecedents and concomitants, and that in Case IV the lesion went on to a condition like Lupus verrucosus; but the histology lends no support to their being of a warty character, the epidermis changes being trifling compared to the copious cell-infiltration of the corium.

Their extreme indolence, both in development and course, indicate that they are no ordinary inflammation, though they have a tendency to involute centrally and extend *pari passu* peripherally. In two of the cases there was a family history of tuberculosis, but the number is too small to argue from.

I am not aware of any cases in dermatological literature, except that of Pringle, which correspond with this form of disease. I was at first tempted to include Dubreuilh's case of a chronic circinate eruption of the

* Brit. J.Dermat., *14:*1, 1902.

hand as another example, but the absence of any distinct mention of the rings being composed of more or less distinct nodules and the different histological character of the lesions have made me hesitate to do so. Dr. Dubreuilh himself, while considering that his case approaches nearest to Lupus erythematosus in nosology, identified his case with those of Colcott Fox and Galloway, which the latter has called Lichen annularis.

These cases also form rings on the hands, but the rings appear to develop from a single papule which enlarges peripherally whilst involuting centrally, and there is no nodular character to be observed, the border being only slightly raised and flat. Galloway's histology also is quite different to mine.

To conclude, we have here an eruption with definite clinical characters in which semi-coalescing indolent nodules tend to form rings or segments of rings situated chiefly on the upper extremities or nape, and which clinically and histologically appears to correspond with the pathological condition we call Granuloma.

Paul Gerson Unna

Seborrheic Dermatitis

PAUL GERSON UNNA was born in Hamburg in 1850. He was the son of a medical man, and was educated at the Universities of Heidelberg, Leipzig and Strasbourg, receiving his M.D. in 1875. After a few years of general practice he became interested in dermatology, and in 1881 began a clinic in Eimsbüttle, a suburb of Hamburg. Always a sort of free lance, connected with no special University (there was none in Hamburg at that time), Unna gathered about him a group of devoted students, and from his busy clinic there flowed a constant stream of publications of the highest merit.

Unna's output was tremendous; his publications number over 600. His first loves may be said to have been histopathology and histochemistry, and he was undoubtedly the greatest of the pioneers in these branches of dermatology. He also made valuable contributions to dermatologic therapy, and to the study of seborrheic dermatitis; the modern concept of the latter is based largely on his observations. His views on the microbic origin of eczema prevailed for some years until wider and more exact research showed that they were untenable.

As might be gathered from his list of publications, Unna was one of the most indefatigable workers the specialty has known. He drove his pupils to the limit, but asked no more from them than he did from himself. Leslie Roberts has described a day at his clinic:

"The day began with a visit to the in-patients in the clinic, followed by the ambulatory clinic in Hamburg. The morning work would often be concluded by a clinical lecture from Unna. The afternoon was devoted to histological and bacteriological work, special attention being paid to the staining reaction between the dyes and the dead tissue."

"Later in the afternoon a second visit was paid to the in-patients. After dinner Unna slept for an hour and retired to his study, where he wrote till midnight or later."

Unna died January 29, 1929 after 60 years of active professional life.*

---

* Roberts, H.: Brit. J.Dermat., *41:*157, 1929.

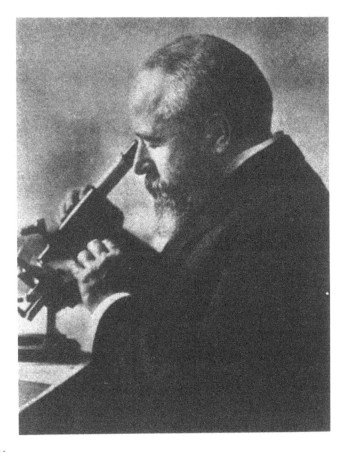

Figure 44 Paul Gerson Unna

SEBORRHEIC DERMATITIS

Seborrhoeal Eczema*

I will today present at some length the clinical side of one of the most important of my types of eczema, *viz.,* eczema seborrhoicum.

The starting point of almost all seborrheal eczemas is from the scalp. Very rarely the affection begins with a corresponding affection of the margin of the eyelids, or upon one of the well-known surfaces rich in sudoriparous glands, such as the axilla, the bend of the elbow and the cruro-scrotal fold.

Upon the head it exists mostly as an affection of scarcely noticeable onset, and it is only after possibly months or years of existence that a sudden increase, a loss of hair, an unusual amount of scaliness, a collection of crusts, severe itching, or, finally, a circumscribed moist spot, or an evident eczema, leads the patient to consult a physician. The affection begins then as a latent catarrh, the first traces of which manifest themselves by an agglutination of the epidermic scales which are thrown off in large lamellae, and, further, as a faulty distribution of the skin's fat, in that the hair becomes abnormally dry from a closing up of the

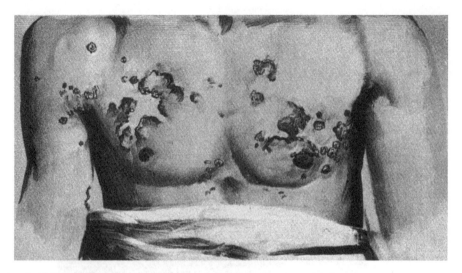

Figure 45 Seborrheic dermatitis. From Unna's paper

opening of the hair follicle, while the epidermis itself and the exfoliating scales become abnormally fatty (from the secretion of the sudoriparous glands).

From this point the process may take one of three characters on the scalp. Either the scaly masses may be simply increased in quantity, but remain white and only moderately fatty, while little by little an increase in the loss of hair is noticed, and the well known and characteristic baldness of alopecia pityrodes appears, and the scalp becomes less and less movable in the regions which are growing bald. The scaliness decreases, and finally ceases entirely, when the scalp is quite bald, to make way for a hyperidrosis oleosa.

In another class of cases the scaliness so increases and persists, that during the whole duration it forms the principal symptom. The scales heap themselves up into fatty crusts between the hairs, which they cause to fall out. There is also a corona seborrhoica, which gives a typical appearance to the patient thus affected. Later on the affection usually extends to the temples, over the ears to the neck, or skips over to the region of the nose and cheeks. In this form also a decided falling of the hair is frequently seen.

The third form is that in which the catarrhal appearances are the most pronounced, and in which "weeping" occurs, especially about that portion of the temporal region lying next to the ears, and following a simple pityriasis, with its attendant itching, tension and redness. The fatty scales are lost, and, as is always the case in eczema, the dark red, moist and shining basal horny layer comes into view. In increased weeping, erosions may appear at different points, and the rete be laid here. Almost always the ears, or at least their outer edges, are affected, accompanied by oedema, swelling of the external auditory canal, and the subjective symptoms usually present in all eczemas of the ears. In children, and especially infants at the breast while teething, the disease attacks the cheeks and forehead, because the habitual hyperemia of these parts produces a favorable soil. The moist condition is not always present upon the whole scalp, and often a simple pityriasis occupies the middle and posterior parts of the head, while the neck and face present the appearance of an eczema madidans.

---

* J.Cutan. Dis., *5:*449, 1887.

The first of these three forms or grades of seborrheal eczema is the ordinary pityriasis capitis, which usually slowly leads to alopecia pityrodes; the second is the so-called seborrhoea sicca capitis; and the third includes a large number of different affections which have heretofore been classed together as eczema chronicum capitis. I shall call these three forms, for the purpose of simplification, the scaly, the crusty, and the moist.

Proceeding downward from the head, we come to the next favorite spot for the eruption in the sternal region. Here the crusty form is found almost exclusively; much more rarely the scaly, when the hair grows thickly on the parts; and still rarer the moist, in conjunction with a moist seborrhoeal eczema of the whole upper portion of the body. The crusty eczema of this whole region had already been described by different authors as a distinct affection. So only recently by Colcott Fox, under Wilson's name of lichen annulatus serpiginosus, and by French writers as eczema marginatum. It has quite a characteristic appearance, and is, indeed, the most clearly defined form of seborrheal eczema. Round or oval spots of the size of the finger nail are grouped together, partly coalescing, and hence forming plaques about the size of a thaler, having a contour made up of segments of circles. A many-leafed variegated flower is thus suggested by the sharply defined outer border and the shadings of color.

Each patch is of a yellow color, and has an outer border of quite a fine red color when the scales are removed from it. This is the most common form of the affection in the sternal region when of slight development. We find it more often where there is a fat deposit upon the trunk, and quite long hair is produced, than where the skin is soft, thin and hairless.

If the affection here assumes considerable dimensions, the point of departure changes into a yellow colored, quite smooth but slightly scaling center, about whose periphery fresh outbreaks of the eruption appear with the characteristic raised papules and yellowish white or yellow crumbling fatty scales of the original. At times this fresh eruption is irregularly distributed, and at times appears in the form of a bow with the convexity always towards the outer side. This last form of the affection is found mostly upon the back, and especially in the interscapular furrow.

In the axilla, on the other hand, crusts are almost never to be seen, and even the yellow color of the central portion of the patch is absent. There is a tendency here to assume the moist form, and to spread with the usual rapidity of an eczema over the thorax.

From the shoulders it spreads down upon the arms almost always in the crusty form, and seldom as a moist eczema. Here a decided predilection is shown for the flexor surface. This, and the tendency to appear upon the surfaces in contact with each other, is explained by the role which the coil glands play in eczema seborrhoicum.

The backs of the hands, and especially the backs of the fingers, are often affected with a moist eczema, when on the head appears a crusty eczema seborrhoicum, and a moist eczema occupies the regions of the ears and face, the trunk and arms escaping.

The affection takes on a peculiar form when it is localized upon the palms and soles. That it makes its appearance in these situations at all is of itself a strong argument that the affection is entirely independent of the sebaceous glands. Here are found little heaped up masses of scales corresponding to individual coiled glands, and resembling psoriasis guttata. Later the epidermis peels off and a geographical appearance is produced. There is no weeping. Upon the lower part of the trunk, the buttocks and hips, we mostly find the crusty form in rings and advancing in serpiginous circles leaving behind yellowish and later on brownish pigmented patches.

The cruro-scrotal fold and the approximating surfaces of the thigh and scrotum are favorite locations for the disease, which forms no small part of the conditions passing under the name of eczema marginatum of Hebra, which term undoubtedly includes at the present day a great variety of distinct germ diseases.

The thigh and extensor surface of the knee are but little affected, while the popliteal space and leg often are. At first we find here only the large papular and thick crusty forms.

I have reserved the face until the last, and until we had passed in review the principal forms found upon the body. Here we find the scaly form, when a beard is worn, as a diffuse pityriasis on the one hand, and on the other as circumscribed, somewhat reddened, exceedingly itchy patches in the moustaches and whiskers, but loss of hair never follows. In women the diffuse scaly form is rare; here are found mostly circumscribed, scaly, yellowish gray slightly elevated patches which can often only be made out on careful examination. These patches occupy mostly the forehead, cheeks, and nasolabial fold, and extend to the side of the neck.

Red papules, from the size of a mustard seed to that of a pea, appear oftentimes upon the forehead, cheeks and nose in congestive conditions of the face. They are free from scales, or covered with fine yellow ones, and between the papules the skin becomes reddened, and causes a slight burning sensation. Unless cured, a true rosacea is developed from this beginning, and it is this form which I have named the eczematous. Seborrhoeal eczema is indeed the most frequent cause of roseola in women, and many cases of roseola begin to improve the moment the causative seborrhoeal eczema of the scalp is cured.

So in men the use of alcohol is frequently the remote [cause] and an over-looked seborrhoeal eczema of the head, the more direct cause of a rosacea.

Extremely seldom do young children have the thick, crusty form upon the face, but the fatty crumbling form of crust. Patches of seborrhoea are often seen about the mouth and nose in old people, which are well known to be the starting point of carcinoma *(Volkmann's Seborrhoeal Carcinoma)*.

The face is a favorite location for moist eczema seborrhoicum, especially in childhood, and only in adults when associated with moist eczema of the neck and head. Itching is not severe. Vesicles are never seen, but eczema rubrum is present so soon as the fatty crusts are raised from the surface.

The affection develops just as well in the Meibomian glands as in the coiled glands, and upon the eyelids is very obstinate. Usually the affection of the scalp has preceded it. The crusts are dry and fatty, and the lashes are seldom shed. Chronic conjunctivitis of the lids is often a concomitant affection. All these forms are found in the ear passages. In almost every case of eczema seborrhoicum of the scalp, a simple scaliness of the ear is observed, accompanied by dryness and itching.

Usually there is an abundant secretion from the coiled glands of the ear canal, i.e., of the fat glands of the ear.

The rarer crusty form is usually transformed into the moist.

The nails are seldom attacked, but seborrhoeal eczema may lead to the formation of verruca acuminata and condylomata.

Let us now look at the course of the disease. Eczema seborrhoicum advances slowly from the periphery, and often years pass and a patch remains in the spot on which it has begun, giving rise to slight symptoms. Beginning upon the head, as a rule, its spread is downward over the ears, face, neck, sternum and interscapular furrow, and upon the arms. This choice of location is so characteristic of the affection as to be considered pathognomonic. No other eczema and no psoriasis has this course.

For the most part over large surfaces the skin is quite free, so that the tendency of the affection to assume disc and ring forms produces a variegated appearance. This is lost in certain rare cases, where, after many years' duration, the whole surface becomes literally covered over. In such cases it resembles pityriasis rubra, but is distinguished from it at the first glance, aside from the difference in odor, by the thickness, yellowish color, crumbling nature and fattiness of the scales, and, further, by its benignity.

Seborrhoeal eczema ends after appropriate treatment in recovery, and does not cause relatively great itching. In the scaly and crusty forms the patients experience only slight itching, and occasionally slight pain at the periphery of the patch.

Charles Quinquaud

Folliculitis Decalvans

CHARLES EUGÈNE QUINQUAUD was born in Paris in 1841. He began his medical studies at Limoges, and received his M.D. in Paris in 1874. In 1878 he became a Médicin des Hôpitaux, and in 1888 became affiliated with l'Hôpital Saint Louis, with which institution he remained until his premature death in 1894. He was greatly influenced by Bazin, and was associated with him during his training.

Quinquaud was a well trained chemist, and in his research applied his special knowledge in this field to dermatologic problems, particularly in the study of the roles of toxins, nutrition, and uric acid in skin disease. In addition, he made a wide range of contributions to clinical dermatology, numerous publications on leprosy, pemphigus foliaceus, syphilis, glanders, chancroid, and many more. He is best known for his description of the scarring alopecia known as folliculitis decalvans (Quinquaud's disease), given below.

Quinquaud was a powerful speaker with a vibrant voice and full command of his material, and was for this reason greatly sought after by students. He was habitually preoccupied and pensive looking when not on the podium.*

FOLLICULITIS DECALVANS

Folliculite Destructive des Regions Velues*

The very poorly understood group of folliculites takes in a number of distinct affections, the causes of which are essentially different; among these lesions is one which causes a very special alopecia, constituting a disease apart, and simulating mycotic pelade.

Clinical Characteristics. The usual site is in the scalp; more rarely it involves the beard, the pubis, and the axillary regions.

The patches of alopecia, more or less numerous, are: 1. Irregular and not exactly circular. 2. They are almost smooth, glossy, presenting granular areas at the periphery. 3. The skin is discolored, white, as with atrophy, and shows a slight redness in some areas; they are disseminated, in area the size of a franc piece, and between them greyish areas of healthy scalp are found, with tufts of hair which offer normal resistance to epilation. 5. With the naked eye, better with a lens, one may clearly distinguish both a dermal depression

---

* Hallopeau, H.: Bull, de la Soc. Fran. de Dermat. et de Syph., 5:7, 1894.

Photograph: Wallach, D., Tilles, G.: Dermatology in France, p. 440, 2002.

and a pseudocicatricial appearance. The fundamental characteristic of the morbid state is found at the periphery of the plaques, or in the islets of healthy skin. These are follicular lesions of different types. Most often one sees purulent points, miliary abscesses, as it were, pinhead sized, or even less voluminous, punctiform, from the center of which a hair emerges which can be pulled out easily on traction with epilating forceps, and which almost always falls out spontaneously. The repetition of this same *processus epilant* in many small islets produces the pseudocicatricial patches of alopecia indicated above; these hairs are feebly adherent. One may see tiny crusts lying on a red base, scarcely moist; or again there may be simple punctiform areas of redness, isolated, with or without secondary desquamation; or there may be a red follicular projection. There are no demonstrable tubercles, no favic scutulae, and no seborrheic changes.

The evolution of the disease is quite distinctive; in the first place one notices an alopecia, but in following the course one sees that the alteration begins at isolated points seated in the area of the hair follicles; a reddish projection is seen there, from the center of which emerges a hair which is shed spontaneously in eight to 15 days. We are dealing, then, with an acute, rapid, *epilating,* folliculitis; often, moreover, but not always, the perifolliculitis is suppurative; it produces outbreaks of small pustules at the base of the hairs; the number of these purulent points is always relatively small; they can be counted; they are isolated one from another; they do not become confluent or eczematous as one sees so often in ordinary folliculitis of the beard or other regions; a great abundance of crusts is not observed; the lesion progresses tidily, dryly, without oozing.

The attacks in the first months are more severe than the later attacks; often, even, there is only a single severe one; the others are more trifling.

Thus the affection may last a long time; I have seen it persist for three years in a young child 15 years old, who, thanks to a special treatment, has been clear for two years; in consultation at l'Hôpital Saint Louis this year I have observed two other cases, one in a child of 12 years, the other in an adult; the affection had begun 18 months previously.

---

* Bull, et Mém. de la Soc. Méd. des Hôp. de Paris, 5:395, 1888.

James C.White

Keratosis Follicularis

JAMES C.WHITE was born in Belfast, Maine, July 7, 1833. At the age of 16 he entered Harvard and in 1853 began his medical education at Tremont Medical School which had a semi-official connection with Harvard. He served a term as house pupil at the Massachusetts General Hospital, and received his M.D. in 1855. A European postgraduate tour, during which he worked under Oppolzer, Sigmund, and Hebra, was completed in 1857. After an early interest in toxicology and chemistry, White turned to dermatology exclusively, and in 1863 became Professor of Dermatology at Harvard, the first chair in this specialty to be established in this country.

Throughout his life White was an enthusiastic naturalist; his botanical knowledge, along with his training in chemistry, added much to the value of his most important work, *Dermatitis Venenata* (1887). As America's first academic dermatologist it is difficult to overestimate the contributions he made to the specialty in this country, particularly from the clinical and educational standpoints. The account given below brings out well his clinical acumen.

White was by nature truthful, fearless, and confident, most necessary attributes in that day when specialization was in its infancy. These qualities exposed him, however, to the criticism of being dogmatic and controversial.

He died January 5, 1916.*

KERATOSIS FOLLICULARIS

A Case of Keratosis (Ichthyosis) Follicularis*

There appeared lately at the clinic for cutaneous diseases at the Massachusetts General Hospital a patient whose skin presented the following extraordinary manifestations: The whole surface, with the exception of the palms and soles, the genitals, and some portions of the flexor aspects of the arms, was thickly occupied by a variety of lesions, which may be thus analyzed.

1. Minute papules, the size of a small pin's head, smooth, firm, and not differing in color from the surrounding skin.

---

* J.Cutan. Dis., *34:*339, 1916.

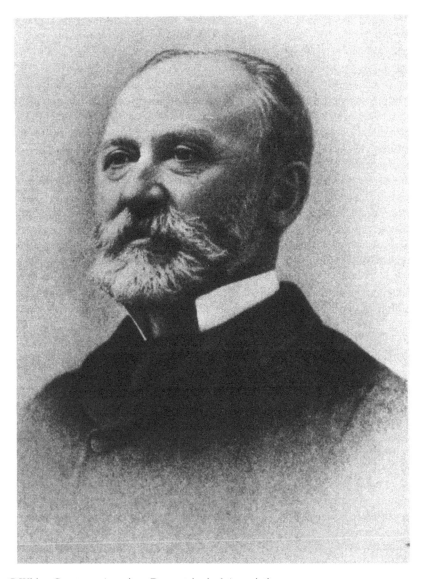

Figure 46 James C.White. Courtesy, American Dermatological Association

2. Papules somewhat larger than the above and slightly hyperaemic in appearance.

Lesions 1 and 2 closely resemble those of keratosis pilaris, but are, perhaps, not so sharply conical as the latter often are.

3. Still larger papules, of flattened hemispherical shape, with smooth or polished, dense coverings of nail-like consistence, and varying in color from dull-red to purplish, dusky-red, brown, and brownish black. At a little distance they strongly resemble the lesions of lichen planus. The tips of some of them have been excoriated by scratching and are covered by hemorrhagic crusts.

All of the above three forms are discrete and are surrounded by apparently normal skin.

4. Extensive elevated areas formed by confluence of the above lesions, presenting uneven surfaces, covered by thick, yellowish or brownish, flattened, horny concretions.
5. Elongated, horny masses, from one-half to one-third of an inch in diameter, and from one-eighth to one-half an inch in height, of irregular outline, with blunt, truncated apices, yellowish in color, of dense consistence, and compactly crowded. They may be removed with little difficulty, and then show bases of corresponding area, considerably elevated above the general surface, hyperaemic, and moist.

All these lesions thickly occupy the trunk and limbs, with the exception of some portion of the inner surfaces of the arms. The smaller discrete papules are distributed over the flanks and the lateral thoracic regions, the flexor surfaces of the arms, and some parts of the legs. The larger forms, and the uniform areas made by confluence of the same, occupy extensive tracts upon the extensor portions of the arms, the anterior and posterior aspects of the trunk and nearly the entire lower extremities. On the lower legs they form thick plates, completely encircling the limb, broken by deep fissures and shallow ulcerations. The most prominent horny prolongations are seated upon the median spaces of the trunk, front and back, and are most pronounced over the sternum and   pubes. *See* accompanying plate from a photograph by Mr. Chadbourne, medical house pupil.

6. Smooth, flattened, blackish, elevated plates, forming a continuous covering upon the backs of the feet, and resembling the condition called by some French writers, *icthyose noire cornée* (*vide* Baretta's model No. 4).
7. Enormously dilated follicular openings, distended apparently by firm, slightly projecting concretions, forming hemispherical elevations. These occupy nearly the whole surface of the upper parts of the face.
8. Small, sharply pointed, conical horns, curved at the tip, protruding one-eighth of an inch from a few of the above distended follicles. These are situated below the eyes.
9. A few large circular elevations with blind central depressions, nearly one-half inch in diameter, closely resembling a crateriform epithelioma, seated upon the temples.
10. Large papilloma-like excrescences, almost fungoid in appearance, nearly filling up the space behind the ears, and separated from each other by deep fissures.

Upon the scalp are some sparsely scattered, medium sized, firm elevations. The hair growth is everywhere normal. The integument of the palms, soles and genitals is but little changed from its natural condition. The nails are coarse, slightly thickened, and jagged at their free edges. A few firm, small, papular projections are seen upon the hard palate.

The skin is nowhere over-sensitive or painful on pressure, excepting about the ulcers on the lower legs. There is a nearly universal pruritus, which leads to almost incessant violent scratching, in consequence of which the horny elevations are frequently torn away, to be in turn slowly reproduced. An intolerable stench is given off by the patient, especially from the lower legs, characteristic of decomposing epithelium. The clothes are saturated with it.

The patient gives the following account of himself: He is an American, 49 years old. His parents and an older brother are in good health. None of his family are known to have had any cutaneous disease. His skin was always natural until after entering the army in 1862, at the age of 22. He underwent the usual inspection on enlistment, and no marked disorder, at least on the skin, was noted. The first sign of the affection observed

---

* J.Cutan. Dis., 7:201, 1889.

by him was the appearance of a "rash" upon the shoulders beneath the knapsack after a long march. He says that it looked like the smallest lesion now present. During the following two or three years "it spread a good deal" upon the trunk, but "no crusts appeared upon the pimples" until after this period, and then they began to form upon the back and front chest. Two or three years later the limbs began to be affected. Since that time there has been a gradual extension of the lesions over the whole integument, with progressive changes in character up to the present time.

The patient's general health has always been good, although suffering much throughout the disease from itching, and in later years also from the ulcerations upon the lower legs. The horrible odor emanating from the skin has lately kept him from free intercourse with his fellow-men.

What disease do all these extraordinary and multiple manifestations represent? It is easy to trace the intimate connection between the various lesions by their progressive development from the minute primary papule to the largest masses of horn-like concretion. At the beginning of the process we have no lesions in no way to be distinguished from those of simple keratosis (lichen) pilaris, while the other extreme is characterized by formations resembling well-marked ichthyosis cornea. The disease is then, evidently, in all its phases a keratosis, or primarily a hypertrophy, or modified cornification of the epithelial layers. It is also evident that its starting point is in or about the follicular openings.

It is a wholly different affection from ordinary ichthyosis in the location of the primary process, in the character of its individual lesions and entire sequence of appearances from first to last, as well as in the history of its progress. If this indeed be an example of hystricismus, presenting, as it does, opportunity for the study of its anatomical characteristics in every stage of development, it suggests the adoption of the more appropriate names ichthyosis follicularis or keratosis follicularis.

J.J.Pringle

Adenoma Sebaceum

JOHN JAMES PRINGLE was born in 1855 in Borgue, Kirkcudbrightshire, Scotland. After medical schooling in Edinburgh he spent several years in Vienna and Paris attending the clinics of Hebra and Kaposi as well as Vidal and Fournier. His life long association was with Middlesex Hospital in London, where he was chief of the dermatology section.

Pringle wrote comparatively little. In the report below he recorded a case of adenoma sebaceum, a disease to which his name was attached, initially because it was the first case to be published in England, and later because it was felt to be a unique type of adenoma sebaceum. We have selected his summary since it affords such a graphic succinct account of the disease. In addition, Pringle wrote sections on dermatology in various medical encyclopedias. He was editor of the English edition of Jacobi's famed *Portfolio of Dermochromes* (1903).

Pringle was widely known and well liked. He took the keenest interest in teaching and diagnosis. His sense of humor and kindness added to his popularity. Among his special attainments were an unrivaled sartorial elegance, an extraordinary command of the French language (acquired by nightly attendance at the Comédie Francaise for six months), and a considerable knowledge of music and painting. His gaiety and *insouciance* concealed from all but his intimates his fierce 20 year struggle with tuberculosis. He died on December 18, 1922 in Christ Church, New Zealand while on a world voyage in search of health.*

ADENOMA SEBACEUM

A Case of Congenital Adenoma Sebaceum*

A number of cases may be grouped together under the name of Adenoma Sebaceum, first proposed for them by Dr. Balzer.

In all the essential element is an hypertrophy of sebaceous glands.

The seat of election of the disease is the face, and especially those parts of it where the sebaceous glands are normally present in greatest abundance.

The condition is always either congenital or observed in early life.

---

* Little, G.: Brit. J.Dermat., *35:*43, 1923.

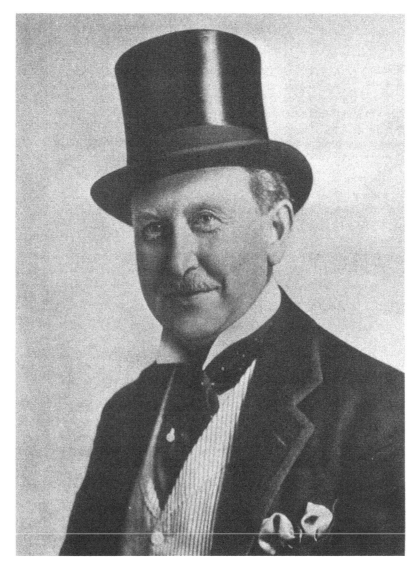

Figure 47 J.J.Pringle. Courtesy, *British Journal of Dermatology*

It is frequently aggravated at the commencement of puberty, or the patient's attention to it may be aroused at that age when "le désir de plaire" is naturally nascent in the mind.

It may be associated with other sebaceous disorders prone to develop at that period, but such association is by no means constant or essential.

There is always a certain amount of concomitant vascular hypertrophy or telangiectasis, but the amount present varies within very wide limits, being in certain cases so inconspicuous as to attract no attention, whilst in others it constitutes the main feature of the disease.

Telangiectases often coexist in regions other than those affected by the sebaceous changes, and to this clinical type the additional epithet "telangiectatic" may reasonably be applied.

Other degenerative or "naevoid" conditions of skin are often also present (warts, true naevi, molluscum fibrosum, pigment changes, etc.), the association being so frequent as to suggest their possible dependence upon a common cause.

The subjects of the disease appear to be generally intellectually below par; all those cases hitherto observed have been in members of the lower orders.

Apparently females are more frequently affected than males.

The disease is absolutely benign, and unattended by subjective symptoms unless complicated by other affections.

Its tendency is to increase up to, and remain stationary after, puberty; or to disappear slowly, leaving shallow, atrophic scars which ultimately fill up.

It can be removed by operative procedures, but may afterwards recur *in loco*.

---

* Brit. J.Dermat., *2:*1, 1890.

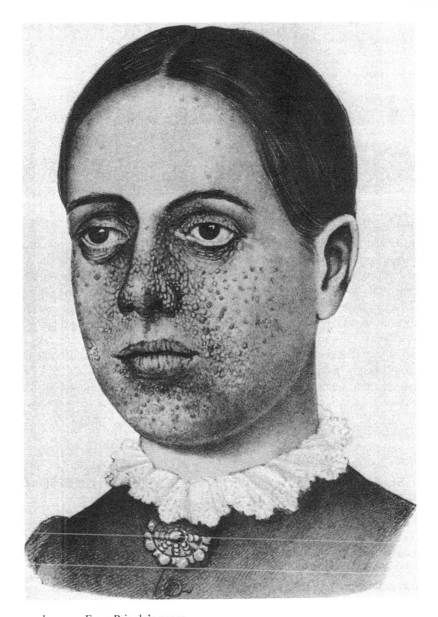

Figure 48 Adenoma sebaceum. From Pringle's paper

Thomas Colcott Fox

Erythema Gyratum Perstans

THOMAS COLCOTT FOX was born in 1848 in Broughton Hants. He was educated at University College School and was graduated as M.B. London in 1876. His first medical appointment was that of super-intendent of the Fulham Smallpox Hospital. The meteoric success of his talented older brother, Tilbury, attracted him irresistibly toward dermatology, and he was early in his career appointed Physician to the Department of Diseases of the Skin at Westminster Hospital, a post he held until his death in 1916.

He was not a prolific writer. His contributions to dermatologic literature were chiefly clinical in nature, with the notable exception of his mycologic research in which he confirmed and added to the work of Sabouraud. In addition to the disease the account of which is given here, he added much to the knowledge of the tuberculids, dermatitis factitia, and pityriasis rosea.

Fox was unassuming and sincere; he was an enthusiastic sportsman, an admirable skater, and a better than average golfer.*

ERYTHEMA GYRATUM PERSTANS

Erythema Gyratum Perstans in the Two Elder Members of a Family*

George W.T., aged 19½ years, and his sister, Sarah Ann T., aged 18 years, are affected in a precisely similar manner with an erythematous eruption of the skin from which they have never been entirely free since its onset in each case at about the age of three or four years only. The exact age of origin is a little doubtful but it was in infancy. The patients are the two elder children of a family of five, who are all alive and healthy. The family history is quite devoid of any facts throwing light on the case.

The description of the eruption in one case will serve for both, although the attacks are rather more severe and extensive in the brother. The eruption begins by the evolution of scattered, isolated, slightly raised, erythematous papules, about the size of a millet seed, effaceable temporarily by pressure, accompanied by the most intolerable itching, which at its height destroys the sleep and much distresses the patient. These papules quickly extend centrifugally, whilst the central hyperemia as rapidly subsides, so that in a few hours after the appearance of a papule we observe a circular area of skin pigmented but otherwise normal, ever enlarging in exact ratio with the narrow, slightly raised, advancing erythematous border. Such areas

---

* Pringle, J., and Adamson, H.: Brit. J.Dermat., *28:*93, 1916.

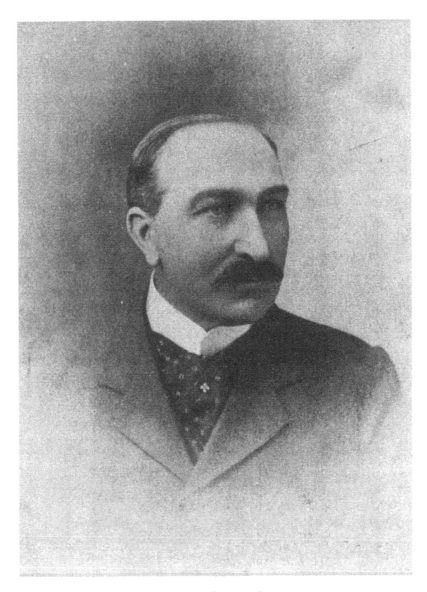

Figure 49 Thomas Colcott Fox. Courtesy, *British Journal of Dermatology*

complete their desquamation so rapidly that there is only a ragged cuticular fringe adherent to the inner edge of the advancing erythematous border of the ring, but this white fringe constitutes a very curious and conspicuous feature. Now as these rings continue to enlarge, which they may do up to about the size of the palm of the hand, they meet other adjoining similar rings and fuse together, and so in time large tracts of skin are covered with festooned and gyrate figures. The skin over which the erythema has travelled resumes in a few days its normal condition, excepting as regards the pigmentation. Both patients are subject to recurrent non-febrile outbreaks of greater or less intensity, which occur at least every three months, and last

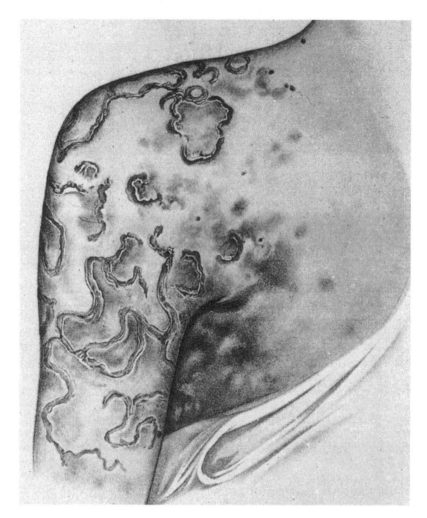

Figure 50 Erythema gyratum perstans. From Fox's paper

from 10 days to six weeks according to the severity, and then the greater part of the trunk, with the extremities, especially their extensor surfaces, may be attacked; but in the intervals also between these outbreaks there is a continuous evolution of papules here and there, particularly over the shoulders, the thighs and buttocks, and in the girl the popliteal spaces, so that I have never yet seen the skin absolutely free; and thus it has been, the patient informs me, ever since they were about four years of age. The palms and soles, the face, neck, and scalp are never attacked, and rarely the dorsal surfaces of the hands and feet. The patients associate the special outbreaks with changes in the season or in the weather, and they say the disease is always less intense in the winter. The male patient further notices that the eruption will start from the region of any scratch or cut, and experience teaches him that an attack will quickly and certainly follow any irregularity of living.

The patients have been under my observation from time to time ever since. The eruption has presented but few variations, and these have been due to the greater or lessened intensity of the evolution.

I do not think the name, *Erythema gyratum perstans,* which I chose, a good one, but until further experience accumulates it will perhaps be best not to coin another for this remarkable persistent circinate pruritic dermatitis.

---

* International Atlas of Rare Skin Diseases. Hamburg, 1891, Part XVI.

Ernst Schweninger

Multiple Benign Tumor-like New Growths of the Skin (Schweninger-Buzzi Anetoderma)

ERNST SCHWENINGER was born on June 15, 1850, in Freistadt, Germany. He received his medical training in Munich, and from 1870 to 1879 served as assistant to the pathologist, Buhl. His academic connections were severed in 1879, following which he attained publicity and fame by proposing a fluid restriction weight reduction diet which bears his name.

In 1884 he was called to Berlin as Bismarck's personal physician, and concomitantly was made Professor of Dermatology at the University of Berlin. This political appointment of a man ignorant in the field of dermatology was strongly protested by the faculty, but to no avail. Schweninger assumed control, and with a frequently changing staff of army physicians he developed an active skin clinic at Charité Hospital.

He was a dynamic individual, expounding his ideas with vigor, and constantly disagreeing with the faculty. For over 14 years he was Bismarck's friend, confidant and physician. As such, he actively entered into political life, at times assailing classical academic medicine. His interest in dermatology gradually declined, although he continued to publish a number of articles, including the selection below. Not until 1902, four years after Bismarck's death, was the faculty successful in partially deposing Schweninger. At that time he accepted a post in general pathology, therapeutics, and the history of medicine. This marked the termination of his role in dermatology.

During the ensuing years, he sought to found a naturalistic school of medicine. This project was bitterly opposed by academic physicians, and in 1906 he left Berlin, later returning to Munich where he remained until his death. He died on January 13, 1924 after a long lingering illness.*

ANETODERMA (LOCALIZED ELASTOLYSIS)

Multiple Benign Tumour-like New Growth of the Skin[†]

Mrs. A., 29 years of age, does not remember ever having been ill. Has been married eight years. Six months after marriage some little white flat elevations appeared on the upper part of her back which according to her account became somewhat rapidly enlarged and more numerous. Though the patient felt no inconvenience from the "white things" she nevertheless consulted a physician who prescribed arsenic and sea salt baths. This treatment which was continued for several months had no perceptible effect. Subsequently the small elevations increased slowly but surely especially between the shoulder blades. Four years ago the disease spread to the shoulder blades, somewhat later to a slight degree to the upper part of the arms and at the end of 1887 the chest was suddenly attacked with from 20 to 30 elevations. In consequence of the appearance of

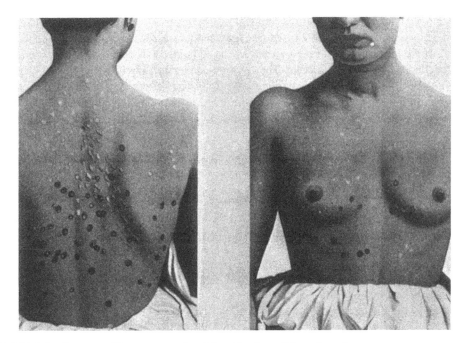

Figure 51 Multiple benign tumor-like new growths of the skin. From Schweninger's paper

a similar formation below the chin the patient in 1889 applied at the University polyclinic for skin disease in the Charité Hospital of Berlin.

Present State. The plates show fairly well the topography of the multiple formations though those on the arms and the one on the chin are not visible. On the back the formations extend over the dorsal region while the lumbar region is free. They are most numerous and dense between and above the shoulder blades and are distributed irregularly. Several also exist along the spine while on each side they become fewer in number and have a linear arrangement according to the natural furrows of the skin. There are also some 30 irregularly scattered on the chest.

These formations are of a size from a lentil up to a sixpence and have a more or less rounded contour. They are quite round on the chest and on the middle line of the back, oval with the longest diameter towards the lines of cleavage on the sides of the thorax. The colour is usually more or less white but with a slightly blue tint. The dilated orifices of the follicles appear prominent in most cases as thick black points. The lanugo hairs on the formations are as well developed as those on the surrounding skin. Some of the formations on the upper part of the chest and back are of a peculiar slate colour with delicate interlaced vascular dilatations. On these parts one sees and feels instead of an elevation a distinct depression, a change which according to the patient has occurred spontaneously.

The smallest formations, about a lentil in size, look like vesicles, the larger ones like somewhat withered bullae. Stretching the surrounding skin removes this appearance, leaving at the most a whitish mark with the dilated orifices of follicles. By pressure most of the formations can be forced into the deeper skin producing

---

* Hoffman, E.: Dermat. Zeitschr., *40:*252, 1924.

† International Atlas of Rare Skin Diseases. Hamburg, 1891, Part XV.

on the surface a shallow pit. Soon after the removal of the finger the swelling reappears like an umbilical hernia. This phenomenon occurs chiefly in the smaller elevations and where the skin is freely movable such as on the side of the thorax. Some of the formations on the interscapular and sternal regions are somewhat hard to the touch and cannot be pressed in. They appear as elevations only when viewed with a side light, while to the touch the actual elevation is hardly perceptible. The patient assures us most positively that the larger elevations spring from the smaller ones, and our own observations confirm this view. In the process of extension they become flatter, less white but harder and consequently less compressible. The formations never exceed a diameter of 2 cm. and when they reach the maximum size a process simulating involution begins at the same time as the other changes. Other formations remain stationary, that is to say, white, small and vesicular looking.

The patient states that she feels no subjective local or other symptoms during the appearance of the formations. There is no tenderness or pain either, when pressed, and tactile sensation is normal. When squeezed only a trace of sebum can occasionally be forced out of the follicles. In every respect the patient is healthy both as regards the skin and other organs with the single exception of frequent herpes labialis during menstruation.

None of the known changes in the skin are in any way similar to this case, but nevertheless it is of importance because little is known of the value of the elastic tissue and its changes as well as its attachments and distribution.

This case is also of much value for the scientific investigation of tumours as regards their origin, course and development. Without any primary local disturbance of circulation, simply by a passive change of the tissue an active change in other tissue results in a manner formerly unknown. The passive change is atrophy by retraction of the elastic tissue, and the active changes consist in the proliferation of the sheaths of the glands and vessels as well as the glands and vessels themselves without mentioning other less remarkable changes. These facts justify us in giving no better title for the case than that of "Multiple benign tumor-like new growths of the Skin."

Sigmund Pollitzer

Acanthosis Nigricans

SIGMUND POLLITZER was born on Staten Island, New York, November 1, 1859. He was graduated from the College of the City of New York, with honors, in physics, astronomy, and mathematics. In 1882 he took his master's degree at the same institution. His first publication, a manual of logarithmic computation, enjoyed considerable success. He next entered Columbia and took his M.D. there in 1884 submitting as his thesis an original piece of research, *Temperature Sense,* which was later published in the *British Journal of Physiology*. Following his graduation, Pollitzer went abroad where he worked in Heidelberg, Wiesbaden, and Berlin, doing research in physiology, bacteriology, and general medicine. When the war between Serbia and Bulgaria broke out, in 1885, he volunteered for service with the Serbians and after heading two of the base hospitals was discharged as a major at the close of hostilities.

Returning to the United States, Pollitzer practiced general medicine for three years with indifferent success and, turning his attention to dermatology, again went abroad where he studied with Unna, became that master's favorite, and later worked with Malcolm Morris. After a stay in Paris, where he formed a close association with Darier, Pollitzer returned to the United States, and became Professor of Dermatology at the New York Post-Graduate Medical School and Hospital, which post he held until 1915.

Pollitzer was not a prolific writer; his early basic science training is reflected in all his meticulously worded papers. Besides the definitive account of acanthosis nigricans we have presented below, he wrote of hydradenitis destruens suppurativa, parakeratosis variegata, and the xanthomas. He was one of the first to use arsphenamine in the treatment of syphilis, and was an early worker in the serodiagnosis of that disease. In 1920 he translated his friend Darier's *Précis* into English.

A lively participant in discussion and a keen critic, his comments were pertinent and a little sharp. His insistence on regular parliamentary procedure often involved him in polemics from which he emerged more frequently in defeat than victory.

His death in 1937 brought to a close a 47 year career in dermatology.*

ACANTHOSIS NIGRICANS

Acanthosis Nigricans[†]

The following case was admitted to Dr. Unna's Clinic for Skin Diseases in Hamburg in July, 1889, and by him very kindly entrusted to me for study and publication.

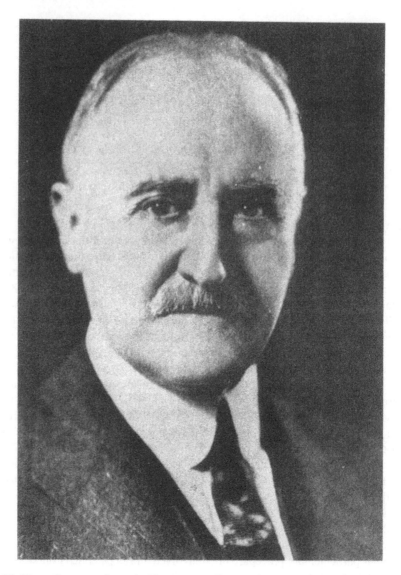

Figure 52 Sigmund Pollitzer. Courtesy, *Journal of Investigative Dermatology*

Mrs. J., aged 62 years, widow. No history of tuberculosis or of syphilis. Patient has always enjoyed excellent health. The disease for which she consulted Dr. Unna had existed for about eight weeks, and attacked all the affected regions at about the same time. There was at first everywhere except on the hands a slight pricking sensation which ceased in the course of a few days; at the commissures of the lips the affection began as, and was at first thought by the patient to be, a simple fissure or "crack." Status. The disease affects the upper extremities, the neck, the mouth, part of the trunk and genito-crural regions. The skin of the hands is in general of a dirty brownish colour; on the dorsum manus there are patches of a bluish-grey, somewhat deeper in colour along the course of the veins. The normal areas of the cuticle are very prominent, standing out somewhat convex and with a glassy shimmer. Some of them show several glittering points corresponding to the smaller sub-divisions of the cuticular areas. The natural furrows are deeply marked, the skin of the entire hands looking as if it were too large for them. On the back of the proximal phalanx of the thumb there is a patch the size of a shilling in which the dirty discolouration and the prominence of the cuticular areas are especially marked, giving the patch the appearance of a diffuse flat wart. The skin of the entire hand is rough and unelastic. The palms are slightly darker than normal, their furrows and folds are strongly marked and the skin feels dry, hard and thickened.

On the anterior surface of the lower one-third of the fore-arm the peculiar discolouration is very striking and numerous small brownish patches (like ephelides) are to be seen. On the dorsal surface of the fore-arms the discolouration is especially marked over and along the course of a vein. On the upper arms there are several lentil-sized warts which are said to be of recent development.

The neck appears as if encircled by a dirty greyish band which sends irregular offshoots downwards towards the sternum, clavicles, shoulders and scapulae, and upwards toward the face. The skin here shows the changes described as existing on the hands, but in a much more marked degree. Some of the cuticular areas project above the general level almost like papillae, others are flatter; the whole running together to form a diffuse, discoloured warty surface. Similar changes are seen in both axillae and under both breasts, only that here the colouration is rather greyish-white. On the abdomen there are a few horizontal streaky indications of a similar condition. The crurogenital folds and the large labia show the same changes in a marked degree. The entire region presents a greyish discolouration and diffuse warty prominences, the latter especially marked in a greyish-white patch the size of a florin, to the right of the vulva.

There is a slight indication of the disease on the chin and on both auricles.

From the beginning the tongue and mouth have been painful. The anterior one-half of the hard palate is covered with fine granulations resembling small venereal warts but softer to the touch than those growths. A few outlying patches of a similar growth are seen on the posterior half of the palate. The upper surface of the tongue, especially in the middle line is covered with more or less prominent condylomatoid growths, the marked process sparing only a narrow strip on each side extending from behind forwards to a point about 2 mm. from the tip. These lateral strips are free from prominences, smooth and of a bluish white colour; and at their borders, as they merge into the affected region, there are numerous small discrete papillary growths. Underneath the plate of artificial teeth the depressions for the teeth on the lower jaw are seen to be occupied by similar warty growths. A like condition is seen on the mucous membrane of the upper lip and extends for about 2 mm. beyond the commissures of the lips, as an irregular prominent greyish mass.

The affection on the hands and other parts was treated with daily inunctions of soft soap, and washing with a soda solution. Under this treatment the discolouration and the thickening became markedly less, and the skin of the hands resumed an almost normal appearance.

The improvement in the condition of the skin and mouth was progressive and by the end of February, 1890, the patient was practically well, so far as the peculiar affection of the skin and mucous membrane was concerned. At the same time, however, the oedema of the feet was becoming more marked and the patient complained of great general feebleness. Repeated examinations of the urine showed neither albumen nor casts, but it was observed that the daily quantity was under the normal. From about the beginning of February the oliguria and the anasarca gradually increased and considerable meteorism was noticed together with a little abdominal ascites. The daily quantity of urine steadily diminished—no albumen or

---

* U.J.W.: Arch. of Dermat. and Syph., *37:*499, 1938.

† International Atlas of Rare Skin Diseases. Hamburg, 1891, Part X.

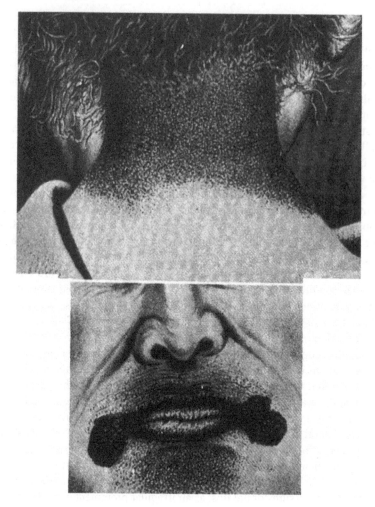

Figure 53 Acanthosis nigricans. From Pollitzer's paper

morphological renal elements being at any time present—till on the 8th of April complete anuria supervened, death resulting from heart failure, without signs of uraemia, on April 14th. A post-mortem examination was not permitted. The diagnosis of Dr. Michael and Dr. Bülau, who met him in consultation, was that of Carcinoma occultum.

No case bearing a close analogy to this has been recorded. That, which perhaps most nearly approaches it, was published by Hardaway in his monograph in *Papilloma cutis* under the title of *General idiopathic papilloma,* which occurred in an infant of seven months. The points of divergence however are more striking than those of similarity.

I concur in Dr. Unna's opinion, that the term Papilloma and its derivative Papillomatosis are unhappily chosen, Virchow having long since insisted that the adjective papillary was a permissible epithet for a growth, but not the substantive Papilloma. The denomination, *Acanthosis,* derived from Auspitz's group of Acanthomata has therefore been applied to this disease by Dr. Unna in his demonstrations of the case. The qualifying adjective *("nigricans")* was selected as descriptive of the blackish colour of the affected regions.

Ernest Besnier

Atopic Dermatitis

ERNEST HENRI BESNIER was born in Honfleur in 1831. He studied in Paris, and was a celebrated pupil of Hardy and Bazin. Having been graduated in 1857, he turned his attention exclusively to dermatology, and by 1872 had become a chief at l'Hôpital Saint Louis. He left in 1896.

Besnier was active in all phases of dermatology. Although essentially French in his diathetic thinking, he was responsible for translating Kaposi's text into French, with masterful annotations by himself. His monograph on psoriasis, his work on atopic dermatitis (the prurigo of the piece included here), and his work on eczema entitle him to his place as the leading French dermatologist of his time. Great as were his contributions to clinical dermatology, his highest attainment was as a teacher. At his death in 1909 a pupil, J.J.Pringle, noted:

"No one who ever attended his clinics can forget the tender thoroughness with which every patient was examined, the grace and accuracy of the language in which all points were demonstrated or elucidated, the unflagging and disinterested zeal of the master's labour, and the delicate—and withal affectionate—irony which he displayed toward his pupils."*

ATOPIC DERMATITIS

Première note et observations préliminaires pour servir d'introduction a l'étude des prurigos diathésiques*

The multiform, pruriginous, chronic, exacerbating, and paroxysmal dermatitis which the illustrious Hebra described in unforgettable terms under the name "prurigo," and which we call the prurigo of Hebra, is not the only one to which we may apply the spirit, if not the absolute letter of his description.

Several species of this dermatologic genus, or if you wish, several forms of this disease or syndrome do not fit into the much too narrow group outlined by the Viennese master, and have strayed into the composite groups of a series of banal dermatidides in the first order of which is found the lichen of the authors who preceded Hebra, and of several of the contemporary and present teachers of the French school, and into the chronic eczemas although they are, in any case, neither lichens nor true eczema, but always multiform

---

* Brit. J.Dermat., *21:*226, 1909.

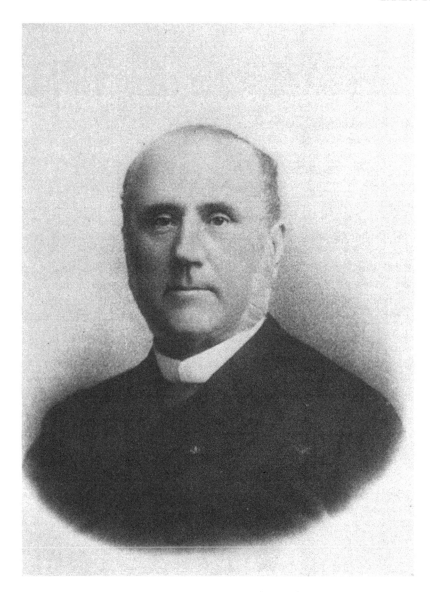

Figure 54 Ernest Besnier. Courtesy, *Annales de Dermatologie et Syphiligraphie*

dermatidides in which eczematization or lichenification dominates different periods of the disease, being important lesions of it, but not the essential ones.

The time has come to put an end to these ambiguities and confusions, to purge the lichen group, and proceeding to the eczemas, to remove the various species that have strayed there, and re-classify them in natural groups.

The first group which it is urgent to place with the affections which we designate by the name prurigos diathésiques can be, henceforth, based upon a group of features the unity of which is glaring, and separates them from the groups in which they have been misplaced. Its first symptom and prime symptom is pruritus, intense pruritus, remitting, exacerbating, with nocturnal paroxysms, with seasonal remissions and exacerbations. Usually it appears in infancy or childhood, but also at other ages, often in an insidious and almost always larvate manner. It is an absolutely fundamental characteristic that none of the lesions that accompany it or are provoked by it is specific; in infancy it may be any one of the numerous varieties of infantile erythemas, the urticarias, or pseudo-lichens, or one of the forms of eczematization or lichenification of the skin commonly known as milk scab.

Later, when the disease is established, one may still see one of these forms reappear, but usually lichenifications are seen which may be papular, in plaques or in large sheets and, with the paroxysms, eczematization in a variety of forms— figured, diffuse, impetiginous, etc.

When the disease begins in infancy it may stay within narrow limits, remain incomplete, abort, or, after several years duration, go into an intermission which is more or less long, or even permanent. In many of the cases the process abandons the skin, temporarily or permanently, for visceral sites, producing later, as its predominating manifestation, emphysema, bronchial asthma, hay fever, and more rarely gastrointestinal troubles.

In all the cases in which it has been established for a time, even when it has had an external provocative agent, the disease becomes a marked property of the individual, a pruritic diathesis; it may attenuate or diminish, but it is rebellious to all medications; if it clears up or burns out one may never say that he was responsible for curing it. It is a true pruriginous diathesis with multiform lesions, about which one can do no more than give it a name; it is a prurigo in the true sense of the word, a prurigo diathésique.

---

* Ann. de dermat. et syph., *3:*634, 1892.

H.G.Brooke

Epithelioma Adenoides Cysticum (Trichoepithelioma)

HENRY AMBROSE GRUNDY BROOKE was born in Lancashire in 1854. He received his medical education in Manchester and London. After qualification he spent two years in Vienna and Paris studying dermatology, and diseases of the ear and throat. He returned to Manchester to accept the post of physician to the Manchester and Salford Hospital for Skin Diseases, soon built up a tremendous practice in the Midlands and North of England, and became known as "Brooke of Manchester."

Brooke is most remembered for his identification of epithelioma adenoides cysticum given below, and for his work on arsenical eruptions, keratosis follicularis contagiosa, seborrhea, and allergic skin diseases. His interest in the latter was stimulated by a marked sensitivity he himself had to eggs.

He was an accomplished amateur musician, and an excellent judge of painting. His mordant wit and gift for making epigrams were well known. Of a pompous contemporary he said: "*Blank's* papers usually begin with a quotation from Herbert Spencer and end with lead lotion."

He died in Manchester in 1919.*

EPITHELIOMA ADENOIDES CYSTICUM

Epithelioma Adenoides Cysticum*

The affection presents itself in the form of small tumors, varying in size from the head of a pin, projecting very slightly above the surface, to that of the half of a small pea. They are at first of the color of the surrounding skin, or may be a little darker, as if some minute body of neutral tint were imbedded beneath the epidermis. As the growths increase in size, they become often shining and translucent, but hardly sufficiently so to suggest that they really contain fluid. Some have a faint yellowish or bluish tinge. Nearly all contain one or more minute milium-like bodies, which are plainly visible to even a casual inspection. The size of these bodies bears no marked relation to that of the lesions in which they occur, some of the larger nodules presenting no external signs of containing any, whilst a small nodule here and there seems to be nearly filled up by its white contents; again, two or three may occur in one nodule.

As regards the feel of the papules, all the writers are unanimous. They are firm without being hard, and if taken between the fingers can be felt to lie in the skin and to move with it.

---

* Little, G.: Delib. 9th Cong. Dermat., Budapest, *4:*144, 1935.

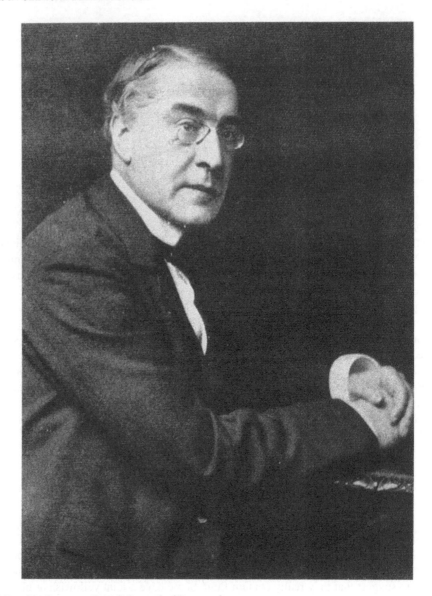

Figure 55 H.G.Brooke. Courtesy, *British Journal of Dermatology*

The sites of predilection were the space between the eyebrows, the root of the nose and neighboring area of the cheeks, the upper lip, and to a less extent the chin. In these situations they become so thickly grouped together as to form raised lumpy patches of most disfiguring appearance. They also occurred on the back, in the middle line between the shoulders, and later on they were found scattered as solitary papules about the rest of the face, on the scalp, especially the front portion, and in one case (Mrs. E.) freely on the tragus and auracephalic furrow, where they formed thickly grouped masses as on the face. They were strewn thinly

* Brit. J.Dermat., *4:*269, 1892.

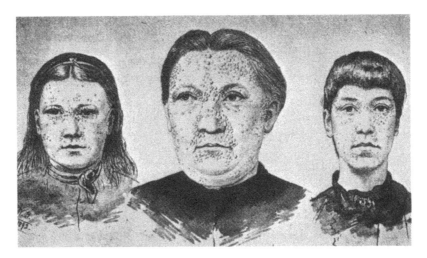

Figure 56 Epithelioma adenoides cysticum. From Brooke's paper

over the shoulders and upper part of the back, on the neck and upper part of the arms, and slightly on the chest.

The course of the affection is always slow, but may vary at times, taking on a sudden acceleration even after many years' duration. It begins in youth, for the most part between the tenth and fourteenth year, so far as the insidious and inconspicuous origin of the growth will allow the patient to judge. The lesions either persist unchanged for years or increase until they reach the size of a small pea, a limit which they never exceed.

The symptoms, if any are present, are very slight, at most a little pricking when the skin is hot, or an occasional itching.

William F.Milroy

Hereditary Edema of the Legs (Milroy's Disease)

WILLIAM FORSYTH MILROY was born December 28, 1855; in New York City. He was educated at the University of Rochester, Johns Hopkins, and Columbia, taking his degree at the latter institution in 1882. Two years later he moved to Nebraska, and began practice in Omaha, where he remained until the late 1930s.

When Milroy arrived in Omaha in 1884, medicine was not of the high caliber to be found there now. He contributed much to the establishment of progressive practice in the young city. Besides the account of the disease named for him, given here, he did important work on typhoid fever and its relation to the water supply of the area. He was President of the old Omaha Medical College, and in 1894 wrote the first and only complete record of pioneer medical history in Omaha.

The last few years of his life were spent in California. He died in 1942.

It is interesting that some years after he had seen Milroy, the patient described below had occasion to consult a London physician, and was told that he had "Milroy's disease."*

HEREDITARY EDEMA OF THE LEGS

An Undescribed Variety of Hereditary Edema*

On August 20, 1891, Mr. H. presented himself for examination for life insurance. He was an American, a clergyman, 31 years of age, six feet and one-half inch in height, and weighed 178 pounds. His habits were the best, and he had never been sick in his life. With regard to longevity, his family history was excellent. Physical examination revealed nothing abnormal with regard to the thoracic or abdominal viscera. The applicant called my attention to his lower extremities. I found a condition of oedema involving the feet and extending up the legs to the knees. It was, and the patient states had always been, somewhat more marked in the left extremity than in the right. Upon inspection, the leg presented a slightly rosy hue, extending around its whole circumference and involving the whole extremity, gradually disappearing near the knee. When lightly pressed, the color disappeared, but returned quickly when the pressure was removed. Scattered thickly over this base were white spots about the size of a pea. These also were found over every part of the leg as far as the rosy color extended. This appearance of the leg, according to the statement of the applicant, is constant. There were no varicose veins and no evidence of bad nutrition, nor was there any tendency to

---

* Tyler, A., and Auerbach, E.: History of Medicine in Nebraska, p. 217. Magic City Printing Co., Omaha, 1928.

ulceration in any part of the leg. The circumference of the calf of the leg at its largest part was 17 inches, and the smallest circumference of the ankle was 14 inches. Deep pressure with the finger over the crest of the tibia, at a point near its middle, produced a depression which was distinctly apparent to both touch and sight 10 minutes after the pressure was removed. This will convey an idea of the well-marked character of the oedema. The pitting on pressure was quite evident as far up as the tubercle of the tibia, but not over the patella or above it. Mr. H. stated that this oedematous enlargement had existed from birth. As he had grown in stature, the oedematous parts had grown so as to preserve the same size relative to the remainder of the body. It had always been free from pain, showed no disposition to ulcerate, and in short had never given him the least inconvenience. In the evening, if he had been on his feet a good deal during the day, the swelling seemed somewhat greater than in the morning, the skin appearing rather tense.

The applicant stated that this enlargement of the extremities was a family characteristic which he had inherited from his mother. Fortunately for the purpose of this study, the family of Mr. H's mother is one which has been long in America, and has been productive in New England. In 1883 a member of the family published a neat volume, giving the family history in America for a period of 250 years. It should be remarked, however, that the peculiarity now under discussion seems to have entered the family by marriage about 1768. With the aid of this volume and the assistance of members of the family still living, I am able to offer the facts which I present, feeling that they are thoroughly reliable, though not at every point as complete as could be desired.

It thus appears that in the six generations of the family, comprising 97 individuals, there have been 22 cases of this deformity, or about 23 per cent of the whole number. Of the 22 cases, 12 were males, seven females, and three unknown, appearing to show that it is rather more common among the males than females of the family. In the later generations the percentage of cases is about as large as in the earlier, but there is a decided decrease in the extent of the oedema in most of them.

Atavism is frequently apparent in the development of the family peculiarity. I have not been able to learn that treatment has been undertaken for the cure of the affection in any case.

The invariable characteristics of the disorder have been: 1. Congenital origin with a steady growth corresponding to the normal growth of the body until adult size is attained. 2. The limitation of the oedema to one or both lower extremities, the area involved varying. 3. Permanence of the oedema. 4. Entire absence of constitutional symptoms, or local symptoms aside from those described.

---

* New York Med. J., *56:*505, 1892.

Émile Vidal

Keratosis Blennorrhagica

ÉMILE VIDAL was born in Paris, June 18, 1825, received his medical training at Tours and Paris, completed it in 1855, and entitled his thesis *Considerations on Chronic Progressive Rheumatism*. After an early interest in general medicine and pediatrics, which he never completely lost, he took an appointment as physician to l'Hôpital Saint Louis in Paris in 1861, and profiting from his association with such men as Bazin, Hardy, and Laieller, soon acquired a service of his own. Vidal was a prolific writer on all aspects of dermatology, and was one of the earliest workers in cutaneous pathology. He was especially interested in lupus vulgaris and the lichens, being the first to bring real order to this difficult latter group. His studies culminated in the masterful work of his pupil Brocq on neurodermatitis circumscripta.

He was charming personally, fond of society, and popular in the salons. His pupils regarded him almost as a father, and frequently in their early struggles they got from him material as well as spiritual aid. Brocq said of him:

"The penetration of his mind was truly marvelous. He examined the patient with a vivacity and dexterity which was not soon forgotten. He left nothing unexplored, discovering the decisive point with an almost uncanny rapidity. He pronounced a word and the diagnosis was made. His pupils had on numerous occasions admired this almost infallible diagnostic ability. One felt himself to be in the presence of a born clinician. It was in the midst of his patients, surrounded by his pupils and visiting physicians, indefatigable, animated, excited by his successes, that one should see him, follow and observe him, in order to understand the worth of such a man, his devotion to science, his ardor in relieving those who entrusted themselves to his care."

He died in 1893, universally respected in medical circles, having devoted some 30 years to the advance of his chosen specialty.*

KERATOSIS BLENNORRHAGICA

Éruption Cornée d'Origine Blennorrhagique[†]

Observation. C.—, Alphonse, age 24, book binder by profession, is a man of average build, of a nervous temperament.

---

* Beeson, B.: Arch. of Dermat. and Syph., *22:*115, 1930.

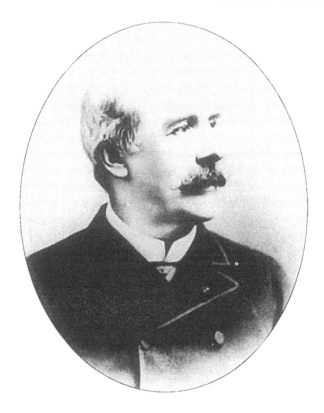

Figure 57 Émile Vidal

At the age of 18 contracted gonorrhea and soft chancre. The gonorrhea cleared up rapidly with no complication. The chancres cicatrized in less than three weeks.

On the 25th of February 1890 he noticed a new attack of gonorrhea which was quite acute; this was the beginning and the origin of the infectious symptoms which obliged him to spend several months in the hospital. In the first few days in the month of May sharp pains in the right knee forced him to enter the Charity Hospital.

Several joints became painful; on May 12th the left knee was attacked as well by typical gonorrheal arthritis.

In the first few days of April, without the patient being able to indicate the exact date, he quickly developed, on the skin of the anterior part of the right knee, crusts which persisted even several weeks later, and of which we will speak in describing the cutaneous lesions at the time of entrance into l'Hôpital Saint Louis.

Toward the end of April, crusts of the same type formed on the feet and on the hands, much more abundant in the plantar and palmar regions. The patient says that these crusts were preceded neither by vesicles nor bullae.

[†] Ann. de dermat. et syph., *4:*3, 1893.

This eruption brought him to l'Hôpital Saint Louis; he was admitted to my service (Devergie Ward no. 44), 27 May, 1890.

Present condition. The patient is pale, emaciated, profoundly cachectic, and condemned to dorsal decubitus by the prolonged suffering from gonorrheal polyarthritis.

The right knee is still very tumefied, and immobilized by pain. The right scapulo-humeral articulation is painful. The middle finger of the right hand is swollen, red, and painful at the level of the articulation of the first and second phalanges. This small articulation is also the seat of a gonorrheal arthritis.

The skin attracts the attention because of an extraordinary dermopathy, a symmetrical and generalized eruption of hard, horny, dry scales without a trace of moisture or oozing. Small and disseminated on the head, on the face, and on the trunk, these scales become larger on the trunk, and are proportionately more abundant as one approaches the extremities, especially the lower extremities.

The right hand is much more involved than the left. The palmar surface shows yellow brown crusts, some isolated, others confluent, some flat, others projecting, imbedded in a very thickened epidermis, strongly adherent, and bearing a very great resemblance to the cornified syphilid.

The fingers are unequally involved, discrete crusts on their external, internal and anterior surfaces. They are more abundant toward the end of the fingers, where they run together to form a thick horny crust enveloping all the end of the finger, and lifting the nail which is already almost detached. Pressure causes drops of pus to ooze out from the subungual tissue. These horny productions are surrounded by a shiny reddening.

The left hand, much less affected, presents only three small horny crusts, yellowish, on the palmar surface. The last two fingers are unaffected. The crusts elevate the free edge of the nails of the first three fingers.

The arms and forearms are very little affected. Small disseminated horny crusts are seen there, which resemble small droplets of yellow wax, both in their coloring and semi-transparency. They are in general discrete; one finds them grouped only at the external margin of the right forearm.

While around the left knee very few crusted elements are seen, on the anterior surface of the right knee (seat of a gonorrheal arthritis) the crusts are more abundant, larger, yellowish in appearance, waxy, forming conical projections from 1 to 3 mm. above the level of the skin, arranged in two groups, one superiorly situated, just above the patella, and one inferiorly, made up of smaller elements.

The right foot is less involved than the left. The skin of its dorsal surface is normal.

That of the dorsal surface of the last three toes is covered over by a yellow brown horny envelope, thicker on the prominences of the inter-phalangeal articulations.

The extremity of the last three toes is capped by a horny covering which is beginning to elevate the nails. A veritable cutaneous horn, which is somewhat transparent, and forms a cone a centimeter and a half high, with a base not more than a centimeter in diameter, stands on the dorsal surface of the fifth toe at the level of the articulation of the first phalanx with the second.

The plantar surface of the foot, on all the parts that rest on the ground, is covered by a horny crust in the form of a horse shoe, concave toward the internal margin. This horny plaque is thicker and harder under the heel and the base of the toes. In these regions it is partly broken up and exfoliating, lifting up in large, thick and hard scales.

The lesion goes beyond the plantar surface of the foot, and extends a little over the edges.

On the left foot the same lesions are found, but are more accentuated.

The extremities of all the toes are covered by a horny crust, more complete and thicker than those on the right hand. All the nails appear elevated.

There is a conical crust the diameter of a 50-centime piece, completely cornified, along the internal margin. In detaching it, a papule is exposed to view which is a little moist and papillomatous.

Another similar crust is seen in the area of the external malleolus.

On the anterior surface of the chest, on the back, and on the abdomen, crusts are present which are small, convex, dry and hard, and which for the most part do not exceed the size of a millet seed. Generally isolated, they are at some points grouped together. Reddish macules, some pigmented, indicate sites previously occupied by crusts which have fallen off.

On the face and on the ears some small crusts are seen.

There are some, a little larger, on the scalp.

Vittorio Mibelli

1. *Angiokeratoma*

2. *Porokeratosis*

VITTORIO MIBELLI was born February 18, 1860, in Portoferraio on the island; Elba. He began his studies in Siena, and after further training in Florence returned to Siena as a prosector at the anatomical institute, and later an assistant at the dermatologic clinic in that city. Qualifying as a dermatologist in 1888, he spent the next year in Hamburg at Unna's clinic. After two years in Cagliari he was called to Parma, and held the Professorship in Dermatology there until his death, April 26, 1910.

From his early anatomical training and his time with Unna, Mibelli acquired a great interest in histopathology, and many of his publications deal with this phase of dermatology. He was particularly interested in hydroa vacciniforme, fixed drug eruptions, acne keloid, and the keratoses. A skilled mycologist, he was one of the early proponents of the theory of plurality of the trichophyton group. We have selected the two disease descriptions for which he is most remembered, porokeratosis and angiokeratoma, both of which are sometimes known as Mibelli's disease. Other of his important clinical works deal with urticaria pigmentosa, the etiology of alopecia areata, and exfoliatio linguae areata.

Mibelli was an ideal teacher for the beginning student in dermatology, as well as for the most advanced. His thorough knowledge of his material, and his careful and well organized presentation, without histrionics or verbosity, made him the easiest of lecturers to understand.*

ANGIOKERATOMA

Angiokeratoma[†]

Louise Palazzi, 14 years old, from Rosignano Maritlimo (Italy), residing at Siena in St. Catherine Pension, has had the following affection for some years.

On the dorsal surface of the fingers, especially on the middle and terminal phalanges, several small transparent tumors are to be seen, of the size of a hempseed, some almost spherical in shape, others larger and longer. They are lead coloured, but some are violet or dark red, with still darker superficial points. Their surface is rough and sometimes prickly. These tumours are of the consistence of horn, and are sharply defined from the surrounding skin which does not manifest the slightest sign of inflammation. Scattered between them are small spots almost of the size of a grain of corn, the centres of which are of a darker red colour than the periphery. The epidermis covering them is hard, almost horny, but smooth and without a trace of desquamation. Here and there are seen transition-forms between the spots and the tumours described above. The peculiar colour of the spots and tumours disappears completely under pressure.

Similar lesions are observed upon the dorsal surface of the toes, but are not so numerous nor so well formed as those on the fingers. There are no constitutional disturbances and no local subjective symptoms. The girl suffers every winter from chilblains, but otherwise is perfectly healthy.

The cutaneous affection is not congenital; it appears to have developed slowly, and has manifested itself in its present form only within the last five years.

The patient has been visited frequently for a year and a half and no noteworthy change in the general appearance of the lesions has been perceived. The chilblains which appear during the winter were situated only on parts of the skin otherwise healthy and had no influence on the affection. In winter the fingers were usually cold, and the spots and tumours seemed to be harder, and their colour darker than in summer. Occasionally, however, the presence of small red spots could be seen, which resembled telangiectases and were covered already by a slightly elevated and horny epidermis. The gradual development of these spots into the small tumours was observed.

For the purpose of studying the disease no treatment was employed beyond the excision of some of the tumours for histological study. More than a year has passed since these tumours were excised, and there is no sign of recurrence.

The external appearance of the small tumours suggested the diagnosis of keratoma. We must however distinguish what I call Angiokeratoma from simple keratoma (verruca vulgaris). The differential diagnosis is easy when the peculiar colour of the angiokeratoma is considered—a colour which disappears under pressure and immediately reappears when the pressure is removed, and also the changes which the colour undergoes under the influence of cold.

POROKERATOSIS

An Uncommon Form of Keratodermia: Porokeratosis*

Richard Bozzani, 21 years old, unmarried, of a well-to-do family of Parma, is a young man of strong constitution (height 1.78 meters) well proportioned in skeletal and muscular development, with regular features and in a good state of health. His skin is coarse, dark in colour, on the face ruddy brown; beard deep chestnut; hair of the head almost black and slightly curling, not too abundant; eyes clear, visible mucous membranes rosy.

The most important and most characteristic lesions are seen on the backs of the two hands and on the postero-internal surface of the right forearm where they extend to a little below the elbow.

Left hand. Patches of varying size and irregular form, sharply limited by a kind of small peripheral "dike" sinuous but uninterrupted; of a colour varying from red or whitish red to dirty white and but little different from that of the healthy skin; raised as a whole on the surface of the surrounding healthy skin but more frequently depressed in the centre as compared with the small peripheral dike; dry, hard, rough without trace of scales or crusts, giving to the touch the feeling of a harsh and almost horny body. The small peripheral dike which is the most striking feature in all the patches, and the dryest and hardest part of them, is always well developed and distinctly marked in the shape of an elevation resembling a truncated cone or section,

---

* Ullmann, J.: Archiv für dermat. und syph., *103:*566, 1910.

† International Atlas of Rare Skin Diseases. Hamburg, 1891, Part V.

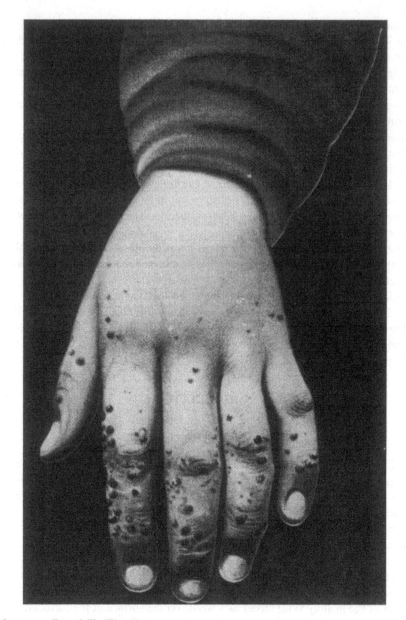

Figure 58 Angiokeratoma. From Mibelli's paper

measuring two millimeters in height and three millimeters in area at the base which bears on its summit a small whitish crest, dry, sharp and of horny aspect.

Having regard to the different keratosis development of the small peripheral dike and of the surface of the patches, two different degrees can be distinguished in the lesions above described. Some among them indeed are but little developed, measuring scarcely from 5 to 6 mm. in diameter; they have the same colour as the healthy skin (some of them rather more coloured) and present in the centre only a greater accentuation of the normal folds of the skin, absence of hairs and follicular orifices, some small whitish conical elevations of a horny aspect like the point of a pin; nevertheless they show a small peripheral dike though not greatly developed always well defined and surmounted by the small thin and dry crest already described. Others are much more developed having a diameter of 1 to 2 cm. They are much more raised and the largest are depressed in the centre, the small peripheral dike being more pronounced; they are dry and hard like a thick callosity and harsh to the touch. The more developed and hardest ones correspond to or are situated in the neighborhood of the cutaneous folds, made by movement as follows: On the postero-internal surface of the little finger near the articulation of the first with the second phalanx, at the root of the same finger over the metacarpal-phalangeal articulation of the same digit. Others less developed exist on other points of the backs of the fingers as well as on the back of the hand properly so-called and on the extensor surface of the forearm.

Right Hand. Patches similar to those of the left hand. Here also those corresponding to the joints of the fingers are much developed. One can be seen corresponding to the articulation of the first with the second phalanx of the fourth finger, another near the articulation of the first with the second phalanx of the index finger, a third a little below the metacarpo-phalangeal articulation of the same finger and a fourth near the metacarpo-phalangeal articulation of the thumb. Others less developed exist on the back of the thumb, ring, and little fingers, and only two on the back of the hand. No changes in the third finger of the right hand nor in the second of the left hand.

Again on the back of the right hand is seen a wide space prolonged upwards in the form of a broad band on the posterior surface of the forearm to 2.5 cm. below the olecranon where the skin is a little smoother and thinner than the surrounding healthy skin and altogether bare of hairs. This zone of skin bears a singular likeness to a geographical map, for it is sharply limited by a line standing out in relief in the form of a dike, sinuous and irregular, which describing a closed uninterrupted line from the back of the hand (2 cm. from the metacarpo-phalangeal articulations of the third and fourth fingers) is directed upwards along the ulnar border of the forearm and from 2 to 5 cm. below the olecranon and turning in the opposite direction comes back to the dorsum of the hand.

This kind of limiting dike presents the same character as that already described as bounding the isolated patches, and this border is itself the most remarkable feature of the lesion of the right forearm, for the area of skin which it encloses is, over the greater part of its surface, only slightly smoother than the healthy skin and it is destitute of hairs (no moisture, scales, or crusts). Nevertheless there are to be seen in the space referred to small conical elevations, whitish in colour, acuminated and hard like pin's points; elsewhere conical elevations with truncated summits and measuring about 2 mm. in diameter; in other places, especially above, there are in the large spaces larger islets very varied in form marked out by a thin peripheral collaret of a dirty white colour. Outside the large space and close to the outer limiting line are also seen other isolated spaces resembling those on the backs of the hands.

The flexor surfaces of the forearms as well as the palmar surfaces of the hands are normal in appearance. Only on the palm of the left hand there is a small callosity similar in appearance to ordinary callosities.

History. The beginning of the disease was noticed when the patient was two years old and it was neither preceded nor accompanied by any other symptoms. There was noticed at first without any previous changes a small isolated disc on the back of the right hand in the place which is now occupied by the large marginated space. From this primary centre the change spread gradually, and within a period of three years came to occupy all the part of the back of the hand and forearm which it occupies at present. From the age of

---

* International Atlas of Rare Skin Diseases. Hamburg, 1891, Part XXVII.

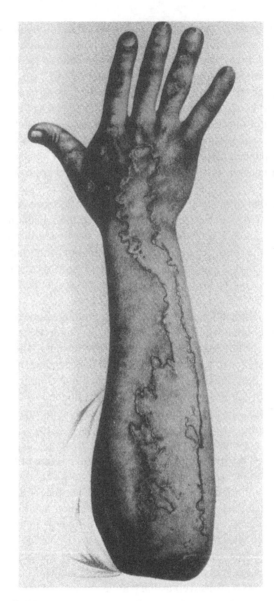

Figure 59 Porokeratosis. From Mibelli's paper

five years the other isolated patches developed on the same hand and in the course of nine years two patches showed themselves on the back of the thumb, three on the index and one on the ring finger. At the age of 14 all the lesions had attained nearly their present development. Afterwards new patches showed themselves on the first, fourth, and fifth digits and in correspondence with the interosseous space between the first and second metacarpal bones.

About the age of seven, similar lesions began to develop on the back of the left hand without any of them showing a tendency to spread like the primary patch on the right hand. At the age of 14 there were only five on the left hand, three of which were near the carpus, one on the thumb and one on the base of the third finger: the others developed during the last few years.

The lesions which have been mentioned manifest themselves in the beginning in the form of a small dry conical projection which slowly increases in size, becoming flat on the top and surrounded by a small raised collaret which afterwards develops further and widens out at the circumference. The lesions on the face show themselves in the form of a slight roughness of the skin and seem to result from the confluence of small acuminated elevations; afterwards they become more individualized by the presence of the thin peripheral border; if the patient tries to pick them off with his nails the part removed is immediately reproduced and the patch widens.

A patch, which showed itself about the age of eight, at the base of the second finger of the right hand after attaining a considerable development began spontaneously to fade away so that at the age of 12 it had completely disappeared.

The dike surrounding the large zone on the forearm has also shown a tendency for some years back to become less prominent and in some places it looks as if it were slowly disappearing without any treatment. Most of the other lesions that have been mentioned have undergone no change for some years; the most recent of them have a tendency to spread and to become more prominent in a very slow almost insensible manner. No subjective phenomena.

No treatment has ever been tried. The patient himself has succeeded in making some of the patches disappear by removing them with a knife. This same procedure has also been employed by us for histological purposes; one of these patches which we partially excised was completely reproduced after cicatrization; the others have shown no sign of recurrence.

Bozzani has always enjoyed the most perfect health: he does not remember having suffered from other diseases except syphilis which he contracted three years ago and which has had no influence on the course of the pre-existing affection of the skin.

There are no hereditary antecedants in the family. A brother aged 24 has had for 16 years the same skin affection as our patient on the backs of the hands; a sister aged 12 has been affected in the same way for two years; the father has noticed similar lesions only within the last two months.

I will add further that I have had the opportunity of seeing another case identical clinically and histologically in an adult man in whom the disease had begun only towards the age of 60 as in Bozzani's father.

For the rest as regards the microscopic examination the case presents itself as a pathologic fact *sui generis,* inasmuch as the principal alteration consists in hyperkeratosis of the sudoriferous ducts; and it is on this account that it deserves to be considered apart under the designation of "Porokeratosis" which I propose provisionally as it has the merits of indicating clearly the anatomo-pathological significance of the alteration itself.

Andrew Rose Robinson

Hidrocystoma

ANDREW ROSE ROBINSON was born in Claude, Ontario, July 31, 1845. He took his M.D. at Bellevue Hospital Medical College in 1868, and did post-graduate work in Toronto, Edinburgh, London, Paris, and Vienna. Always interested in pathology, he was appointed professor of histology and pathologic anatomy at the New York Medical College. The institution in which he was most interested was the New York Poly-clinic Medical School and Hospital. He was one of its founders, and for many years Professor of Dermatology and Vice President.

Robinson was not a prolific writer, but his publications were carefully prepared, and gained for him an international reputation as an authority on dermatology. Besides the original description of hidrocystoma given here, he wrote of pompholyx, ringworm, alopecia areata, and xanthoma diabeticorum. His *Manual of Dermatology* (1884) enjoyed considerable success.

Robinson was absorbed in medicine, and gave little time to social affairs. Because of a certain abruptness of manner, he did not make many friends. He was fond of nature, and in later years spent considerable time at his country estate in Ontario, He died July 8, 1924.*

HIDROCYSTOMA

Hidrocystoma*

All of the cases which have come under my observation, with one exception, have been in women in middle life or older, although there are no reasons, as far as I know, why it should not appear in quite young persons, and perhaps does in some cases. I saw one case this year in a young man, 28 years of age, in whom the eruption was limited to the lower half of the right side of the nose. In the majority of the cases the women have been doing general housework, housewives doing cooking, washing, etc., and whilst some of them did but little if any washing, the rule was that they attributed the eruption, or a great aggravation of an already existing one, to washing, as that kind of work, excessive exercise in a warm vapor atmosphere caused them to sweat very much. I have seen it also in cooks who did no washing, also in persons who did very little cooking or washing, and finally also in those who neither cooked nor washed. In my cases, however, the rule was that the disease appeared in middle-aged women who habitually perspired greatly,

---

* Unsigned Obit.: Arch. of Dermat. and Syph., *10:*333, 1924.

and who did washing over tubs, thus exposing the skin of their face to the action of a warm, moist atmosphere. All of the cases have been worse in summer than in winter, and in many of them the eruption would almost, if not entirely, disappear in winter, whilst in others it would entirely disappear during cold weather. In a case described by Hallopeau, and in whom the disease was limited to the nose, the eruption was more severe at the menstrual period than at other times, and it appeared to him to be much influenced by the condition of the nervous system, an emotional state aggravating the condition. In this case the eruption was also worse in summer than in winter.

The eruption usually occurs upon the regions occupied by it in the accompanying portrait, that is, it appears upon the lower part of the forehead, the orbital region, the nose, the cheeks, and often the upper and lower lips and the skin. I have not seen it upon the lower jaw or neck, or upon the rest of the body. In a case reported by Jamieson, of Edinburgh, the eruption was confined to the nose and right side of the forehead, temples and cheek. The woman was 45 years of age, and perspired freely and easily upon the right side of the body, and only on rare occasions and when much excited, to a slight degree upon the left side. When first seen by Dr. Jamieson, there were large beads of perspiration on the right side of the forehead and corresponding cheek, whilst the left side was absolutely dry.

The lesions are either discrete or situated closely to each other, but it is not usual to find them in any considerable number closely crowded together, especially if they are not very numerous. When perhaps 100 to 200 lesions are present—and I have seen such cases—then the lesions over a greater part of the affected area may be closely situated to each other, but when few lesions are present they are usually discrete.

The individual lesions appear as tense, clear, shiny vesicles, obtuse, round or ovoid in form and varying in size from that of a pin head to that of a pea. They are, at first, always deep seated, that is, their base reaches deep into the corium, but on account of their size they are also usually more or less elevated above the general surface. The smaller ones, especially, bear considerable resemblance to a boiled sago-grain. The larger lesions sometimes have a darkish blue tint, which is most marked at the periphery. This is well shown on the chromo-lithograph. From the drying up of the contents, disappearing lesions may have a whitish appearance like that present in cases of milium. I have not been able to recognize with positiveness the presence of an excretory sweat duct orifice over the central part of an individual vesicle. The skin over the lesions is not inflamed, and there are no signs of inflammation present in any part of the affected region. If the lesion is a large one—slight circulatory disturbance—a mild hyperaemia is often noticed at its periphery. There are no subjective symptoms, or the eruption may be accompanied by a slight sensation of tension or smarting.

The contents of the vesicles are clear and never change to a yellowish color, but dry up and the lesion disappears, unless mechanically injured, without rupture, often lasting one, two or several weeks, leaving the part in a normal condition or followed by a slight temporary pigmentation. In the late stage of evolution the dried up contents sometimes appear whitish, like in milium. If the vesicles are ruptured the contents are found to be always slightly acid and never alkaline.

---

* J.Cutan. Dis., *11*:293, 1893.

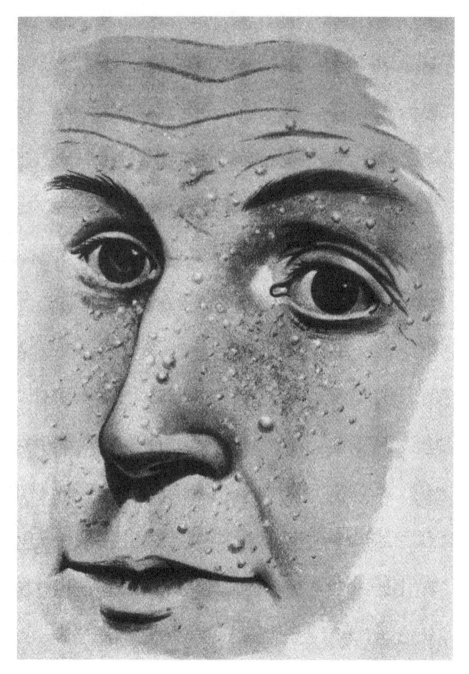

Figure 60 Hidrocystoma. From Robinson's paper

John Addison Fordyce

1. *Angiokeratoma of the Scrotum*

2. *Pseudo-colloid of the Lips*

JOHN ADDISON FORDYCE was born in Guernsy County, Ohio, February 16, 1858. After a common school education he did his undergraduate work at Adrian College, received his M.D. in 1881 from Northwestern University Medical College, and interned at Cook County Hospital (Chicago). After three years in general practice he journeyed to Europe and studied in the great medical centers of Vienna, Berlin and Paris, devoting most of his time to the study of dermatology, chiefly under Kaposi in Vienna.

He returned to the United States and set up practice in New York City, became chief of the skin department at Bellevue Hospital Medical College and later at Columbia.

Fordyce built up a tremendous practice. He was a prolific writer, making many important contributions to his fields of special interest— syphilology and dermal pathology, as well as to dermatology in general. He was extremely active in teaching, editorial and organizational work at a time when the specialty was undergoing its greatest expansion in this country.

Personally he was lenient, tolerant and kind. MacKee said, "He lived in an atmosphere of culture and refinement surrounded by etchings and paintings and a voluminous and varied library, all of which were very dear to him. It was a treat to spend an evening with this gracious, versatile host and his happy family. He enjoyed good music, humor, high class theatrical productions, literature, history and most of the things that are conducive to the happiness of educated, cultured persons."

Although customarily a healthy and strong man, Dr. Fordyce was stricken in 1925 in his 67th year with appendicitis, and although an appendectomy was performed he did not survive.*

ANGIOKERATOMA OF THE SCROTUM

Angiokeratoma of the Scrotum[†]

The patient, a male, aged 60, was admitted to the City Hospital in the Spring of 1894 for some urinary trouble. He was somewhat feeble, both mentally and physically, and could give little information regarding the eruption which was present on his scrotum, except to say that he had had it for a number of years.

He feared that some harm would come to him if he remained in the hospital, and demanded his discharge before a careful study could be made of the interesting skin lesions which he presented.

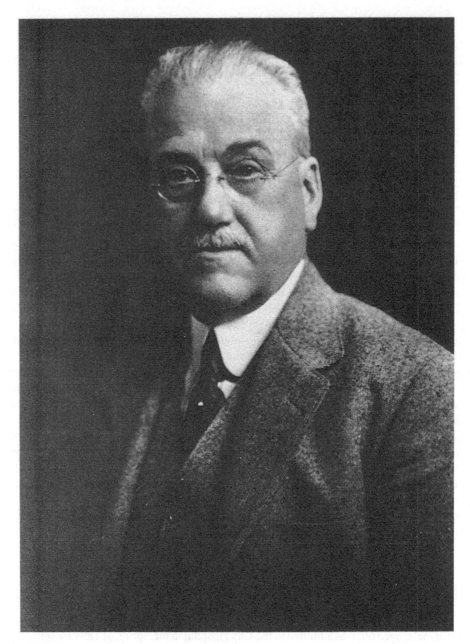

Figure 61 John Addison Fordyce. Courtesy, Dr. Homer Swift

An opportunity was afforded, however, of excising a number of the small tumors for microscopic purposes, and of having made the coloured sketch, which is reproduced in connection with the present article.

The skin covering the thighs and lower part of the abdomen was the seat of a number of patches of vitiligo. The patient was also affected with a double varicocoele, which is interesting in connection with the superficial vascular dilatation. His hands and feet were free from any skin affection, and he denied having suffered with chilblains. The scrotum, especially on its lateral and posterior surfaces, was the seat of a great number of small, spherical-shaped, dark purple tumors. They were arranged in a linear manner as if following the superficial vascular supply of the parts. The small growths were from a pinhead to several times that size, their dimensions being pretty uniform. Pressure caused the color of the majority of the tumors to disappear. In some of them, however, the color was only partially lost.

The small growths were distinctly elevated above the surface of the scrotum, seeming to rest on it rather than to be imbedded in the skin. Some of them were covered by a slightly thickened horny layer, under which minute dark red points could be seen, which gave the tumors a warty-like appearance.

Composite lesions were formed by the union of two or more of the smaller ones, which, however, preserved all the characteristics of the original growths. No pain, pruritus or other subjective sensation were complained of by the patient. Puncture of the tumors with a needle was followed by slight hemorrhage.

In cases heretofore reported, the eruption has been, with few exceptions, confined to the extremities.

PSEUDO-COLLOID OF THE LIPS

A Peculiar Affection of the Mucous Membrane of the Lips and Oral Cavity*

In the Autumn of 1895 I presented to the New York Dermatological Society a physician who had consulted me for an affection of the mucous membrane of the lips and oral cavity. The patient's attention was first attracted to the condition about two years ago by a symmetrical fading of the vermillion border of the upper lip, extending from the corners of the mouth almost to the median line, leaving only a narrow margin free next to the skin and a wedge-shaped area in the center of the lip. The two patches were connected at the inferior median line, where the lips come in contact, by a segment of a circle, making three patches, all of uniform color, with well-defined borders and areas slightly elevated. When first noticed the color was but a shade lighter than normal. The appearance otherwise did not seem abnormal, but by putting the tissues on the stretch, small, irregular, closely aggregated milium-like bodies of a light yellow color just beneath the surface of the epithelium were plainly visible and completely covered the patches. While the borders appeared as well-defined lines, a chain of from one to three milium bodies could occasionally be seen in advance of the main patch, but not disconnected. The two sides have progressed symmetrically. On the lower lip was a parallel line of similar bodies extending horizontally through the center. The patient is unable to state positively whether there has been any extension of the condition since it was first noticed. He is positive, however, that the color has become lighter within the past six months. This he thought might be due to the fact that the bodies have become more closely aggregated. The subjective symptoms have been very slight. The patient experiences at times a slight immobility of the upper lip, which he is inclined to attribute to a dryness just above a nerveless tooth. This feeling preceded the onset of the above condition by several years. Within the past year he has felt a slight burning and itching of the upper lip, accompanied by some stiffness, as though the lip was swollen. This is only an occasional feeling, and may be due to errors

---

* MacKee, G.: Arch. of Dermat. and Syph., *12:*268, 1925.

† J.Cutan. Dis., *14:*81, 1896.

* J.Cutan. Dis., *14:*413, 1896.

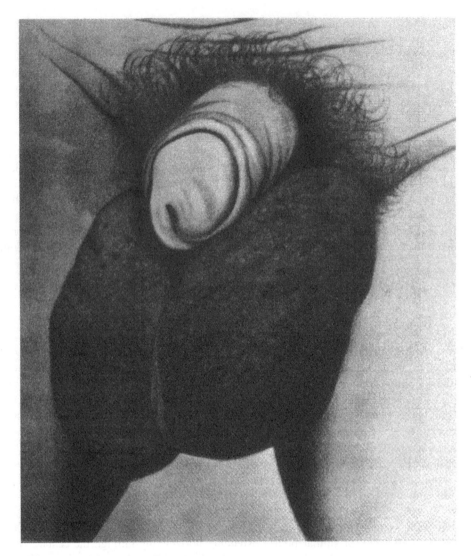

Figure 62 Angiokeratoma of the scrotum. From Fordyce's paper

of diet. The patient does not use tobacco or alcohol. His family as well as his past history is negative, and he is in good health at present.

An examination of the mucous membrane of the mouth revealed a similar condition extending along the line of the closed teeth from the angle of the mouth backward to a point opposite the last molar teeth. The lesions within the oral cavity were lighter in color and in places somewhat elevated and papillomatous in character.

On the lips the minute yellowish-white bodies imbedded in the mucous membrane suggested the ordinary milium seen on the face. An endeavor was made to remove them by incising the skin and picking them out with a needle. They were, however, found to be firmly adherent, and could with difficulty be detached from the surrounding tissue.

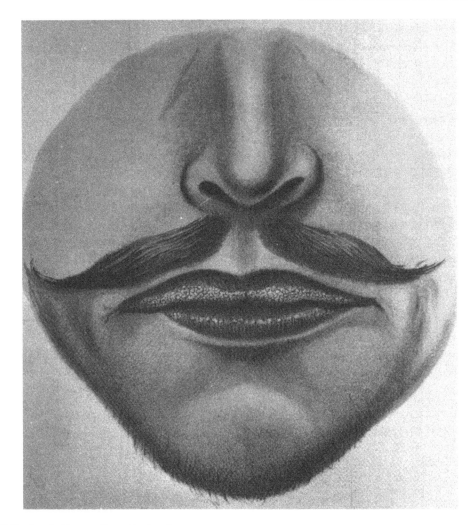

Figure 63 Fordyce's disease. From Fordyce's paper

The lesions were rendered much less noticeable for a time by the use of the curette. When the superficial layer of the epithelium was scraped away, some of the bodies could be pressed out by the blunt edge of the instrument, but as a rule a portion of the discoloration remained, as if only the upper part of the affected tissue had been removed. When the epithelium was restored a marked improvement was noted in the appearance of the lips, but after a few weeks it became less perceptible, gradually assuming the same yellowish white granular appearance that was present before interference.

I report the affection as an example of a mucous membrane change, which while apparently not uncommon, has hitherto escaped observation.

Henri Rendu

Hereditary Hemorrhagic Telangiectasia (Rendu-Osler-Weber Syndrome)

HENRI JULES MARIE RENDU was born in Paris in 1844. The son of an Inspector of Agriculture, he was first intended to follow in his father's footsteps, and studied for two years in the Agronomic School in Rennes, where he acquired a taste for physical science, especially geology and botany. He won a Doctor of Science degree for an important work on the tertiary strata in the neighborhood of Rennes. Turning to medicine, he became an externe of the Paris hospitals in 1867, and after winning several prizes for scholarship, took his M.D. in 1873. His thesis dealt with the paralyses occurring with tuberculous meningitis. He remained associated with l'Hôpital Necker in Paris until his death in 1902.

Rendu was one of France's leading internists. A prolific writer, he was especially interested in diseases of the heart and liver; he is most remembered for his account of hereditary hemorrhagic telangiectasia, presented below, as well as for the hysterical intention tremor and the camphor menthol treatment of tuberculous peritonitis which bear his name.

Rendu was a religious man, and led a simple life. He spent his holidays perambulating France in search of plants to add to his botanical collection.*

HEREDITARY HEMORRHAGIC TELANGIECTASIA

Epistaxis Répétées Chez une Sujet Porteur de Petits Angiomes*

On my service I have just observed a patient who in certain respects recalls to mind the history of a case of hemophilia presented a few months ago by M.Chauffard.

Since these cases constitute a rarity as yet, I feel I ought to recapitulate the principal features of this observation.

S—, 52 years of age, a terrace maker, entered the Bouley Ward on the 28th of last September. He is a large and well muscled man, but pale and weak, with a yellowish color, almost sub-icteric. He feels extremely weak, and is capable of no effort without experiencing palpitations. When he stoops over and stands erect quickly, he is the victim of vertigo. His appetite is good, however, and he has no fever.

The anemic appearance, and the debilitation of the patient are the result of a double series of symptoms. For two months he has had frequent attacks of diarrhea which have exhausted him, and which recur in an

---

intermittent fashion, one after another, sometimes for a week. This diarrhea, however, presents none of the characteristics of dysentery, and has never given rise to intestinal loss of blood. The abdomen is supple and non-painful; no swelling nor appreciable lesion can be demonstrated. Moreover, at this time the patient has perfectly regular digestion, and is not troubled by his disorder.

The predominating symptom at present is the quotidian disposition this patient shows to bleed from the nose. For three weeks epistaxis episodes have followed one another daily, and even several times a day. They usually appear in the morning, and even during the second half of the night; it is rare for the patient not to be awakened by the sensation of nasal hemorrhage appearing unconsciously during his sleep. During the daytime they are more rare, and appear only rarely when the patient is in open air.

These hemorrhages are ordinarily not very copious, about 40 to 50 gms. each time, but in several attacks they have reached 200 to 300 gms., and even without being copious their repetition weakens the patient considerably. The anemic appearance, the yellow color, the vascular troubles, and the vertigo are due to these losses of blood.

Examination of the organs provides no explanation for these epistaxes. There is no congestive tendency in this man. He is subject neither to habitual headaches nor to hot flashes; he is not alcoholic, and leads a very sober life. He has no cardiac nor vascular defect, no threat of arteriosclerosis at present. Urines examined from the point of view of possible interstitial nephritis revealed no suspicious particulars; there is no polyuria, no pollakiuria, no albuminuria. The spleen is not enlarged. In short we are faced with an epistaxis apparently essential, the cause of which eludes us.

In investigating the personal and hereditary antecedants of this man we have found several indications, if not of true hemophilia, at least of a certain tendency to hemorrhage easily.

The father died of dysentery with repeated attacks of melena, at 55 years of age; the mother, it appears, was subject to nose bleeds. A brother, dead of albuminuria it is true, had frequent and copious epistaxes.

He himself had his first nose bleeds at the age of 12 years, and throughout his youth he was subject to them, chiefly in the spring and in the warm season. This disposition, far from attenuating with advancing age, became considerably aggravated, and since the age of 35 the hemorrhages have become very frequent, always in the form of epistaxis. Indeed, he has never had hematuria, purpuric spots, or gingival hemorrhages, and it is interesting to note that when he injures or cuts himself he loses no more blood than a normal person. He has had two teeth pulled without having had notable consequent hemorrhages. This is, therefore, no true hemophilia, in spite of the ease with which he loses blood from the nose.

A particularity which recalls to mind the case described by M.Chauffard explains, perhaps, this peculiar localization of the hemorrhages and their frequent repetition.

On the skin of the nose, the cheeks, the upper lip, and the chin, there are small purple spots as large as the head of a pin; the largest reach the size of a lentil; they are true cutaneous hemangiomas, produced by a dilatation of the superficial vessels of the skin. Pressure causes them to blanche, but not to disappear; the blood flows back immediately when compression is released. Angiomas of the same nature are scattered over the neck and chest; there appear to be none on the extremities.

This anatomic disposition is not limited to the skin; it extends also to the mucous membranes, and this fact is of considerable interest from the point of view which concerns us. Indeed, small vascular dilatations, true telangiectatic foci, are present on the inner surface of the lips and the cheeks, on the tongue, and on the soft palate, with characteristics identical to those on the integument, but with a very bright color, owing to the decreased thickness of mucous epidermis.

---

* Gaz. des Hôpitaux, *69:*1322, 1896.

In the nostrils we have not demonstrated these punctiform angiomas, but it is not irrational to suppose that there are similar ones on the nasal septum or in the nasal fossae. It would then be understood why it is always the nasal mucous membrane that is the seat of the hemorrhages, and why they are so recurrent and copious.

Antonin Poncet

Pyogenic Granuloma

ANTONIN PONCET was born March 28, 1849, in Saint-Trivier-sur-Moignans. An Interne des Hôpitaux in 1869, he became a chief in the clinic of Desgranges in Lyon in 1874. His great talent for surgery soon became manifest, and at the early age of 34 he was named Professor of operative medicine in the medical school at Lyon. He held the position of surgeon-major at l'Hôtel Dieu de Lyon until his death September 17, 1913.

Poncet, with his pupil Dor, did the original work on botryomycosis (pyogenic granuloma) in humans, although it had been noted in horses some years before. We have reproduced his original case. He was a pioneer in surgery of the thyroid, appendix, stomach, and urinary bladder, and an early advocate of the aseptic principles of Lister. His greatest work was in elucidating the clinical and pathological picture of tuberculous rheumatism, and this entity has since been known as Poncet's disease. His name is also connected with a number of operative procedures: lengthening the Achilles tendon for talipes equinus, perineotomy, and perineal urethrostomy.

Poncet was a tremendously energetic man, and an active teacher. He was tall in stature, with a sonorous voice, and though kind and even tempered, he had a sharp and piercing glance.*

PYOGENIC GRANULOMA

De la Botryomycose Humaine*

Jeanne-Marie P., 55 years of age, born at Maclas (Loire), entered l'Hôtel-Dieu de Lyon, Saint Anne's Ward, No. 16, June 26, 1897. Three months previously the patient, who is free from pathological symptoms, noticed on her right hand, more or less in the area of the digito-palmar fold of the little finger, a red spot which was indolent but pruriginous. In progressing, this spot soon reached pinhead size. It ulcerated due to movement of the hand and then bled very easily. Its growth was slow until, six weeks before her admission to l'Hôtel-Dieu, the patient applied an empirical ointment with a caustic base. Since then her tumor has increased greatly in size, and has reached, as we have already indicated, the size of a hazel nut. It is, moreover, the seat of lancinating pains which radiate into the wrist and forearm.

---

* X.D., Lyon Méd, *121:*557, 1913.

At the time of admission, a large ulcerating reddish nodule is noted in the region cited, very much like a large, fleshy, exuberant pimple of long standing. This mass is renitent and elastic to the touch. One part of it appears to be covered by a cornified malpighian layer no different in color from the rest of the neighboring skin, except that it is a little reddened. If this vegetation is lifted up, and only then, a short and very slender pedicle will be seen fixing it to the subjacent tissue, and giving it completely the form of a mushroom with a short thin stalk. Around the pedicle the skin is pinkish and painful to pressure; undoubtedly due to the ill timed application of the ointment employed, these inflammatory symptoms are not unexpected. The underlying bone and joint are unaffected.

June 27. Local anesthesia with cocaine. Section of the pedicle with scissors, wide excision of it by an oval incision made with the bistouri.

We have recently seen this woman again, and she has remained well.

---

* Lyon Méd., *86:*217, 1897.

Domenico Majocchi

Purpura Annularis Telangiectodes (Majocchi's Disease)

DOMENICO MAJOCCHI was born August 5, 1849, in Roccalvecce, a town near Rome. After preliminary education in his native city, he entered the seminary at Bagnorea in preparation for a career in philosophy. His thoughts turned to medicine, however, and he matriculated at la Sapienza, taking his degree in 1873. After a year in general practice in Roccalvecce, he returned to Rome, and devoted himself entirely to the study of dermatology and syphilology.

Under Scillingo at the Ospedale di S.Galligano, Majocchi had access to a tremendous amount of clinical material; it was his assiduous study at this period that laid the foundation for his remarkable skill in all branches of dermatology. In 1880 he was made Professor of Dermatology at the University of Parma, and later held the same position at the University of Bologna.

Majocchi was the first Italian dermatologist of note. From his pen came many fine laboratory and clinical reports, the latter usually with detailed histological studies, for he was an especially expert microscopist. His writings on granuloma tricofitico, on osseous syphilis, and purpura annularis telangiectodes are particularly well known. His account of the latter condition, often called Majocchi's disease, is given below. He was, in addition, greatly interested in medical history, and wrote accounts of the ill starred campaign of Charles VIII in Italy, of Marcello Malpighi, and of prehistoric medicine.

Majocchi was kind and generous, and beloved of his many pupils. He was a popular figure at social gatherings. Fond of music, he particularly admired Wagner. In 1920 he retired, after 40 years of service, and died March 7, 1929 at Bologna.*

PURPURA ANNULARIS TELANGIECTODES

Purpura Annularis Telangiectodes*

The descriptions of the cases just given show on all points such agreement as to the morphologic individuality of the dermatosis that we can compile the following general characteristics:

---

* Diasio, F.: Med. Life, *39:*597, 1932.

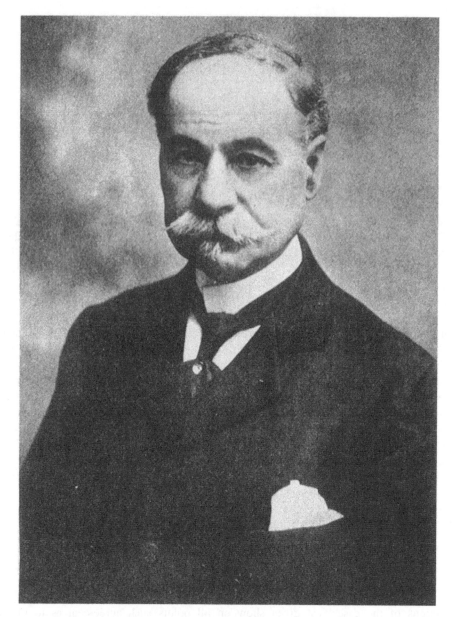

Figure 64 Domenico Majocchi. Courtesy, Froben Press, New York

1. Rose-colored and livid red spots made up of capillary ectasias with subsequent hemorrhages, without preceding hyperemia, without perceptible infiltration of the skin, and usually in distinct association with the hair follicles.
2. Slow development and extension of these.
3. Constant eccentric growth of the spots.

4. Symmetrical distribution of the dermatosis.

5. Primary location always on the extremities, particularly on the lower.

6. Usually absence of itching and disturbances in sensation.

7. Termination in slight atrophy and achromia of the skin, together with alopecia.

But, if these are the general symptoms of the dermatosis, it is also necessary to observe the order in which they develop and within what limits, and it is necessary to study the history of the development of the disease itself. Thus, one can determine from comparative study of the foregoing cases that the disease runs through several stages, although the cycle is not always regular. We can divide these stages into three:

1. **Telangiectatic Stage.** In relation to time, the first appearance of the illness is characterized by rose-red punctate or streak-forming spots which occasionally are serpiginous or slightly branched, and made up of capillary ectasias which because of their increased size may be seen with the naked eye, although better with a lens. Under a transparent plate which is alternately pressed on and released from the ring-forming lesions one can get a better idea of their composition, and also differentiate easily the hemorrhagic lesions from the capillary ectasias. They are located particularly at the follicles, as one can determine from the presence of a small hair in the center of nearly every spot. They persist for a very long time, until by gradual enlargement they unite with one another, either by becoming confluent or contiguous, and in this way produce the ring-forms described above. Pruritus is usually lacking throughout the entire course of the dermatosis; only rarely does the patient experience minor annoyance with the eruption of the livid red spots, and this soon yields.

2. **Hemorrhagic Pigmented Stage.** This frequently accompanies the telangiectatic stage; however, extravasation of blood does not take place from every ectasia, although it appears at different points. For this reason the hemorrhages do not form an essential stage of the dermatosis, but are only a feature of it.

Further, the punctate and lenticular hemorrhages form at the follicles or in their neighborhood and persist for a long time, so that one may see in their midst tiny ectatic vessels. After a more or less protracted existence they resolve into pigmentations which disappear completely in time.

3. **Atrophic Stage.** After the disappearance of the pigmented spots, or even during their presence, an important change in the lesions of the disease takes place. The hairs thin out, that is, become colorless, atrophic and fall out; also, the follicular openings disappear, and only with the aid of a lens can one detect them as tiny points. But after several months one sees no trace of either hair or follicular opening. The skin in the ringed lesions becomes somewhat thinner, shiny, loses its pigment and is traversed by delicate wrinkles. This is the atrophic stage, but also during this time the lesions are growing through eccentric extension of the perifollicular capillary ectasias, at the expense of the neighboring follicles.

Course and Outcome. Although the number of cases I have collected is limited, one can still determine with certainty that the development of the dermatosis reported here is extremely slow; only one of the cases showed a truly rapid development. Usually the livid red spots appear gradually, as discrete lesions, and their arrangement in circular forms also manifests itself with steady slowness. But what is noteworthy in the course of the disease is the lack of sudden or intermittent paroxysmal-like eruptions as occur frequently in purpura hemorrhagica. But the slow development is not so surprising as, in contrast to purpura hemorrhagica, the long duration and persistence of the spots. As proof of this, we present in evidence the second and third of the cases above. As already said, these livid red spots terminate usually in pigmentation

---

* Archiv für dermat. und syph., *43:*447, 1898.

and atrophy. But what is the final outcome of this affliction? The difficulty in keeping patients under observation for a longer period of time has not allowed us to observe the last stage of development of the dermatosis.

Henri Hallopeau

1.   Lichen Sclerosus et Atrophicus

2.   Acrodermatitis Continua

FRANÇOIS HENRI HALLOPEAU was born in Paris, January 17, 1842. A brilliant scholar, he entered the Paris Medical school at 24 and three years later was second among a large number of candidates for Parisian internships. His thesis, submitted in 1871, dealt with convulsive symptoms in disorders of the spinal cord. He became affiliated with the Tenon and Saint Antoine hospitals, and later, in 1884, with l'Hôpital Saint Louis, where he remained until his retirement in 1907.

Hallopeau took up dermatology only after he had acquired quite a reputation as a pathologist and neurologist, yet the amount of work he turned out is prodigious, over 800 publications. In addition to the description of acrodermatitis continua for which he is best known, and *lichen plan atrophique,* which we now know as lichen sclerosus et atrophicus, both of which we have included here, he added much to our knowledge of mycosis fungoides, eczema, trichotillomania, leprosy, and lupus vulgaris. He was one of the early workers in the evaluation of arsenic in the treatment of syphilis.

Hallopeau was a most affable man, and became known in later life as "le Père Hallopeau." Although retired in 1907, he continued consultant work until 1919 when almost blind and barely able to walk he gave it up; a few months later, on March 20, 1919, he was dead.*

LICHEN SCLEROSUS ET ATROPHICUS

Lichen Plan Atrophique*

In contrast to the preceding variety we must describe, as a new form, a *lichen plan atrophique.*

In the case we present to you, we have observed simultaneously lichen papules and cicatrices which present characteristics not attributable to lupus. Here is a resumé of the history of this patient, compiled with the aid of M.Lefèbvre, *interne du service.*

Mlle, de T. is a neuropath; she frequently experiences sensations of numbness and burning in the extremities, cramps, and insomnia; she believes that she has attacks of fever; she feels depressed, and weak. In 1884 she began to suffer from an extremely troublesome vulvar pruritus. The eruption that brings her to the hospital today began in August 1885; the lesions appeared on the forearms; since then they have

---

* Beeson, B.: Arch. of Dermat. and Syph., *23:*730, 1931.

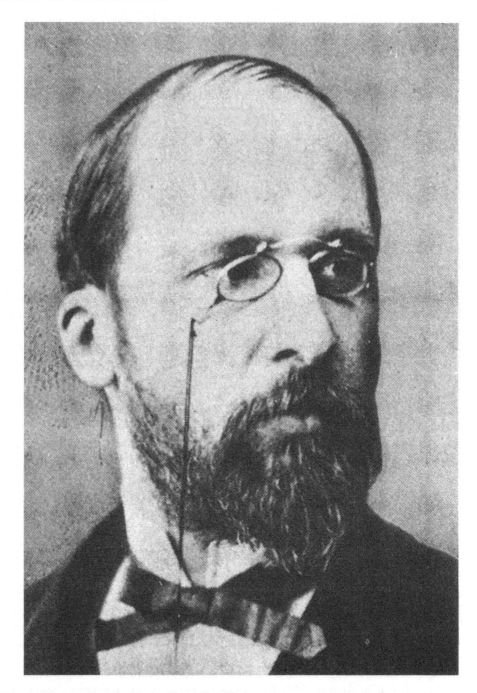

Figure 65 Henri Hallopeau. Courtesy, Froben Press, New York

persisted, and new eruptions have appeared successively, provoking itching and needle pricking sensations. The patient entered l'Hôpital Saint Louis in February, 1887, Henri IV Ward, No. 42; age around 45 years, somewhat obese; Mlle. X had no troubles with the general health other than those nervous phenomena mentioned above. Her cutaneous affection occupied chiefly the forearms, the back, and the inguinal folds.

On the palmar surface of the left forearm, toward the lower part, a plaque is seen which measures some 5 cm. vertically and 3 cm. transversely. Its sinuous and slightly raised contours appear to be formed from conglomerated papules; two of these papules are clearly isolated, round, a little raised and 2 to 3 mm. in diameter; they show in their centers punctiform depressions which evidently correspond to glandular orifices or to hair follicles, and are identical to those seen in ordinary lichen planus. Similar depressions, very pronounced, are seen in considerable numbers over the entire surface of the plaque; they are encircled by a slight epidermal projection; the plaque is discolored, white, shining, with cicatricial appearance; numerous folds traverse it and intersect with one another forming a quadrillage. Around this plaque several isolated lenticular spots are seen which present the same characteristics and the same punctiform depressions.

On the corresponding part of the right forearm there is a plaque which is somewhat similar; its contour is more irregular; at its periphery the same papular projections are found, and the same punctiform depressions with exaggeration of the folds of the skin; it is evident that the plaque was formed by the confluence of papules similar to those which are as yet isolated.

In the area of the elbow crease on the left, analogous lesions are seen which are, however, less advanced in their evolution. The plaques are less extensive; they effect a transverse direction, and are parallel to the folds in the skin; the same depressions with epidermal collarettes are to be noted there, the same exaggeration of the cutaneous folds that has been indicated above. These plaques are pale rose colored. On the under surface of the same arm one finds a large plaque blending inferiorly with the preceding, and presenting the same characteristics; it has a light scale; the same type of plaque, shiny and slightly elevated at its borders, over the sternum; it is formed of small elements which are isolated at the periphery, confluent at the center, and which represent involuting papules. The characteristics of the lesion in this case are clearly shown in the dorso-lumbar region; indeed, several large cicatricial plaques analogous to the preceding are seen along with more recent papules, raised, flat, shining, rose colored, covered with punctiform depressions, similar, in a word, to those of lichen planus. The patient still feels troublesome sensations in the region of the plaques at times. The patient mentioned an intense vulvar pruritus, and examination of the vaginal regions shows considerable thickening with exaggeration of the folds of the skin.

In summary, *lichen plan atrophique* begins with the formation of papules which are similar at first to those of ordinary lichen planus, although less highly colored, and, which, like those, give rise to a sensation of pruritus, become pale, involute promptly and form, then, white spots with a cicatricial appearance which are remarkable for the presence of punctiform depressions; these eruptive elements become grouped and confluent in such a way that they produce plaques several centimeters in diameter; their surface is checkered, and riddled with punctiform depressions; their contours are irregular; isolated papules are seen at their periphery, some discolored and involuting, others still rose colored and active. These plaques are disseminated over the extremities and the trunk. The eruption progresses by successive attacks.

---

* Union Méd., *43*:742, 1887.

ACRODERMATITIS CONTINUA

Des Acrodermatitis continues*

It is probable that causes diverse in nature are able to produce acrodermatitis; the clinical picture, in fact, permits us to distinguish a vesicular form, a pustular form, and a bullous form. It is probable that each of these is due to one or several different causative agents; we are able to group them together in a single description because of their usual location in the same region, and because of the common features that result from them.

We will consider the three forms successively.

Vesicular form. Cause unknown; it is observed in adulthood and old age; it appears without other morbid phenomena; the subjects which it affects are not neuropathic; a previous eruption or traumatism may be the starting point; in the case of M.Audrey it followed the appearance of blisters on the anteroexternal surface of the thumb. In one of our recent observations it followed an irritation provoked by the penetration of and inflammation from a particle of phosphorus under one of the nails. In two of our cases the eruption remained localized to one of the fingers; in a third, after remaining circumscribed on one of the middle fingers for nearly five years, it extended to other fingers.

This eruption consists of vesicles seated on a red surface; these vesicles are isolated and persist for a certain time after their eruption; each finger is only partially involved at first; the eruption may spread here and there on the palm of the hand, which it affects only as part of its extension.

When the isolated vesicles break, they leave excoriations which soon become covered either with crusts or lamellar scales which are more or less thick.

The underlying skin is red and tumefied.

When the scales become detached, the epidermis appears thin, smooth, and shiny; in other areas, on the contrary, the thickness of the skin becomes altered through an exaggeration of the folds.

The nail suffers in its nutrition; it loses its polish and becomes deeply grooved and furrowed vertically; moreover one sees transverse flattening of the nails, and also numerous punctiform depressions measuring a few millimeters in diameter.

The patients describe a troublesome smarting sensation, but no itching.

The progress of this dermatosis is continuous; thus, as the vesicles become excoriated or dry up and give rise to the formation of crusts or scales, others appear, usually within the area of the affected portion, sometimes at its periphery.

During the long period in which it is limited to one finger, it is localized on one phalanx for a great while at first, and then progressively involves the greater part of the whole; it may gradually reach a neighboring finger, and also spread to the palmar surface of the hand; in one of our cases most of the fingers have been involved successively in this manner; the dorsal surface may also be affected, but here the eruption is less pronounced.

In no case have all the fingers been involved simultaneously, and usually a part of the affected fingers remain free of disease.

As yet we have not seen this form develop on the toes.

This affection is essentially rebellious to treatment.

---

* Rev. Gén. de Clin. et de Thérap., 1898, p. 97.

Suppurative form. As in the preceding, this form is produced at times, but not always, as a sequel to trauma, either on the palm of the hand or on the end of the finger.

In our first patient the appearance of the suppuration was preceded by local asphyxial phenomena of a year's duration.

Usually the initial lesions appear in the area of periphery of the nail. In M.Frèche's case a partial smoky coloration of the nail was noted at first, in the form of spots, or diffuse.

The border of the nail soon becomes reddened and tumefied, becomes painful, elevates and detaches; there is discharge of pus; the suppuration then extends to part of the first phalanx, usually to its palmar surface; it may involve the other phalanges successively; the skin reddens and becomes the seat of numerous suppurating points which vary in size from that of a pea to that of a franc piece.

Usually several other fingers are involved in their turn, as well as several toes; similar alterations appear on the palms of the hands; beginning at isolated sites they become confluent to form large plaques from the surface of which the epidermis has been lost; on the bright red base, numerous flat suppurative areas of variable dimensions with polycyclic contours stand out clearly because of their whitish color; in the cases of M.M.Stowers and Frèche the borders of these surfaces were formed by an elevation of the epidermis. In places islets of epidermis persist within the area of the plaques. The suppuration dries up quickly, forming crusts. These are renewed continuously for months, and even years without going beyond the limits of the hand, and predominating always on the ends of the fingers.

As in the vesicular form, and to a greater degree, the nails suffer in their nutrition; several times we have seen some of them cast off with subsequent suppuration of the matrix.

When they persist they are usually elevated by a friable mass, incompletely keratinized. These same masses form at the sites of cast off nails; they are thick, yellowish, and infiltrated with meliceric concretions, with an uneven and rocky surface, and have neither the shiny appearance nor the longitudinal striations of the normal nail.

These same alterations may be produced without suppuration.

The evolution of the suppurations is often very rapid: in one of our cases they dried up so very quickly that punctures performed too late failed to produce a flow of fluid from them; the epidermis was then surmounted either by a crust or a thick scale.

The disease proceeds, thus, by continual extension over a period of years.

It may remain localized to the extremities, or may be accompanied by generalized eruptions.

These eruptions may be erythematous. These secondary extensions, the simple erythematous and the pustular variety, are always distributed symmetrically; their sites of predilection are the neck, the groin, the elbows, the wrists, the scrotum, the knees, the lower parts of the legs, and the instep; the head is not always unaffected; the erythematous and pustular manifestations appear on the scalp, the forehead, in the beard, behind the ears, and on the auricles; at other times a simple furfuraceous desquamation leads to an erythema which is rapidly effaced.

The quantity of liquid exuded from these pustules is so scanty that they dry up in a few hours; one sees in their place, usually a simple furfuraceous desquamation; if true crusts are present, which is exceptional, they are somewhat thick, and of a yellowish color.

The desquamation from the erythematous surface may take the form of large fragments, and may be plentiful enough to fill the bed, as in the case of exfoliative dermatitis. When the disease is complicated with secondary suppuration it presents features similar to those of impetigo herpetiformis; the prognosis becomes almost necessarily fatal, and it merits the name, *infection purulente tegumentaire* which we have given to it in a recent communication to the *Société de Dermatologie;* the acrodermatitis in such cases is only the initial manifestation, isolated for a long time.

Mixed form. We are familiar with only one case, that of M.Audrey. The eruption began with large recurrent blisters on the palmar surface of thumb; the fluid, serous at first, soon became purulent; it was subsequently complicated by a recurrent and localized eruption on the thumb of vesicular and purulent elements; since then it has presented the features of acrodermatitis continue.

The prognosis in all the forms is poor because of the indefinite duration of the disease, and because of the obstacle it presents to manual work.

Benjamin Robinson Schenck

Sporotrichosis

BENJAMIN ROBINSON SCHENCK was born in Syracuse, New York on August 19, 1872. He received his M.D. at Johns Hopkins Medical School in 1898. Following a three year residency in Gynecology and several years as an instructor, he left Hopkins to practice in Detroit, Michigan. At the Detroit College of Medicine he held the title of Associate Professor of Gynecology. In 1916 he was forced to retire to Colorado to fight a pulmonary disease which eventually led to his early death on June 30, 1920.

Schenck's contribution in dermatology is the original clinical description of sporotrichosis which appears below. The dateline bears noting. Here is a classic description in clinical dermatology accomplished by a keen observant medical student.[*]

SPOROTRICHOSIS

On Refractory Subcutaneous Abscesses Caused by a Fungus Possibly Related to the Sporotricha[†]

The patient gave the following history: Age 36. Marked family history of tuberculosis. Patient has suffered from phthisis for the past 12 years.

During the latter part of August, 1896 (three months before visit to the Johns Hopkins Hospital Dispensary), while working at the iron worker's trade in St. Louis, the patient scratched the index finger of right hand, on a nail, while reaching into a red lead keg. Shortly after this a small abscess formed which was opened with a pin. A slight amount of watery fluid escaped, which patient thinks did not look like pus. In about three weeks the ulcer between the second and third metacarpal joints appeared. This was treated at the St. Mary's Dispensary (St. Louis). The inflammation traveled up the arm, and in about seven weeks after the infection seven similar abscesses had formed. These were opened, and a watery discharge escaped. About this time a "waxen kernel," size of a walnut, appeared in the axilla. It was not especially tender and disappeared in two days. While in St. Louis the arm was bandaged daily with bichloride and carbolic dressings. The patient thinks he had no fever, and says the pain was very moderate. Being unable to work he returned to his home in Baltimore late in November.

---

[*] Kelly, H., and Burrage, W.: Dictionary of American Medical Biography, New York, Appleton, 1928.

[†] Johns Hopkins Hosp. Bull., *9:*286, 1898.

Physical examination on entrance showed evidences of advanced tuberculosis of the lungs, and the sputum contained numerous tubercle bacilli.

The infection involving the hand and arm proved very refractory to treatment, the last lesion, at point of primary infection, not granulating until late in February, 1897.

The organism which was assumed to be in etiological relationship to the above-described lesions was obtained in three cultures from two different foci of the disease: Once from one of the lesions in the forearm, admixed with the skin coccus, and twice from one of the lesions in the arm, in pure culture.

Caesar Boeck

Sarcoidosis

CAESAR PETER MOELLER BOECK was born September 28, 1845, in Lier, Norway. After graduation from medical school in Christiania (Oslo) in 1871, he practiced general medicine for several years. In 1874 he spent a year on the continent studying dermatology and histology, particularly in Vienna. He returned to Christiania as an assistant physician at the Rikshospitalet and later joined the staff of the University of Norway. In 1895 he was made Professor of Dermatology.

He was an outstanding teacher, clinician and diagnostician. His clinics were exceptionally popular, in part due to his resounding enthusiasm and his skill in therapy. Author of over 100 articles, many of which appeared in numerous foreign periodicals, he is best known for his brilliant work on tuberculides and sarcoidosis. He was among the first to see clearly the relationship between a large group of obscure dermatoses and tuberculosis. In 1880 he described a case of papulo-necrotic tuberculid, being the first to record the histologic findings. In the later years of his life his investigative talents were focused largely on sarcoidosis. His original account of sarcoidosis was published simultaneously in the American and Norwegian literature. Interestingly enough, the patient described below died recently at the age of 80, and at autopsy was found to have no trace of sarcoidosis.

Boeck was accorded many high honors, and the esteem in which he was held internationally is reflected in the *Festschrift* issue of the *Archiv für Dermatologie* which appeared in 1911 in honor of his sixty-sixth birthday. He was an exceptionally industrious worker, unselfish, and always a wise and kind counsellor. A connoisseur of fine paintings, he possessed a magnificent collection himself.

In 1915, Boeck retired at the age of 70, pleased to see his protegé, Bruusgaard named as his successor. Always a man of robust health, he died on March 17, 1917 shortly after a coronary attack.*

SARCOIDOSIS

Multiple Benign Sarkoid of the Skin[†]

The skin affection here described is, so far as I am aware, not generally recognized. I have seen two cases in Norway; one in a female many years ago of whose case I have no notes, and the example which forms the subject of this paper. A typical case in a male was presented at the *Dermatological Congress in London* (1896), but I do not know by whom. A majority of the experienced observers present failed to recognize the condition, so that I am not far wrong in saying that the disease is a rare one.

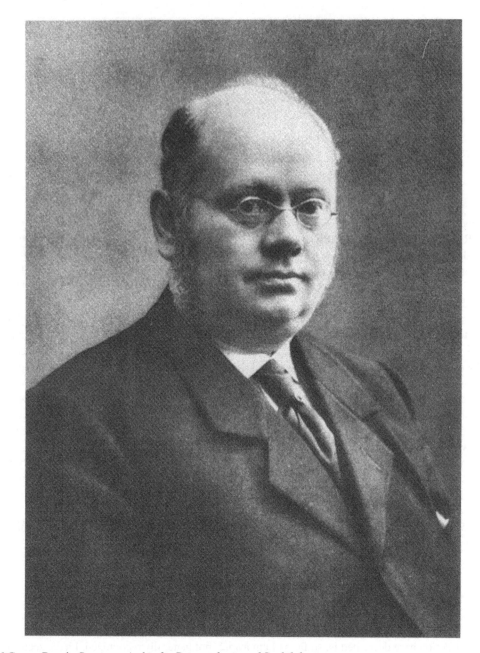

Figure 66 Caesar Boeck. Courtesy, *Archiv für Dermatologie und Syphilologie*

The only clinical description known to me which bears any resemblance to my case, is given in a recent paper by Jonathan Hutchinson in his *Archives of Surgery,* October, 1898. I dare not say that the skin affection there described as "Mortimer's Malady" is identical with my case, since the latter shows some very marked clinical features not found in Mortimer's disease, and since Mr. Hutchinson has had no opportunity to examine his cases histologically. Nevertheless, I am inclined to believe that they are only variant types of the same group of diseases and perhaps, later on, they may be found to represent benign forms of so-called pseudoleucemic affections of the skin. I shall return to this discussion after having given an account of my own case.

The patient, a policeman, was presented first at the University Polyclinic in September, 1894, and the disease was almost in the same condition then as two years later, when he came to me privately. He was 36 years old, and stated that he had always been in good health, and especially that he had never suffered from any scrofulo-tuberculous affections nor from syphilis. His children were healthy. The skin disease appeared first on the brow, spreading to other parts of the face from there. It made its appearance gradually on the scalp, trunk and limbs.

Present Condition. The patient looked a little pale, but felt tolerably well, and his functions were normal. On the forehead and temples a number of characteristic spots and patches were visible, although they were of somewhat different appearance, varying with the stage of development they had reached. Their size ranged from that of a small pea to a large bean, and were slightly elevated above the skin surface. At first glance, therefore, one might believe that they were only slightly infiltrated, but when grasped between the fingers they were felt to penetrate deeply and to form well defined nodules and infiltrations. The surface of the smaller efflorescences was of a uniform yellowish-brown color, sometimes slightly scaling. Somewhat larger nodules showed a slight central depression of a bluish-red tint, sharply contrasting with the border. As the growths increased in size and became large, flattened, irregularly contoured patches, the depressed centers deepened in color and the border became narrower until it was reduced to 1 mm. in breadth. The large patches with their apparent atrophy could by palpitation be determined to form well defined, deep infiltrations of the skin. On close inspection a network of dilated capillaries could be seen in the central area; the interpapillary lines and lanugo hairs were also distinct. As remarked before, these patches, with their irregular contour, bluish-red center and yellow border, presented so characteristic an appearance that they can be mistaken for no other known skin disease. Similar areas were found on the radix nasi, in front of the ears, on the cheeks, in the beard, and even in the sub-maxillary region.

On the hairy scalp there were visible everywhere a great many lesions of varying size but not so sharply outlined here as on the face. The infiltration of the skin was also less marked, at all events more difficult to demonstrate. It was only on close inspection that the patches could be made out at all. As in the beard, the growth of hair was in no way interfered with. On the neck, only three small areas could be seen on the right side below the ear, and on the left a single symmetrical spot.

The whole anterior surface of the trunk was entirely free from lesions. Between the axillary lines on the right side two small brownish spots could be detected. On the upper part of the back, to the superior limit of the lumbar region, a great number of disseminate nodules and patches, varying in size from a pea to a bean, were to be seen, which were sometimes elevated above the skin level, sometimes not (Plate II). The likeness of these lesions to the nodules of leprosy was quite close. Grasped between the fingers, the more recent were found to be infiltrated, the older not so much so. Lumbar and sacral regions were free, but on the buttocks, again, there were a number of efflorescences of the same color as those on the back.

The eruption was confined to the extensor surfaces of the upper extremities, both forearms and upper arm. They were numerous pin-head size and larger, varying in size from a hempseed to a bean, and showed

---

* Haarvaldsen, J.: Dermat. Wchnschr., *65:*763, 1917.

† J.Cutan. Dis., *17:*543, 1899.

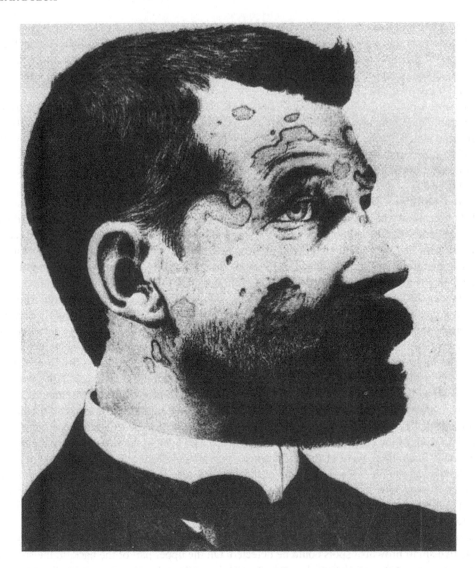

Figure 67 Boeck's sarcoid. From Boeck's paper. Courtesy, American Dermatological Association

irregular outlines. It was easier to follow evolution in this situation than anywhere else. The beginning lesions, the nodules, deep-seated in the skin, already hard and dense, were rose-red in color; they became darker later and showed some of yellowish-brown appearance at the periphery. The capillary network mentioned above appeared here also, especially in the center of the eruptive elements. Near the shoulders, very small yellowish lesions appeared, scarcely the size of a pin-head. They were connected with the hair-follicles, were superficial and palpable with difficulty. The hands were free.

The thighs showed no signs of the disease except that on the internal surface of the left extremity and behind, just under the nates, it appeared in the form of groups of numerous, very small bluish or brownish-red flat papules. Here and there they were quite confluent, as in lichen ruber, and slightly scaling as well.

These small lesions seemed to be connected with the hair-follicles. On the left thigh just above the patella a dense, hard giant nodule was visible. Over the right patella there was a flattened infiltration of irregular form and blue color, developed partly in and around an old cicatrix of 20 years' standing. It seemed evident that it was the previous lesion which had determined the outbreak in this locality. On the legs, from knee to ankle, there were only a few large, dark brown, atrophic spots resulting from the disappearance of large nodules. On the left calf there were three such areas. On the right leg patches of an oval form occurred on the anterior and inner side of the tibia. The feet, like the hands, were entirely free.

Lymphatic System. The cubital lymph nodes were enormously swollen and were easily felt in size and shape, like Spanish nuts, along the inner side of the biceps from the cubitus for half the length of the arm. The axillary glands were tumefied, but relatively not to so great an extent. Submaxillary glands were not swollen, and the cervical very little. The femoral nodes were so enlarged as to be visible in the fovea ovalis when the patient stood upright; the inguinal glands were not so increased in size. The spleen was never found enlarged.

The blood. I regret to say, was not so thoroughly studied as it should have been. I can only say that the number of leucocytes was a little greater than normal, especially in the case of the mononuclear cells. The number of eosinophiles was not notably increased. The urine contained no albumen or sugar.

After this description it will hardly be necessary to give *in extenso* the copious notes taken during the two or three years following, when the further development and final recovery occurred. A short summing up will be sufficient.

In October, 1896, administration of arsenic in granules (each containing 1 m. of arsenic) was begun, and in six weeks the dose was raised to 18 pills per diem, when a very rapid decrease of the swollen femoral glands was noticed, even by the patient himself, although no effect on the skin eruption could be detected as yet. At this time an obstinate diarrhea, very likely occasioned by the arsenic, had set in, and so the drug had to be stopped and could be resumed only after a lapse of some weeks. Wine of iron and quinine, and in the spring cod-liver oil, were also given with the arsenic.

The last development of a new nodule in the skin occurred in the middle of December, 1896, and in January, 1897, the first evidence of beginning involution was noted. The superficial lichenoid eruption on the inside of the left thigh was rapidly fading. In April of the same year the first of the large patches began to disappear under arsenic, iron, and cod-liver oil very slowly. The large patches on the face underwent retrogression in the period from June to October, the central area growing paler and the yellow margin fading. During this process the declivity from margin to center became perpendicular, and the sharply drawn line so formed was often seen as a minutely denticulated zig-zag. No infiltration of the skin could be felt anywhere, but in many situations involution had left marked loss of substance. Since August, 1897, when the arsenic was stopped, the patient has taken no medicine. On April 7, 1899, I made the following note: The patient looks rather stronger than before, and feels pretty well. On the face the disease has left slightly depressed but sharply defined white cicatrices, which redden with the heat of exertion. The loss of substance on the extremities is marked and deep, the skin being thin and atrophic, following disappearance of larger lesions; in the case of the smaller it is not so noticeable. On the upper arms the trace may be somewhat hyperemic; on the back, they are yellowish; on the legs, dark brown, pigmented and very atrophic. The cubital glands are very large, though a little reduced in size. They are quite soft. The patient has pursued his occupation during the whole course of the disease. I found him sound and healthy for the last time on July 8, 1899.

PART IV

THE EXPANDING UNIVERSE

Jean-Louis Brocq

1.   Pseudopelade

2.   Keratosis Pilaris

3.   Neurodermatitis Circumscripta

4.   Congenital Ichthyosiform Erythroderma

5.   Parapsoriasis

JEAN-LOUIS BROCQ was born at Laroque-Timbaud, February 1, 1856. At the age of 20 he went to Paris to begin his medical studies, and in 1882 presented his doctoral thesis on exfoliative dermatitis. This thesis was a masterpiece, so greatly enlarging and clarifying the clinical picture of the disease to which Erasmus Wilson had called attention some years before, that it has since been known as Wilson-Brocq's disease.

The greatest influence on the young Brocq was undoubtedly Emile Vidal. It was Vidal who persuaded him to adopt dermatology as a specialty, and the disciplined observation and elegance of language of the master are clearly reflected in the pupil.

After rather rocky tours of duty with Fournier and Quinquaud at Saint Louis, Brocq left to become chief at La Rochefoucauld, and later, with great success at l'Hôpital Broca. In 1905 he was recalled to l'Hôpital Saint Louis, 14 years after he had left under unpleasant circumstances.

Brocq's health was never good. As early as age 27 he had been thought to have incurable tuberculosis. Throughout his life he suffered from incessant attacks of asthma and bronchitis. In 1921 he resigned his service at Saint Louis, gave up his huge private practice and retired. During these last eight years he made but a handful of personal appearances, although he worked steadily at his writing almost to his death December 18, 1928.

Brocq's contributions to dermatology were immense. The number alone of his publications is staggering, and the scope of them is Dermatology itself. His greatest achievements were along three lines—his work in clarifying that difficult group of diseases we know as parapsoriasis, his superb conception of neurodermatitis, and his detailed investigations of the pruritic vesicular eruptions. We have included the first two here; the third has been overshadowed by the equally fine investigations of Duhring in this field. We have also brought together his notable descriptions of congenital ichthyosiform erythroderma, pseudopelade, and keratosis pilaris.

Pautrier, a pupil of his, made the following observation:

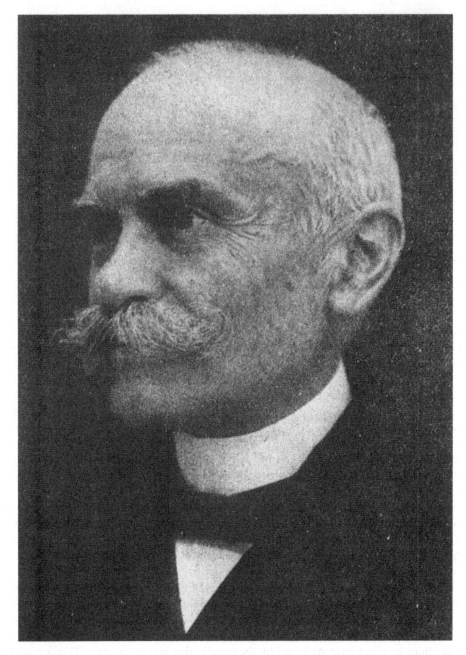

Figure 68 Jean-Louis Brocq

"He impressed those seeing him for the first time as being cold and distant; he retained, from his southern origin, besides the pungency of his gascon accent, a vivacity of spirit and almost petulance in discussion which made him a remarkable speaker, and a redoubtable opponent in debate."*

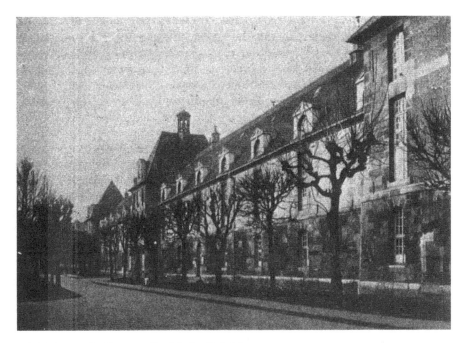

Figure 69 L'Hôpital Saint Louis. Courtesy, Dr. Marion B.Sulzberger

PSEUDOPELADE

Des Folliculites et Perifolliculites Decalyantes*

The first variety is extremely rare; it simulates pelade, with which it has probably been confused so far—whence comes the name *pseudo-pelade* which I propose to give to it.

1. The follicular and perifollicular inflammatory process is very moderate here, for it is characterized only by a mild tumefaction, and a slight pinkish color of the scalp around the affected hair.
2. If one applies moderate traction to the hairs he finds that they come out very easily, and that the root very often shows a sheath which is more or less thick, translucent, and quite similar to those that encase the hairs in favus; no parasites, however, can be demonstrated.
3. After the hair has been pulled out, or has fallen out spontaneously, the inflammatory process subsides, but it has produced complete atrophy of the papilla, and nothing is left but white, smooth, ivory-like scalp which looks atrophic, and on which there is no longer vestige of hair or down.
4. The affection reaches neighboring hairs without following any regular outward course; on the contrary, it sends out prolongations, very bizarre in form, into normal areas; here and there small, completely isolated patches of alopecia may even be found.

---

* Pautrier, L.: Ann. de dermat. et syph., *10:*133, 1929.

I have seen only two cases of this type. I mentioned one for the first time in my correspondence to the *Journal of Cutaneous Diseases* (February, 1885, p. 50), and at that time I was well aware that this was no special form of pelade. Indeed, here is a translation of the passage referring to this affection:

"I myself have just seen a patient who was attacked more than a year ago with an alopecia of this particular form, which several physicians had already diagnosticated as an alopecia. In fact at first glance it looked like an alopecia in patches, especially marked toward the vertex, at the level of which the integument appeared white, smooth, waxy like, altogether like a true alopecia; no seborrhea, no scale, no crusts upon any portion of the hairy scalp. In examining it with more care, I discovered in two or three points, where the hairs still remained, a light rosy erythematous tint, a little more marked around each hair. The hairs which were surrounded by the erythematous areola were not at all adherent, the least traction sufficed to detach them, and it is certain that they would have soon spontaneously fallen out; on the contrary, the adjoining hairs around which the derma had not the red coloration were still perfectly solid. The condition might have been regarded as an erythematous lupus of the hairy scalp, but the lesion had not the circumscription, the aspect, the distinct appearance of this disease; the alopecia parts did not present the least trace of a cicatrix; there were neither scales nor crusts. It was evidently produced by a sort of slow inflammatory process acting especially upon the hair follicles, and resulting finally in complete, total and definitive atrophy of the follicle, and an irremediable alopecia. It was then, if the term be preferred, an acne or better a folliculitis decalvans, for there was not an actual papular and pustular acne, distinctly and frankly inflammatory. On the other hand, we should not confound cases of this kind with ordinary alopecias."

Since then I have examined another case, also a patient from the city, who was sent to me by one of my friends who had called it rebellious pelade. Again I became convinced that I was dealing with a process entirely different from pelade. The hair is not atrophied or dead looking as in pelade; unlike that disease no more slender, drier, broken or unbroken hairs are to be found at the edge of the patch; the hairs are normal in almost all characteristics—volume, length, and appearance. However, I don't wish to be too assertive on this last point, for I have observed my two patients on only a few occasions and in a rather superficial manner. I have not had the opportunity to study them as I would, had I had the good fortune to meet with them in the hospital. I believe that I am able only to affirm that true pustules are never produced in these cases, because physicians caring for them concluded they were dealing with pelade, and because, moreover, the alopecia was irremediable, for in those regions involved for more than two years, and treated during that time with all known remedies for pelade, not the least vestige of downy hair nor hair follicles can be seen, either with the naked eye or with a lens.

KERATOSIS PILARIS

Pour servir a l'Histoire de la Kératose Pilaire*

It is common knowledge that a great number of persons show on the posterior part of the arms, and on the internal surface of the thighs, small elevations the size of a pinhead, dry, cornified, formed around the hair follicle, the hair of which is almost always atrophied. This deformity of the skin, which is more or less developed depending on the subject, is accompanied by a certain state of dryness of the integument in the area in which it exists.

---

* Bull, et Mém. de la Soc. Méd. des Hôp. de Paris, 5:400, 1888.

When it is mild it is not ordinarily accompanied by any coloration, and the papules are white or greyish white or blackish; we designate it then by the name *kératose pilaire blanche*.

Sometimes, even when the elements are few and disseminated, it presents a rose color, fiery red, or bluish red, livid; certain can be colored while others in their vicinity are not. These colorations are almost always accentuated in proportion to the intensity of the cutaneous lesion of which we are speaking. We then call it *kératose pilaire rouge*.

This affection may not be limited to the extremities; it is present in some cases on the trunk and on the face. These last manifestations are much less known than the first. On the face in particular the rose or red tint which accompanies the little papules may be very well developed, and the disease in involving the eyebrows, forehead, chin, lateral parts of the cheeks, may succeed in producing true deformities, extremely difficult to get rid of.

Keratosis pilaris of the trunk and limbs, these cutaneous lesions are very frequent. All dermatologists are acquainted with them, yet until now they have been described in a rather imperfect manner, undoubtedly because of this very banality.

In almost all the classic works they are described only very briefly as small circumpilary elevations, whitish or light brownish, which are met with so frequently on the posterior part of the arms, the forearms, the external regions of the thighs and legs, and which give the sensation of a rasp when one passes the hand over these regions.

Keratosis pilaris of the arms consists (as the classical authors have said) in its most banal form, and to our mind the most attenuated, of a small solid elevation the size of a small pinhead, the color of the surrounding skin, developed around the hair follicle, the hair of which is rolled up or atrophied, and bearing often a dry scale on a summit which is rounded or acuminate; there may even be no papule, properly speaking, and the keratotic element thin, as has been written, only a simple accumulation in the follicle of dry epidermal scales which disappear on washing with soap, and which reappear however little one neglects his toilet.

But in its most striking form keratosis pilaris of the arms is an entirely different thing. It is then basically constituted by a true papule which washing with soap will by no means make disappear. This papule is quite uniform in size in the same region: it can, however, vary in mass from that of a small to that of a large pinhead. It forms a more or less marked projection on the skin of the area (we will see that this projection may be completely lacking); in certain cases it reaches a height of a quarter, a half, and even a millimeter. It will be understood that it conveys to the touch the very marked sensation of a rasp, moreover that it bears almost always on its summit a dry and hard scale, visible spontaneously or following scratching. This scale may, however, be absent. The papule is quite regular in form; its base is rounded or a little oval, sometimes a little polygonal. Its summit is acuminate, or more often, blunted in the form of a dome or cup, especially when one lifts off the scale which covers it.

Its coloring is extremely variable. We have just seen that the keratotic element, even when it is clearly papular, can be of a shade similar to that of the neighboring integument, or may well be tinted a blackish brown by dirt; but this type which we have designated by the name *kératose pilaire blanche,* and which is most frequent, is met with only in cases of mild intensity. When the affection is of real importance the papules are colored, taking on a rose shade, a bright red, dusky red, or violet red; certain are even fiery red, but then they appear to be frankly inflammatory; they are large, projecting, have a central crust and an acneiform appearance. Even though there are very numerous exceptions, one can state as a rule that the intensity of the red color is in direct relation to the size of the papule, and the intensity of development of

---

* Ann. de dermat. et syph., *1:*25, 1890.

the affection. Almost always, especially on the lower extremities, the red is mixed with dark brown; this dark brown shade often becomes livid on the buttocks, thighs and legs.

Whatever the intensity and the quality of this coloring, it always disappears completely, or almost completely, on pressure with the finger. It increases when one makes friction on the affected parts.

Pilous system. The hair situated in the center of the typical papules of *kératose pilaire rouge* is almost always atrophied. It is often completely destroyed; frequently it is broken off even; only a vestige of it is seen in the form of a little black point; sometimes (especially on the calves), it forms a small black projection and contributes in its way to the exaggeration of the rasp-like sensation; sometimes it is small, slender, dry, and rolled up upon itself under the scales in the follicle in such a way that when one scratches off the summit of the papule it may be seen to unroll. This fact has been known a long time and has been pointed out by almost all the classic authors. More rarely it is frizzled, bent, or quite large, blackish; still more rarely it is intact in all its features.

Such is the typical papule of *kératose pilaire rouge* in its complete development.

In the great majority of cases the patients affected with keratosis pilaris do not experience the slightest subjective phenomena. A certain number, however, are plagued with itching which is quite intense, intermittent, and as soon as they begin to scratch, all the little papules become the seat of a very distressing pruritus.

From the preceding description it appears that one might be able to propose in principle that the localizations of keratosis pilaris should be governed by the localizations of the pilous system. This is only partly true. On the disposition of the pilous system depends the seat and the frequency of the keratotic elements of a given region, consequently the appearance and form of the lesions vary depending on the size of the hairs, and depending on the distance to which they are implanted, but one ought not presume that keratosis pilaris will always be abundant chiefly in the regions of the body normally the most hairy in subjects with normal skin. On the contrary, in the majority of cases it is absent in the regions where considerable hair exists, such as the scalp, the axillae, the pubis, the internal superior parts of the thigh, the internal part of the legs; it attacks only the lanugo hair follicles, and although there may be exceptions to this rule, they are very rare.

NEURODERMATTTIS CIRCUMSCRIPTA

Notes pour servir a l'Histoire des Nevrodermites*

Despite some differences in details, the preceding observations present such an *air de famille* that one does not hesitate for an instant to group them together. In all, the picture is of an eminently pruritic circumscribed affection giving rise to the formation of circumscribed plaques, constantly and absolutely dry, characterized by thickening and infiltration of the skin, great fixedness and a chronic evolution.

This stated, we begin detailed study of the cases.

Analysis of Cases

Etiology. In our nine cases one finds four men and five women. The disease we are speaking of appears then to affect the two sexes with almost equal frequency; however, from our personal notes which do not appear to be precise enough to be published, we are willing to believe that it is a little more frequent in women.

The ages of the patients at the time of onset were variable; they were exactly: 32, 34, 31, 38, 48, 24, 63, 33, 23. The affection appears therefore to be chiefly a disease of adults; our other documents led us likewise to think that it attains its maximum frequency during the most active period of existence, that of 20 to 50 years.

The family histories which one finds noted in our observations are not very detailed, but from those we have seen we believe we are able to say that with regard to the forebears of the patients one finds the following three great disease categories: *arthritism, alcoholism, nervousness.*

In personal histories, chronic bronchitis, emphysema, pseudo asthmatic attacks, rheumatic pains, sciatica, prolonged outbreaks of furuncles, leucorrhea, hemorrhoids, etc. have been noted. We have several times observed diabetes in subjects affected with lichen simplex chronicus. But the thing which seems especially to dominate in these cases is a marked nervous condition; sometimes it consists of a simple impressionability, keener than that of the great majority of persons; sometimes it is a very pronounced tendency to fly into furious rages for the most trifling reasons, and even without reason; sometimes it is a pre-disposition to cry for the least cause, to have gloomy ideas; sometimes it is a true neurosis well characterized by nervous crises, hysterical choking sensations, hemianesthesia, attacks of hystero-epilepsy, etc.

It appears that sedentary professions predispose to this affection; in fact among our patients are several seamstresses, a paste-board maker, a brandy merchant, a shoemaker, and a lawyer. This tallies well with the preceding facts, I mean with the influence which nervousness appears to have in the genesis of this dermatitis.

Frequency. Lichen simplex chronicus is a relatively frequent affection, at least in France. In several months during which one of us replaced our excellent and most honored master, Dr. E.Vidal at l'Hôpital St. Louis, he was able to observe some 10 cases on this service alone. The constantly increasing frequency of nervous diseases makes us believe that this dermatosis cannot but have a tendency to become even more common.

Symptoms

Mode of onset. When one considers only the patients' accounts of it, it is difficult to understand how the affection begins. Usually they do not know what to answer when one questions them in this regard, and this is understandable since they have most often been affected for several years. We find, however, the mode of onset indicated in our observations III, IV, V, and VII. In observation III it began with pruritic papules; in observation IV with a small pruritic plaque, but in observations V and VII, it is expressly noted that *the affection began exclusively with pruritus alone, without preceding cutaneous lesion;* the pruritus induced scratching after which the eruption appeared. These documents are, as one will see later on, of greatest importance for conception of the true nature of lichen simplex chronicus.

Location. The involved sites vary greatly with the subject; the same patient may have one (Obs. I) or several plaques (Obs. VII, Tennison). Here are the regions which have been involved in our nine cases: the palm of the right hand (once), the right forearm (once), the left forearm (once), the right elbow (once), the axillae (once), the nape of the neck (twice), the lateral part of the abdomen toward the anterior superior iliac spine on the right (once), and left (once), the left greater trochanter (once), the anus, the intergluteal cleft and genital organs (twice), the internal and superior part of the left thigh (three times), the internal and superior part of the right thigh (four times), the popliteal fossa (twice).

---

* Ann. de dermat. et syph., *2*:97, 1891.

The lichen simplex chronicus of Doctor E.Vidal is constituted in typical cases by plaques which are usually oval, the long axis of which varies in size from 5 to 15 cm., and in which one can distinguish the following three zones:

1. An external pigmented zone or zone of beginning papillary hypertrophy, which may be absent in certain cases and which is characterized by a color varying from light coffee to light brown, by a group of small compact squares formed by two series of parallel ridges crossing each other at right or acute angles, by a papillary hypertrophy which is not too marked, giving to the integument a velvety appearance.
2. A middle papular zone, which may be missing in certain cases, or even, on the contrary, which may at times be the external zone when the preceding zone is not present; it is made up of a series of small papular elements, irregular in form and contour, rather poorly circumscribed, pale rose or greyish, acuminate, rounded or flat, of a size that varies from that of a small pinhead to that of a large one, and which appear to be due to a papillary hypertrophy quite advanced in degree.
3. An internal zone or zone of infiltration which is the essential or constitutive part of the lichen plaque and which can exist alone, especially in those cases in which the affection has not progressed far; it is characterized by a pale rose or more or less pigmented color, by a marked infiltration and thickening of the integument, by a mesh work of more or less large and regular squares figured by a hatch-marked design, and finally by absolute dryness of the lesion.

The pruritus is the most important phenomenon of the affection; it exists prior to the cutaneous lesions; it is the originating factor in these lesions, thanks to the traumatism that it provokes; in fact, when one puts a sealed dressing on the diseased areas one can cause them to involute, but one cannot bring about the disappearance of the pruritus.

To understand well the true nature of this affection one must go further than the cutaneous lesions and consider the disease as a whole. Supported by, 1. The nervousness of the patients affected. 2. The constant pruritus that dominates the morbid scene, at least during the onset and development. 3. The circumscription of the eruption in plaques. 4. Its distribution in concentric zones in the typical cases. 5. Its absolute dryness. 6. The papillary hypertrophy, papular projections, dermal infiltration and pigmentations that characterize it objectively. 7. Its chronic course and its tendency to recurrence, one can consider it as a distinct dermatosis, meriting its place in the nosologic framework. It is, in reality, a sort of *nevrodermite circonscrite,* but one should keep for it the name under which it has already been described by the older authors, that of *lichen circumscriptus;* this is the *lichen simplex chronique* of Dr. E.Vidal.

CONGENITAL ICHTHYOSIFORM ERYTHRODERMA

Érythrodermie Congénitale Ichthyosiforme avec Hyperépidermotrophie*

If one reads the preceding observations with some attention he will be struck from the very first by the chief characteristic, of primordial importance, that this affection makes its debut, as it were, at birth, that it is also congenital, that it persists afterwards without great modifications, without troubling the general health to any great extent for many years. It presents, therefore, the character of perpetuity most distinctly. However, it appears able to attenuate, and also to become modified in certain of its symptoms in proportion to the patient's advance in age. Thus in the bullous variety the appearance of bullae may become more and more uncommon, and they may even gradually cease to be produced as the patient reaches adolescence and adulthood. It is no less true that we have known no case to be cured. Congenital origin, perpetuity, these are, then, the two major characteristics of this curious affection.

From the objective point of view, the *generalized redness of the skin* predominates, a redness sometimes little marked, especially in certain regions, such as the face, the thorax, the abdomen, and which may be light enough not to attract the attention of observers. There is a tendency not to take this much into account, for we have reported it in our three cases, and in two among those of eminent dermatologists who neglected to mention it in their accounts of the symptoms, although they noticed it.

Sometimes this redness is intense, especially in certain regions, such as the neck, the articular folds, the extremities; it can be sufficient to lead to the diagnosis of pityriasis rubra pilaris or pemphigus foliaceus. It appears gradually to attenuate, at least in some cases, as the subject advances in age.

There exists moreover, in certain regions, a *considerable exaggeration* of the *papillary projections*. This symptom, which is absent, or which appears macroscopically to be absent, from the face, from the anterior part of the thorax, etc., is especially accentuated on the neck, toward the nape, and the large articular folds. It attains in these latter places an extraordinary development at times, resembling with exaggeration, acanthosis nigricans, with the difference that the colour of the integument is frankly red, and the colour of the scales that cap and bristle on the papillary projections arranged in a linear fashion is whitish grey, sometimes a little brownish.

This striking symptom results from a *generalized accentuated hyperkeratosis* which gives the patient at first glance the appearance of an ichthyotic, and even of a subject affected with ichthyosis cornée hystrix in places; this is almost always the first diagnosis proposed, but one soon perceives that the articular folds are greatly involved, also that the disease appears to reach its maximum development there, in such a manner that its maximum development is in localizations exactly the inverse of those of true ichthyosis; this is an anomaly of greatest importance; moreover the generalized redness of the integument does not permit us to group this dermatosis purely and simply with simple ichthyosis.

The hyperkeratotic process may affect the palms of the hands, and the soles of the feet to such a degree that it constitutes there an enormous mass of cornified material with a yellowish appearance, almost villous, nearly amber coloured, recalling the most developed arsenical hyperkeratosis.

All our patients presented a *very abundant seborrheic secretion* in the scalp area; this was also present, but to a much lesser extent, in the area of the median part of the face. On the scalp this secretion is sometimes so exaggerated that on some days it forms a sebaceous layer dense and adherent, several millimeters thick. Beneath it, in the case of the patient of E.Vidal, the dermal papillae were hypertrophied, almost papillomatous; they bled easily.

Another most extraordinary symptom is the *rapidity of growth of the epidermal appendages, of the hair and nails* which one is obliged to cut two or three times as often as in the healthy individual. In certain cases the hair of the body, particularly the extremities, developed excessively in places; the nails are arched; they have a certain tendency to grow crooked with respect to their length. It is this rapidity of growth of the appendages that persuaded the late E.Vidal to propose for this dermatosis the name, hyperepidermotrophy. But we must add that these patients may have rather sparse hair, though these scanty hairs grow with true rapidity. So in this case rapid lengthening of the hair does not always indicate a bushy and luxuriant growth.

We have seen that in certain of these cases, not in all, *bullous elevations of the epidermis,* irregular in form, containing an opaline serosity, and flaccid in appearance are produced, either in a continuous manner, especially in the first years of life, or sometimes in an intermittent manner, more and more seldom as the

---

* Ann. de dermat. et syph., *3:*1, 1902.

subject grows older. They recall to mind quite well the bullae of pemphigus foliaceus. These epidermal elevations, which are not accompanied by pruritus, but with simple pain due to the vesication of the integument, are formed especially on the extremities, in particular on the lower extremities, the calves and the feet.

Thus it appears that it is possible to have two forms of this dermatosis, one bullous, the other dry.

As to the pathogenesis of this affection, nothing is more obscure. We have been able to determine only a single influence which appears perhaps to play a certain role; this is hereditary syphilis. But if syphilis counts for anything in the genesis of this disease, it must certainly do so in an extremely indirect manner; indeed, one would not be able to consider it as a direct manifestation of hereditary syphilis modifiable by antisyphilitic treatment.

PARAPSORIASIS

Les Parapsoriasis*

During the past few years work has appeared from time to time on a relatively rare group of dermatoses characterized essentially by redness of the skin and by more or less marked dry desquamation; the elements are more or less widespread; in certain cases they have scarcely the dimension of a pin head, or of a lentil; in other cases they approach the size of the palm of the hand and even larger. Their colour is more or less accentuated. But as a general rule they have the following common characteristics: 1. Little or no infiltration of the integument. 2. Little or no pruritus. 3. Very slow evolution. 4. Little tendency to involution.

This group of dermatoses is evidently very closely related to psoriasis. The affected patients are even almost always considered to have an abortive or anomalous form of psoriasis. However, certain forms rather resemble lichen planus, others pityriasis or psoriasiform seborrheides, accounting for the diversity of the names that have been given to these affections.

Let us say immediately that we have chosen for the group of cases the very debatable but short and hitherto unused term *Parapsoriasis*. It has the advantage of indicating that these dermatoses have a real affinity to psoriasis; they cannot, however, be considered as simple varieties of that affection. We have seen from the analysis of work already published, and we shall bring it out again in analysing our personal observations, that certain among them have a very striking resemblance to lichen ruber, and that consequently these varieties might just as well be named *paralichens*. One could, if one wishes, conserve that name to designate them in a very precise manner. But, in the end, when one considers the whole group together, one is quickly convinced that most of the varieties are related chiefly to psoriasis and the seborrheides: therefore we prefer for the general denomination the word parapsoriasis to the word paralichen. Surely the word parapsoriasis is quite vague and it may certainly be applied to a multitude of dermatoses other than those we are studying, in particular to the pityriasic and psoriasiform seborrheides. But it will not be at all repugnant to us to see the seborrheides form a part of this new group, especially since between the pityriasic seborrheides and the psoriasiform seborrheides on the one hand and our *érythrodermie pityriasique en plaques* on the other, there is, one may say, no definite line of demarcation: these morbid groups are linked closely together by an imperceptible bridge of transitional cases.

---

* Ann. de dermat. et syph., *3:*433, 1902.

Clinical Classification of Parapsoriasis. When we consider in the broad perspective, the series of clinical cases which we have seen, and which have been reported in this morbid group which we have undertaken to study, we see that one can divide them into three principal varieties.

First variety (very closely related to psoriasis)—*Parapsoriasis en gouttes* (Jadassohn's cases are very probably of this type).

Characterized objectively by a macular and flat papulosquamous eruption without notable dermal infiltration, varying in colour from dusky pink to brownish red, not showing, on scratching, the hemorrhagic punctae and smooth and shiny surface of psoriasis, but having sometimes a certain tendency to bleed on scratching, resembling on the whole an eruption of secondary syphilis without infiltration, or an abortive guttate psoriasis, localized chiefly on the trunk and limbs, leaving the face and extremities almost always unaffected, slow in evolution, and offering great resistance to local treatment.

Second variety (intermediate between lichen and psoriasis)—*Parapsoriasis lichenoides* (this is the parakeratosis variegata of Unna, the lichen variegatus of Radcliffe Crocker).

Characterized objectively, in the beginning, by minuscule papules of pin head size, flat, shiny, and thus resembling the papules of abortive lichen planus, except for the colour which is very bright, sometimes depressed and having an atrophic appearance, sometimes with light scales, never demonstrating the scratch characteristics of psoriasis, causing little or no pruritus, having a tendency to form networks the component lines of which are more or less narrow, sinuous and irregular, encircling larger or smaller zones of healthy or nearly healthy skin, forming also, in certain cases, irregular plaques which are more or less extensive, and in this event constituting forms transitional to the third variety, having variable colours, pale pink to bluish red depending on the localization, and consequently giving on the whole a generally mottled appearance to the patient, localized chiefly on the trunk and limbs, almost always leaving the face unaffected, evolving very slowly and offering great resistance to local treatment.

Third variety (very closely related to the psoriasiform seborrheides)— *Parapsoriasis in plaques* (these are our érythrodermies pityriasiques en plaques disseminées—and those cases of J.C.White).

Characterized objectively by circumscribed plaques, rather well demarcated, two to six centimeters in diameter, scattered here and there over the integument, varying in colour from pale reddish to dusky or livid red depending on the subject and on the localization, presenting a fine pityriasic desquamation more or less marked depending on the patient, but which may be lacking, never demonstrating the scratch characteristics of psoriasis, appearing sometimes to be made up, in certain places, of aggregates of small flat papules and in this event able to be considered cases transitional to the second variety, without appreciable infiltration of the skin to the sight or touch, attacking the face only very rarely, giving rise to little or no subjective sensations, evolving with extreme slowness, and offering very great resistance to local treatment.

Such is the clinical classification of the three varieties.

Edvard Ehlers

The Ehlers-Danlos Syndrome

EDVARD EHLERS was born in Copenhagen, March 26, 1863. The son of the mayor of that city, he had all the advantages of money and position. After an early and thorough classical education he turned to medicine and took his medical degree in 1891, entitling his thesis, *Extirpation of the Primary Lesion of Syphilis.* On completion of a period of dermatologic study in Berlin, Breslau, Vienna, and Paris, he began practice in Copenhagen. From 1906 to 1911 he was Chief of the poly clinic for skin diseases in the Fredericks Hospital, and from 1911 to 1932 he directed the special service at the Kommunhospitalet in Copenhagen. He died in 1937.

Ehlers was a clinical dermatologist *par excellence.* Not satisfied to wait in his clinic for cases of those diseases which interested him particularly, he struck out for their endemic areas. Thus many of his finest publications deal with leprosy, which he studied first hand in Iceland and the Antilles, and with mal de meleda, which he explored thoroughly on a journey to Adriatic waters. He was a student of syphilis, both in its clinical and social aspects, and was instrumental in the founding of the Danish Welander asylum for the treatment and rehabilitation of congenital syphilitics. His best known clinical description is his account of the disease known as the Ehlers-Danlos syndrome, given here.

Ehlers was a confirmed Francophile. He spoke the language perfectly, made frequent trips to France, and was as much at home in Parisian dermatologic circles as in his own. The French were extremely grateful for the care he accorded French prisoners of war in the murderous influenza epidemic which followed the first World War. He inherited more than the wanderlust from his Viking ancestors. He was tall, blond, and blue eyed, with a penchant for proposing toasts.*

THE EHLERS-DANLOS SYNDROME

Cutis laxa, Neigung zu Hemorrhagien in der Haut, Lockerung mehrerer Artikulationen[†]

The patient I will show to you here was kindly sent to me by Dr. Kjoer. Like me, he had not the least idea as to what was really wrong with the patient. It is never difficult for me, whether faced by colleagues or patients, to admit that I know nothing about a given case, and I always wonder about colleagues who insist on fastening a label on every disorder. It is much more important to classify, mark, and define diseases on the basis of etiology than to label them as isolated, rare, and hitherto unobserved cases.

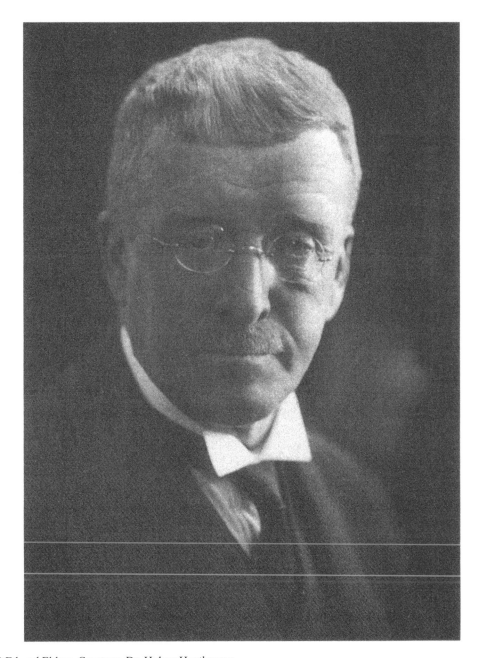

Figure 70 Edvard Ehlers. Courtesy, Dr. Holger Haxthausen

In the case in question, for which, until now, the patient has not consulted a specialist in skin diseases, I wonder whether it is possible to find out what the trouble is. To my way of thinking, his disease process has entered the self-healing stage, to be sure only after he has carried off sore wounds from the battle; it is possible, however, that at an earlier time perhaps the diagnosis could have been established.

Our colleagues in Bornholm who have cared for the patient up to now have assured him that it "will disappear with the years"; they did not find it necessary, however, to ask the opinion of other colleagues.

The patient is a 21 year old law student. His father is living, and, except for the fact that he suffers severely from gout, is healthy. The mother has had an Ulcus cruris for 20 years. Three sisters and three brothers are living and well. No disposition to hemophilia. No chronic infectious disease, in particular no syphilis, revealed in the anamnesis.

Throughout his entire development the patient has always been rather delicate, and in particular began to walk very late; he was told that he had had rickets. When he was two years old his nurse let him fall, whereupon he developed a large swelling which resorbed only with difficulty.

Later, until his eighth year, the patient was beset by the formation of hematomas which arose with the most trivial trauma, resorbed only with difficulty, and left behind persistent discolored hematoma residua, especially on the elbows, the knees, and the knuckles.

Around the eighth year the patient became more developed, and gained considerably in strength; his limbs became stronger, and he walked better, so that he was in better condition to protect himself from trauma. But even today there exists an excessive disposition to the formation of hematomas which dominate the disease picture, as well as discolored hematoma residua over all those bony prominences beneath the skin which are exposed to contusions.

Another prominent symptom is the drawn, pale, and wrinkled skin. It recalls to mind perfectly the skin of myxedema patients, which looks like the skin of a baked apple. It feels cool; nowhere can the ruddy color of blood be seen shining through, and it can be so markedly folded over the insensible subcutaneous tissue that on the fingers and knuckles, for example, enough skin is present to wrap half again around the finger. The hands are flabby and thin, with atrophy of the thenar, the hypothenar, and interossei. The fingers can be subluxed outwards without hindrance, indeed almost to a right angle. The patient has frequent spontaneous luxations of the knee which he has to reduce by walking.

No claw formation nor loss of limbs. All knuckles are covered with brownish discolored skin, due to hematoma residua. No sensation abnormalities, except for a permanent feeling of coldness in the skin of the extremities.

There are no other signs of myxedema present; the intelligence in particular is completely unimpaired; the speech is free and not dragging; movements are as energetic as the habitus of the patient will allow. He cannot be said to be strongly built. No changes are noted at the site of the thyroid gland. The face has the same pale color as the rest of the skin which, despite the considerable cicatricial changes in the upper layers, is able considerably to be moved over the substratum. The eyebrows are thin; the hair growth is good. The eyes are healthy; the rest of the sense organs are in good condition. A marked keratosis pilaris is seen on the arms.

The secretion of sweat is increased, which speaks for myxedema. The gait is a little ataxic, waddling. Patellar reflexes are strong. Besides the hematomas on all places in which there are lesions, small isolated xanthoma-like papules are noted in the region of the shoulder blades. On the elbows, in addition to the numerous hematoma residua, a great number of small papules are seen which are grouped in rings, and which turn one's thoughts instinctively to syphilis. There are, however, no other signs of that disease.

---

* Simon, C.: Ann. de dermat. et syph., 8:458, 1937.

† Dermat. Zeitschr., 8:173, 1901.

George Henry Fox

Fox-Fordyce Disease

GEORGE HENRY FOX was born at Ballston Spa, New York, October 8, 1846. The son of a clergyman, he was educated in private schools, was graduated from the Rochester University in 1867, and took his M.D. at the University of Pennsylvania in 1869. He served his internship at Blockley Hospital, Philadelphia, following Duhring. As was customary in his day, he traveled to Europe for further training, and studied with Virchow in Berlin, Bazin, Hardy and Vidal in Paris, Tilbury Fox and Jonathan Hutchinson in London, and notably with Hebra in Vienna.

In 1873 he began practice in New York City and after a number of preliminary appointments became in 1880 Professor of Dermatology at the College of Physicians and Surgeons of New York. For many years he was attending physician to the Skin and Cancer Unit of the New York Post-Graduate Medical School and Hospital.

Dr. Fox was the longest surviving member of the six founders of the American Dermatological Association. His contributions to dermatologic teaching were unmatched. His writings were numerous and outstanding, including the first photographic atlas of skin diseases (1880).

Pusey said of him: "Not the least of Dr. Fox's admirable qualities was his personality. He had a strong social instinct and enjoyed his friends, which was one among many other qualities that made him popular. He was rather short, well proportioned, without superfluous flesh, erect, quick and active, with a friendly expressive face. He looked the scholar and man of dignity, but without a trace of self importance."

He died suddenly at the age of 91 on May 3, 1937.*

FOX-FORDYCE DISEASE

Two Cases of a Rare Papular Disease Affecting the Axillary Region*

The first patient who presented the peculiar eruption which I wish briefly to describe, entered the New York Skin and Cancer Hospital in January 1899. She was 28 years old, unmarried, and born in Russia. The eruption was mainly confined to the axillary region, had existed for a year or more and caused no little distress. The itching was intense and of a paroxysmal character, robbing her of sleep and impairing her

---

* Pusey, W.: Arch. of Dermat, and Syph., *36:*361, 1937.

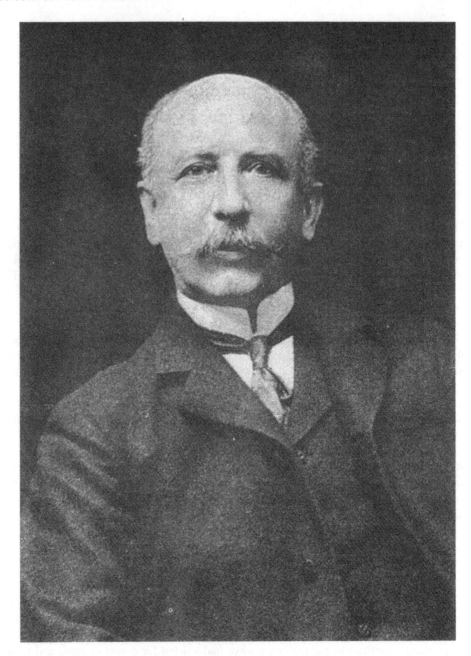

Figure 71 George Henry Fox. Courtesy, Dr. Fred D.Weidman

general health, in a marked degree. The patient was thin and of a highly neurotic temperament and it was not easy to determine to what extent the impaired health was a cause or result of the distressing dermatosis.

The eruption was of a papular character and the lesions were numerous, small, firm, smooth and rounded. The skin was deeply infiltrated and slightly fissured. The aggregated papules were of normal color or but slightly reddened, although the scratching produced at times a considerable amount of congestion and excoriation.

Over the pubic region were a number of small rounded papules, evidently of the same nature as those in the axillae, but not accompanied by such intense pruritus. Upon other portions of the body no sign of eczema or other disease was noticeable.

Upon the assumption, after my first examination of the patient, that the eruption was either a chronic lichenoid eczema or one which would at least yield to the usual treatment of such a condition, a variety of local applications were successively employed. Nitrate of silver, oil of peppermint, tar and chrysorobin were alternated with ichthyol, zinc ointment and carbolated vaseline, and I may add that never in my experience have I seen a case in which local treatment has had less beneficial effect.

Bromides and trional were found necessary to relieve the persistent insomnia, while arsenic and iron, together with compulsory exercise in the open air, were prescribed for their tonic effect. At times slight improvement both general and local was noted, but after eleven months in the hospital the patient was finally discharged in a condition which clinical accuracy compels me to characterize as "unimproved."

I have met with one other case of this rare, obstinate and distressing affection. This occurred in a young man who was extremely neurotic and suffered much from the intense pruritus as in the case above reported; the eruption consisted of small, rounded, aggregated and almost colorless papules. It was confined to the axillary region and resisted the ordinary methods of treatment.

---

* Fox, G., and Fordyce, J.: J.Cutan. Dis., *20:*1, 1902.

Abraham Buschke

Scleredema Adultorum

ABRAHAM BUSCHKE was born in Nakel (Poland), September 27, 1868. He studied in Breslau, Berlin, and Greifswald and was graduated in Berlin in 1891. After an assistantship at the surgical clinic in Greifswald under Helfreich, at the dermatology clinic in Breslau, under Neisser, and in Lesser's clinic in Berlin, he became Chief of the dermatologic section of the city Urban-Krankenhaus in Berlin. He remained with the Virchow hospital in that city until 1933. A victim of Nazi tyranny, he died in the concentration camp in Theresienstadt (Czechoslovakia) in 1943.

Buschke put the tremendous amount of clinical material at his disposal (400 dermatologic beds) to good use. His publications deal with all phases of dermatology, clinical and laboratory. He was particularly interested in the problem of immunity in syphilis, the social aspects of venereal disease, hereditary syphilis and the yeast mycosis. With Busse he did the original work on Cryptococcosis (Busse-Buschke's disease). Best known of his clinical descriptions is his account of scleredema adultorum, given below.

He was driving and energetic, a strong personality and an independent thinker. William and Helen Curth said of him:

"His assistants loved his great vitality, although it was not always easy for them to work out to his satisfaction dermatologic problems which he handed them in the morning in the form of cryptic notes scribbled down during the night."*

SCLEREDEMA ADULTORUM

Ueber Scleroedem*

The patient is a 46 year old wagon painter.

In February of the year 1900 he became ill with influenza, with symptoms of fever, chills, angina, and bronchitis. He took quinine internally and, apparently due to this, developed spots on the skin which were partly roseola-like and partly urticaria-like, and which disappeared quickly. The influenza subsided gradually, yet the patient did not feel entirely well. He noticed a certain weakness in the extremities, felt unable to stir a finger. Especially troublesome to him was a stiffness of the nape of the neck which hindered movement of the head. In the course of the next few weeks this stiffness spread gradually and continuously

---

* Curth, W., and Curth, H.: Arch. of Dermat. and Syph., *52*:32, 1945.

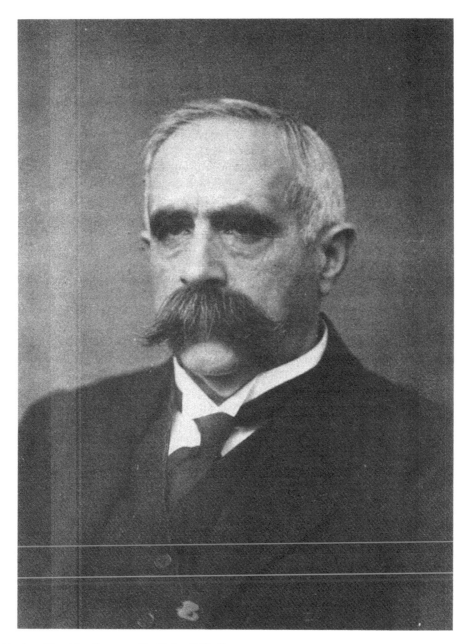

Figure 72 Abraham Buschke. Courtesy, Dr. Helen O.Curth

from the nape to the face, the scalp, the anterior part of the neck, the thorax to the abdomen, and the upper extremities as far as the fingers, the back down to the gluteal regions. The stiffness of the skin was so severe that for a long time breathing was extremely difficult for the patient. In the course of time these manifestations involuted somewhat; they were, however, still very considerable when the patient was seen for the first time in the Poliklinik on April 27, 1900:

Examination of the internal organs of this strong, muscular, well nourished man reveals no disease aside from a mild bacterial cystitis which has so far caused the patient no difficulty. The skin is, in the areas mentioned, altered in such a way that it appears greatly swollen; to palpation it is woody hard, and it is impossible to make an indentation even with the strongest pressure, nor is it possible to pick the skin up in folds; only here and there—especially at the edges of the diseased areas—can the skin be pinched into small folds. Otherwise the surface of the skin is normal, and conveys only the impression of skin tightly stretched. Particularly at the edges of the diseased area, one can feel clearly that this is an infiltration deep in the cutis, the subcutaneous tissue, and perhaps also in the musculature, while the upper layers of the skin are unaffected, both in appearance and to the touch. Examination of the skin with reference to its sensation and electrical conductivity revealed no deviation from normal. The skin feels cooler than in the normal areas, and appears white, anemic, smooth and shiny; the borders of the diseased zones show no inflammatory manifestations. The patient feels pain in the affected parts neither spontaneously nor on pressure, although he mentions that he experiences from time to time abnormal sensations such as prickling.

The skin of the back of the neck is affected in the manner described, so that movement of the head is difficult. From there the skin changes spread out in a continuous fashion over the neck, the chin area, the face (especially the cheeks), the scalp, the thorax down to the umbilical region, the back to the gluteal region, and the arms to the elbow region. Because of the infiltration of the skin of the face, the facial expression has a staring and mask-like quality, as in scleroderma. The involvement of the skin of the chest and back makes breathing difficult for the patient, even with great exertion.

The course of the illness was such that with the employment of massage it improved very slowly. It took almost a year for the skin changes on the body and extremities to disappear. Not until later did the infiltration disappear from the nape, the anterior part of the neck, and the head; and examination of the patient on July 24, 1902, showed that, with the exception of the face, the previously diseased skin had become normal, but for a slight diminution in its elasticity; on the other hand, the skin on both cheeks had lapsed into an apparently permanent state of stiffness and solidification which is most similar to elephantiasis, except that in this case the surface of the skin is in no way altered; it shows neither atrophy nor pigmentation.

---

* Berl. Klin. Wchnschr., *39:*955, 1902.

Martin Feeney Engman

Infectious Eczematoid Dermatitis

MARTIN FEENEY ENGMAN was born in New Orleans on August 20, 1869. After study at the Universities of Kentucky and Virginia, he received his M.D. from New York University in 1891. Following this he did postgraduate work in London, Paris, Berlin, Hamburg and Heidelburg, and in 1894 was appointed lecturer in Dermatology at the New York Postgraduate School. He later moved to St. Louis, Missouri where he began practicing in 1897. He was appointed Clinical Professor of medicine (dermatology) at Washington University in 1905, later holding an emeritus title. His other major appointment was that of Chief of Staff at Bernard Free Skin and Cancer Hospital in St. Louis.

Engman published widely in the fields of cancer, syphilis, and clinical dermatology. He also published a number of basic investigative studies. He was a member and one-time President of the American Dermatological Association and held memberships in numerous societies in this country and abroad. He initiated the founding of the National Leprosarium in Carville, Louisiana.

One of his preceptees was his son, Martin F. Engman, Jr. who enjoyed a distinguished dermatologic career in St. Louis following his father's death in 1953.*

INFECTIOUS ECZEMATOID DERMATITIS

An Infectious Form of an Eczematoid Dermatitis*

There is a catarrhal inflammatory condition of the skin, which, to me, seems to be a distinct clinical type, distinctive through its etiologic factors, objective symptoms and clinical history. In all textbooks upon diseases of the skin, it is included in the eczema group, one form under the name of eczema impetiginodes, impetiginous eczema and sometimes scrofulous or tuberculous eczema.

Since the idea of the parasiticity of eczema was brought so prominently before the profession by Unna, in 1890, the role of micro-organisms in that group of affections has been energetically investigated by many observers, with the result there is at present some confusion as to just what is meant by the term eczema. This is the battleground, one might say, of modern dermatology. Is "eczema" a purely vesicular disease, or should the term include various other forms of inflammatory lesions and catarrhal conditions? The majority of investigators have found the initial and earliest eczema vesicle sterile, while all of them admit the

* Obituary: Arch. Dermatol. *70:*392, 1954

important pathologic role played by staphylococci later on in the process. Through this confusion of names and what is meant by them, and since modern investigations have not isolated the specific cause of the eczema vesicle and the common forms of this catarrh, we are therefore compelled to take seriously the definition of Norman Walker: "Eczema is the term used to designate all inflammations of the skin, whether moist or dry, of which the observer does not know the cause or nature."

From these few remarks you will admit our wisdom in speaking of the condition which we will attempt to describe as a "dermatitis"; an "eczematoid dermatitis," because in its course we have papules, vesicles, pustules, a reddened scaly surface, from which oozes a sticky liquid that stiffens linen and forms crusts.

You can discern that we wish to call your attention to a condition which is from clinical observation, apparently, infectious, characterized at the height of the process by a crusted, weeping or scaly inflammatory patch (or patches) which extends at the periphery by the formation of vesicles or pustules, but more commonly by the splitting up or undermining of the peripheral epidermis. Insensible or sensible weeping forms a scaly, crusted or discharging surface as it thus progresses, dependent probably upon the particular chemotactic power or character of the organism and the reaction of the patient's tissues. There is never any attempt here to central involution, as in many other dermatites, as, for instance, in impetigo circinata.

From a close study of this affection a vesicle, pustule or an erythematous, scaly, crusted or weeping spot, seems to be the primary lesion. These points may coalesce into a patch, if closely placed, or individually spread from an initial point. When the dermatitis has been too energetically treated, irritated, or if the infection is of great sero-tactic power, a condition indistinguishable from an eczema rub rum of the ordinary type supervenes.

In these cases, if the patient is carefully questioned, a history of preceding trauma or infection can generally be elicited. The trauma may be in the form of a blow, surgical wound, bite of insects (*Pediculus capitis* or *P. vestimenti*), irritation of a simple pimple, chemical or thermal irritation; scratching, especially in complication with certain symptomatic prurituses and lichen tropicus, or any factor which may break or assist in rendering the epidermis vulnerable. In this group may be included various ulcers and vaccinia ulcers, about which this eczematoid dermatitis often occurs, especially frequently is it a complication of the former; in fact, the majority of the so-called varicose eczemas are of this type, the organism readily gaining access and virulence through the ulcer, invading the vulnerable, sodden and poorly nourished epidermis.

The most aggravated form of this dermatitis often occurs after a surgical or accidental wound or recent irritation of an old ulcer as a rapidly spreading, discharging surface, extending with sharply defined, irregular borders over great areas of skin, undermining or raising the peripheral epidermis by the attraction of a sero-purulent discharge for one-eighth of an inch to three inches from the denuded surface border; thus, in a few days to as many as weeks stripping the whole hand or foot of its epidermic covering. There is sometimes in these virulent cases slight edema of the subjacent tissues. The surface thus denuded is covered by a sticky sero-purulent discharge which oozes from points, and when not too profuse dries into thin crusts. This fluid teams with white or yellow staphylococci, or both, and can be pressed out, when profuse, in drops from under the loosened epidermis at the border; but, when it is not so freely attracted, the disease progresses slowly with just enough moisture to detach the peripheral epidermis, which unites with it and with the debris to form crusts upon the reddened surface thus left in its wake. The older part may slowly undergo restitution by the cessation of the discharge and the formation of new epidermis; this new covering may again be attacked and destroyed in the same manner, a procedure I have seen repeated several times. In

* Amer. Med., *4:*769, 1902.

this form of the eczematoid dermatitis, vesicles or pustules never form, as the organism's chemotactic attraction is so powerful that the epidermis becomes soaked, then lifted up en masse as it were, and is in several cases washed or broken away before the flow of serum, which thus actively attracted also prevents the formation of crusts to any marked extent, but in the slower or less virulent forms these features are of less degree; we may have a slowly progressive, spreading inflammation, taking weeks to destroy the epidermis of the back of the hand, to a rapid, virulent, profusely weeping type, taking only a few hours to accomplish the same result, when, the soaked and sodden epidermis is detached in sheets of a dirty, creamy-white color, breaking upon slight traction and readily detachable, flush with apparently healthy skin.

Theodor Escherich

Erythema Infectiosum

THEODOR ESCHERICH was born November 29, 1857, in Ansbach, Germany. His medical studies were pursued at the Universities of Strassburg, Kiel, Berlin, and Würzburg, and he took his degree in the last named city in 1881. After preliminary work in Gerhadt's Klinik he turned his attention to pediatrics, became an assistant at the University Kinderklinik in Munich, under von Ranke, in 1885, and qualified in pediatrics the following year. At the early age of 33 (1890) he became Chief of the Kinderklinik in Graz. After the death of Wiederhofer in 1902 he went to Vienna for nine years of intense scientific and organizational activity. He enlarged the clinic there by establishing an infant and new-born division and laid groundwork for the pediatric clinic. He was a zealous worker for child welfare.

In addition to the administrative achievements he found time to do the fundamental work on the bacterial flora of the gut, describing the *B. coli* which has since been named for him. He clarified the picture of cholecystitis and streptococcal enteritis in infants, and made important contributions to our knowledge of infant tetany, diphtheria, tuberculosis, and infant feeding. He died February 15, 1911.*

ERYTHEMA INFECTIOSUM

Demonstration zweier Fälle von Erythema contagiosum*

The illness always occurs in epidemic form, usually in connection with measles epidemics at intervals of several years, and is usually seen in siblings, schools, kindergartens, etc. Most of the cases are children between the ages of four and 12 years; the youngest was 14 months old. It appears to spread through a contagion to which, however, no great susceptibility exists. The incubation period in well followed cases is six to 14 days. The onset is sometimes accomplished by slight malaise, lassitude, and sore throat. Usually, however, the well being of the child is not disturbed throughout the entire illness, and the eruption is the only symptom. This latter occurs exclusively on the outer integument. Constant mucous membrane changes are not observed. The eruption begins on the face with an intense redness and turgescence of the cheeks which erysipelas-like sharply demarcates itself at the nasolabial folds and thereby stands out clearly from the pale chin and oral areas. Rarely one finds macular and gyrate lesions. The swelling and redness disappear toward the ears and end there in a scalloped or sinuate line. This appearance, which is sometimes

---

* Fischer, I.: Biog. Lex. der Hervor. Ärzte, Berlin, Urban and Schwarzenberg, Berlin, 1932, p. 375.

not only not recognized as an illness by the mothers but even interpreted as the picture of glowing health, is the most constant and characteristic form of the disease. In addition, discrete large patches of a bluish red color occur on the forehead and ear regions and are essentially the same as those which by this time have appeared on the body and extremities. The extremities are involved to the greatest extent. The patches which can still be distinguished clearly on the flexor surfaces of the arms usually become confluent on the extensor surfaces. On the lower extremities, the gluteal region is most heavily covered by the large patchy, superficial papular eruption which extends downward predominantly over the flexor surfaces of the legs. The patches are relatively sparse and late appearing on the trunk, which not infrequently remains entirely clear.

The exanthem is visible for six to 10 days. It fades out first on the face and trunk, and lasts longest on the extremities where the sharp borders and papular quality of the patches fade out gradually and give way to a pale map-like or reticular pattern similar to cutis marmorata. This remains visible for a long time in isolated places as the last remnant of the eruption, and stands out clearly on irritation, as from the warmth of bed, etc.

---

* Wiener Klin. Wchnschr., *17:*631, 1904.

Josef Jadassohn

1.   *Macular Atrophy*

2.   *Granulosis Rubra Nasi*

3.   *Cutis Verticis Gyrata*

4.   *Pachyonychia Congenita*

JOSEF JADASSOHN was born September 10, 1860, in Liegenitz, Schleisen. His medical studies were pursued at the Universities of Göttingen, Heidelberg, Leipzig, and Breslau. He took his degree in the latter city in 1887, and remained there as an assistant to Neisser until 1892. In 1896 he was called to Bern as Professor of Dermatology, and after 20 years work in that city, he returned to Breslau where he stayed until his retirement in 1931.

Although Jadassohn was a fine clinician, and made many contributions to the clinical dermatologic literature, his most notable accomplishments were in the application of laboratory methods to the study of skin diseases. It is to him that we mainly owe the development of the study of immunology in its relation to dermatology. His work in this connection on tuberculosis and trichophytosis is classical. He was also one of the leading dermatologic editors, and served in this capacity, not only with the *Archiv für Dermatologie und Syphilis,* but also in compiling the great *Handbuch der Haut-und Geschlechtkrankheiten* (1929).

Jadassohn was quiet and unassuming; he was at his clinic from early morning until late at night, sparing only a few hours for his private practice, and available always either to direct the most advanced research; or to help the most elementary student with the same interest and courtesy. He died March 24, 1936.*

MACULAR ATROPHY

Ueber eine eigenartige Form von "Atrophia maculosa cutis"[†]

A.Z., 23 years old, had measles and whooping cough in childhood; no eruptions, no glandular disease. Both parents living and well, also an only sister. No skin or nervous system disease in the family. Patient herself has had no headaches, nervous symptoms, nor hysterical symptoms.

At the age of nine, she burned both hands with boiling water, large bullae which healed (with scarring) in about three months.

In her eighteenth year the patient noticed "red spots" without pain, itching, or other subjective symptoms on both elbows, which increased very slowly, chiefly in these areas. In about a year, a few more spots appeared on the arm, and then also on the forearm, the patient herself noted that very soon there appeared a

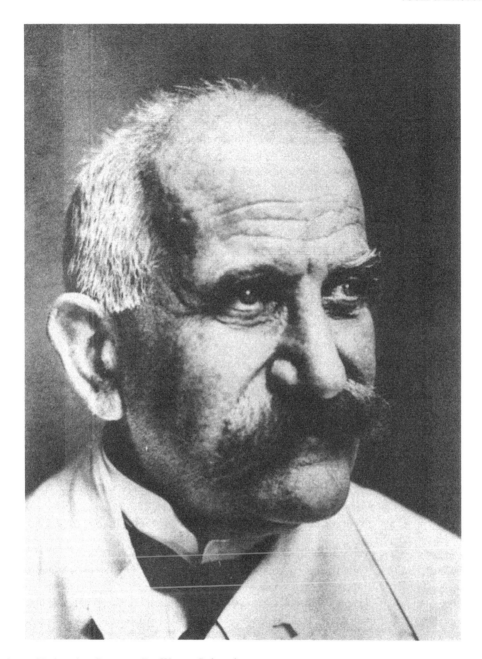

Figure 73 Josef Jadassohn. Courtesy, Dr. Werner Jadassohn

"sinking in," a depression of the skin in the reddened area; the spots on the arm and forearm increased gradually but continually. At about age 19 the skin on the backs of the hands became thinner, wrinkled, and light red.

Two years after the onset of the disease she noted "stinging" here and there, "as if it were coming out of the bones," especially with the changes in the weather, sometimes more frequently, sometimes almost daily, but never to the extent that the night's rest was disturbed; never any itching. These symptoms localized chiefly to the elbows, less commonly to the arms and hands. In the course of a year they became more marked, and more frequent, but were never on the whole of much importance. The patient is not able to give any more definite information concerning the times of appearance of the spots, etc.

Since August 1, 1899 has had a Tumor albus of the right knee. The patient believes she has become thinner in the past two years. In the meantime the Tumor albus has healed sufficiently, with an ankylosis, not to cause the patient any difficulty. No sign of lues.

Status praesens. A completely healthy looking well nourished girl. No bodily abnormalities except for the Tumor albus of the right knee; on the thighs are a number of white streaks which are moderately well developed and look exactly like ordinary Striae.

Only the upper extremities are remarkable. The skin on the back of both hands is thin, smooth, and shiny. Large and small veins show through very clearly; the skin is on the whole somewhat brownish colored—in contrast to its otherwise white color. These changes, which the patient attributes to the burns, do not have sharp borders.

The really characteristic efflorescences that concern us here are localized mainly to the extensor surfaces of both arms. They begin at the wrist and extend to the deltoid region. They have no particularly regular arrangement. We must differentiate between the following forms; they correspond to different stages in development:

1. Definite round or more irregular, lentil to 10 Pfennig piece sized, bright, livid red spots which are covered by a slightly wrinkled epidermis, and which appear to be slightly depressed; on palpation, however, one notices that the skin on these places is somewhat thinned, and that the examining finger sinks in, as if into a shallow hiatus filled with soft tissue.
2. Dark bluish red, entirely irregular, larger (to a mark-piece in size) spots, limited to both olecranons, from which a few streaks lead off in various directions; these last give the impression of being a bit raised, and are usually covered with a somewhat scaly epidermis as well. On pressure they seem to be empty, and the epidermis over them feels somewhat wrinkled.
3. More streaky, light red, irregular efflorescences, remaining grouped together, and at least in the beginning, looking more like striae ovale.
4. Lastly, on the inner surface of the arm, very fine white lines comparable to long established striae.

The picture on both arms is strikingly similar, the symmetry being very marked.

In describing the individual areas I must add that follicle openings are not clearly to be seen—the lanugo hairs are but very little developed, the red color of the first mentioned forms disappears completely on digital pressure, and when one picks up individual spots with smooth surfaces between the fingers, the epidermis falls into small, fine folds.

---

* Goodman, H. Notable Contributors to the Knowledge of Dermatology. Medical Lay Press, 250, 1953.

† Verhandl. der Deutsch. Dermat. Gesell., Kong. zu Berlin, 342, 1891.

GRANULOSIS RUBRA NASI

Ueber eine eigenartige Erkrankung der Nasenhaut bei Kindern (Granulosis rubra nasi)*

The clinical picture, as far as I can develop it on the basis of the seven patients I have observed, is as follows:

On the tip of the nose and on the alae nasi, always on the cutaneous part in my cases, a rather intensive, not sharply demarcated erythema is found, which is readily effaced by pressure. Discrete papules which have a deeper red color arise in this area. They are often minimal, pinpoint size, and scarcely raised above the surface; they sometimes become pinhead sized, and they then stand out more clearly. They are rather more acuminate than flat topped, arranged in no particular pattern, and not confluent. It is impossible clinically to determine whether they are localized at the sebaceous openings or at the sweat gland pores. No firm infiltration can be demonstrated; on pressure they blanche out (no yellowish brown color). The test in which one attempts to insert a blunt probe into them (as in Lupus vulgaris) is negative. From time to time they become transformed into very small pustules which dry up quickly.

The skin of the nose feels cool. Telangiectasias were usually insignificant, occasionally none at all; they were sometimes quite prominent. Scaling was almost completely absent. In one case a very insignificant symmetrical atrophy appeared to me to be present in the skin of the tip of the nose.

In the majority of the cases, at any rate in all those I have been able to observe for some period of time, a hyperidrosis was present which varied in intensity in different cases, and also in the same patient at different times, and which was almost completely limited to the nose, although it might involve the rest of the face to a slight degree. It was usually present without external cause, or appeared with very slight stimuli (including psychic).

The course of the disease was very uniform, although the symptoms varied within rather wide limits; at times the erythema was more marked, at other times less; in one case it disappeared completely, so that the papules were located on entirely normal skin; these latter were at times numerous, and at other times scanty, or even hardly distinguishable; occasionally they appeared quite suddenly in rather great numbers.

Differences in winter and summer are not striking, but I have been able to follow the cases only for a small part of several seasons; in one case it appeared that the redness might have been more marked in the Spring.

The localization on the nose was present in all cases. In one child solitary papules were found from time to time on the cheeks, in another on the upper lip; still, the question as to whether these were the same efflorescences on the nose remains undecided.

In every case the localization on the cutaneous part of the nose is especially characteristic.

All my patients were children, six girls and one boy; whether or not this sex incidence was fortuitous must be left for further observation to decide. It is, however, no coincidence that this disease was present exclusively in children. Despite the fact that I have naturally been looking especially for it, no truly similar disease picture has as yet turned up in adults.

The children ranged in age from seven to 16 years; the parents declared repeatedly that the redness of the nose had been present for many years,—for example, in a girl who came under observation at 16 years, since the eighth year. In this case I am convinced of it, for after one and one-half years (when the girl was 16½ years old) the disease subsided, for the most part, spontaneously.

---

* Archiv für dermat. und syph., *58:*145, 1901.

The children were weakly, for the most part; hereditary factors were not evident. The boy was epileptic; one child showed a bilateral enlargement of the external ear which from a rhinologic standpoint was probably on a tuberculous basis; there was no reaction to tuberculin, however. No organic illness was to be found in the other children. Several of them were tested with tuberculin injection, but no reaction took place.

CUTIS VERTICIS GYRATA

Eine eigentuemliche Furchung, Erweiterung, und Verdickerung der Haut am Hinterkopf*

The skin disorder this man shows is surely of no practical significance at all. I should like to secure its entrance into our dermatologic realm only as a small increment to our factual knowledge. Although I cannot remember having seen anything similar described or portrayed, neither have I had the time to look for it. Perhaps something can be found regarding it in older dermatologic or anthropologic works.

The anomaly (I should like to designate it as such) consists of a peculiar furrowing of the skin over the occiput. In a well defined, rather sharply demarcated, on the whole irregularly roundish area, reaching from the vertex to the region of the hairline at the nape, and laterally to the region over the muscles of the ears, a peculiar disposition of the hair is the first thing that draws one's attention. Instead of the natural downward course in this region, a tendency of the hair to separate into irregular channels running in different directions is noticed; usually these have a longer or shorter straight or curved longitudinal axis. The hairs here seem also to be less thick; they are, however, completely normal and firmly implanted as well. On closer inspection, especially where the hair is cut short, it is seen that this behaviour of the hair results from a peculiar condition of the scalp. This is normal in color and consistency, but is not, however, as smoothly stretched as usual; it is disposed instead in irregular folds which are at least three-fourths to one and one-half cm. thick, shallowly arched, and run straighter from above downwards in the lateral areas, and more obliquely and irregularly in the central areas; they anastamose with one another, as it were, and are sharply separated from one another by narrow deep furrows. These furrows produce small continuations into the folds here and there. The whole reminds one of the gyri on the surface of the brain. To palpation the skin feels thick, is easily slid over the underlying structures, and may be picked up in folds; if one pushes together the skin on both sides of the head, it appears in great volume, and the previously visible furrows stand out very clearly. When it is released it returns rather quickly to its original position. The sensibility of the rest of the scalp is entirely normal. The galea also slides easily over the rest of the skull. The first patient affected with this anomaly, and the one I am presenting to you, was a 40 year old man who (like the others) knew nothing of it. He has a thyroprivic habitus, but his intelligence is not that of a cretin. Since then I have seen the same thing in two men in whom it was not so well developed and lesser in extent, but in the same region—in a 45 year old patient from my private practice, a thick-set, somewhat corpulent, nervous, but otherwise physically normal man, and in a 40 year old clinic patient in whom psychic anomalies were not prominent.

This material is quite sufficient to demonstrate the actual picture of the anomaly as I have met with it, but it is not, of course, sufficient to determine the conditions under which it occurs. This must be left to a later collecting and statistical project.

---

* Verhandl. der Deutsch. Dermat. Gesell, Kong. zu Bern, *9*:451, 1906.

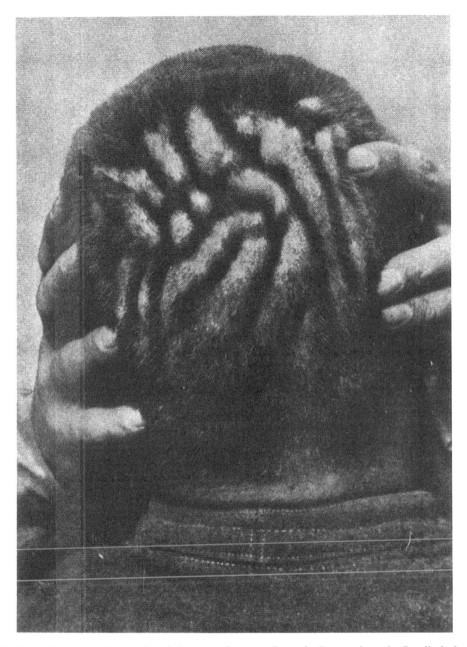

Figure 74 Cutis verticis gyrata. From Jadassohn's paper. Courtesy, *Deutsche Dermatologische Gesellschaft*

PACHYONYCHIA CONGENITA

Pachyonychia congenita*

We have reproduced only the nail changes from the case reported here, and we shall consider these first; the

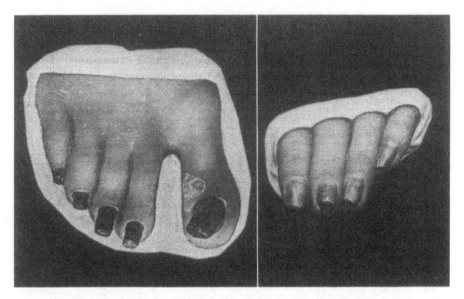

Figure 75 Pachyonychia congenita. From Jadassohn's paper. Courtesy, Urban and Schwarzenberg, Berlin

other findings on the skin and mucous membrane will be considered later in detail.

E.C., a 15 year old girl, admitted on June 15, 1905, for a fungating tuberculosis of the skin had, besides this, an alteration of the nails which is the feature we are most interested in here; moreover there were well marked peculiar keratinization anomalies of the skin and of the tongue. The malformation of the nails has been present since birth. The patient can tell us nothing about the skin and tongue. The parents and seven sisters have no similar disease; one brother does (see below).

Status praesens. The nail plates of all the fingers and toes are extremely thickened, and so hard that they cannot be cut with scissors; the father has to trim them with a hammer and chisel. The fingernails are of normal length and width (rather long and narrow), shiny and smooth on the surface, and show dry whitish streaks here and there at the free edges. They are translucent on the whole, and only at the very tip of the fingers are they colored greyish black. At the distal parts, especially, they are much more strongly arched transversely than normal; some are also somewhat more curved in their long axis toward the volar surface. They become thicker toward the free border, measuring three to five mm. in thickness there. For this reason they project quite markedly on the dorsal aspect, but at the same time they lie on a greatly thickened nail bed; this is, as it were, enveloped by them and compressed from the sides toward the middle so that it stands out on the free edge as a small addition to the thick sickle shaped plate.

The toenails are also greatly thickened, especially those of the great toes (resembling onychogryphosis). Their surfaces, however, are not flat but rather irregularly furrowed transversely, and are heaped up stump-like in the distal portions over the nail bed which latter is normal, as in the nail fold. The consistency is the same as on the fingers. The growth of the nail is not particularly rapid. No keratinization anomaly in the nail bed can be demonstrated. The nail changes cause the patient no trouble (nor does trimming them). Neither is she hindered apparently in doing fine work.

---

* Ikon. Dermat., *1:*29, 1906. Jadassohn, J., and Lewandowski, F.

The hairy scalp is clear; on the face there are intensely red, somewhat acuminate, pinhead sized, firm papules, only on the nose and the furrow of the chin, and amongst them, especially on the nose, are very discrete, water clear vesicles with sterile alkaline contents. The number of these efflorescences varies greatly at different times, and the vesicles especially are more numerous at higher environmental temperatures.

There is hyperidrosis of the skin of the nose, the palms, and the soles; on the latter there are marked pressure point callosities which have become whitish colored with maceration. In the summer (rarely in the winter) extremely painful large bullae form beneath these, containing a water clear alkaline liquid, and staphylococci and streptococci, as well as an unidentified bacillus.

On the elbows and knees a few papules are present which are not distinctly grouped, apparently follicular, hempseed sized, slightly raised, and a bit reddened; they have a scarcely projecting central horny plug, the removal of which leaves a crateriform pit.

The surface of the tongue has a coating which is firm, sharply and irregularly circumscribed here and there, thick and white. At its edges are found permanent strikingly white and irregular streaks which encroach on the under side, and are in part unevenly elevated. The rest of the mucous membrane of the mouth is normal. Nothing in the internal organs, and especially in the nerves, which can be linked with the skin anomaly.

Some four weeks after the admission of the patient, an affection of the skin of the body appeared, which has since persisted, but has changed considerably in intensity and extent. On both scapulae, in the neighborhood of the axilla, as well as in the gluteal region, irregularly disseminated efflorescences are found which correspond in part to those on the elbows and knees. Some of them, however, appear as pinhead to split pea sized papules with an intensely reddened base, and with a thick whitish to greyish yellow central horny mass which, usually in the form of a laterally curved cone one to four mm. in length, is raised above the surrounding area, or less commonly, in the form of a flat plate, is fixed in the skin. After removal of this horny mass a pit is left which bleeds slightly. The skin between the individual papules looks normal.

The brother mentioned above (four years old), who looks very much like the patient, is completely healthy except for the dermatosis; he shows on the nails, the soles, and the tongue a completely analogous picture. The skin changes on the nose, the furrow of the chin, the elbows, knees, and the body were the same, except that here and there they had a more comedo-like appearance because of their darker color.

Eduard Jacobi

Poikilodermia Vascularis Atrophicans

EDUARD JACOBI was born in Liegnitz on January 20, 1862. After completing studies in Freiburg, Breslau, Würzburg and Halle, he returned to the University of Freiburg in 1889 to organize a Department of Dermatology. Within six years he was appointed Professor, a post which he held until his death in 1915.

Jacobi pioneered the development of dermatology at Freiburg. He was held in high esteem by the faculty, and a large group of students came to know him as a distinguished, energetic, and conscientious teacher. At meetings he had a keen interest in making his point, but was at once tactful and reserved.

His publications covered a wide field; in addition to the selection below, he is best known for his *Atlas der Hautkrankheiten* (1904). This latter was the first dermatologic atlas to be printed with a four color process.[*]

POIKILODERMIA VASCULARIS ATROPHICANS

Fall zur Diagnose (Poikilodermia vascularis atrophicans)[†]

A 30 year old farmer, no hereditary disease.

The disease began seven years ago with swelling of the eyelids and intense itching, and spread gradually over the body and the extremities. In the year 1902 the patient came to the medical clinic where the diagnosis of scleroderma (?) was made. The patient was admitted to the dermatologic clinic in February 1906; since then his condition has changed little except that the skin now appears somewhat lighter. No changes in the internal organs could be ascertained, although an increase in the area of liver dullness can now be demonstrated—in March the patient had a marked purpuric eruption on both lower extremities.

At first glance the face appears somewhat darkly colored, the eyelids rigidly edematous. On the hairy scalp, the skin is atrophic, especially in the occipital region; it is not easily moved, and shows numerous telangiectasias with a few firmly adherent scales. The skin of the neck is reddened. On the chest and back are net-like white atrophic areas in which the follicle stands out clearly as a reddish brown point. The area around the atrophic site is darkly pigmented, the skin in general somewhat thinned, but not much sclerosed, not easily moved; similar areas are found on the abdomen and in the sacral areas, to a lesser extent on the

[*] Buschke, A.: Deutsch. Med. Wchnschr., *41:*29, 1915.

[†] Verhandl. der Deutsch. Dermat. Gesell, Kong. zu Bern, *9:*321, 1906.

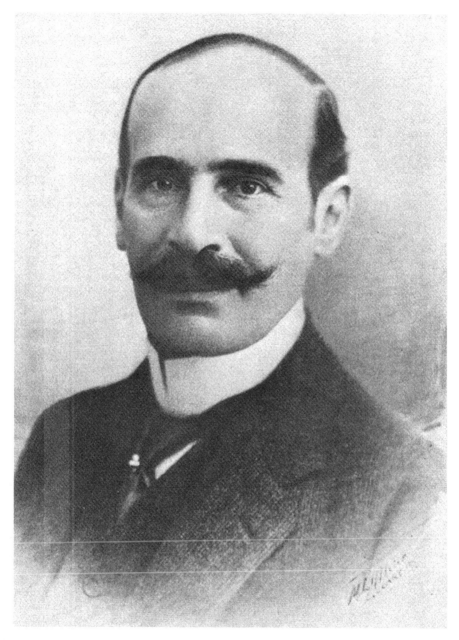

Figure 76 Eduard Jacobi. Courtesy, Dr. A.Stühmer

arms and legs, as well as on the hands and feet, the nails of which are unaltered, although the nail beds are atrophic and permeated by telangiectasias. The atrophic sites described developed from a light red marmoration which enclosed islands of normal skin, and which was composed of telangiectasias and hemorrhages in the skin.

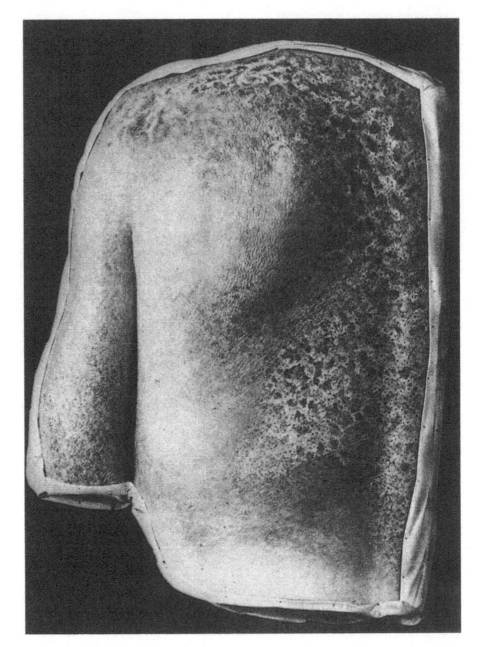

Figure 77 Poikilodermia vascularis atrophicans (Jacobi's case). Courtesy, Urban and Schwarzenberg, Berlin

A marked hypertrichosis of both forearms should be mentioned, less on the feet, as well as changes in the mucous membranes of the cheeks which resembled those on the skin.

The presenter is not able to identify the case with any known disease picture. The most analogous situation is presented by an affection described by Petges and Cléjat (Clinique Dubreuilh) under the name

Sclérose atrophique de la peau et myosite géneralisée (Annales de Derm. June 1906), yet even here there are a number of differences. In consideration of the mottled color (which most closely resembles the picture of a Roentgen burn), the presenter would like to propose the name "Poikilodermia vascularis atrophicans."

Felix Pinkus

Lichen Nitidus

FELIX PINKUS was born on April 4, 1868, in Berlin. He received his medical education at the University of Freiburg, and was graduated in 1893. After several years of research, he became an assistant to Neisser, in Breslau. It was during this period that he acquired a basic knowledge of dermatology, and at the same time his research talents were employed in investigations of the anatomy of the skin. He continued his dermatologic training as a student of Jadassohn in Bern, and did further postgraduate work at l'Hôpital Saint Louis in Paris.

From 1898 to 1938 Pinkus practiced dermatology in Berlin. By 1915 he had received the rank of Associate Professor of Dermatology at the University of Berlin. In 1939 he left Germany, and after a brief stay in Oslo, Norway, he came to the United States to live with his dermatologist son, Hermann, in Monroe, Michigan. It was here that he pursued his histologic studies until his death on November 19, 1947.

Pinkus published over 150 scientific articles, and several books, including a textbook of dermatology. His monumental contribution was a volume on the anatomy of the skin in the Jadassohn "Handbuch." His best known contribution to clinical dermatology is perhaps his description of lichen nitidus, which is given below.

Pinkus was a modest, friendly man. His intelligence and integrity won for him world wide esteem and admiration. Aside from his profession, he had many interests and skills. Sketching was paramount among these, and one could always see him at meetings deep in the absorption of capturing the likeness of the speaker in his sketch book.*

LICHEN NITIDUS

Ueber eine Neue Knoetchenfoermige Haut-Eruption: Lichen nitidus[†]

As early as 1897, during my assistantship at the University of Breslau clinic for skin diseases, I saw a striking skin affection which after a most exact analysis could not be fitted into any known disease picture, and which after an attempt to clarify matters by histological examination, proved to be a new entity in its structure as well. After long and repeatedly futile experiments to determine whether or not it might be related to lichen planus, which is most similar to it, or to one of the known granulomas, I must conclude finally that it is unknown. I have followed it zealously during the succeeding years, and accordingly have gotten a large number of observations together. I believe that I have found the proper place here to report them.

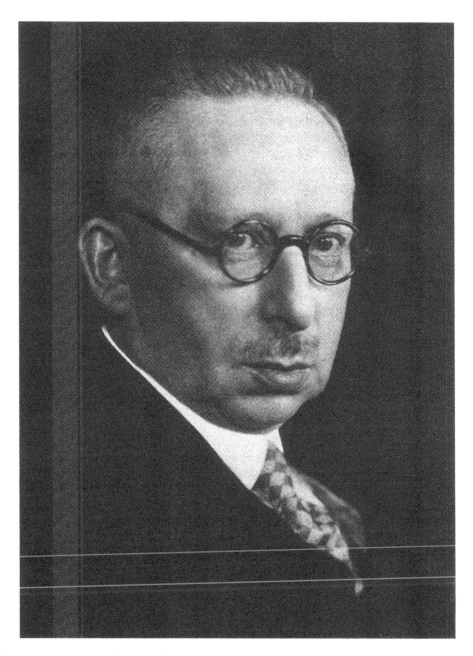

Figure 78 Felix Pinkus. Courtesy, Dr. Felix Pinkus, Jr.

I feel that a distinct portrayal of the disease which I propose to designate by the name *Lichen nitidus* is best accomplished through presentation of the findings I have brought out in the individual cases.

Case I. University Polyclinic in Breslau. A young otherwise healthy male was under treatment for a minor venereal affliction. On inspecting the penis I found an eruption of closely set glistening papules which covered the prepuce, and even a large part of the shaft of the penis. The papules were about the size of a pinhead or slightly larger, closely set, but not so crowded that neighboring ones became confluent. They were not distinguishable in color from the surrounding skin, although they appeared somewhat lighter because of their sheen. They resembled the large follicles so frequently encountered in these parts of the penis, but differed from them in several characteristics. First, they did not have the yellow color of these follicles, which is certainly due to a rudimentary hair follicle and a ring of sebaceous glands about it shining through the epidermis, and which is seen as a lob ate structure when the skin is stretched. They form, rather, a structure which lies close beneath the epidermis and is almost joined to it, and they do not become much more distinct on stretching the skin; secondly, they do not have the point projecting up as a small plug which is always recognizable in these glands, and which is similar to a small comedo; thirdly, their borders are not so indefinable as those of the glands. While in the latter no sharp line is recognizable as the border, and the skin stretches over them uninterruptedly, a distinct fine border line may be recognized at the edge of the lichen nitidus papules.

They resemble small warts, from which, however, they may be differentiated by several peculiarites. To begin with, they do not lie on the surface of the skin forming as it were a single structure with the epidermis; they are more deeply emplanted beneath the epidermis. Further, they have a round or oval plug centrally which, as we have just noted, is differentiated from a follicle orifice by its irregularity. Moreover, they were too numerous to be verrucae vulgares, and not so granular as juvenile plane warts. Their surfaces were either smooth, not so rough as normal skin, or still showed, at least in the peripheral parts, the normal folds and furrows of penile skin.

The patient was observed for a long time, and during this period no change of any kind was noted in these manifestations. We finally lost sight of him.

After this case, during my assistantship at Breslau, I saw two more identical cases, but since I have no exact data on them I will not discuss them further.

The fourth case was a man some twenty-five years of age who came under my care for gonorrhea in the year 1900. On his penis we found a wonderful crop of the papules we have described, differing however from the first case in a way which we often later observed.

The whole penis, from the prepuce to the belly insertion, was covered with polygonal or roundish, flat, shining papules. They varied greatly in size from points scarcely visible, recognizable only with a lens, to the size of a pinhead. There were some forty of the largest in one square centemeter, but if one included all of them, the smallest as well, there were about a hundred in this area. Within the small space of a grid the distribution was irregular, but taking the entire member into consideration, it was apparently quite uniform. The penis looked as though it were covered with tiny shiny spangles. A linear arrangement was not everywhere to be seen. Most of the papules had a flat surface, without the central opening which was so striking in the first case, and corresponded to the peculiar microscopic findings. A few of these, however, showed a central depressed point.

The color was the same as the surrounding skin, although in certain light the shininess gave the

* Michelson, H.: Arch. of Dermat. and Syph., *58:*92, 1948.

† Archiv für dermat. and syph., *85:*11, 1907.

appearance of a lighter shade. Under the lens (Zeiss 10x and binocular Zeiss-Greenough Loupe) the surface was smoother than the flat velvet-like roughness of the normal surrounding skin.

The affection was so pronounced that it was easy to get a plaster cast and wax moulage from it.

Carl Leiner

Leiner's Disease

CARL LEINER was born in Flöhau, Bohemia, January 23, 1871. He studied in Vienna and Prague, and took his degree in the latter city in 1896. Following his graduation he worked in the Hautklinik and the Pathological Institute of Vienna and became an assistant at the Caroline Hospital for Children. In 1912 he qualified as a lecturer in pediatrics. From 1920 until his death, April 24, 1930, he served as Primarzt at the Mautner-Markhofschen Children's Hospital in Vienna.

Leiner's chief contributions were in the field of pediatric dermatology; he was one of the earliest workers in this field. The account given here is his best known work. Of his many publications his most important was, perhaps, the *Hautkrankheiten in Säuglingsalter* (1930), in the famed *Handbuch der Haut-und Geschlechtkrankheiten*. Infectious diseases were also his special province; he was the originator of the intracutaneous vaccination.*

LEINER'S DISEASE

Erythrodermia Desquamativa (Universal Dermatitis of Children at the Breast)[†]

I wish to draw attention to a peculiar disease of the skin, which spreads itself all over the body, but which, however, must be distinguished from the specific forms of eruptions in infants, from the dermatitis exfoliativa Ritter, from the slight form of this disease the pemphigus contagiosus neonatorum, and also from the various other diseases of the skin; eczema, prurigo, etc.

This dermatitis, about which I am reporting, presents a special type for itself, and it is of the greatest importance to be able to recognize it, for with few exceptions it only attacks children at the breast. This disease, far from being harmless, very often is even extremely dangerous for the infants, and death from this form of dermatitis is not at all infrequent.

During the last five years I have made it my special task to study this form of dermatitis, and during this time I have closely observed 43 cases of it in the Carolinen Children's Hospital in Vienna. Forty-one cases were in children nourished at the breast, and two with the bottle. Twenty-eight were cured and 15 died from the disease.

---

* Fischer, I.: Biog. Lex. der Hervor. Ärzte, Berlin, Urban and Schwarzenberg, 1932, p. 884.

† Brit. J.Dermat. *5:*244, 1908.

As a rule the children are brought for advice when the illness is already at its height, that is to say, at the end of the second or the beginning of the third month of life, seldom later. The children then present the picture of a universal dermatitis, which in all these specific cases bore the same aspect. The head presents the same appearance as in the case of seborrhea. It is covered like a cap with thick yellow fatty scales and crusts, which may be easily removed from the slightly inflamed but in no wise ulcerated skin. The hair is sparse, on some spots matted. The eyebrows also present the same appearance as the scalp.

The rest of the face is almost entirely slightly inflamed and covered with thin yellow scales. Only the tip of the nose and the nostrils and the neighboring parts of the cheek still bear a normal appearance, and it is only at the later stage that these parts are attacked by the eruption. The trunk is intensely red and at first covered with whitish grey opaque scales, which later become lustrous. They may be easily removed from the slightly inflamed epidermis. The dorsal aspects of the extremities are more thickly covered with scales than the flexor. The hands and feet are red, but only in circumscribed spots. The nails also are affected by the disease and show various deformities, transverse and longitudinal grooves and small prominences and cavities of irregular form. The nail bed is often hyperkeratotic, causing an abnormal convexity of the nails. In the folds of the skin and on the flexion sides of the joints no scales are formed. Here the skin is of a dark red colour and oedematous. Only in the depths of the folds a covering of a dirty white colour is to be seen. Examination of the other organs proved them to be quite normal. The glands are only slightly swollen, about to the size of a cherry stone; suppuration of the glands never occurs. The general health of the child is quite good, and the sleep is but little disturbed, this being due to the absence of itching. At this stage I could find no increase of temperature. On examination the urine proved quite normal. The mucous membrane of the mouth showed no remarkable changes. Changes are only to be found at this stage in the digestive organs and in almost every case, so that this seems to be one of the symptoms of this particular skin disease.

I have already mentioned that the disease cannot always be cured; about one-third of the patients die from it.

In spite of continuing the breast feeding the intestinal troubles come more and more to the front, the decrease in weight becomes more and more evident, so that the little sufferers are so terribly changed that they do not bear the slightest resemblance to the normal child at the breast.

The little one is emaciated and appears as if suffering from a severe illness. It is in a state of collapse, the face and extremities are of cyanotic colour and the former is drawn with pain. The extremities become hypertonic; the whole skin is so dry that it often looks like parchment, and is covered with thin dry scales and traversed with fine rhagades. These rhagades are most severe round the mouth. On account of the infiltration of the lips and dryness of the skin, the act of suckling becomes very difficult or even impossible. Continual increasing cachexia and fever, associated with diarrhea, soon cause death.

Grover Wende

Erythema Figurata Perstans

GROVER WILLIAM WENDE was born April 6, 1867, on a farm in Erie County, N.Y. His early education was in public schools and he took his M.D. at the University of Buffalo in 1889. After three years postgraduate work, chiefly in Europe, he began practice in 1892 in Buffalo.

Wende was a well rounded dermatologist, thoroughly competent in all phases of his specialty. As a clinician he had few equals. He was especially interested in the dermatologic aspects of bacteriology and pathology. He conducted a tremendous practice for years, and drawing on this material he became nationally known for calling the attention of American dermatologists to the rarer dermatoses. He was a skilled photographer and over the years gathered together a collection rivalled only by Fordyce's.

Wende was a most public spirited citizen and was often called upon for help and leadership in all movements for the betterment of his city.

Pusey noted that he "was much more than a leader in a narrow field; his interests were catholic, and his energy and ability made inevitable his participation in the widest variety of activities. He was a recognized leader of the medical profession of his city and of his state."

He was struck by a street car February 9, 1926 and died on the way to the hospital.*

ERYTHEMA FIGURATA PERSTANS

Erythema figurata perstans*

Such cases as are considered in this paper are few in number, but are sufficiently characteristic to be described as a distinct variety under the title of erythema figurata perstans. Some of the cases possess anomalous features, suggesting a type of erythema multiforme, yet not sufficiently distinctive to place them in that group.

The disease under consideration begins with scattered and isolated papules, which tend to fade at the center while extending peripherally, thus forming circinate erythematous outlines. The outer half of the advancing margin is smooth and slightly raised, the inner edge scaly and desquamating—a marked feature. The surface over which the disease has traveled is sometimes slightly scaly and pigmented. The larger lesions vary in size from a 25 cent piece to the palm of the hand, occasionally larger. The rings assume

---

* Pusey, W.: Arch. of Dermat. and Syph., *13*:401, 1926.

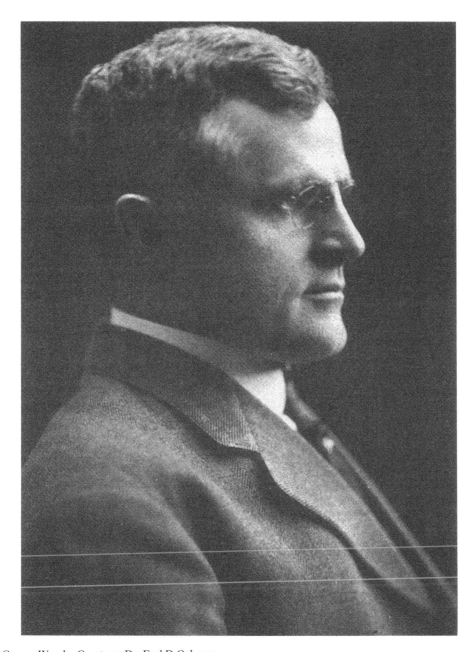

Figure 79 Grover Wende. Courtesy, Dr. Earl D.Osborne

circinate, annular, discrete, confluent, gyrate or zigzag forms. In certain instances, the lesions, whether evanescent or of long duration, do not develop the ring form. Two observations have been made in which the lesions formed within the area occupied by the disease followed the lines of evolution established by the first. Subjective sensations may or may not be felt.

In these cases, clinically considered, the erythema presents a peculiar type, different from any other form. This difference is further confirmed by the inflammatory character of the lesion, with an absence of pronounced infiltration in the fresh foci. The arrangement of the skin lesions constitutes the most important clinical feature.

The rate of development of the lesions of erythema figurata perstans varies widely. In some instances the ring lesions extend as much as a half inch in a couple of hours, while in others the same growth requires an indefinite period. Exacerbations vary with the case, sometimes occurring three or four times a year, or oftener. As a rule, the body does not entirely clear up during the intervals. The outbreaks are in some cases said to be influenced by changes in temperature.

There is no special sex or age predisposition. The disease asserts itself in earliest childhood as well as in later life. In rare instances it begins at birth and may be regarded as congenital. The patients are generally in good health; in a few instances the disease is reported to begin with constitutional disturbances. The etiology of this peculiar skin affection is meager and unsatisfactory, and necessitates a careful study from a purely medical standpoint. It is fair to assume that the manifestations in the alimentary tract indicate the presence of an irritant circulating in the blood which, acting on the cutaneous vessels, produce this peculiar result.

---

* Trans. Cutan. Med. and Surg., 1908, p. 75.

Jay Frank Schamberg

1. *Schamberg's Disease*

2. *Grain Itch*

JAY FRANK SCHAMBERG was born in Philadelphia, November 6, 1870. His early education was in local schools, and he received his M.D. from the University of Pennsylvania in 1893. Although he spent a year in Europe preparing for the practice of dermatology he was essentially of the American school, taking his inspiration from such leaders as Duhring, van Harlingen, Stelwagon, and Hartzell. He became Professor of Dermatology at Temple Medical School, Jefferson Medical School, and the Graduate School of the University of Pennsylvania.

Schamberg made contributions to many aspects of dermatology but was particularly interested in the exanthems, especially in the public health problems occasioned by these diseases. He is best known for the two original accounts given below, and for the important part he played in foreseeing a shortage in World War I of arsphenamine, almost exclusively imported from Germany, and in working out a satisfactory production method for it in this country.

Schamberg was tall with black hair and eyes, a handsome face and courtly manners. He was a polished speaker and always well dressed.

After two years of failing health he died on March 30, 1934, of heart disease, leaving his son Ira a dermatologic heritage for Philadelphia.*

SCHAMBERG'S DISEASE

A Peculiar Progressive Pigmentary Disease of the Skin*

P.C., aged 15, a robust lad of 120 pounds, has had the usual diseases incident to childhood, but has never suffered from a serious illness. In 1896, four years ago, "spots" were noticed upon the anterior surfaces of the tibial region of both legs. These did not give rise to any subjective symptoms, but were conspicuous enough to attract the attention of the boy's mother. The affection slowly spread, so that one year later the patches occupied irregularly oval areas, about three inches by two in diameter, in the middle third of both legs anteriorly. The patches were not elevated, of a diffuse reddish brown colour, and covered with a shining epidermis showing an exaggeration of the natural furrows of the skin. About the same time the

---

* Friedman, R. A History of Dermatology in Philadelphia. Froben Press, 1955.

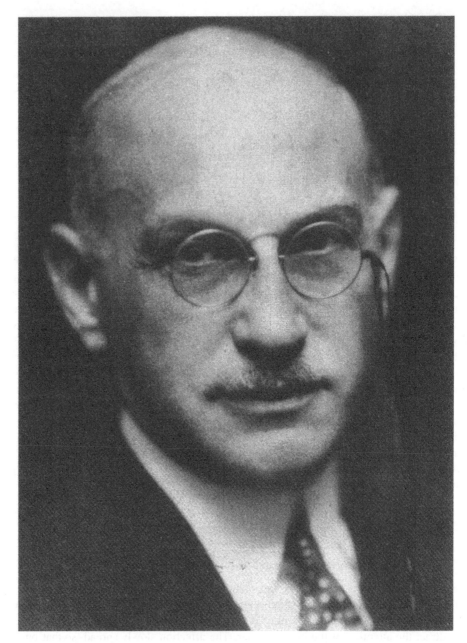

Figure 80 Jay Frank Schamberg. Courtesy, Dr. Donald M.Pillsbury

process was noticed to commence upon the flexor surface of the left wrist. In about one year it presented the following appearances: upon the left wrist is a sharply marginated patch of a reddishbrown colour, four inches by two inches in diameter. Beyond the border are visible a number of small outlying macules of the same colour and of the size of pin-heads. The skin is soft, wrinkled, and possibly thinned. There is over the entire area an exaggeration of the natural folds of the skin. Through the centre of the patch is a thickened, linear scar which is of a paler tint than the rest of the patch; this is said to have been produced some years ago by the accidental insertion of a meat hook.

During the past three years the disease has been slowly spreading. The patches upon the legs have extended upwards, going beyond the knees, and downwards involving the ankles and feet.

Notes made upon April 6, 1900, read as follows: Upon each leg is a patch extending three or four inches below the knees to one or two inches above. The patches are irregular in shape, smooth, non-elevated, and of a reddish-brown or burnt sienna colour. The border of the patch is made up of pin-point to pin-head sized reddish puncta, closely resembling grains of cayenne pepper, although perhaps of a slightly darker tint. They have somewhat of a telangiectatic appear-ance. The middle third of both legs, the seat of the disease primarily, is almost normal, exhibiting merely a slight diffuse brownish-yellow staining. Upon the angles and feet is a punctated "cayenne pepper" eruption, with moderate brownish-yellow pigmentation between the lesions. The patch on the left wrist retains the same characters of a year ago, with the exception that the borders are somewhat extended.

The right wrist is the seat of about one hundred "cayenne pepper" points, surrounded by slight areolae of pigmentation. These are for the most part discrete, although some are aggregated in groups. This manifestation upon the right wrist dates back but six months, but appears to be pursuing the same course of gradual extension.

It will be noticed by the title of this paper that no attempt has been made to class this case under any hitherto described dermatosis. In some features there is a resemblance to the "angioma serpiginosum" described by Hutchinson, and later by Crocker. The primary lesions of the disease are reddish puncta, barely elevated above the level of the skin. These are quite like the "cayenne pepper dots" which are seen in angioma sepiginosum. Then again, the manner of spreading (described by Hutchinson as infective) and the slow progressive course are strikingly analagous to that seen in angioma serpiginosum. The latter differs from this affection, however, in its onset in the first years of childhood (although Jamieson's case occurred in a boy of 15 years), in its constant tendency to form circinate patches, in its absence of marked pigmentation and in the different histological picture.

White's case of angioma serpiginosum was proven to be of the nature of an angiosarcoma.

We have here, then a disease which begins as pin-head reddish puncta or dots forming irregular patches, which slowly extend by the formation of new lesions upon the periphery. The puncta in the course of time disappear, leaving behind a brownish, brownish-yellow or reddish-brown pigmentation, which slowly fades. The process is, however, so slow in some regions, as upon the left wrist, that patches may remain practically unchanged for several years. The disease involves distant areas of the integument, the four extremities being at present affected. The disease is progressive, a constant spread having taken place during almost five years. Spontaneous involution occurs in the oldest areas, and it would seem from present appearances that a complete restoration to the normal condition of the skin may in time take place. There is entire absence of subjective symptoms.

---

* Brit. J.Dermat., *13:*1, 1901.

GRAIN ITCH

Grain Itch (Acaro-Dermatitis Urticarioides): A Study of a New Disease in this Country.*

In the late spring of 1901, there appeared in Philadelphia and its vicinity an unfamiliar eruptive disease occurring chiefly in household epidemics, which attracted the attention of the various skin specialists of the city. Having had an opportunity of studying about a dozen of these cases, I published in the *Philadelphia Medical Journal,* July 6, 1901, several photographs of the disease and a brief description under the title: "An Epidemic of a Peculiar and Unfamiliar Disease of the Skin." Since 1901, cases of the same character have been encountered each year in Philadelphia, usually between the months of May and the beginning of October. The cause of the disease remained obscure and undetermined despite careful interrogations designed to ascertain the cause of the affection and the explanation of the household epidemicity.

In the spring and summer of 1909, this peculiar eruptive disease became quite prevalent in Philadelphia and neighboring towns. An outbreak among 20 sailors upon a private yacht docked in the Delaware River attracted the attention of both the city and the federal health authorities. The Surgeon-General of the United States Public Health and Marine Hospital Service delegated Dr. Joseph Goldberger, Past Assistant Surgeon, to proceed to Philadelphia to make an investigation of the disease. Being already engaged in a semi-official study of the outbreak myself, Dr. Goldberger and I concluded to continue the inquiry jointly.

After carefully examining the 20 sailors who had been sent to the hospital, we visited the yacht whence they came and made a searching examination of the conditions aboard. Our attention was directed to the fact that a number of new straw mattresses had been received and that the disease was confined to those who had slept upon these mattresses or had placed their clothes upon them. Eleven officers and members of the crew who did not sleep upon the new mattresses remained entirely free of the disease.

At about the same period information was received concerning a similar eruptive disease prevailing among the sailors of four other boats, plying along the Delaware River. Investigation disclosed the fact that these boats had also received new straw mattresses, and, furthermore, that only those were attacked who slept upon the mattresses or otherwise came in contact with them.

In addition to these cases among sailors, we examined or received authentic information concerning 70 other cases of the disease occurring in 20 different households in Philadelphia and its vicinity.

In practically every instance we were enabled to determine that the patient had either recently slept upon a new straw mattress or had freely handled the same. Where only one person in a household was affected, it was found that he was the only one to occupy a bed supplied with a new straw mattress. We were able to trace all of the incriminated mattresses to four leading mattress manufacturers.

Careful investigation warranted us in excluding from consideration the ticking of the mattresses and the jute or cotton topping contained therein. The cause of the disease was, therefore, circumscribed to the straw. Repeated inquiries elicited the information that all the manufacturers had received at the time the disease-producing mattresses were made up, wheat-straw from a dealer in Salem County, in southern New Jersey. One manufacturer had used straw from this source exclusively in the infested mattresses.

Finding of a Parasite. Dr. Goldberger and the writer sifted the straw from a mattress through the meshes of a fine flour-sieve upon a large plate glass over white paper. Close scrutiny of the siftings under strong electric illumination soon detected some slight motion. The moving particles were touched with a needle

---

* J.Cutan. Dis., *28:*67, 1910.

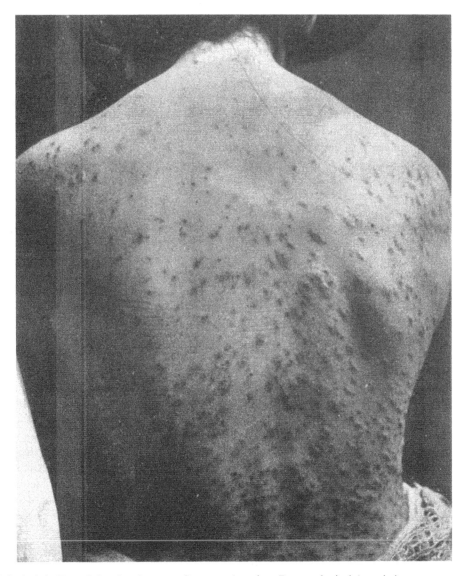

Figure 81 Grain itch. From Schamberg's paper. Courtesy, American Dermatological Association

moistened in glycerine and transferred to a glass slide. Search with a microscope disclosed the presence of a mite of very minute dimensions. This mite was identified for us by Mr. Nathan Banks, expert in acarina of the United States Bureau of Entomology, as very close to, if not identical with the *Pediculoides ventricosus*.

In order to demonstrate experimentally the aetiological relationship of the suspected straw mattresses, Dr. Goldberger exposed his bared left arm and shoulder for one hour between two mattresses. At the end of about 16 hours, a number of characteristic lesions appeared upon the arm, shoulder, and chest. Later, three volunteers slept upon the mattresses, and each one developed the eruption at the end of about the same period.

Dr. Goldberger later took some of the sifted straw, divided it into two portions and placed it in two clean Petri glass dishes. One of these was applied for one hour to the left axilla of a volunteer. At the end of 16 to 17 hours, the characteristic eruption was present in the left axilla to which the Petri dish of straw siftings had been applied.

The second portion of the straw siftings in a Petri dish was exposed to the vapor of chloroform under a bell jar with a view to killing any insect or acarina that might be present. These siftings were then applied to the right axilla of the same volunteer to whose left axilla the untreated siftings had been applied. The chloroform evidently destroyed in the siftings the agent that was producing the eruption, for no lesions appeared after the application of the chloroformized siftings.

Dr. Goldberger further fished out of some straw siftings five minute mites, and, placing them in a clean watch crystal, applied the crystal to the axilla of another volunteer. At the end of about 16 hours following this application, five of the characteristic lesions appeared on the area to which the mites had been applied.

Eruption. The disease is characterized by an eruption consisting of wheals, many of which exhibit at their summits a central pin-point-sized vesicle. This is the peculiar lesion of the disease, and is so characteristic as to immediately suggest this affection. The contents of the vesicle are clear but for a brief period of time and then become lactescent or distinctly puriform, constituting a well-marked pustule. Instead of frank wheals, the efflorescence may consist of barely elevated, erythemato-urticarial spots or papulo-urticarial lesions. The latter are oedematous in character, but have the size and shape of papules. The lesions generally vary in size from a lentil to a fingernail, and are rounded, oval, or irregular in shape. They are oedematous like the wheals of ordinary urticaria and are not infrequently elevated 1 to 2 mm. above the level of the skin. The color is usually a warm rose tint; only rarely do the lesions exhibit the pinkish-white anaemic area seen in ordinary "hives." The central vesicle or pustule is usually minute, not exceeding in diameter 0.5 mm.; in many cases it is pin-head in size (about 2 mm.); exceptionally the vesicle or pustule may reach a diameter of 3 mm. In such cases, the large vesicles situated upon an erythemato-urticarial base present a strong resemblance to the lesions of chicken-pox. In many patients the tops of the lesions are so excoriated by scratching that no vesicles are seen; instead the wheals are surmounted by punctiform, dark red blood crusts.

The eruption varies in extent in different subjects; usually it is profuse, involving the neck, chest, abdomen, and back, and in a lesser degree the arms and legs. The greatest number of lesions is observed upon the trunk. The face is often free, although at times scattered lesions are present. The hands and feet are nearly always exempt. The extent of the eruption and the size of the individual lesions are apt to bear an inverse relation to each other. In the most profuse eruptions, 10,000 or more lesions may be present.

In rare instances, the eruption may undergo modification and take on the characteristics of the macular type of erythema multiforme. I noted this especially in the sailor patient shown in Figure 6. The eruption on the face of this man was profuse and there was an erythema involving both of the lower eyelids. In another patient there was, in addition to the usual eruption, a partial scarlatinoid rash involving the anterior and lateral surfaces of the chest. This patient had fever, nausea, chilliness, and vomiting.

There are, therefore, three varieties of the eruption. In the order of their frequency they are: 1. Urticaria-vesiculo-pustulosa type. 2. Varicelloid type with large central vesicle or pustule, and 3. Erythema multiforme type.

The eruption is usually accompanied by the most intolerable itching. This is worse at night and seriously interferes with sleep. The itching leads to violent scratching with the consequent production of excoriations and blood crusts, and at times pyogenic infection of the skin.

Systemic Symptoms. During the early days of the attack the patient may experience chilliness and in some cases nausea and even vomiting. Mild rigors may recur throughout the course of the next few days.

The temperature may be elevated from 100°F. to 102°F., or higher, with corresponding acceleration of the pulse rate; this pyrexia may continue for several days. It is, however, a very variable symptom and is often lacking. Some patients, although afebrile, complain of malaise and anorexia; others do not admit being ill at all. Indeed, even the patients with some elevation of temperature are not inclined to seek their beds. There is at times a moderate enlargement of the superficial lymphatic glands.

Louis Queyrat

Erythroplasia

LOUIS QUEYRAT was born in 1856, in France, in the Department of Creuse. The son of a country physician, he received an intensive and well rounded medical education in Paris before turning to dermatology as a specialty. In 1898 he joined the staff of the Ricord Hospital in Paris (Cochin-annexe), and was so successful in renovating the clinic of that hospital that it became a leading dermatologic center. He remained there until his retirement in 1923.

From his many publications we have selected Queyrat's well known and definitive report of erythroplasia.

A true student of syphilis, he was particularly interested in the congenital form of the disease and wrote much on its clinical, laboratory and epidemiologic features. He founded one of the first hospital poly clinics for the care of syphilitic mothers and children.

Queyrat was large in stature, wore great old fashioned moustaches and an imposing beard, and had a mischievious eye. He maintained a lively interest in art and literature, collected poetry, and at one time compiled a Creuse dictionary. He died suddenly on October 18, 1933, the victim of a stroke.*

ERYTHROPLASIA

Erythroplasie du Gland*

The patient I am presenting to the Société de Dermatologie is interesting for several reasons: he is affected by a lesion of the glans which has not to my knowledge as yet been described.

We have here a chronic affection characterized by the appearance and persistence of red plaques, non-painful or a little sensitive, accompanied by a slight infiltration of the dermo-muqueuse, and able in some cases to eventuate in epithelioma.

V.Ferdinand, 62 years of age, admitted to my service at l'Hôpital Cochin-annexe (Ward 7, No. 14) on January 16, 1911.

He denies any venereal disease, syphilis in particular. I must add immediately that despite his denials his serodiagnostic test, done by the Bauer technic, is clearly positive.

---

* Gougerot, H.: Bull, de la Soc. Franc. de Dermat. et Syph., *40:*1375, 1933.

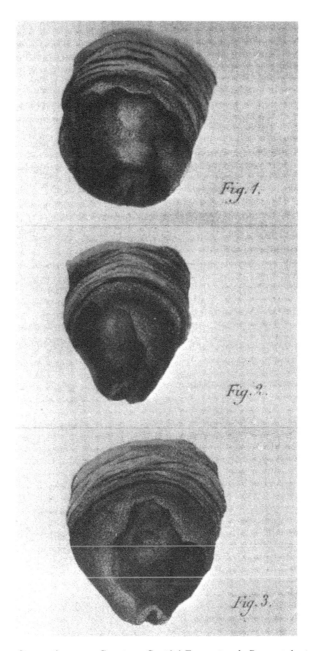

Figure 82 Erythroplasia. From Queyrat's paper. Courtesy, *Société Française de Dermatologie*

By chance, two years ago, he noted the presence of a red, shining, and absolutely painless plaque on the left part of the glans. The plaque enlarged progressively and the patient, finally becoming a little upset, consulted me about the matter.

On the superior and lateral surfaces of the glans a large plaque is seen which is bright red (see Plate I, Figures 1 to 3), has the dimensions of a franc piece, and extends distally to within a few millimeters of the meatus. The base of it is smooth, glazed, a little moist, and shows four small ulcerations which are as large as a hempseed, irregular, non-pustular, do not bleed on pressure, and are paler in hue than the rest of the plaque; two of them are immediately behind the meatus; the other two are located in the central part. The borders of the plaque do not stand out in relief, but are clearly demarcated by the change in color.

Palpation produces neither pain nor serous discharge, but reveals a slight infiltration of the epidermis. On each side of the frenulum four small plaques are found which are the size of a pinhead, and are absolutely comparable in all respects to those on the dorsal surface.

No penile lymphangitis; there is slight inguinal adenopathy, more marked on the right. The general condition of the patient is excellent. Detailed examination of his organs reveals no lesion; there is no sugar in his urine, and only a very slight trace of albumen.

Despite the absence of exact signs of neoplastic transformation I was concerned over the persistence of the small ulcerations which had been present for five or six months; I asked my colleague Michon to perform a biopsy, which he did on February 4th.

It was then apparent that we were dealing with a *parakeratotic lesion of the glans with epitheliomatous transformation,* a lesion that had developed on the surface of a glazed, shiny, red plaque which had begun two years before.

I have had the opportunity to observe three analogous cases.

Because of the color, the infiltration of the tissue, and the similarity to leukoplakia, a similarity which holds again in its epitheliomatous evolution, I propose to give to this lesion the name, érythroplasie du gland.

---

* Bull, del a Soc. Franc. de Dermat. et Syph., *22:*378, 1911.

J.E.McDonagh

Nevoxantho-Endothelioma

JAMES EUSTACE RADCLYFFE MCDONAGH was born in London on October 17, 1881. After medical training at Bedford College, St. Bartholomew's Hospital, and a period in Vienna, he returned to London, as a surgeon, and became associated with the London Lock Hospitals. He became the Director of the Nature of Disease Institute at its founding in 1929, and published many papers on pathology, microbiology and clinical medicine. His account of nevoxanthoendothelioma is of especial interest to dermatologists. Author of numerous books, including a textbook on venereal disease (1915), he also published *The Universe in the Making*. He continued to engage in medical research and consultation into his 70s.

NEVOXANTHO-ENDOTHELIOMA

A Contribution to our Knowledge of Naevo-xantho-endotheliomata*

In June, 1906, a child was brought up by its mother to St. Bartholomew's Hospital under the care of Dr. Morley Fletcher, to whom the author is indebted for the case, for some "yellow swellings" which it had scattered about the body.

The face was the part most affected, especially the eyelids. There were two swellings in the neck, one on the left arm, one or two on both legs, and a few scattered about the trunk. To look at they were bright yellow, slightly depressed in the centre, and had a glazed surface resembling very closely Xanthoma planum. The edge of each swelling was reddish where vessels could plainly be seen.

The tumours in size varied from one-fourth inch to one-half inch in diameter. They were raised about 3 or 4 mm. above the surface, were of firm consistency and moved with the surrounding skin, which was in every way normal. In other respects the child was quite healthy.

What urine could be obtained was carefully examined, but nothing abnormal was discovered, no sugar, bile or albumen. These swellings were present at birth, and the following account is taken from Mr. Woodman's notes, who attended the confinement.

Born April 7, 1906. L.O.A. position. Weight 10½ lbs. About the body were scattered brownish-red swellings, raised well above the surface of the skin, of firm consistency, elastic, almost cartilaginous. The surface of the tumours was quite smooth and showed numerous small injected capillaries.

---

* Brit. J.Dermat., *24*:85, 1912.

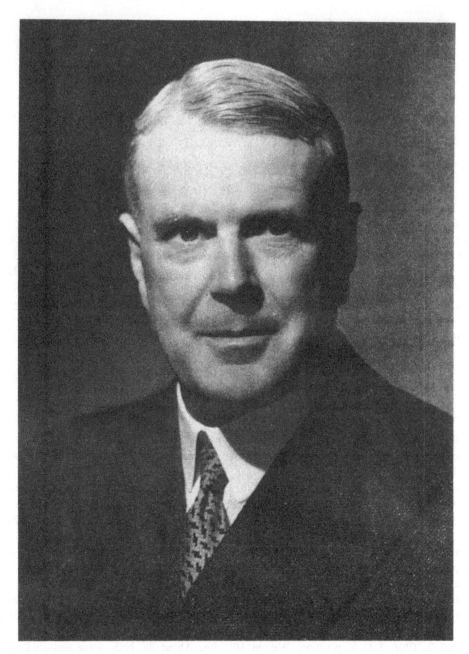

Figure 83 J.E.R.McDonagh

In June, 1906, some of the nodules were removed for microscopic examination, and a painting was made (*see* Figure 1). I did not see the child again for a year. When in April, 1907, I wrote and asked the mother to bring the child up to hospital, I found that the swellings were of the same size, not such a bright yellow in colour, and quite flush with the surface of the surrounding skin. The lesions still had the glazed appearance,

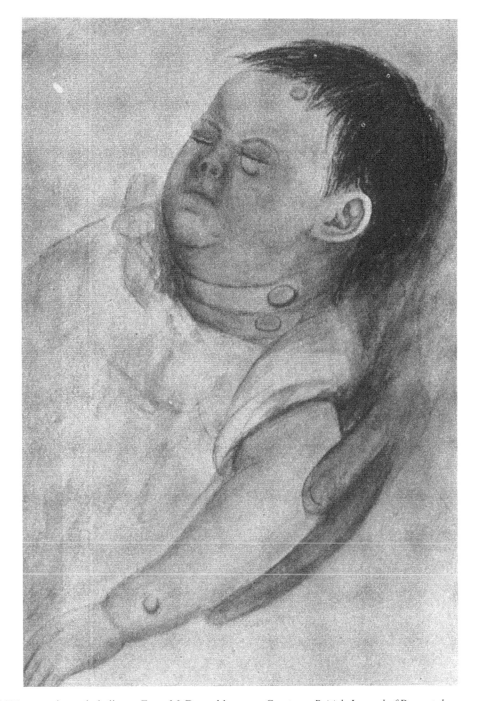

Figure 84 Nevoxantho-endothelioma. From McDonagh's paper. Courtesy, *British Journal of Dermatology*

the central depression had disappeared, the edges were of the same colour as the rest of the swelling and showed no dilated capillaries. Urine quite normal.

Some more nodules were removed for microscopic examination.

Owing to my being abroad I was unable to see the child again till June, 1909, when I was surprised to find all the swellings had disappeared. The old scars resulting from the biopsies were scarcely visible and there was no keloid formation in them. The scar over the right eyebrow had, according to the mother, given the child a good deal of pain, which has for a few months past quite disappeared. I searched the legs where I knew there had been some swellings and all I could find in their place was a piece of skin which was whiter and of a more glazed porcelain-like appearance than elsewhere; so slight was the difference that had I not known that something had been there I should have overlooked any change. The mother had had 14 children; this child was the thirteenth, but none of the others had a similar condition and no member of the family had ever suffered from any "swellings of the skin."

John T.Bowen

Chronic Atypical Epithelial Proliferation (Bowen's Disease)

JOHN TEMPLETON BOWEN was born in Boston, July 8, 1857. He attended the Boston Latin School, was graduated from Harvard University in 1879, and took his M.D. at the latter institution in 1884. After three years study abroad, in Berlin, Munich, and Vienna, he returned to the United States and began practice in Boston. An assistant physician at the Massachusetts General Hospital in 1889, he became an instructor in dermatology at Harvard in 1896, and in 1902, with the retirement of James C.White, he was appointed assistant professor. He became the first Edward Wigglesworth Professor of Dermatology in 1907.

Bowen was not a prolific writer. Most of his contributions were made to the "systems of medicine" so popular in that day. The two notable exceptions were his well known and remarkable study, *The Epitrichial Layer of the Skin* (1889), and his famous account of the precancerous dermatosis to which his name has been applied (at Darier's suggestion). The clinical section of the latter paper appears below.

A bachelor, Bowen held membership in many of the Boston social clubs. Yet he was quiet and retiring; lecturing was almost a torture to him. Following his retirement in 1927 he became somewhat of a recluse, and died December 30, 1940, after a long illness.*

BOWEN'S DISEASE

Precancerous Dermatoses: A Study of Two Cases of Chronic Atypical Epithelial Proliferation*

Case i. Lesions of the Buttock of Twenty Years' Duration. The first case which I have to describe is remarkable on account of the length of time the affection had already lasted. The patient was admitted to the skin ward of the Massachusetts General Hospital at three different times during the years 1909, 1910, and 1911, so that abundant opportunity was offered for a thorough study of his case.

He was first admitted on April 16, 1909. The man was of English birth, a native of Fall River, Massachusetts, 49 years of age, a weaver by occupation, and a man of considerable intelligence. He declared that the affection had first appeared 19 years previously when he was 30 years of age. The first appearances were those of a good sized "pimple" on his gluteal region, which was accompanied by slight itching, but of which he took no notice for several years until he became conscious that it was gradually

---

* White, C.J.: Arch. of Dermat. and Syph., *43*:386, 1941.

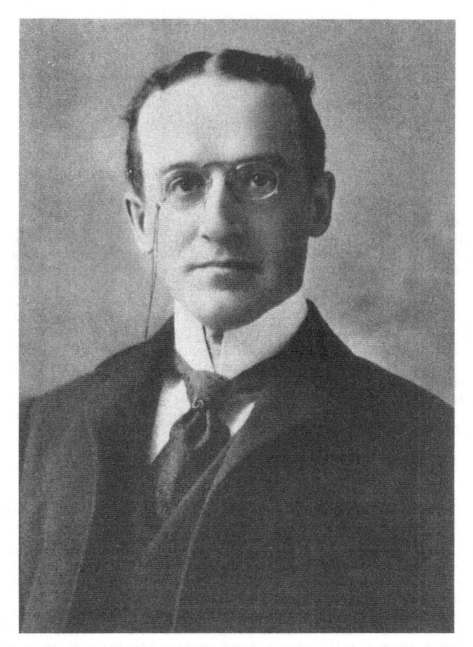

Figure 85 John T.Bowen. Courtesy, *Archives of Dermatology and Syphilology*

increasing in size. He complained of some pain in connection with the lesions, chiefly noticeable when seated or after walking, and especially marked at times when the lesion became excoriated and showed a discharge. The inconvenience and pain were chiefly noticeable in warm weather. During the past 19 years he had used many external applications and at one time he had one treatment of X-rays without producing any marked reaction or results.

The patient was a man of small stature, weighing only in the neighborhood of 105 pounds. His appearance, however, was that of a person in fair health. Nothing of importance could be found in the family history. He had two brothers and one sister living and well, and could give no history of any preceding affections except congestion of the lungs 12 years ago. He denied venereal disease. He was not addicted to the use of alcohol.

Nothing abnormal could be detected on examination of the internal organs. When stripped, the patient presented the appearance of an undersized, thin, but not cachectic man. In the right lumbar region there were scars which the patient said were derived from an abscess which he had when a boy. An interesting feature was the presence of quite numerous small angiomata, scattered over the abdomen and back, from the size of a pin's head to that of a small pea. These lesions he had never observed with any care but they had probably been present for many years.

The affection of the skin for which he sought relief was situated on the left buttock. The area invaded was irregularly rounded and measured about four inches in diameter. The isolated lesions were represented by papules and tubercles slightly raised above the surface, flattened at the top, and generally rounded at the circumference. These isolated lesions varied in size from an eighth of an inch to half an inch in diameter; they were generally situated at the outer borders of the patch, and at the extreme edge they took on often an annular arrangement, or in some instances they formed almost serpiginous figures. The centre of the patch was made up of more or less confluent lesions, although there were many partially defined, separate lesions. A small amount of cicatricial tissue could be seen interspersed between papules and raised, confluent areas.

The color of the lesions and confluent patches was a dull red. The lesions were moderately firm, but not hard to the touch. The surface of the lesions was somewhat uneven. In places there was a papillomatous tendency. The surface was, in places, scaling and crusted, and here and there were marks of a slight exudation. The crusts were always extremely superficial.

On the possibility that these lesions might be of syphilitic nature the patient was put upon iodide of potash. Some improvement was noted under this treatment during the first few weeks, but as the improvement seemed to be at a standstill, curetting was resorted to, small areas being treated at a time, as the patient was extremely sensitive and refused active surgical intervention. Under the curette the lesions bled freely and were extremely painful.

On the 5th of June he was discharged, much relieved. A large portion of the tissue had been mechanically destroyed by the curette, although there were still a number of areas which had not been entirely removed.

During his stay in the hospital the patient's condition was extremely good. Examination of the blood and secretions showed nothing abnormal. Several pieces of tissue were removed for microscopical examination. The findings will be referred to later.

Just about a year later, on April 4, 1910, the patient was readmitted to the hospital. During the interval since last seen he had worked quite steadily at his occupation. Practically no treatment had been followed with the exception of some in different ointments. He appeared again at the hospital because the lesions in the affected area had considerably increased in number and sitting and walking had again become painful.

On examination it was found that the lesions were still much less pronounced than when he had first applied for treatment, but that there had been a considerable increase within the last year. The extent of the area had slightly increased, new lesions having appeared at the lower border of the patch. Considerable

* J.Cutan. Dis., *30:*241, 1912.

smooth cicatricial tissue was to be seen in the centre of the patch, which represented the site of the lesions that had been removed by the curette. The confluent areas that had previously been present no longer existed.

At this time it was decided to treat the lesions by freezing with carbon dioxide snow, as the patient was still extremely sensitive, and refused active surgical treatment. The lesions were deeply frozen with firm pressure for 60 seconds, the area and lesions being treated piece-meal, a few at a time.

The patient remained this time in the hospital six weeks and when he left, the skin over the patch had been converted into a smooth cicatrix with only here and there the remains of a lesion.

Again, on September 27, 1911, the patient was admitted to the hospital. In the interval of 15 months, during which time no treatment had been followed, there had been a considerable recurrence at the edge of the area, and also here and there in the midst of the cicatrix caused by treatment. Some of the new lesions had a papillomatous appearance clinically, and bled rather freely upon being handled. None of the lesions was as large as the largest individual ones described previously. Many of these lesions were distinctly nummular in shape and varied in size from that of a three-cent piece to that of a half dollar. The largest ones were raised one-eighth of an inch above the surface of the skin. The nummular patches were situated chiefly along the lower border of the affected area and were more or less confluent, forming polycyclical figures along the lower edge.

The pinhead to pea-sized angiomata over the body and extremities had not increased in numbers apparently, and presented the same appearances as before.

The patient's condition was practically the same. He asserted that although not precluding work, the lesions made it hard to get about, especially in hot weather. He also declared that no lesion had disappeared spontaneously, so far as he could determine, but that all improvement had been from mechanical interference. The patient was again treated by the freezing method and remained in the hospital nearly two months. At the time of his discharge practically the whole area had been transformed into a cicatrix and only a slight infiltration was left at the site of some of the lesions that had resisted the freezing more than the others.

Case II. Lesions of the Lower Leg of Nearly Ten Years' Duration.

The case that has just been described immediately recalled to mind a similar case that had been observed at the out-patient department of the hospital at intervals for several years. The man was 52 years of age, a native of Scotland, a cooper by trade, residing in the suburbs of Boston.

He first came to the hospital September 6, 1907. The history was that the lesions had existed for some four to five years. He presented, on the outer side of the calf of the right leg, an area resembling in a marked degree the appearances that have just been described as occurring on the buttock in the previous case. The area was from three to four inches in diameter and consisted of nodules from the size of a pin's head to that of a bean, many of which were confluent, others discrete and well bounded from the sound skin. They were raised about one-eighth of an inch above the level of the skin, were flat on the surface and many of the larger lesions showed a papillomatous element. The color was a pale red. Some of the lesions were covered with crusts and a slight oozing occurred when these were removed. In some parts of the patches the lesions had joined to form irregular plaques and portions of rings. According to the patient's story, none of the lesions had ever disappeared spontaneously. The patient's general condition was good and beyond some pruritus and tenderness the lesions were not especially sensitive.

This patient presented himself rather irregularly and it was not possible to study his case so carefully as the preceding one. The lesions proved resistant to many forms of treatment. At one time they seemed to be improving under the iodide of potash but this improvement soon came to a standstill. Finally freezing with solid carbon dioxide was resorted to as in the preceding case with good results, but the lesions had not entirely disappeared when the patient was last seen. Fortunately it was possible to obtain a generous amount of tissue for microscopical examination.

Benjamin Lipschuetz

Ulcus Vulvae Acutum

BENJAMIN LIPSCHUETZ was born on October 4, 1878, in Brody, Galicia (Austria). He received his medical education in Vienna, and was graduated in 1902. Following this he studied widely, spending some time with Missen in Breslau, and also a period at the Pasteur Institute. In 1915 he was made chief of the skin clinic at the Children's Hospital in Vienna. He was made Professor only a few months before his premature death, on December 20, 1931.

Lipschuetz was a discerning and critical clinician, a capable virologist, and histologist. Most of his research centered about virus diseases of the skin, and the investigation of the possible role of viruses in skin diseases of unknown origin. We have given below a clinical excerpt from his paper on ulcus vulvae acutum, for which he is best known.*

ULCUS VULVAE ACUTUM

Ueber eine eigenartige Geschwuersform des Weiblichen Genitales (Ulcus vulvae acutum)[†]

In attempting to compose a coherent picture of this peculiar ulcerative entity with respect to its clinical appearance on the basis of the cases thus far observed, we should note to begin with, and a study of the case histories will bring it out, that there are certain variations in almost every case. Nevertheless, a clinical picture is formed by a group of symptoms common to all. Despite the limited number of cases described so far, the clinical picture of this ulcerative disease seems to have two different forms. At times the ulcers appear acutely, "overnight," accompanied by fever, fits of shivering, and smarting burning pain on the external genitalia. With respect to course these ulcers, which are usually of different sizes and are found on the inner surface of the labia minora, increase rapidly for two to three days; the process extends more deeply into the tissues, and the base becomes covered by a pseudo-diphtheritic membrane which in the beginning is strongly adherent. At this stage the ulcers are very tender to touch, and give rise to a peculiar odor which is stale, but not foul. In the next few days the strongly adherent greyish yellow crust begins to separate from the periphery,

---

* Dermat. Wchnschr., *94:*318, 1932.

[†] Archiv für dermat. und syph., *114:*363, 1912.

whereupon healing of the disease process begins; the temperature returns to normal; the pain disappears, and in two weeks at the most the ulcers heal completely leaving delicate scars.

In another series of cases the onset of the disease is more subacute or insidious, and the disease is prolonged for several weeks. Accompanied by mild subjective difficulties and a temperature which remains normal, superficial, shallow, or deeply penetrating ulcerations appear in the vestibulum vaginae, the labia minora, and majora. The borders of the ulcers may be irregular and undermined; the base is covered with pus. These ulcers may heal up completely, while new ulcers with similar clinical characteristics appear in the vicinity; in this manner, in the case R.Chr., the disease pursued a tedious course.

The first type of this ulcerative disease reminds us of a sort of nosocomial gangrene of the genitalia; the second disease picture mentioned above bears a great resemblance to the many venereal ulcers, and we were persuaded to make this diagnosis at first in two of our cases. The microscopic investigations, however, furnish us with proof that this is a special sort of infection, in that we could find neither fusiform bacilli nor thick spiraled spirochetes in the first named cases, nor Ducrey bacilli in the last mentioned form; this fact certainly establishes our ulcerative entity as separate from the several variants of Ulcus molle and nosocomial gangrene. However, it might appear odd at first glance that two ulcerative types so different in clinical appearance and course should be thought to owe their origin to a single cause, and we must come back to this later in detail.

No particular reason for the appearance of these ulcers could be established from the anamneses of our cases (and this should be particularly stressed with regard to the cases observed in Finger's clinic in the year 1904). Four cases involved young girls from 14 to 17 years old in whom poor care and uncleanliness could scarcely be blamed for the appearance of these peculiar ulcerations. That very small mucous membrane injuries on erosions appearing with a slight leucorrhea might be held responsible for the beginning of the affection cannot, of course, be ruled out.

Coitus could be excluded in three patients who were virgines intactae; in the case of R.Christine the last marital coitus had taken place four months previously, while in Case II the last sexual intercourse had occurred more than two months before. Against the postulation of an infection from sexual intercourse a series of particulars can be cited. First, we were in a position to observe the appearance of new ulcers in the case of R.Christine during her long hospital stay; further, the rarity of the ulcerations—which we should meet with much more frequently in the very abundant venereologic material of a large city. Finally, the postulation, later found to be plausible, of the facultativeparasitic characteristics of the bacilli, the detailed report of which is given below.

The general condition was constantly affected in the disease form which showed the gangrenous ulcer picture, so that the patients give the impression of being very ill, what with their high fevers (up to 40.1°C.) and the chills which usually occur initially; on the other hand the general condition was not disturbed at all in the mild ulcerative disease type, and the temperature was always normal.

An important symptom was the marked painfulness of the inflammatory process in the first disease type; it was greatly increased by walking or when the labia were touched during examination, while in the form of ulceration which was not unlike the Ulcus venereum the painfulness was very mild, but very annoying to the patients nonetheless.

An important characteristic common to all cases is the purely local character of this ulcerative process; we were unable to demonstrate the appearance of lymphangitis or inguinal adenopathy, or any other sequellae.

Richard L.Sutton

1. *Periadenitis Mucosa Necrotica Recurrens*

2. *Leucoderma Acquisitum Centrifugum (Sutton's Nevus)*

RICHARD LIGHTBURN SUTTON was born in Rockport, Missouri, on July 9, 1878. After receiving an M.D. both from the University Medical College in Kansas City and from George Washington University, he took postgraduate training in London, Paris, Hamburg and Berlin. He returned to Kansas City where he was successively assistant, associate and full Professor of Dermatology, at the University Medical College during the period from 1907 to 1912. Following this, he held similar appointments at the University of Kansas. In 1940, an Emeritus Professor, he retired from practice to live in McAllen, Texas. During the last two years of his life he suffered through six major operations. On May 18, 1952 his death came as a result of a coronary occlusion.

Sutton was a member of the American Dermatological Association as well as numerous other societies. He wrote on various aspects of clinical dermatology, and, with his distinguished son, was the author of several textbooks, including his famed encyclopedic volume, *Diseases of the Skin*. Sutton's name has been linked with several dermatoses which he first described. We have included his accounts of leucoderma aquisitum centrifugum and periadenitis mucosa necrotica recurrens.

A most interesting side of Sutton's career was his world wide explorations. As a representative of the Natural History Department of the University of Missouri, he made expeditions to Africa, China, India, Australia, New Zealand, South America and the Arctic. Concerning these adventures he wrote a number of popular books, including *An*

PERIADENITIS MUCOSA NECROTICA RECURRENS

Periadenitis mucosa necrotica recurrens*

The following case, which was seen in consultation with Dr. Frank J.Hall, a pathologist of this city, and which was later referred to me for treatment, represents an affection which is new to me and also to various other dermatologists with whom I have communicated concerning it.

The patient, A.G.L., was a male, a student, 16 years of age.

Since early infancy the patient had suffered from a peculiar, recurring, localized inflammation of the lingual and buccal mucous membranes. About once every fortnight a slightly elevated, sharply circumscribed, red nodule (occasionally two, or even three, are present at the same time), varying in size from the head of a pin to the top of an ordinary lead pencil, appears on one of the above named surfaces. In

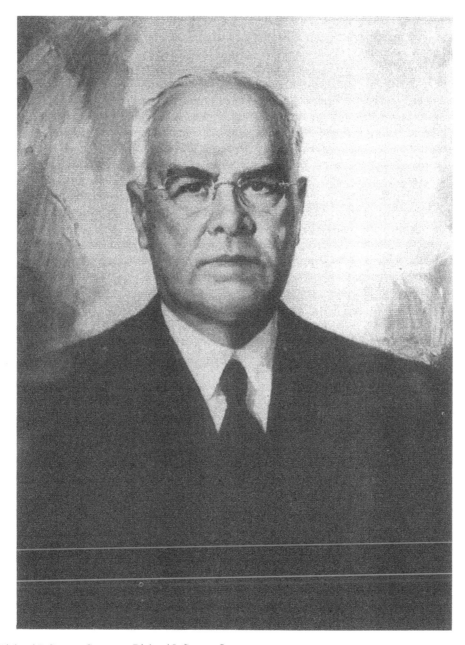

Figure 86 Richard L.Sutton. Courtesy, Richard L.Sutton, Jr.

African Holiday (1924), *Tiger Trails in Southern Asia* (1926), and *An Arctic Safari* (1932).

the course of three or four days the intense congestion is followed by sloughing, and a solid mummified-like plug separates, leaving a crateriform depression which extends well down into the corium. The ulcer then bears a considerable resemblance to an inflamed lingual chancre with a depressed centre. While the lesions are in course of development they are smooth, hard, and resistant to the touch, and quite painful, and the associated lymphatic glands are enlarged and tender. There is some elevation of temperature during the course of an attack—100° to 101°F.—and the pulse averages from 96 to 100 per minute. There is apparently no suppuration, and no pus can be squeezed out when the nodules are incised. No haemorrhage results when the plug is thrown off. The lesions heal within six or eight days, leaving smooth, pliable, grayish scars, from one-half to one centimetre or more in diameter. These cicatrices bear very little resemblance to the whitened areas seen in leukoplakia. They are irregular in outline and imperceptibly fade into the healthy contiguous tissue. Apparently trauma, such as the slight injuries received when cracking nuts between the teeth or while masticating hard or rough articles of food, plays but little part in the aetiology. The sides and under surface of the tongue are attacked more often than the dorsum. The mucous surfaces of the cheeks and lips are affected with about the same degree of frequency. During the course of an exacerbation the patient is mentally irritable, and somewhat restless, and the tongue becomes covered with a heavy, light-brown coat. The appetite is not particularly impaired, however, and the boy continues his school work as usual. The gingivitis appears to bear no relation to the accompanying disease. The size and severity of the lesions vary somewhat with the seasons of the year. As a rule, they are worse in the Spring and Fall than at other times.

LEUCODERMA ACQUISITUM CENTRIFUGUM

An Unusual Variety of Vitiligo (Leucoderma Acquisitum Centrifugum)*

Recently I have encountered two cases of vitiligo which presented some unusual features, both clinically and histologically.

Case Reports. The first patient was a housewife, aged 22, referred to me by Dr. T.J.Beattie, of Kansas City, in October, 1915. The personal and family histories were negative. There was a single rounded lesion, located on the right cheek. The spot measured a little more than 2 cm. in diameter, and had been present three months. There was no history of trauma. Exactly in the centre of the patch was a minute, rounded, slightly elevated, brownish maculopapule which had been present only since the onset of the attack. The hyperpigmented areola commonly found in vitiligo was absent. The lesion had developed slowly, and has never given rise to subjective symptoms of any kind. The patient was somewhat sensitive regarding the blemish, and objected to having it photographed. Permission to perform a biopsy also was refused. A one per cent solution of mercuric chloride in alcohol and water was prescribed, to be applied frequently to both the central portion and the margin of the patch, in order to lessen the disfigurement. Shortly afterward the young woman removed to Southern California, and I had no further opportunity to study the case.

The second patient was a schoolgirl, aged 16, referred to me by Dr. W.F. Fairbanks, of Kansas City, Kansas, in 1915. The disorder had first become apparent three years before, but the earliest patch, which was located on the right side of the forehead, had gradually regained its normal color, and at the time of consultation was scarcely discernible. A second small patch in the left clavicular region also was very faintly defined. Two other lesions, in the right and left scapular regions respectively, had changed but little, however, since attaining their present size, and stood out sharply as snowy, oval plaques with normally pigmented borders. The centre of each spot was marked by the presence of a small, roundish, brown maculopapule. The patient's mother said that the lesions had begun as minute, brownish points, which were

---

* J.Cutan. Dis., *29:*65, 1911.

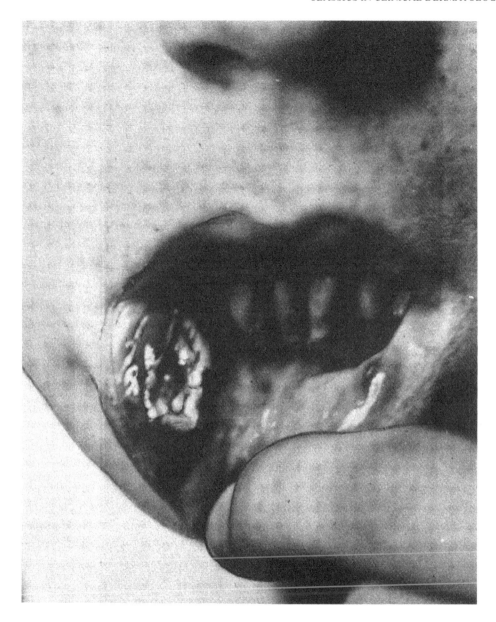

Figure 87 Periadenitis mucosa necrotica recurrens. From Sutton's paper. Courtesy, American Dermatological Association

usually, but not invariably, sufficiently elevated to be perceptible to touch. There was no history of trauma, or of preexisting naevi. The family history was negative. A careful physical examination of the patient revealed nothing abnormal. There was no reaction to tuberculin, and both the Wassermann and luetin tests gave negative results.

The second case here described has now been under observation for more than one year, and during that time the appearance of the lesions has changed but little, if at all, despite the frequent employment of various chemical and actinic irritants, calculated to hasten the formation of pigment.

---

* J.Cutan. Dis., *34:*797, 1916.

C.Guy Lane

Chromoblastomycosis

CLARENCE GUY LANE was born in Billerica, Massachusetts, on October 21, 1882. He graduated from Harvard Medical School in 1908 and entered general practice in Woburn until 1914. Following service with the Army Medical Corps in World War I, he became a member of the dermatology staff at Massachusetts General Hospital in 1919. Having been associated with the Department of Dermatology at Harvard from 1925, he was made Clinical Professor of Dermatology in 1939, and held the title of Emeritus Professor from 1947.

Dr. Lane was a member of numerous societies, and was President both of the American Dermatological Association, and the American Board of Dermatology and Syphilology. His writings in dermatology included works on industrial dermatoses, radiation therapy, and basic investigative studies. The selection below represents the first clinical description of chromoblastomycosis. Dr. Lane died on March 12, 1954.*

CHROMOBLASTOMYCOSIS

A Cutaneous Lesion Caused by a New Fungus (Phialophora Verrucosa)[†]

J.P., 19 years old, Italian, living in East Boston, was referred to the Dermatological Department of the Boston Dispensary by the Surgical Department for the failure of an abscess on his buttock to close within a reasonable time after operation. He had lived in East Boston for the last year and a half, and for a year previous to that he was in Detroit most of the time, making one trip as far west as Denver. Previous to that he had lived in Boston and Revere since coming to this country, when he was seven or eight years old.

Past History. Negative, except for an operation at the Boston City Hospital nine years ago, when a gland was removed from the right side of his neck.

Present Illness. About a year ago there appeared on the right buttock a small "pimple," which he squeezed and from which he obtained some material. A scab formed and the process was repeated. There has been comparatively little discharge and the lesion has gradually increased in size. He has had no pain and it has not been tender. About 7 or 8 cm. away from this lesion he noticed, about six months ago, a rather hard, painless lump, about as large as a marble, which gradually became softer without giving pain.

---

* Obit.: Arch. Dermatol., *69:*763, 1954.

† J.Cutan. Dis., *39:*840, 1915.

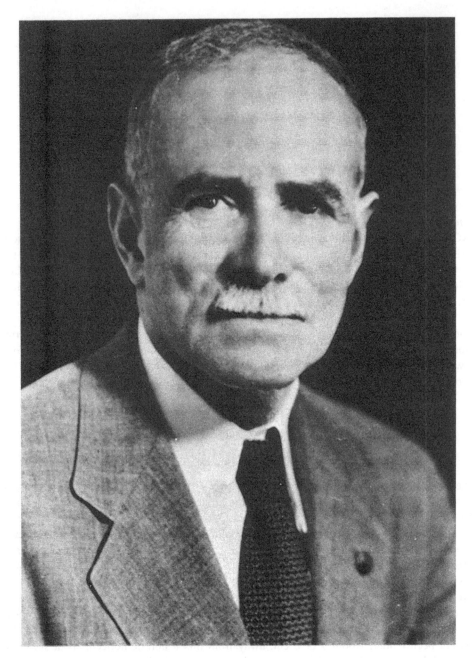

Figure 88 C.Guy Lane

He thought it was ready to be opened and came to the Surgical Department, where it was incised under local anaesthesia and a diagnosis of furunculosis of the buttock recorded.

Examination of the first lesion showed a small tumor in the skin, just outside the ischial tuberosity. It was about 2.5 cm. by 2 cm., purplish in color, raised about 3 mm. above the surface, rather soft, not tender, with an irregularly papular surface, the top of which in places was slightly grayish. There were a few grayish scales on the lesion. There was no discharge at the time of examination. The second lesion was the one which had been operated upon in the Surgical Department. This showed, at the time when he visited the Dermatological Department, a purplish, slightly raised, rather soft area about 2 cm. in diameter, freely movable and not tender. From a small crater-like opening in the centre there could be expressed a slightly gray, somewhat cheesy substance mixed with a little blood.

The lesion, with its color and sharply localized, irregularly papular growth, seemed to resemble a tuberculosis of the verrucous type. Of course, it was an unusual position for such a lesion and the picture presented was not exactly typical of a tuberculosis verrucosa, but it seemed to resemble this more than any other condition and this was the diagnosis which was made. With this diagnosis in mind, excision of the discharging lesion was recommended. Under local anaesthesia (one per cent cocaine solution) an oval incision about the lesion was made and the tumor was removed intact. The wound was closed with horsehair, a dry, sterile dressing applied, the stitches removed on the eighth and ninth days, and the wound healed by first intention.

Max Winkler

Chondrodermatitis Nodularis Chronica Helicis

MAX WINKLER was born in Hitzkirch, Switzerland, on June 9, 1875. After studying in Geneva, Munich and Berne he received his doctorate in 1901. A student of Jadassohn, he later settled in Lucerne.

He served as attending dermatologist at the Lucerne Kantonspital. His interests covered a wide field and his writings included papers on venereal diseases, industrial hygiene, tuberculosis and tumors of the skin. All of his contributions were characterized by sound practical thinking. Active to the end, he died on January 27, 1952.*

CHONDRODERMATITIS NODULARIS CHRONICA HELICIS

Knoetchenfoermige Erkrankung am Helix[†]

Since beginning practice in Lucerne in the year 1905 I have had the opportunity to observe an affection of the outer ear which until now has failed to attract the attention of dermatologists, and, apparently, otologists. The disease, however, appears to be of sufficient practical importance to merit discussion. I have seen eight cases so far. Twice the patients consulted me only because of the disease of the ears; in the other six the affection was an incidental finding.

We are dealing then with an affection of the outer ear which clinically is manifested by pea to cherry sized tubercles which are usually covered by a central crust. The tubercle is as a rule quite firm in consistency; the borders are a little raised and are the color of the surrounding skin or somewhat whitish and translucent so that in the first case a probable diagnosis of epithelioma was made. The crusts are sometimes quite firmly attached to the underlying structure; at other times they may be relatively easily removed. If one tries to scrape off the crust intense pain results. After removal of the crust one sees a small sharply circumscribed ulceration with a red base and no covering. The borders are of irregular contour and undermined here and there. The tubercle is fixed to the underlying tissue.

From time to time more marked inflammatory changes are found in the papules. The lesion swells, reddens; there is a little pus formation and in a few cases marked bleeding on scraping of the crust. The inflammation subsides spontaneously, by degrees, only to flare up at various intervals. At the time of

---

* Miescher, G.: Der Hautartzt. *3:*287, 1952.

[†]Archiv für dermat. und syph., *121:*278, 1916.

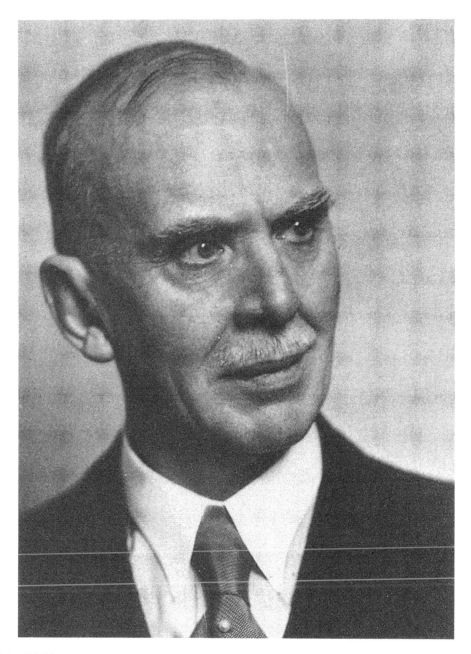

Figure 89 Max Winkler

intense inflammatory swelling the patients experience pain, especially when they lie on the affected ear, so that they may be disturbed in their sleep. The affection has a chronic course. I have not yet been able to determine whether complete healing occurs spontaneously, but in any case I have observed remissions a year in duration.

The disease is situated on the helix, usually on the margin near the upper pole. Twice the affection was bilateral; it was localized on the left three times, on the right three times. So far the youngest was 28 years old, the oldest 65; it appears, then, preponderately in adult males. There does not appear to be any occupational influence. My patients belonged to different occupational groups. No patient admitted having had chilblains. Also freezing was noted only in one case observed, and this was a questionable one. One of my patients told me that the affection first appeared in the winter and exacerbated in the wintertime; others, on the contrary, asserted with certainty that the disease is of equal intensity summer and winter. For the present the etiology remains obscure.

Jean Darier

1.   Darier's Disease

2.   Pseudo-xanthoma Elasticum

3.   Erythema Annulare Centrifugum

FERDINAND-JEAN DARIER was born in Budapest, in 1856. After preliminary education at the College of Geneva, he moved to Paris where he became an Externe des Hôpitaux in 1878, and an Interne in 1880. Graduated in 1885, he did further work with Ranvier, Malassez, and Fournier, and became chief of service successively at La Rochefoucauld, Pitiée and Broca hospitals. In 1909, he joined the staff of l'Hôpital Saint Louis and headed a service there until his death, June 4, 1938.

Darier was a master of all branches of dermatology, but before everything he was a microscopist. His international fame rested to a large extent upon his skill in this specialty. An assessment of his contributions to dermatology is difficult, so great were they. From his many publications we have presented clinical material from his works on keratosis follicularis, pseudoxanthoma elasticum, and erythema annulare centrifugum. Other important works deal with atrophic lichen planus, hypodermic sarcoid, and the tuberculids. His admirable *Précis de Dermatologie,* translated into English by Pollitzer, and German by Jadassohn, became the breviary of dermatologists the world over.

Darier was ever the progressive, the healthy skeptic, ready to put to the test all new material and discovery. He was among the first to use radiotherapy, chemotherapy, and vaccines. This continued interest in the new made him one of the most notable of teachers, and he attracted a larger number of pupils than any man of his generation. Perhaps the greatest achievement was in infusing into these pupils a genuine enthusiasm for the basic research we so badly need.

Graham-Little said of him: "He was of middle height and of slender figure, which he retained to the end, as well as an undiminished head of hair. He wore a small and well-kept beard. His face was dominated by a noble Roman nose, truly symbolic of his character in its Roman simplicity and thoroughness. He gave one throughout his life the impression of abundant energy, vivacity, and those indefinable personal qualities summed up in the word 'charm.' Like his life-long friend, Pringle, whom he resembled in many respects, he cultivated a certain elegance in his dress, and was a collector of beautiful objects."*

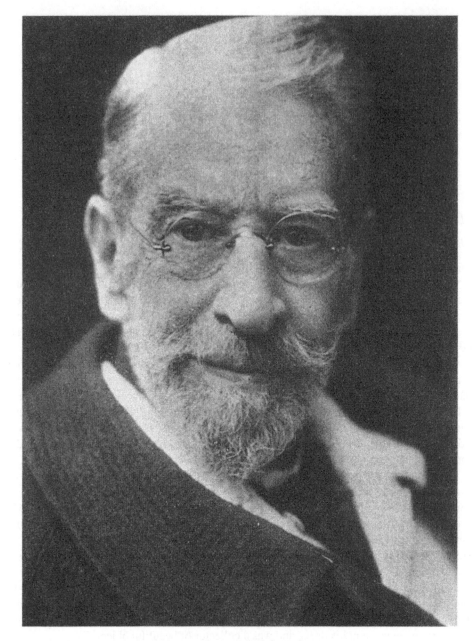

Figure 90 Jean Darier. Courtesy, *Annales de Dermatologie et Syphiligraphie*

DARIER'S DISEASE

De la Psorospermose Folliculaire Végétante[†]

The disease the anatomo-pathologic description of which I will take up under this title appears to be quite rare. I have observed only two examples of it at l'Hôpital Saint Louis on the service of M.M.Fournier and E.Besnier; but the lesions which the two patients presented formed such a characteristic clinical picture, and the results of the histological examination in the two cases were so absolutely concordant and so special that I believe the present facts suffice to secure for the disease a separate place in the framework of cutaneous nosography.

The lesions of follicular psorospermosis extend over most of the surface of the integument, but there are points of predilection where they attain their maximum development or at least confluence; these are the scalp, the face, the presternal region, the flanks, and especially the inguinal regions.

In its first stage the elementary lesion is a small papule surmounted by a blackish or greyish brown crust. This thin projecting crust is hard and dry to touch; if one tries to pick it off one finds that it is extremely adherent to the integument; after one has succeeded in removing it one sees that it is actually a little horn encased in an infundibuliform depression with a conical or cylindrical extremity, dirty white in color, semi-soft in consistency, and a little greasy to the touch.

The depression in the skin which receives this extremity is a small funnel, a little raised at the edges, papular; it corresponds evidently to the dilated orifice of a pilosebaceous follicle. Indeed, sometimes a hair is found after removal of the crust. In the confluent areas there is a dull or brownish colored layer on the skin, more or less greasy to the touch; a series of very serrated and irregular projections is found there, and to the hand it feels very rough. After removal of this layer by scraping one finds an uneven or rugose skin riddled with the little funnel orifices; the epidermis is intact, and there is no oozing of blood.

Such were the lesions of the patient of *Observation I* in Mr. Thibault's thesis, who had been afflicted for three years. In the case of the man of *Observation II,* and in the case of the patient of M.Lutz in whom the affection had been present seven and eight years, were found, in addition, hypertrophic elements which were much more developed. They consist of reddish projections the size of a lentil, a pea, or even larger; the summit presents a depression, a crateriform opening circumscribed by an annular border, thick and shiny. At certain points this border has lost its epidermis and appears ulcerated; pressure on the mass causes sebaceous matter, pure or mixed with pus, to issue from the orifices. These elements, grouping and becoming confluent, form very bulky masses, veritable tumors.

They are encountered in the principal areas of confluence which we have indicated. It is in the hypogastric region, the folds of the groin, and the anal region that the tumors of which we have spoken are found.

PSEUDO-XANTHOMA ELASTICUM

Pseudo-xanthoma elasticum*

I wish to say at the outset that I believe that this supposed elastic xanthoma is a disease apart, very rare it is true, but well characterized. It is of certain interest:

1. Because of the confusion that has arisen between it and xanthoma.
2. In that it is a special morbid entity, as I will attempt to show.

---

* Graham-Little, E.: Brit. J.Dermat., *50:*384, 1938.

† Ann. de dermat. et syph., *10:*597, 1889.

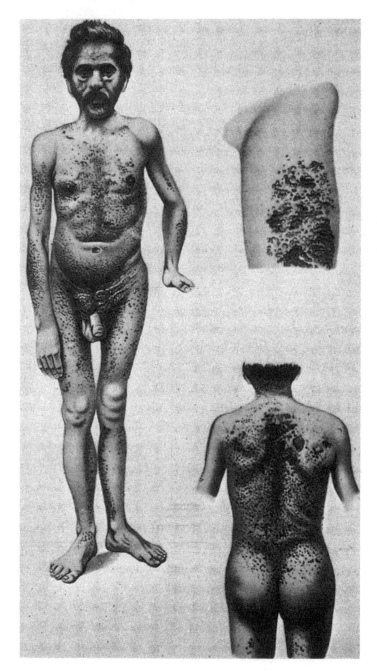

Figure 91 Keratosis follicularis (one of Darier's original cases). Courtesy, College of Physicians, Philadelphia

The first author who stressed alterations of the elastic tissue in xanthoma is my colleague and friend, Balzer.

Indeed, he observed an extremely remarkable case of which he made a careful study; he has allowed me to represent the principal features of it.

A man 49 years of age, having had intermittent fevers, and being affected with third degree phthisis, had had abundant plaques of xanthelasma since early childhood. They were flat, pale yellow, located on the neck, in the axillae, the elbow creases, the folds of the groin, the abdomen in the region of the umbilicus as well as the popliteal fossae, in a word they occupied the flexor folds and were almost absent in other regions.

At autopsy were found, besides pulmonary tuberculosis and a fatty liver, yellowish white spots in several places on the endocardium.

A second observation exists which alone, to my knowledge, merits comparison to the preceding case; Chauffard presented it to the Société Medicale des Hôpitaux. It is a case that one might call *historic* because M.M. Besnier and Doyen honored it by reproducing it *in extenso,* and because of the discussion which it has occasioned. I am personally much obliged to Chauffard for having called me to see his patient and to study the lesions histologically; in this first examination I found alterations in the elastic tissue identical to those Balzer indicated.

Recently I had the good fortune to come across this patient again, and to be able to arrange for his admission to the service of my excellent teacher, M.Besnier. This made it possible to have made the colored moulage by Baretta and the photographs of Méheux which I present to you; I have also studied the cutaneous lesions anew, and in addition have now completed and rectified my first conclusions in part.

I will be brief in the clinical history of the patient; thanks to Besnier all the dermatologists have the text of it in hand.

This man, at present age 42, without notable family history, had typhoid fever at age 23, an alcoholic gastritis with repeated hematemesis and jaundice, as well as marsh fever. Moreover, he shows in both pulmonary apices signs of an induration which is probably tuberculous. His blood is normal; his urine has never shown sugar.

At the age of 26 he noticed the appearance, in the flexor creases of the elbows, of livid spots which were a little pruritic and which quickly took on a yellow color which they have since kept. The other diseased regions were affected shortly after, and since then the affection has progressed continually. At present it occupies symmetrically the flexor folds of the trunk, and the large joints of the extremities; that is, it is located on the neck and clavicular regions, the axillae, the creases at the elbow, the abdominal region, at least in its sub-umbilical portion, the inguinal femoral regions, the inferior surface of the penis, the intergluteal cleft and the popliteal fossae. It consists of large spots or plaques, xanthomatous in appearance, scarcely raised, of a uniform yellowish or light café au lait color. The one on the left elbow measures 5 cm. in width by 10 cm. in length. If one examines these plaques closely one sees that they are formed by the confluence of small creamy white miliary or lenticular spots standing out from a reticulated background of a violaceous or lilac shade. The skin in this area is smooth to the touch, a little doughy in consistency, like wet velvet; it is, moreover, manifestly loose and less elastic than normal. At the periphery of the plaques the lesion breaks up into small yellowish papules surrounded by an areola and centered by a brown pigmented follicular orifice; these papules, very similar to those of certain "diabetic xanthomata," become smaller and smaller in proportion to their distance from the plaque.

The back, the sternal region, the extensor surfaces of the extremities, the hands and feet are unaffected. The same could be said of the head, except for a small miliary yellowish spot on the palpebral commissure

---

* Trans. Internat. Cong. of Dermat., London, 1896, p. 289.

of one eye, and another on the edge of the upper lip; the mucosa of both lips and that of the inner surface of the cheeks is marked by spots of an opaque white, confluent in certain areas, on a richly vascular background.

Conclusions. There exists a disease of the skin, probably very rare, having clear cut and well defined clinical and anatomical characteristics, a disease which one may call *Pseudoxanthoma elasticum*.

Clinically this disease consists of yellowish spots, plaques, or papules which resemble those of xanthoma greatly. They are distinguished by their almost exclusive localization on the flexor folds of the large joints of the extremities and trunk, also by laxity and loss of elasticity of the skin in the affected regions.

Anatomically it is characterized by fragmentation, with swelling and finally complete disaggregation of the elastic network, a lesion which merits the name *elastorrhexis*. The specific alterations of xanthoma (xanthoma cells, fatty granulations) are lacking in this disease.

Until now there has been no precise data on the pathogeny and the nature of pseudoxanthoma elasticum; it appears in childhood or in adulthood in subjects prone to multiple intoxications and persists indefinitely. It seems logical to group it with the cutaneous atrophies, with atrophia cutis maculosa (Jadassohn), for example.

This pseudo-xanthoma merits, in any case, a separate place in that it furnishes a remarkable example of a predominating and apparently primary alteration in the elastic tissue.

ERYTHEMA ANNULARE CENTRIFUGUM

De l'Érythème Annulaire Centrifuge*

An eruption characterized by large annular lesions, and festooned or arciform infiltrations, reddish, elevated, and firm to touch; which cover large areas of the body; which advance eccentrically, and which change in location quite rapidly so that at the end of eight or 10 days the pattern formed by them may be completely transformed; which after a certain time break up, and are replaced by new elements of the same type, a procedure which may occur over many consecutive months. Here, certainly, we have a surprising clinical picture, and one which forcibly draws the attention.

I had the opportunity, nearly 20 years ago, to observe a case of this type. It seemed to me that I was dealing with a form of erythema; from all the evidence it did not seem simply to be that eruptive modality, polymorphous erythema, mentioned in all dermatologic treatises under the name erythema annulare.

L..., age 26, an artist, came to me on May 15, 1898, to find out whether or not he had syphilis, as he had been told by several other physicians whom he had consulted.

I found on examining him an eruption of circular and annular lesions, abundant on the lumbar regions, on the buttocks, and on the posterior surface of the thighs, a few on the lateral aspects of the back, on the anterior surface of the thighs, and on the forearms, and which were nearly symmetrically distributed.

Having questioned the patient on several subsequent visits over a period of two or three months, I have been able to assure myself that this topography has been constant; the head and neck, the upper part of the chest, the axillary folds, the groin and genitalia, as well as the feet and the hands have always been unaffected, as have the mucous surfaces. Exceptionally some elements have appeared on the arms in the vicinity of the elbows, on the left wrist, on the abdomen, and on the upper part of the legs.

---

* Ann. de dermat. et syph., *6:*57, 1916.

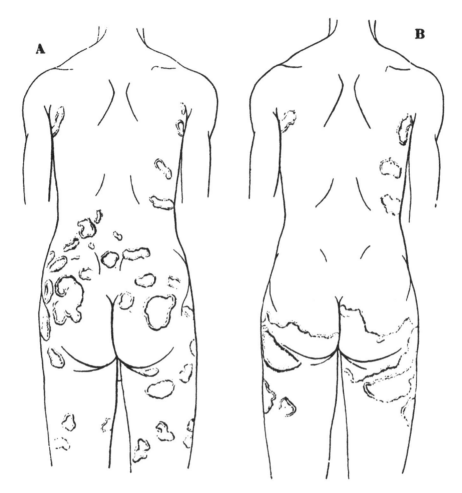

Figure 92 Erythema annulare centrifugum. A and B portray evolution of lesions in 10 day period. From Darier's paper. Courtesy, *Annales de Dermatologie et Syphiligraphie*

At any given time one finds, simultaneously, elements of different ages, and successive examinations have made it possible for me to follow their evolution.

They appear in the form of a pinkish papule, a half to one centimeter in diameter, flat, or sometimes depressed in the center from the beginning, and marginated. On digital palpation one perceives an induration of the whole which is quite often already *en bourrelet*. Soon the border extends eccentrically in the form of a ring 4 to 6 mm. wide and 2 to 3 mm. in height, conveying to the touch the sensation of a hard cord; at the same time the central area becomes depressed to the level of the neighboring integument, and regains its normal appearance, except for a light pigmented or violaceous color which persists for several weeks. The eccentric extension of the initial papule is so rapid that in a week the resulting ring reaches the dimensions of a franc piece, or even of a silver 5 franc piece. Subsequent involution varies with the lesions. Some, having reached 3 to 5 cm. in diameter, and a round or oval form, progress no further; they persist eight to 15 days, then disappear, leaving a pigmented macule. Others, meeting in their extension a neighboring element, join with it *par interference,* that is, by effacement of the separating wall with formation of festooned bands enclosing polylobate areas. Some rings, finally, often more or less festooned, extend until they encircle areas of skin as large as the palm of the hand, or of the entire hand, taking in the whole of some large region. The rings which are several centimeters in diameter are sometimes open at a point in their circumference, through disappearance of the infiltration, producing "C" forms or forms *en cross;* the largest break up into numerous arcs which continue eccentric progression on their own. The evolution of these last elements takes several months.

Gustav Riehl

1.   Tuberculosis Venrucosa Cutis

2.   Riehl's Melanosis

GUSTAV RIEHL was born in Vienna on February 10, 1855. He studied in Vienna, and received his doctorate in medicine in 1879. A student and assistant of Kaposi for several years, he became Professor of Dermatology in Leipzig in 1896. In 1902 he returned to Vienna as Kaposi's successor.

His contributions to the literature were numerous, covering a wide range of topics. The tremendous span of his literary life is indicated by the wide separation of the two selections we have chosen. One of his fields of especial interest was the radiation therapy of skin diseases. He maintained a lifelong interest in tuberculosis of the skin, and also wrote much on this. Riehl was a distinguished gentleman in dress and manner. He was agreeable, pleasant, and an excellent lecturer.

Following a statutory age retirement in 1926, he assumed the role of international consultant for 17 years, and after seeing three generations of dermatology, he died at the age of 88 on January 7, 1943.

TUBERCULOSIS VERRUCOSA CUTIS

Tuberculosis Verrucosa Cutis*

One of us (Riehl) during his assistantship had the opportunity to see, in the ambulatorium of this dermatologic clinic (Prof. Kaposi), a series of cases of a skin disease which differs essentially from the dermatoses thus far known and described, both in its symptoms and its course, and which offers, moreover, interesting characteristics in its histologic and etiologic aspects.

To begin with we wish to present in brief, in the following, a picture of the symptoms and the course of this affection based on these observations.

In persons of both sexes, although more often in the male, one sees plaques which occur sometimes on the dorsal surfaces of one or both hands, occasionally on the extensor surfaces of the fingers or on the interdigital folds, rarely on the vola manus or on the adjacent parts of the forearm, which would at first glance be taken for Lupus verrucosus, or which might strike one as an inflamed irritated group of warts.

When completely developed, these pea to thaler sized plaques show, for the most part, a roundish, sometimes almost circular or more oval outline, or present serpiginous forms when a number of them

---

* Riehl, G. and Paltauf, R.: Vierteljahrschr. für Dermat. und Syph., *13:*19, 1886.

become confluent, as frequently happens. Enlargement of the plaques always takes place through the appearance of new primary manifestations on the convex border of the original diseased part of the skin, so that in progressive lesions the most recent morphologic manifestations are regularly to be found at the border, while in the central parts of the plaques are seen the manifestations of the acme and involution. One has almost no opportunity to observe the first appearance of the illness on previously normal skin, and we are forced to determine the appearance of the initial stage of the process from the new lesions at the peripheral parts of the older plaques.

The outermost border of an advancing area forms an erythematous band in various stages of development, usually only a few millimeters wide, in the form of a circle partially surrounding the plaque. It has a bright red color which disappears completely on digital pressure. The level of this outermost border is scarcely elevated above the neighboring normal skin; it is, however, raised above the central zone. Its surface is flat and sometimes more shiny than the normal epidermis. Glandular orifices and hair follicles are clearly recognizable in the area.

In the enclosed zone one notices frequently a series of small millet seed, or at the most hempseed sized pustules with a thin covering which are consequently easily broken, seated very superficially and irregularly scattered, or one sees numerous little roundish crusts and scales, their residue, covering the surface.

The colors of this zone are brownish or livid red differentiating it clearly from the bright red of the outermost margin. On pressure these places also blanch out, leaving behind, however, a light yellowish tinge from which the presence of an infiltrate can be recognized, which sometimes can be perceived also by the palpating finger.

The nearer the center the more important the changes. The next zone is rather considerably raised above the general level (2 to 5 mm.), and has an irregular uneven surface which toward the center is formed into warty excrescences with roundish, clubbed, or more pointed ends. These papillomas, which become gradually larger toward the center and form scarcely any elevation at the periphery, are chiefly responsible for the prominence of the plaques and show marked variations in size in some cases, in one and the same plaque. Some reach a height of 5 to 7 mm. The surface of this zone is usually covered with crusts which contain much cornified epidermis in lamellar form; after removal of the crusts the brown red color becomes very prominent.

Between the papillomas, which are frequently crowded thickly together and have on their tips a thick horny layer, rhagades and small erosions or pustules are found. On pressing from the sides one may produce small drops of pus from numerous points between the warty excrescences so that sometimes one gets an impression of pus passing through the openings of a sprinkler or sieve.

Only rarely does one see acute swelling and redness appear in the large part or the whole of the plaques; in such cases the characteristics of this extremely chronic affection give way to the manifestations of acute inflammation for a while, but return, however, as soon as the inflammation subsides.

The papillomas may occupy the whole central part and cover over larger surfaces of 1 to 1½ cms.

The glandular orifices and hair follicles are not recognizable in this stage, although one may find here and there a lanugo hair which is easily pulled out.

With this picture the process reaches its maximum, and the further stages belong to the involution metamorphosis.

Thus, the papillomas on the older plaques flatten toward the center, become less crusted, and lose their rather thick horny layer; the small abscesses between them disappear. In still older plaques the central part is usually flat, with no papillomas, shows a smooth or mildly scaly epidermis, and has an atrophic appearance.

The cicatrix is located only in the upper layers of the cutis, especially in the papillary layer; it is thin and flexible.

In the way of subjective symptoms may be mentioned only a sensitivity to pressure at the height of the process, which may sometimes reach the point of severe pain to light touch.

The patients are usually robust healthy appearing people in the active period of life (19 to 45 years).

Progress is very slow and interrupted by many periods of inactivity, and in the larger plaques occurs almost always only in the fraction of the periphery where the irregular serpiginous contours are seen.

RIEHL'S MELANOSIS

Ueber eine eigenartige Melanose*

In the months of February, March, and April of this year we have seen a number of patients—men, women and children—with a most striking skin alteration, the chief symptom of which is a dark coloration of the skin of the face.

The first impression made by these patients brings to mind the marked browning usually seen in sportsmen who have been exposed to intense sunshine for a long time. Our patients were, however, in no position to acquire a solar dermatitis from a stay in the open air, nor had they any opportunity to do so in these continually cloudy months. A careful consideration of the histories, moreover, makes it possible to rule out light in the form of sunlight, ultraviolet rays, etc. as a direct cause of the disease.

We have found the following changes in our patients—with some variations, namely in intensity: The skin appears deeply browned, the shade varying from weather-beaten bronze to chocolate, and in some places it has a gray lustre. The discoloration extends over the entire face, and is most pronounced on the forehead, and in the zygomatic and temporal regions; in most cases the lateral parts of the face are more affected than the medial, that is, the nose. The same discoloration extends over the ears, neck, and nape of the neck, and for varying distances onto the scalp. The surface of the discolored skin looks dusty or slightly scaly, and over the forehead, cheeks, and ears, shows dilated follicular orifices which appear plugged with horny scales. The diseased skin is quite markedly thickened, somewhat doughy to the feel, its surface faintly roughened. No sign of atrophy nor exudation; almost no hyperaemia. The borders of the affection toward the thorax show a gradual transition of the browness into normal skin; they are nowhere sharp. The diffuse discoloration of the head and neck then breaks up at the margins into discrete lesions in the form of millet seed, almost to hempseed sized spots or slightly raised papules which are usually situated around the follicles. In the outermost zone, toward the normal skin, these efflorescences remain discrete, surrounded by normal skin, and toward the diffusely diseased area they crowd more and more together, finally becoming confluent. From newly erupted isolated efflorescences we may observe that in the beginning they are reddish brown and only later become dark brown.

In some patients we have found, in addition to the localizations mentioned, other parts of the skin affected in a similar fashion, but to a lesser extent—the hands and forearms, specifically the extensor surfaces, the axillary folds, the skin beneath the breasts, the area around the navel, and, in one case, the inguinal region. All these regions appear less deeply brown than the skin of the face, and show the spots and papules.

---

* Wiener Klin. Wchnschr., *30:*780, 1917.

Thus the parts of the skin exposed to light are not at all exclusively involved, although they are, as in other diseases leading to pigmentation, the parts chiefly and most intensively affected.

In no stage does the affection itch; it does not lead to scratching, and produces no pathological sensory changes.

F.Parkes-Weber

Relapsing Non-suppurative Nodular Panniculitis

FREDERICK PARKES-WEBER was born on the 8th of May, 1863, in London. His medical education was obtained at Cambridge, with postgraduate studies in Vienna and Paris. He was physician to the German Hospital in London from 1894. His bibliography of approximately 1000 papers, books, and notes was the fruit of over 60 years of continuous productive work at bedside, laboratory and library. Dermatology was well represented in his labors. His name is attached to a sizeable group of syndromes, including Rendu-Osler-Weber's disease (Hereditary hemorrhagic telangiectasia), the Weber-Klippel syndrome (Hemangiectatic hypertrophy of limbs), Sturge-Weber-Kalischer's disease (Haemangiectatic nevoid conditions of face and meninges), the Weber-Cockayne syndrome (Epidermolysis bullosa of feet), and Weber-Christian's disease (Relapsing febrile nodular non-suppurative panniculitis), his account of which is given below. In addition, Parkes-Weber, with Hellenschmied, first described telangiectasia macularis eruptiva perstans, relating it to urticaria pigmentosa. His later contributions included two volumes entitled *Rare Diseases,* and *Further Rare Diseases*. He continued to work with untiring enthusiasm and at an unslackened pace until he died peacefully on June 2, 1962, aged 99.*

RELAPSING NON-SUPPURATIVE NODULAR PANNICULITIS

A Case of Relapsing Non-suppurative Nodular Panniculitis Showing Phagocytosis of Subcutaneous Fat-cells by Macrophages*

The patient, Mrs. M.R...., aged 50 years, a Russian Hebrew widow, thin rather than fat, was admitted to the German Hospital on January 23rd, 1924, with the history that for the last five weeks she had been laid up with rheumatic pains all over her body, and headache, and that during the same period she had had red patches at the lower part of the back of both legs above the ankles, which on admission felt indurated. She had been subject to constipation and dyspepsia for years. Lately there had been some vomiting. In the hospital there was slight pyrexia at first, up to 101.6°F. and the urine contained a trace of albumin. The chronic inflammatory swelling was at the back of the legs just above the ankles, chiefly in the right limb, and tended slowly to disappear. For rheumatic pains, especially pains and stiffness at the back of the neck, she was treated with small doses of sodium salicylate and sodium bicarbonate and with hot-air baths, and with hot-

---

* Obit.: Arch. Dermatol., 1962.

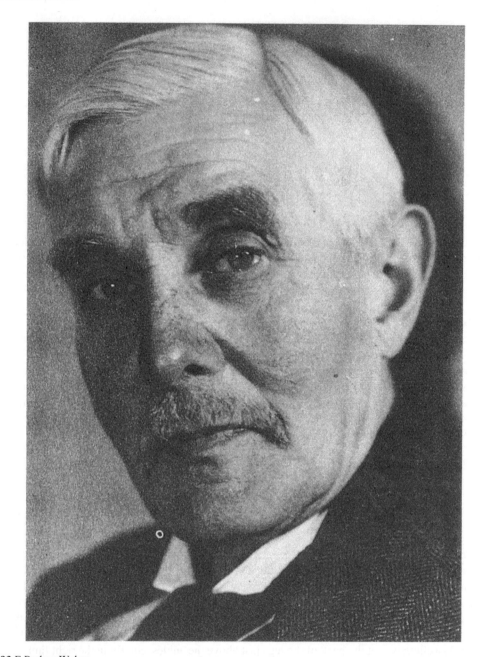

Figure 93 F.Parkes-Weber

air douches for the neck. Small doses of a digitalis preparation were also given. After January 27th, her temperature did not exceed 99°F., except for slight fever in February, which was probably connected with inflammation of sweat glands in the right axilla. Her urine became free from albumin, and the erythematous patches above the ankles nearly disappeared. There was slight gastroptosis, but otherwise nothing special was found by x-ray examination of the stomach, nor by examination of the gastric contents. Brachial systolic blood pressure (January, 1924) 115 mm. Hg. The fundi of the eye were normal. The patient had been operated for cataract in the right eye four years previously. A Roentgen skiagram of the thorax suggested slight hilus tuberculosis. Pirquet's cuti-reaction for tuberculosis was slightly positive, as it is in most adults. It was not thought necessary to take the Wassermann reaction. The patient had had two children —both of whom were living and healthy—and one miscarriage. She left the hospital on February 27th, 1924.

After leaving the hospital she was able to get about in her home, but could do no work, she said. About April 1st, 1924, she began to complain of painful swellings and "inflammation" in both legs, in the right more than in the left. On April 3rd, the legs were said to be very much swollen, and she had to keep to bed. Afterwards she suffered from pains in her upper extremities likewise, and became somewhat dazed or somnolent. On readmission to hospital on April 15th, 1924, she was found to have tender phlegmon-like swellings (involving the subcutaneous tissue and skin) at the back of both lower limbs below the knees, and one or two swellings on the left thigh and buttock. There were likewise reddish tender nodules in both upper extremities—the left more than the right—especially near the elbows; these swellings, which involved the subcutaneous tissue and the cutis, had, I understood, appeared only quite recently. I thought that a bromide-containing mixture which she had been taking might possibly have favoured the development of these nodular swellings.

She soon commenced to improve in every way. The swellings diminished, but without bruise-like coloration of the skin as there would have been in a typical case of erythema nodosum. Some of the swellings on subsiding left hard pea-sized nodules behind them, and two or three such nodules might be left by a single swelling.

After leaving the hospital the patient remained in satisfactory condition till the end of September, 1924, when she commenced to feel ailing and suffered from a subcutaneous swelling over the sacrum. She was readmitted on October 29th, complaining of pain in the shoulders, back of neck, thorax and sacral region. Over the middle of the last mentioned region (slightly more to the left than the right) there was a large circular reddish area of subcutaneous swelling, of about the diameter of a large orange, somewhat tender to palpation. No swellings were found elsewhere in the skin or subcutaneous tissue. She said she felt miserable; the tongue was irregularly coated, and there was slight fever.

She left the hospital on December 8th, 1924, and on May 15th, 1925, I heard that she had had no relapse of the subcutaneous swellings, and that she was doing well.

---

* Brit. J.Dermat., *37:*301, 1925.

Aldo Castellani

Dermatosis Papulosa Nigra

SIR ALDO CASTELLANI was born in Florence, Italy, on September 8, 1876. He was educated at the universities of Florence and Bonn, receiving his M.D. in 1899. He spent some time in the London School of Tropical Medicine, and in 1902 was sent by the British Royal Society to Uganda to study sleeping sickness. He discovered the cause of this disease, a trypanosome which he demonstrated in the cerebrospinal fluid. In 1903 he became Professor of Tropical Medicine and lecturer in Dermatology in Ceylon Medical School, where he remained until 1915. During this period he made basic observations on yaws, lepothrix, copra itch, and pulmonary mycoses. In 1915 he became Professor of Tropical Medicine in Naples, with subsequent service with the Italian Navy during the first World War. After a second period at the London School of Tropical Medicine, as Director of Mycology, he served from 1924 to 1930 as Professor of Tropical Medicine at Tulane University, in New Orleans. During this period he wrote the selection we have chosen. In 1931 he founded the Tropical Institute in Rome, and until 1944 he held the post of Professor of Tropical Medicine at University of Rome. He was Surgeon General to the Italian Forces in Ethiopia in 1935–36. He has been physician to King George of Greece and was medical adviser to the Italian High Command in World War II.

Castellani published over 400 articles in medical journals. Among the books he published were *Manual of Tropical Medicine* (1910), *Fungi and Fungous Diseases* (1918), and *Climate and Acclimatization* (1930). For many dermatologists his name is most readily associated with the carbol fuchsin paint he recommended years ago.

No one should fail to read his fascinating autobiography, "A Doctor in Many Lands" (Doubleday, 1960).

At the time of his death in 1971, Sir Aldo Castellani was Professor of Tropical Medicine in Lisbon, Portugal.*

DERMATOSIS PAPULOSA NIGRA

Observations on Some Diseases of Central America[†]

In Jamaica and Central America I have come across a peculiar dermatosis which does not seem to have been described previously. It is particularly common in natives of Jamaica. In a well-marked case a large number of black or very dark-brownish papules, somewhat cupoliform or flattened, are seen on the face, principally on both malar regions, while they are rare or absent on the lower parts of the face and chin: a few may be present on the forehead. They are not pruriginous and not painful. The maximum diameter of each papule varies between 1 mm. and 4 or 5 mm. At times two or three papules are very close together and seem to coalesce. The first papules appear in youth. I have seen them present in small numbers in boys and girls of 16 to 18 years of age. The condition gradually becomes more marked, and the papules increase in number and size the older the patient becomes, and it is quite common to see middle-aged men and women with their faces studded with these black papules.

---

* The International Who's Who, 15th Edition. London, 1951.

† J.Trop. Med. and Hyg., *28*:9, 1925.

Henri Gougerot and Paul Blum

Pigmented Purpuric Lichenoid Dermatitis

HENRI GOUGEROT was born on July 2, 1881, in Saint-Ouen-sur-Seine. He received his medical training in Paris. From 1910 to 1914 he served first as chief physician, and then as Assistant Professor on the Faculty of Medicine in Paris. After four years with the French army during World War I, he returned to this post. In 1928 he was named Professor of Clinical Dermatology and Syphilology, and Chief of Service at l'Hôpital Saint Louis. During the second world war he served with the French army.

He was President of the French Society of Dermatology and Syphilology, 1933–34. He was an honorary member of 22 dermatologic societies throughout the world, and in 1935 was Honorary President of the Ninth International Congress of Dermatology held in Budapest.

His writings covered the entire field of dermatology and syphilology. In 1936 he co-edited the famed encyclopedic *Nouvelle Pratique Dermatologique*. He wrote extensively on sporotrichosis, sarcoidosis, tuberculosis of the skin, and cutaneous papillomatosis. A second eponymic achievement is the Gougerot-Carteaud syndrome. He died in 1955.

PAUL BLUM was born in Paris on the 19th of August, 1887. After attending medical school in Paris he studied at the Pasteur Institute and later received clinical training under Gilbert. He became an assistant of Gougerot at l'Hôpital Saint Louis in 1928, and held the title of Physician-in-chief at l'Hôpital Saint Lazare and l'Hôpital de Saint-Denis. His writings range over the entire field of dermatology and syphilology.*

PIGMENTED PURPURIC LICHENOID DERMATITIS

Purpura angiascléreux prurigine ux avec éléments lichenoïdes*

This patient shows lesions on both legs which are symmetrical, and which at first give the impression of an ordinary angiosclerous purpura with red purpuric spots on pigmented plaques, but two points in particular caught our attention on closer examination.

The first is the existence of pruritus localized quite exactly to the area of the dermatosis.

The second is the existence of small, red, purpuric, papular, shiny, lichenoid elements scattered over the pigmented background left from former attacks of purpura, and often localized at the periphery of confluent plaques of purpura.

---

* Wallach, D., Tilles, G.: Dermatology in France. Pierre Fabre, 434

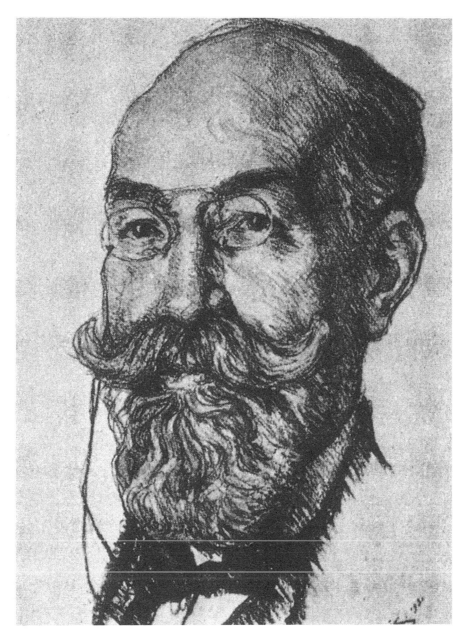

Figure 94 Henri Gougerot. Courtesy, Louis Nékam

The lichenoid purpuric elements are the size of a pin head (around 1 mm.); they are polygonal or rounded, slightly elevated, flat, bright red, shiny, and remain purpuric on vitropression. The impression of lichen is so great that the lesions on the ankle, entirely lichenoid, would lead one to believe this was an atypical lichen planus.

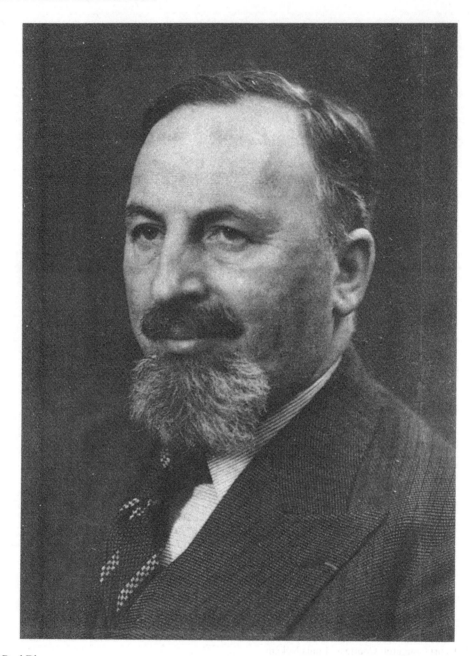

Figure 95 Paul Blum

C..., Carlo, 41 years of age, gas stoker, came to the evening dermatosyphilographic clinic at l'Hôpital Saint Antoine, on March 20, 1925, because of symmetrical lesions on the lower extremities, and angiosclerous purpura of Gaucher and Lacapère, and varicosities of the legs. They have been present for 15 months and are very pruritic. The pruritus appeared early and has been intense. Two pigmented areas are evident immediately, on the medial surface of the middle and lower parts of both legs. These areas are formed from confluent plaques, the islets varying in dimension.

In the center these plaques are pigmented an ochre color, and show an occasional recurrent purpuric papule.

At the periphery of the ochreous plaques there are scattered papules which are small, polygonal, very pruritic, and as large as the head of a pin. On the upper part of the leg the purpuric stippling is clearer. It is also observed to have a linear distribution along the varicose swellings. In addition, several large pale violaceous ecchymoses are noted on the posterior surface of the calves.

On very close inspection, the presence of lichenoid elements can be demonstrated: Small polygonal papules, flat, shiny, slightly elevated, soft to the touch, and remaining purpuric to vitropression. Some, frankly red, are recent; others which are older become pigmented, and somewhat later the purpura disappears, leaving a stippled pigmentation, usually confluent.

In the ankle region, especially over the right internal malleolus, the punctiform elements forming a semicircle have a lichenoid appearance which brings lichen planus to mind.

There are no lichen lesions on the rest of the body, nothing on the mucous membranes; no papules nor pigmented areas on the body.

No purpura is found anywhere but on the legs; we are dealing with a local purpura.

Bleeding time (1½ minutes), and coagulation are normal (2–5 min.). Tourniquet test and cupping glass produce no purpura.

Arterial tension is 16–9 on the Pachon oscillometer.

No visceral lesion found.

Syphilis is not able to be demonstrated, but the patient's wife has had two miscarriages; the Bordet-Wassermann reaction is completely negative, also the Desmoulières.

What is the explanation for these lichenoid and purpuric elements?

Should we suspect an *atypical purpuric lichen planus?* We do not believe so: the lesions are limited exclusively to the lower extremities; there is no trace of lichen planus at any point on the integument or mucous membranes; moreover, there is no pruritus, and the diagnosis of an atypical lichen planus so atypical, and also abnormal in its exclusive localization, would be but a hypothesis.

Can we implicate an eczema, or a pruritus in which lichenified elements have become purpuric under the influence of scratching, thanks to the special varicose terrain with its fragile capillaries? Neither the vesicles of eczema nor the papules of prurigo are present.

A third pathogenesis appears much more tempting: the sanguineous extravasations from capillary rupture (and consequently purpura in the dermatologic sense of the word) give rise to a cellular infiltration which produces the small papules.

The name prurigenous lichenoid purpura appears, then, to be applicable to this new form of angiosclerous purpura.

---

* Bull, de la Soc. Franc. de Dermat. et Syph., *32:*161, 1925.

George Pernet

Symmetric Erythema of the Soles

GEORGE PERNET was born in London in 1862. He received his medical education in Edinburgh, Bonn, and Paris, later returning to London. For many years he was pathologist to the Hospital for Diseases of the Skin, Blackfriars. Later he was assistant at the University College Hospital to Radcliffe Crocker. He also held the post of dermatologist to the West London Hospital. He died January 6, 1940, at the age of 78.*

SYMMETRIC ERYTHEMA OF THE SOLES

Symmetrical Lividities of the Soles of the Feet[†]

In the year 1914, I observed a condition of the soles of the feet to which I gave the above descriptive name, just to pigeon-hole it in my mind. In 1922, I saw an exactly similar looking case. As I do not remember ever having seen such a condition before, and having never met with a description of similar cases in dermatological literature, the details of the two cases maybe of some interest.

Case 1. A girl, aged 13 years, came to my Skin Department at the West London Hospital, July 31, 1914, for morphoea and localized sclerodermia, when the following notes were made: Noticed two or three weeks. On the outer side of right thigh, two sclerosed patches with extensive lilac margin of coarse grained skin. The patient's thyroid could not be felt. I put her on thyroid, 2½ gr. *in die,* and ordered some olive oil to rub into affected areas. She was on this treatment until January 1, 1915, when a note was made that she had improved, the discoloration about left thigh having disappeared. The same treatment was continued.

On April 9, 1915, the patch on the left thigh had become morphoeic and sclerodermic, with distinct lilac discoloration about the border and beyond. For the first time she developed chilblains about ends of fingers. Her circulation was not good. Some of her teeth had decayed badly. Wassermann negative. Later a fresh patch of morphoea appeared about right external malleolus.

We now come to November 12, 1915, when she presented acute symmetrical trouble about the soles of the feet in the shape of bluish-red patches, which had become paler in central parts. The patches were slightly raised and had an oedematous blebby look, but contained no fluid. The borders of these patches were well defined. The symmetrical condition is well brought out in the accompanying photograph.

---

* Unsigned Obit.: Brit. J.Dermat., *52:*95, 1940.

[†] Brit. J.Dermat., *37:*123, 1925.

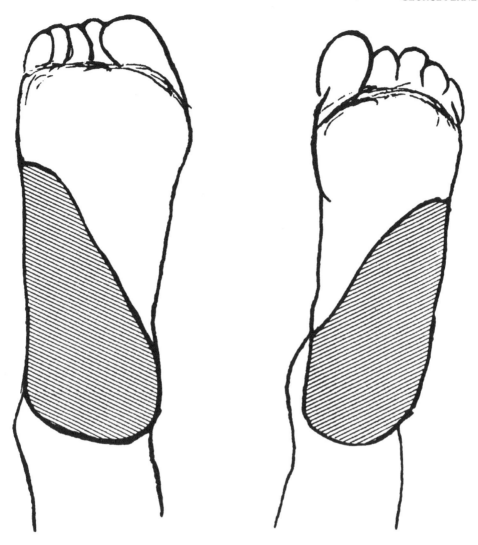

Figure 96 Symmetrical lividities of the soles of the feet. From Pernet's paper. Courtesy, *British Journal of Dermatology*

Hyperidrosis of the rest of the soles was present. I came to the conclusion that the plantar condition was not connected with the morphoeo-sclerodermia, but was a thing apart, probably of chilblainy or hyperidrotic origin. But in any case, I have considered it best to give full details. What struck me most about the plantar condition was the symmetry of the affected areas.

Case 2. In 1922, on October 4, a boy, aged 14 years, turned up in my clinic with the same symmetrical condition of the soles of the feet. Duration, 14 days. Began about plantar area of right heel. Now both soles affected symmetrically. Some hyperidrosis. Pale cyanotic lividities slightly raised above level of skin, and tailing off anteriorly and externally into a somewhat reddened border. The accompanying diagram shows the areas affected. There was nothing else about the boy's skin.

In both cases improvement followed on pulv. sulph. ex lacte internally and lot. calaminae locally.

I have long been interested in symmetrical conditions affecting the skin. In connection with this clinical note, I have again looked up Testut's work *(Leo Testut, De la Symétrie dans les Affections de la Peau, Paris, 1877),* but find nothing like the cases I have just described.

The distribution in my two cases does not fit in with the innervation of the sole of the foot.

Bruno Bloch

Incontinentia Pigmenti

BRUNO BLOCH was born January 19, 1878, in Endingen, Switzerland. At the age of 22 he received his M.D. from the University of Basel. After a period of general medical training under His in Basel, he turned to dermatology and spent four years in the Berlin, Vienna, Paris, and Berne dermatologic clinics. In the latter city he came under the influence of Josef Jadassohn with whom he maintained a life long friendship. Returning to Basel in 1908 he took charge of the University Dermatological Service, and eight years later he took over the newly created Chair of Dermatology in Zurich, which post he held until his death, April 10, 1933.

Like Jadassohn, Bloch was eminently successful in combining intensive laboratory study with fine clinical work. An intimate knowledge of chemistry, physics, and bacteriology fitted him well for the tremendous amount of basic dermatologic research he turned out. His fundamental work in allergy with its direct application to eczema and ringworm, and his revolutionary work on pigment production and the dopa reaction may be mentioned as his most notable successes. From his clinical work we have chosen his short and definitive report of incontinentia pigmenti.

Bloch was also a gifted and inspiring teacher. Despite the great demands his own work made upon him, he found time to take a personal interest in the many students in his clinic, and he had that uncommon faculty of being able to stimulate in them a genuine enthusiasm for close observation and investigation.*

INCONTINENTIA PIGMENTI

Eigentümliche, bisher nicht beschriebene Pigmentaffektion: (Incontinentia pigmenti)†

A two year old girl; the affection has been present since birth and has apparently not changed much since that time (inflammatory manifestations have appeared on the legs from time to time). An enucleation of the right eye was performed a month ago for a retrobulbar glioma *(Professor Vogt)*.

General physical—non-contributory. The pigmentary changes are most pronounced on the lateral parts of the trunk, nearly symmetrical toward the midline anteriorly and posteriorly, forming irregular rings about the mammae, and from the right axilla out to the middle of the forearm, as well as irregular bands from the hips to the ankles. The color of the affection is very distinctive, not a true brown as in pigmented nevi, but rather a dirty brown with a distinct tinge of slate gray, the margins a dirty light yellowish color, especially on the back. The *form* of the pigment spots is most remarkable: They occur in completely irregular splashes

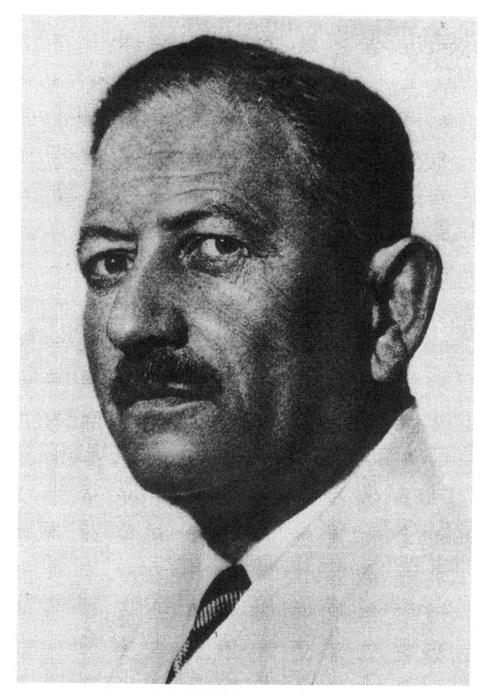

Figure 97 Bruno Bloch. Courtesy, Dr. Guido Miescher

and show figures with spidery projections such as have not heretofore been described in any pigment anomaly. The projecting arms of individual spots join with one another in various ways. The whole picture has something capricious and artificial about it, as if someone had painted completely irregular patterns on the skin.

---

* Unsigned Obit.: Brit. J.Dermat., *45:*269, 1933.

† Schweitz. Med. Wchnschr., *56:*404, 1926.

Francis E.Senear and Barney Usher

Pemphigus Erythematodes

FRANCIS EUGENE SENEAR was born November 5, 1889 in Salamanca, New York. He received his M.D. from the University of Michigan in 1914. After a year as instructor in dermatology at Michigan, he was appointed to the dermatology staff at the University of Illinois. In 1923 he succeeded William Allen Pusey as Professor and head of the department at Illinois, and continued to serve in this capacity for a period of 31 years.

Senear was a member of numerous societies, and was President of the American Dermatological Association, as well as of the American Board of Dermatology and Syphilology.

He wrote widely on clinical dermatology, and we have reproduced the clinical section from his original account of pemphigus erythematodes. When he died in 1958 he was President-elect of the World Congress of Dermatology.*

BARNEY USHER was born on July 1, 1899 in Montreal. He received his M.D. at McGill University. From 1922 to 1924 he did postgraduate dermatologic work at the University of Illinois, under Pusey and Senear. He practiced in Montreal, and was a lecturer in Dermatology at McGill University, as well as being President of the Canadian Dermatological Society. He died in 1978, the victim of a heart attack.*

PEMPHIGUS ERYTHEMATODES

An Unusual Type of Pemphigus Combining Features of Lupus Erythematosus*

A study of the cases shows that the eruption has a predilection particularly for the face, trunk, and scalp. On the face, the nose and adjacent parts of the cheek and the forehead are usually most heavily involved. On the trunk the sternal and interscapular regions are almost invariably the most severely affected, but in several instances the axillae, inguinal folds and inframammary regions were principally involved. The extremities are involved sparsely or not at all.

In some instances the eruption is of the same type on the face and on the trunk, while in others there is a distinct difference in the involvement of the two parts, although transitional stages between the various forms

---

* Blankenship, M.: Chicago Dermatological Society—160 Years of Excellence, 73, 2001

* Crissey, J.J., et *al:* Historical Atlas of Dermatology and Dermatologists. Parthenon Publishing, 132, 2002.

* Arch. of Dermat., and Syph., *13:*761, 1926.

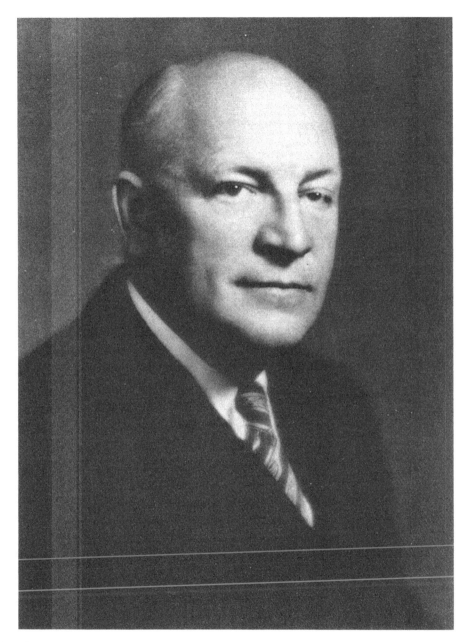

Figure 98 Francis E.Senear

can be traced. On the face the lesions have in some instances appeared as typical lupus erythematosus, in others as typical seborrheic dermatitis. This tendency to evanescence and variability in the eruption on the face has been particularly noticeable in our case.

On the trunk three types of lesions may be found. The primary lesion is unquestionably a bulla, usually of a wrinkled, flaccid appearance, and with a thin roof. These lesions tend to rupture readily, and give rise to

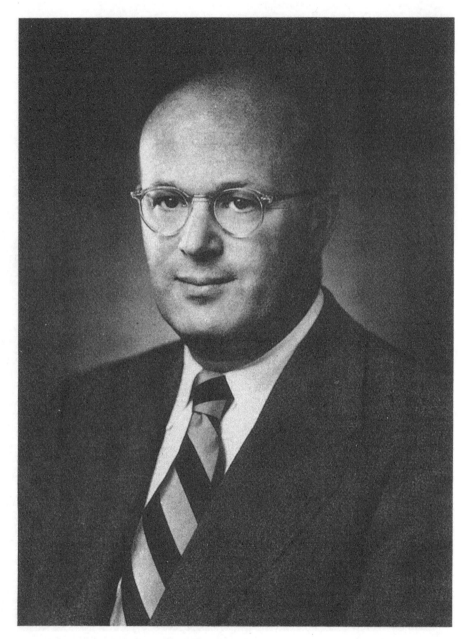

Figure 99 Barney Usher. Portrait by Al.Foreman, Montreal

the other two types. By coalescence or extension of the ruptured bullae, there may result large patches of denuded, raw appearing, sharply defined, oozing dermatitis, often considerably crusted. These lesions tend to disappear spontaneously, and leave reddish or brownish pigmented areas in which fresh bullae may again appear. Here again evanescence and a variability in appearance may be noted. When the ruptured bullae do not enlarge appreciably, they produce what is probably the most characteristic lesion on the trunk, an

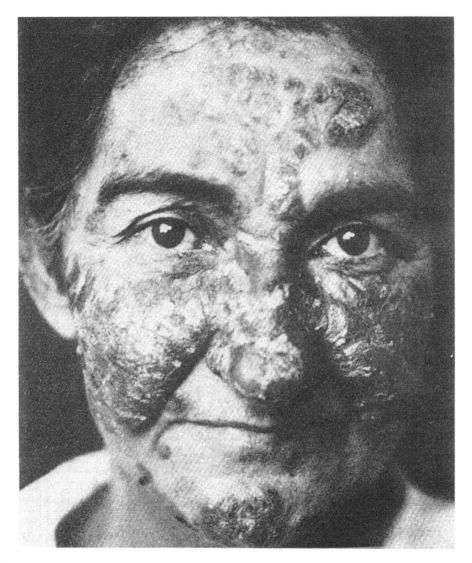

Figure 100 Pemphigus erythematodes. From Senear's paper. Courtesy, *Archives of Dermatology and Syphilology*

inflammatory base covered with a thick crust or scale crust, which is usually of a greasy, seborrheic type, but which may be dry, the lesions then resembling senile keratoses, or they may resemble psoriatic or impetiginous lesions. They may be yellowish, whitish or dirty in appearance. These crusts or scales are usually firmly adherent, and on removal leave a raw bleeding base. The lesions of this type are persistent but tend to involute eventually, leaving brownish stains. These same crusted lesions are seen at times on the face as well as on the trunk, but if present they are usually less numerous and less chronic in course. A patient may show bullae, the large patches, and the crusted keratotic lesions at the same time.

The transitions from the bulla to the crusted lesion are well shown in the histologic sections taken from the different stages.

There is a decided tendency for the bullous lesions to appear in crops, and unless the patient is under close observation for a long period, their occurrence may be discovered only by questioning the patient. The mucous membranes have shown lesions of a bullous type in two cases.

As a rule symptoms have been of little consequence. In seven cases no symptoms have been reported, while in three, mild itching was reported. In our case there was complaint of intense itching, burning and pain, but the patient is excessively neurotic and much of her complaint can be discounted.

As may be surmised from the foregoing description of the eruption, numerous possibilities must be thought of in the differential diagnosis, and this is further borne out by a consideration of the various opinions expressed by a number of dermatologists when the several cases were demonstrated. Among the diagnoses mentioned on these occasions were impetigo vulgaris, dermatitis medicamentosa, epidermolysis bullosa, erythema multiforme, lupus erythematosus disseminatus, seborrheic dermatitis, lupus erythematosus with a pemphigoid eruption on the body, and pemphigus. Study of the course and characteristics of the eruption in this series of cases, however, enables one to exclude from consideration everything but lupus erythematosus disseminatus, pemphigus and lupus erythematosus in combination with pemphigus.

Against the diagnosis of lupus erythematosus disseminatus may be mentioned the distinct tendency in that disorder to involvement of the extremities, which in the condition under consideration are only slightly or not at all affected. In lupus erythematosus disseminatus bullae occur rarely in contradistinction to this disorder, in which they are constantly present. Furthermore, constitutional symptoms are usually present in severe cases of lupus erythematosus, and its course is relatively acute and often fatal. A tendency to atrophy is also commonly seen, while in this disorder it is lacking or but slightly evident. Finally, the mucous membranes are rarely involved, while in our series two of 11 cases showed involvement of the mucosae.

In attempting to establish a diagnosis of pemphigus for this condition, several positive findings may be mentioned. In one case, which was a typical example, the patient's disease followed the usual course of pemphigus, and he died after a little more than a year from the onset of the disease. In no other case did death ensue during the time that the reports cover, but the picture was sufficiently definite in several instances to permit a diagnosis of pemphigus to be accepted by numerous observers, and it is possible that further information regarding these cases would disclose a greater proportion of fatal terminations. Further, the eruption in this condition is primarily of a bullous type, and although the bullae are for the most part flaccid, typical tense bullae have been seen, and these not infrequently arise from a sound skin. Further, confirmation of the alliance of this disease with pemphigus is shown by mention of the presence of Nikolski's sign on three cases, while in the other cases its presence or absence was not noted. The involvement of the mucous membranes cited in two cases should also be mentioned, as should the involvement of the axillae, inframammary and inguinal regions in several instances. While nothing definite could be determined as to a preponderance of patients of Jewish extraction, as is usually found in typical pemphigus, the data are at least suggestive. The race was not stated in four instances, while the remaining seven included two Jewish patients, three Russians, one American born and one Italian. It is probable that some of the unknown or the Russians were of the Jewish race.

It cannot be denied, however, that in several of these cases manifestations occur which are typical of lupus erythematosus and which are not found in the ordinary types of pemphigus. There are, then, two possibilities that must be considered, either that manifestations resembling lupus erythematosus can occur as an atypical feature of pemphigus or that we are dealing here with a syndrome in which pemphigus occurs in combination with lupus erythematosus. Although the former theory cannot be definitely excluded, we believe that the latter conception is the more probable. The opinion is held by a number of observers that a group of toxic eruption exists, including pemphigus, lupus erythematosus, erythema multiforme and other toxic erythema, dermatitis herpetiformis, urticaria, etc., the numbers of which are closely allied from the etiologic standpoint, and they believe that a single toxic agent may produce one of these diseases in one person and another of these conditions in a second person, or that it may produce more than one of these conditions in one person at different times.

If we accept this contention, it is easy to assume that with the syndrome which we are describing may have a common etiologic factor producing at the same time features of both pemphigus and lupus erythematosus. This conception is supported by the fact that in our patient we have been able to observe every gradation between the features of pemphigus on the one hand and of lupus erythematosus on the other.

Erich Urbach

Necrobiosis Lipoidica Diabeticorum

ERICH URBACH was born on June 29, 1893, in Prague. His medical education at the University of Vienna was interrupted by World War I. During the war he served as a lieutenant in the Austrian army, and was twice decorated for valor. Extensive post war training in dermatology and internal medicine led to his appointment as Associate Professor of Dermatology (1929) at the University of Vienna. Here he served as assistant chief under Kerl. In 1938, Urbach came to the United States as a war *emigré*. He was made a member of Stokes's department at the University of Pennsylvania and taught at this institution until his premature death on December 17, 1946.

Two hundred and eleven papers and five books testify to his unflagging energy. Allergy was his forte, and it is in this field that nearly half of his publications lie. He was also greatly interested in clinical dermatology, and from his many publications along this line we have selected his original description of necrobiosis lipoidica diabeticorum.

Stokes has written of Urbach: "He worked himself ruthlessly, contributed cases and disputation, made rounds, taught, wrote and spoke vividly, challenged one's critical faculties and upset one's complacencies and torpors…. His record and achievements speak for themselves and would have graced a much longer life."*

Urbach was another tumours dermatologist who bestowed on our field, a distinguished dermatologic son, Frederick, Professor at Temple University in Philadelphia.

NECROBIOSIS LIPOIDICA DIABETICORUM

Eine neue diabetische Stoffwechseldermatose: Nekrobiosis lipoidica diabeticorum*

Ida St., 44 years old; measles, chicken pox, diphtheria, whooping cough as a child; later frequent sore throats with fever, rheumatic pains. One per cent albumin during pregnancy in 1909. In 1924 the patient noticed an eruption over the entire body which a physician again called measles; about three months later the patient had an attack of fever, headaches, severe diarrhea, and pain in the abdomen, lasting two to three days. Soon after (1925) the patient noted a constant loss of weight, marked thirst, polyuria, lassitude, and increasing nervousness. In 1926 she first consulted a physician who found six per cent sugar. The patient received a high fat, low CHO diet as a result of which the urine sugar fell to three per cent. In 1928 a slowly

---

* Stokes, J.: Arch. of Dermat. and Syph., *55:*545, 1947.

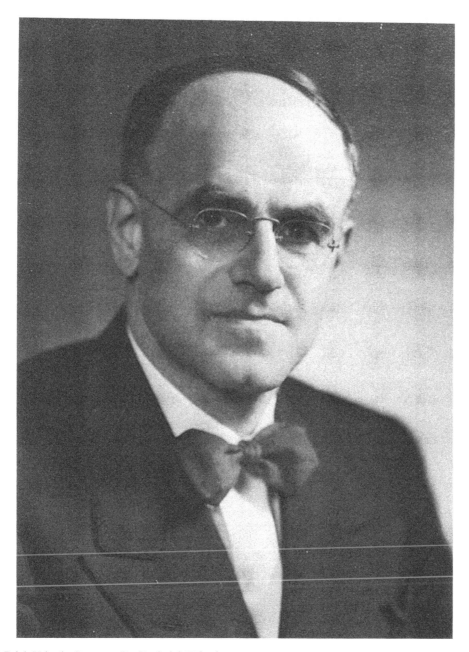

Figure 101 Erich Urbach. Courtesy, Dr. Frederick Urbach

enlarging red spot appeared on the left calf, a hand's breadth below the knee; it was first treated as eczema. A year or so later two new spots appeared on the same leg. The multiple lesions now present developed in the spring of this year; their growth has been gradual. The patient knew nothing of their yellowish color.

Status praesens. December 12, 1931. A rather strongly built woman of average height, with a striking bluish violet color to the cheeks, as is characteristic of diabetics, the same in the area of skin exposed at the neck of the dress; moderate hair loss, slight alveolar pyorrhea, and gum disease; slight enlargement of the thyroid. On the upper half of the left eyelid there is a pea sized, red, firmly elastic tumor, an angioma; similar angiomata between the breasts.

All cutaneous lesions were located on the legs. They appeared as extra-ordinarily sharply demarcated, irregularly contoured, non-painful, very firm plaque-like indurations which were bluish violet at the periphery and yellow in the center. By way of contrast, the more recent smaller nodules showed a slight but definite elevation with an almost normal epidermis, while the older, larger lesions showed an extremely thin overlying skin which was traversed by numerous fine vessel branches, and scaled markedly. No lymph adenopathy.

---

* Archiv für Dermat., und Syph., *166:*273, 1932.

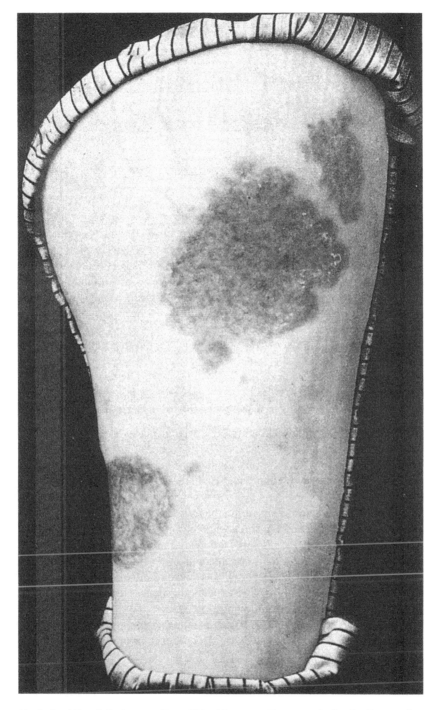

Figure 102 Necrobiosis lipoidica diabeticorum. From Urbach's paper. Courtesy, *Archiv für Dermatologie und Syphilologie*

G.A.Grant Peterkin

Orf

GEORGE ALEXANDER GRANT PETERKIN was born in 1909, and was educated at the Edinburgh University. Following a tetanus immunization he experienced a severe skin eruption. This led to a scholarship in dermatology in Copenhagen. By 1933 he joined the staff of Edinburgh. In 1942 he enlisted in the RAMC and soon was in North Africa recording the first cases of sulfonamide and mepacrine rashes. After the war he returned to Edinburgh, where he remained a clear, no nonsense lecturer and eventually President of the British Association of Dermatology.

He died in 1987, beloved for his warm, gracious personality.*

ORF

The Occurrence in Humans of Contagious Pustular Dermatitis of Sheep ("Orf")[†]

The condition of contagious pustular dermatitis or "orf" in sheep is one exceedingly well-known to veterinary surgeons and farmers, but there appears to be no record of its existence as a disease of mankind.

In sheep the trouble is found in almost every country in the world, but as each country has a different name for it, and as its manifestations can vary, one would therefore expect that other cases in human beings have been noted.

The progress of the disease in humans seems to run the following course: The first lesion to appear is a dark red papule, which grows to any size from threepence to half a crown. This is quite hard and as a rule painless. Gradually the papule begins to resemble a huge red molluscum contagiosum tumour, with a very marked umbilication. This depressed centre is covered with thin white skin and contains clear exudate. This exudate gradually becomes purulent, probably due to secondary infection, and granulations soon heap up. This stage is often painful. If the tumour is dressed with antiseptics, it tends to shrivel up in a few weeks, without any purulent discharge or granulations appearing.

The only difference between the lesions produced in animals experimentally and those found in humans is that there seems to be in the human a tendency for the lesions to be umbilicated.

---

* Biographical History of British Dermatology, 1996

[†] Brit. J.Dermat., *49:*492, 1937.

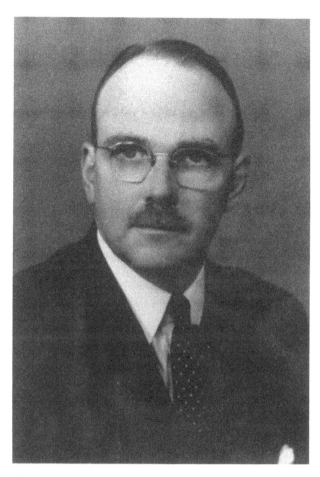

Figure 103 G.A.Grant Peterkin

Marion B.Sulzberger and William Garbe

Exudative Discoid and Lichenoid Chronic Dermatosis (Sulzberger-Garbe Syndrome)
MARION BALDUR SULZBERGER was born March 12, 1895, in New York City. His medical education at the University of Zurich, Switzerland was followed by postgraduate training under Bloch and Jadassohn. From 1929 to 1947 he was Associate Clinical Professor of Dermatology at the New York Post Graduate Medical School of Columbia. In 1947 he became Professor and Chairman of the Department of Dermatology and Syphilology, and Director of the New York Skin and Cancer Unit, affiliated with New York University and the Bellevue Medical Center. In 1960 he "retired" to be Professor at the University of California (San Francisco) until 1975. No one in American Dermatology has ever matched his achievements, as evidenced by his honorary membership in 44 foreign societies. He died on November 24, 1983.

Sulzberger wrote widely in the field of dermatology, contributing numerous papers of clinical dermatology, skin physiology, and dermatologic allergy. His name is linked with both incontinentia pigmenti (Bloch-Sulzberger), and the distinctive exudative discoid and lichenoid chronic dermatitis, his description of which is presented below. His basic studies on sweat retention, initiated during World War II while on active service with the U.S. Navy, have done much to point up the significance of the sweat gland in both local and systemic disease. Among the 16 books which he published are *Dermatologic Allergy, Dermatologic Therapy in General Practice,* and *Manual of Dermatology.**

WILLIAM GARBE was born in Toronto, Canada in 1908. He received his M.D. at the University of Toronto in 1932. From 1934 to 1936 he was in training in dermatology at the New York Postgraduate Medical School, and in the office of Wise and Sulzberger. He practiced in Toronto, and was Chief of the Dermatology clinic of the Mount Sinai Hospital in that city. He died in 1998.*

EXUDATIVE DISCOID AND LICHENOID CHRONIC DERMATOSIS

Nine Cases of a Distinctive Exudative Discoid and Lichenoid Chronic Dermatosis[†]

The outstanding distinctive and constant characteristics which impel us to attempt to delineate and segregate this form of dermatitis are perhaps best illustrated by the report of an actual and representative case.

---

* Crissey, J.T., Historical Atlas of Dermatology and Dermatologists. Parthenon Publishing, 156, 2002.

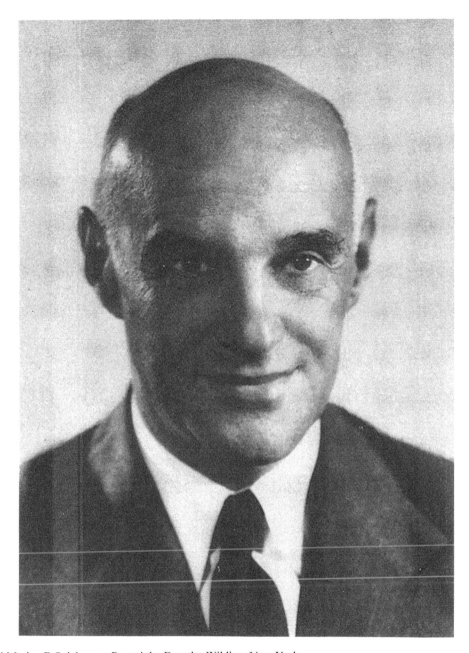

Figure 104 Marion B.Sulzberger. Portrait by Dorothy Wilding, New York

Report of a Case. Case 1. J.R., a Jew aged 42, born in Russia, executive of an insurance company, was first seen in April 1933. There was no history of personal or familial hypersensitivity (no evidence of atopy). There was a history of a severe exudative eczematous eruption which had been of brief duration and confined to the hands. The generalized eruption appeared four years later, and when the patient was first seen by us he had received expert dermatologic treatment for about four months.

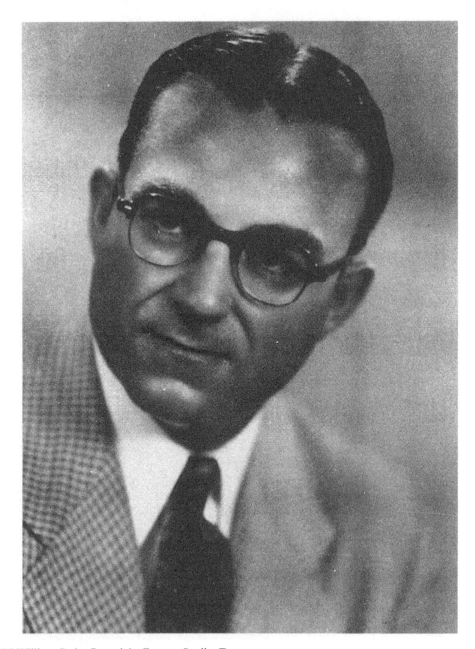

Figure 105 William Garbe. Portrait by Famous Studio, Toronto

We omit the exact description of the dermatosis as it appeared at the first visit for the patient had been employing various topical remedies which had obviously modified the appearance of the eruption.

During our period of observation, which lasted three years and 10 months, the course and appearance of the dermatosis may be described as follows: The principal complaint was severe and often maddening itching. This itching frequently occurred in veritable crisis, and was in general most marked at night. While the exceptional degree of pruritus was certainly the dominant symptom, the patient also complained of frequent sensations of chilliness.

The patient was highly intelligent. He was small and thin and of a nervous and hyperkinetic type, and he evidenced stigmas of a neurotic and cyclothymic personality. When he was questioned he freely admitted that he often scratched without the stimulus of itching (compulsion neurosis?). When the itching was most severe, a crisis developed, taking the form of an evident orgiastic manifestation, with a crescendo of wild scratching followed by rather sudden relief and exhaustion. (As is commonly observed in certain chronic highly pruritic conditions, the patient's fingernails were worn short and smooth and were highly polished.)

An impressive characteristic was the fact that the patient's skin presented truly amazing, rapid and apparently spontaneous changes in appearance. But despite these not infrequent fluctuations in intensity and despite these rapid, almost daily variations in predominant structure, the dermatosis presented certain recognizable phases. While several different types of lesions were as a rule present at one and the same time, we believe that certain efflorescences through their predominance at given periods distinguished the more or less distinct phases of the dermatosis, namely an exudative and discoid phase, a lichenoid phase, a phase resembling the premycotic stage of mycosis fungoides and an urticarial phase.

1. **Exudative and discoid phase.** During this phase the majority of lesions consisted of exudative discoid or oval plaques or patches of different sizes and shapes. These lesions varied from the size of a small pea to plaques the size of a palm and even larger, though such extensive lesions occurred only exceptionally. In shape the lesions varied from small roughly round discs to larger elliptical roughly oval forms. Occasionally they presented more irregular and somewhat bizarre outlines. These discoid or oval lesions were in the main fairly sharply demarcated and even the larger ones showed little, if any, tendency to central clearing. The evolution of these lesions was often that usually regarded as characteristic of true eczema; they passed through the consecutive stages of minute vesiculation, superficial oozing and crusting, and later scaling and lichenification. However, probably because of their fragility and small size, the minute vesicles present in the first stage were never clear-cut or easily discernible on clinical examination, and they were rapidly superseded by serous crusts. Erythema was never marked except after external irritation. The consistency of both the oval and the roughly round lesions underwent rapid changes. At certain times the lesions were distinctly elevated, probably as a result of edema. At other times, the discs were almost flat and flush with the level of the surrounding skin. The crusts covering these lesions were, as stated, of the thin serous type, and frequently the surface presented the minute discrete crusts characterizing the *status punctatus* considered typical of eczema.

The plaques were irregularly scattered over the entire cutaneous surface with the exception of the scalp, palms, and soles. In some areas they were sparsely disseminated; in others, they were closely grouped. The sites of predilection at which these lesions were exceptionally persistent were in the order named: 1. The glans penis, which presented singularly resistant discoid edematous and eczematoid plaques. Occasionally this showed crusting. At times they were moist and denuded. 2. The shaft of the penis and the scrotum, which presented either similar plaques or, occasionally, diffuse erythematous weeping and scaling areas. 3. The circumoral regions which showed small discoid lesions and occasionally exhibited rhagades localized about the mucocutaneous junction and on the skin and vermillion border of the upper and lower lips. 4. The

---

* Crissey, J.T., Historical Atlas of Dermatology and Dermatologists. Parthenon Publishing, 132, 2002.

† Arch. of Dermat. and Syph., *36:*247, 1937.

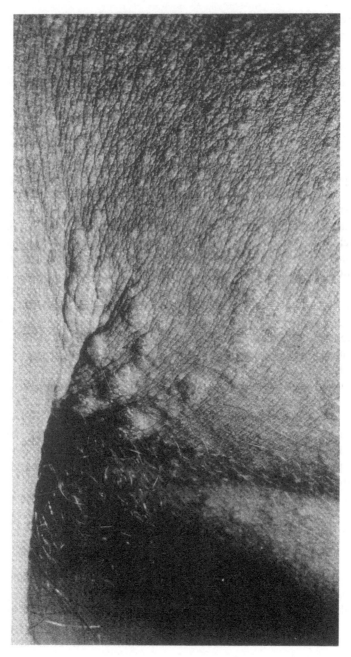

Figure 106 Typical discoid and lichenoid elevated plaques on posterior axillary fold; and typical diffuse lichenification. From Sulzberger's paper. Courtesy, *Archives of Dermatology and Syphilology*

area covering the bridge of the nose. 5. The breasts, particularly the perimamillary region, and even the mamillae themselves. 6. The anterior and posterior aspects of the axillary folds, the hairy apex being spared.

The eyelids and the external ears were somewhat less commonly involved. While these presented occasional ephemeral edema and erythema followed by scaling, the circumscribed discoid lesions were less in evidence. No area of skin could be said to be entirely immune, but there was certainly no sign of predilection for the flexor areas, these being on the whole less affected than the extensor surfaces. In contrast to ordinary atopic dermatitis (diffuse neurodermatitis), the cubital and popliteal spaces were practically unaffected.

On the trunk, the long axes of the oval plaques showed a distinct tendency to follow the lines of cleavage. This was particularly noticeable during the periods of involution and scaling, at which times the dermatosis on the trunk suggested the distribution and sometimes even the appearance of a retrogressing or treated pityriasis rosea.

The discoid exudative lesions characterizing this stage, either disappeared or, more commonly, became lichenified and eventually somewhat infiltrated after going through several exacerbations, the changes leading to the appear-ance not infrequently seen in certain cases of premycotic eczema or in certain forms of leukotic dyscrasia (lymphoblastoma) (phase 3). It must be repeated here that the weeping and oozing of this eczematous phase, while occasionally persisting in a certain number of plaques, was often astonishing ephemeral and often gave way within about a day to a dry or lichenoid phase.

2. **Lichenoid Phase.** In this phase the weeping was either absent or much less marked than in the preceding phase. The discoid lesions either had undergone complete involution or presented a dry and lichenified appearance.

Scattered lichenoid papules appeared on many different areas, some being irregularly distributed and some appearing in larger and smaller groups. The majority of these papules were follicular. While their appearance was suggestive of lichen planus, the papules were generally smaller and less violaceous and did not present the typical striae, umbilication or wax-like sheen. Nevertheless, some of these lesions so closely resembled papules of lichen planus that when they appeared in characteristic localizations (*e.g.,* on the glans penis) the diagnosis of lichen planus was at times seriously considered.

During this phase, as well as during other phases, it was particularly noticeable that an exaggerated cutis anserina developed whenever the patient was exposed to even slight changes of temperature, as when undressing in what was according to normal perception a comfortably heated room. In this connection it may not be entirely irrelevant to mention that the mamillae showed a hyperexcitability, persistent and abnormally marked erection, and even swelling and "burning" sensation being present. These phenomena, how-ever, were not necessarily coincidental with the cutis anserina.

In addition to the isolated lichenoid papules, the entire integument occasionally presented varying degrees of diffuse lichenifications; at times large areas of skin were visually and palpably thickened and showed accentuation of the normal skin markings. There seemed to be not only infiltration, but also latent non-pitting edema, as shown by the rapid changes in consistency. This edema was particularly noticeable on the lower extremities, especially about the ankles. The wrists and dorsa of the hands were frequently the seat of lichenification.

This dry and lichenoid phase was the one most often in evidence, as it was usually of much longer duration than any of the other phases.

3. **Phase Resembling the Premycotic Stage of Mycosis Fungoides.** The patient was twice presented before dermatologic societies by Dr. Paul E. Bechet. At the time of these presentations it was evident that the majority of the discoid and oval lesions showed various degrees of infiltration. The consensus was therefore that the case was one of an early stage of mycosis fungoides.

We, too, subsequently observed the condition passing through similar phases of infiltration and considered the possibility of a premycotic eruption as well as that of some other leukotic dyscrasia (lymphoblastoma).

During these phases the infiltration of the discoid and oval lesions definitely dominated the picture, while the lichenoid papules and the exudative and crusting eczematoid elements were less prominent. These objective observations, combined with the refractiveness to ordinary antieczematous therapy, and the persistence of severe itching, so strongly suggested mycosis fungoides or some other leukotic dyscrasia that it required the repeated reports that biopsy showed only chronic dermatitis to convince us that none of the histologic characteristics of any of the aforementioned dermatoses was then present. Furthermore, the subsequent course, including the variability in the appearance of the dermatosis, the resistance to roentgen and arsenic therapy and the lack of development of the clinical or histological characteristics of true mycosis fungoides, of characteristic changes in the lymph nodes, or in the blood or of other systemic manifestations—all these factors combined to lead us to the ultimate conclusion that neither the diagnosis of mycosis fungoides nor that of any other leukotic dyscrasia could be upheld.

4. **Urticarial Phase.** During the whole course of the dermatosis the patient complained of showers of pruritic urticarial lesions appearing suddenly and lasting from about 30 minutes to several hours. These would appear suddenly, without manifest cause, now on one area and again on another. While they sometimes resembled common hives, the lesions were often smaller and more spherical. They seemed to be more deep seated than the usual urticaria and were of somewhat longer duration, thus bearing some slight resemblance to prurigo papules. As long as the other cutaneous manifestations were present in full force these urticarial papules were but an insignificant and easily overlooked part of the objective dermatologic picture. However, the urticarial manifestations assumed the significance of a distinct phase by reason of the persistence of their appearance in the last four months of our observation, during which time the patient was relatively free from the cutaneous manifestations of the other phases described.

The course of this dermatosis was chronic and persistent, with rapid changes, including apparently spontaneous exacerbations and incomplete remissions of various degrees. There was, however, no period of complete freedom at any time during the entire period of almost four years of observation.

Hulusi Behçet

Triple Symptom Complex (Behçet's Disease)

HULUSI BEHÇET was born in Istanbul, on February 26, 1889. After graduation from the Medical School of Istanbul in 1910, he worked in the clinic of Skin Diseases of the Gülhane Military Hospital until 1914. Following postgraduate studies in Berlin and Budapest in 1918, he returned to Istanbul. In 1933 he was appointed Professor of Dermatology at the University of Istanbul. His contributions to the dermatologic literature included over a hundred papers, and an important textbook on the diagnosis of syphilis.

Most of Behçet's works appeared in the Turkish periodicals, although many were published in the German and French journals. The syndrome, the clinical account of which we have included here, had been studied intensively by him for over 25 years.

Professor ordinarius since 1939, Behçet died in Istanbul on March 8, 1948.

TRIPLE SYMPTOM COMPLEX

Über rezidivierende, aphthöse, durch ein Virus verursachte Geschwüre am Mund, am Auge und an den Genitalien*

The cases which are considered here exhibit the following clinical picture: Lesions in the mouth, on the genitalia, and of the eyes. These lesions are not, however, the same as the *aphthoiden* of Pospischil, nor the as yet but little studied skin lesions frequently met with in children.

When one investigates these relapsing lesions with regard to their localization, it appears that both mouth and genital syndromes may be included in each group. By way of example, in our second case aphthous ulcers appeared from time to time on the genitalia, and at first brought to mind the Lipschütz ulcers or the various forms of ulcers of the mucous membranes (Esthiomène). However, the lesions of the relapses which occurred several times a year appeared either simultaneously or successively in the mouth, on the genitalia, on the conjunctiva, and even as an inflammation of the iris. These manifestations merit special investigation.

In one of the two patients, whom we have observed for 20 years, very painful erythema nodosum-like lesions appeared in association with relapses in the first year. As soon as the aphthous lesions of the mouth and genitalia began to involute, the skin lesions too disappeared. In neither of our cases, which have shown periodic recurrences for 20 and seven years respectively, can one consider these aphthous manifestations as

---

* Dermat. Wchnschr., *105:*1152, 1937.

ordinary aphthae. It is also noteworthy that these recurrent lesions of the mouth or genitalia (on the penis and scrotum in the male, on the vulva or vagina in the female) are associated with inflammation of the conjunctiva. These facts, plus the observation that local therapy was of no help, and that internal therapy succeeded in lengthening the intervals between relapses, make it clear that we are dealing with a disease caused by a general infection, affecting the organism as a whole, and that the aphthous lesions have no relation to ordinary aphthae.

Our first case is a man 40 years old, healthy, with no bodily defect, married and the father of normal children. Our second case is a 34 year old woman, physically normal, and mother of normal children. In this woman (L.D.) the disease began more than seven years ago with lesions on the tongue which spread over the tonsils, the soft palate, and the lips, and after a certain time also involved the genitalia. The mouth lesions, especially those of the lips, reminded one of "Faulecken" (Perlèche), and interfered with the patient's eating and drinking. Because of this the patient wasted markedly with each relapse. Moreover, the aphthous edematous lesions of the genitalia were very painful, and presented here and there a picture of purpura-like ecchymoses. Especially violent relapses evoked corneal erosions and an episcleritis (Igersheimer-Murat Rami). The eruptions lasted from 20 to 30 days, the manifestations then involuted slowly, and the appetite returned so that the patient regained her normal weight.

Howard Hailey and Hugh Hailey

Familial Benign Chronic Pemphigus

WILLIAM HOWARD HAILEY was born on May 17, 1898, in Hartwell, Georgia. He received his M.D. from Emory University in 1920. He practiced as a dermatologist in Atlanta and held the title, Associate Clinical Professor of Dermatology at Emory University Medical School. He was a member of the American Dermatological Association, and wrote on various dermatologic topics. His best known work is that which he did on familial benign chronic pemphigus. We have included his account of this disease, written in association with his brother, Hugh. He died on March 26, 1967.

HUGH EDWARD HAILEY was born in Hartwell, Georgia, in 1909. After receiving his M.D. from Emory University in 1935, he did postgraduate work in dermatology at the Vanderbilt Clinic in New York City, and in 1938 returned to Atlanta, Georgia to practice. During World War II he served on a U.S. Navy Hospital Ship in the Pacific. He was consultant in dermatology at several hospitals, and held the title, Assistant in Dermatology at Emory University. He was active in a score of Atlanta Community affairs. His kindly disposition endeared him to his many patients. He died suddenly on January 14, 1963.*

FAMILIAL BENIGN CHRONIC PEMPHIGUS

Familial Benign Chronic Pemphigus*

A search of the literature fails to reveal any report of a cutaneous condition which has the characteristics of that reported here.

In March, 1936, two white brothers, N.H.B. and S.G.B. came under our care because of recurring lesions of the neck. Their ages were 38 and 35 years, respectively. The older brother was married and the father of a normal child, aged six. The younger brother was single. The older brother was a salesman and the younger brother a banker. They did not live in the same house.

These men were accustomed to better than average economic conditions. Hence their diet and living conditions always had been good. They could afford excellent medical and dental care.

Prior to March, 1936, both men consulted internists and dermatologists of distant cities as well as at home. Various physical and laboratory examinations failed to reveal any information pertinent to their

---

* Steffen, C.: Am. J.Dermatopathol. *25*:256, 2003.

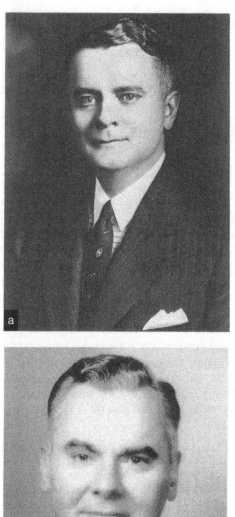

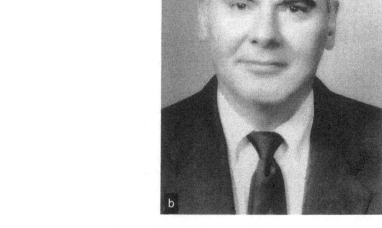

Figure 107 (a) Howard Hailey; (b) Hugh Hailey

complaint. Repeated questioning concerning ingestion of some drug which might have been an etiologic factor elicited negative replies.

The older brother, N.H.B., stated that the eruption began in 1926 while he was in college. Since then he had not been free from it for any prolonged period. The younger brother, S.G.B., first noted the eruption the following year. In neither man had the eruption been influenced by the seasons of the year. They thought perspiration in summer added to their discomfort.

The only subjective symptom was pruritus, which at times was intense, but varied in degree with the different recurrences. The eruption prevented the wearing of a collar, which caused much embarrassment.

The brothers stated that they had been treated repeatedly for ringworm and impetigo contagiosa. Various treatments, including the application of roentgen rays and ultraviolet rays, apparently had not influenced the course of the disease. The number of lesions appearing during the attacks varied from one to many. New "places" frequently appeared while old ones were regressing. They always appeared on the neck and were either bilateral or unilateral. Both patients stated that these focal eruptions began as very small blisters which spread rapidly. They became wet, and in one or more days a crust formed.

Examination on March 5 and on many subsequent occasions showed sharply marginated crusted lesions varying in size from 5 mm. to several centimeters. The crusts were amber colored, and the lesions gave the impression of ruptured flaccid bullous impetigo. At the border of the crusted lesions there was a pellicle of epidermis. It could be torn away with forceps. Nikolsky's sign was present. There was no scarring or other change which suggested the least damage to the skin from previous lesions, although they had appeared and regressed over a period of ten or more years. Some pigmentation marked the sites of recently healed lesions. The lymph nodes were tender sometimes, but this was not a constant feature.

The only other dermatologic condition in either brother was dermatophytosis of the feet and groin in N.H.B. He gave a strongly positive reaction to dermotricofitin, and the treatment of dermatophytosis was supplemented with injections of trichophytin. The injections did not cause any change in the eruption on the neck nor, apparently did they shorten the course of the dermatophytosis. It was hoped that the injections by acting in a non-specific fashion would have a beneficial effect on the eruption.

On October 4, S.G.B. presented three new lesions on his neck. They were from 1 to 1.5 cm. in diameter. One which had not ruptured presented the picture of a flaccid bulla. The sites of recent lesions were marked by areas of pigmentation varying in size.

Both patients presented a most annoying condition with identical characteristics, including a self-limited course.

At the meeting of the Southeastern Dermatologic Society in September 1938, at Charlotte, North Carolina, Dr. G.Richard Allison presented a white man, W.H.H., aged 50, who exhibited a clinical picture that was identical with that found in our two patients except for location. The lesions were present about the axillary folds, groins, legs and body. This patient stated that he had had lesions on his face. At the time of presentation none were present. The lesions were sharply marginated and had amber colored crusts, and their peripheral extension was manifested by separated epidermis. Nikolsky's sign was present. The patient stated that he had had the trouble for 20 years. Pruritus was present. There was no scarring. Pigmented areas were present marking the site of former recent lesions. This patient had a brother, T.H., aged 30, who had had a similar eruption for years. He was in the hospital in December 1936 under the care of Dr. G.Richard Allison, who called a consultant ophthalmologist, Dr. Walter J.Bristow, because the condition involved both eyes. Dr. Bristow rendered the following report: "Mr. T.H. has a keratoconjunctivitis involving the bulbar and palpebral conjunctiva as well as the cornea of each eye. At the time of examination this condition is manifested by the usual signs of redness, swelling, infection and edema of the conjunctiva and by slight

* Arch. of Dermat. and Syph., *39*:679, 1939.

haziness of the cornea, with occasionally a break in the corneal epithelium, such as one sees in herpes of the cornea. I do not recall seeing blebs or blisters of the cornea. There was no iritis or other interocular inflammation.

"I examined the patient's eyes July 18, 1938. He had no evidence of any inflammatory condition at that time, and with a correction for myopia he had normal vision in each eye."

Summary and Conclusion: A report of four cases of a dermatologic condition which has certain constant features is submitted. It is familial and recurs over a long period of years. While simple wet dressings were palliative, apparently no treatment influences the course of the disease. It is benign in that no constitutional signs or symptoms accompany it. Varying degrees of itching are present. The eyes of one of Dr. Allison's patients, T.H., were affected by the condition. After the involvement of the eyes cleared up, both corneas and conjunctivas were normal as in the case of the skin in all four patients.

The individual lesions began as small vesicles, which rapidly became flaccid bullae. Early rupture followed, with formation of an amber colored crust. The peripheral spread was bullous. Nikolsky's sign was present. Possible etiologic factors, such as occupational effect, ingestion of drugs, exposure to sunlight, irritation from clothing or from chemicals and presence of an anatomic anomaly, have been definitely eliminated through repeated taking of histories, through tests, and by protective dressings.

A majority opinion of the dermatohistopathologists who examined the sections supports the clinical diagnosis. Therefore, we submit for consideration this report of what we believe to be dermatologic entity heretofore undescribed —familial benign chronic pemphigus.

João Paulo Vieira

Fogo Salvagem

JOÃO PAULO VIEIRA was born in São Carlos, Brazil, on July 23, 1896. He was graduated from the University of Rio de Janeiro in 1919, having spent a year of interneship in the University dermatology clinic. In 1927 and 1928 he did postgraduate work at l'Hôpital Saint Louis. In 1938 he became Director of a Public Health Division and also of a hospital in São Paulo, both uniquely devoted entirely to the problem of pemphigus foliaceus (fogo salvagem). He conducted numerous clinical and experimental studies on patients with this disease. His account below is the definitive description of this contagious form of pemphigus.

Vieira was a member and founder of several medical societies. As a member of the Sociedade História de Medicine, he wrote an account of the history of dermatology in São Paulo. He was also editor and founder of *Arquivos de Dermatologia e Sifihgrafia de São Paulo*. He contributed nearly 100 papers to the Brazilian dermatologic literature over a period of 30 years.

FOGO SALVAGEM

Pemphigus foliaceus (Fogo Salvagem), an Endemic Disease of the State of São Paulo (Brazil)*

For a number of years physicians practicing in the state of São Paulo, and especially in the city of Franca, reported cases of a rare dermatosis affecting the entire cutaneous surface of each patient and ending in death.

In 1937 and 1938, I made a special study of this type of pemphigus and proposed a classification of its clinical variants, ranging from the abortive to the most advanced type. Pemphigus foliaceus may be easily differentiated now in Brazil from the other types of pemphigus, such as the acute or infectious type, the chronic type, the pemphigus with extensive bullae of Brocq and pemphigus vegetans.

From 1929 to 1937, the spread of the epidemic was so rapid that the legislative assembly of the state of São Paulo appropriated a large sum to assist Professor Adolfo Lindenberg in his research on the disease, and in 1938 the state created an official commission under my direction to study and propose the necessary measures to check the disease.

The census was taken as the first step in this campaign and showed that two-thirds of the state of São Paulo was affected and that the greater incidence of the disease occurred in the territories of Franca,

---

* Arch. of Dermat. and Syph., *41*:858, 1940.

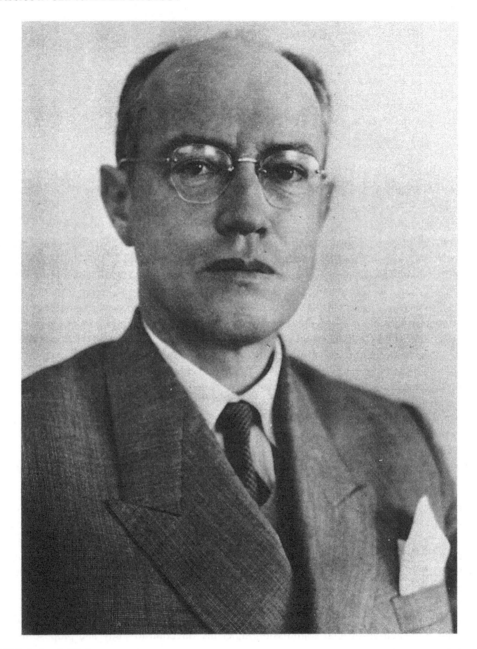

Figure 108 João Paulo Vieira

Ribeirão Preto and Batataes. Other large foci were in São Carlos, Bocaina, and Jaú. In the majority of the new foci of the disease the cases were traced to one or more patients coming from infected zones.

The studies carried out by the São Paulo investigators seem to prove that the disease is infectious, but the etiologic agent has not been isolated. A number of familial cases have been reported. Direct contagion has not been proved, and it seems that a certain predisposition is required and perhaps a carrier or a vector. This may explain why persons living with and caring for patients with pemphigus may remain unaffected, although other members of the same family are sooner or later taken with the disease. I believe that the Brazilian pemphigus foliaceus is a contagious disease, as Lindenberg, Orsini de Castro, Aleixio and other investigators have stated, but exhaustive studies carried out in the Conde de Lara Institute and numerous inoculations in Macacus rhesus monkeys, guinea pigs, rabbits and white mice have failed to demonstrate the etiologic agent.

I have been able to demonstrate that the disease presents several clinical types, ranging from the most benign forms to the most severe, and that, contrary to the usually fatal ending of the European pemphigus, the Brazilian pemphigus foliaceus ends in recovery in about 10 per cent of the cases. The possibilities of recovery are greater with certain clinical types that I have studied, especially with the verrucous and the hyperpigmented type.

The classification of the clinical variants of pemphigus foliaceus (fogo salvagem) is as follows:

A common complication in the cases that I observed was ankylosis of the large joints and osteoporosis and demineralization of the articular extremities of the long bones.

Pemphigus foliaceus *(fogo salvagem)* affects patients of all ages, the youngest one in my series being six years old. More women are affected than men; 67 per cent of my patients were women. In some cases the normal development of the body suffers, creating a special clinical type of the disease, which I have called "dystrophic."

The condition begins usually with bullae on the face and thorax, and gradually the eruption becomes generalized. During the period of invasion a temperature of from 37.5 to 38.5 C. (99.5 to 101.3 F.) is the rule, but in the acute form the temperature may be much higher. The skin is affected uniformly, and Nikolsky's sign is always positive. Subjective symptoms consist of pain and sensations of heat and chills. Alopecia of the scalp, eyebrows and eyelids is common, but after recovery the hair grows back normally, as the skin is never scarred. Up to the present 250 patients have been studied.

Stuart D.Allen and John P.O'Brien

1. Tropical Anidrosis

2. Actinic Granuloma (O'Brien's Granuloma)

STUART DOUGLAS ALLEN was born in Sydney, Australia, February 4, 1900. After graduation from the University of Sydney in 1924, he practiced in that city as a general medical consultant until his retirement. He was a Fellow of the Royal Australasian College of Physicians, and Lecturer in Clinical Medicine in the Royal North Shore Hospital at Sydney. He served in both World Wars, and was a Specialist Physician in the latter. Dr. Allen died on August 11, 1979.

JOHN PATRICK EDWARD O'BRIEN was born in Sydney, Australia in 1914. He was graduated from the University of Sydney in 1938, and during World War II served with the Australian Army as a pathologist. After the war, he held the post of pathologist to the Prince Henry Hospital, and then became postgraduate lecturer in pathology at the University of Sydney. He continued to study clinically, histopathologically, and experimentally the anidrosis he first observed with Allen during the War. In 1975 he described the new clinical entity, actinic granuloma. He died in 2002.

TROPICAL ANIDROSIS

Tropical Anidrotic Asthenia: A Preliminary Report*

The following description is based on the study of the condition of 10 Australian soldiers admitted to an army hospital in the Northern Territory during the months of February, March and April, 1943, and 12 soldiers admitted to a field ambulance in New Guinea during early 1944.

The significance of the first case of tropical anidrotic asthenia was not appreciated until further cases were found which did not conform to either of the two classical disorders of heat regulation (heat hyperpyrexia and heat prostration). Neither hyperpyrexia nor collapse was present. In all cases similar changes were found in the skin, and the majority of patients, as well as having enlarged lymph glands, had suffered from *Miliaria rubra* (prickly heat) shortly before the onset of the condition.

Definition. The disorder is a clinical syndrome observed in tropical areas amongst troops who have suffered from *Miliaria rubra* and is characterized by anidrosis (failure to sweat), changes in the skin and enlargement of the axillary and inguinal lymph glands, with symptoms of exhaustion occurring in the heat. Complete recovery usually takes place in six to 12 weeks.

Symptoms. In 18 out of 22 cases studied the patient gave a history of *Miliaria rubra*. Usually the rash had been severe, extensive and recurrent, but had, as a rule, disappeared three or four weeks before the

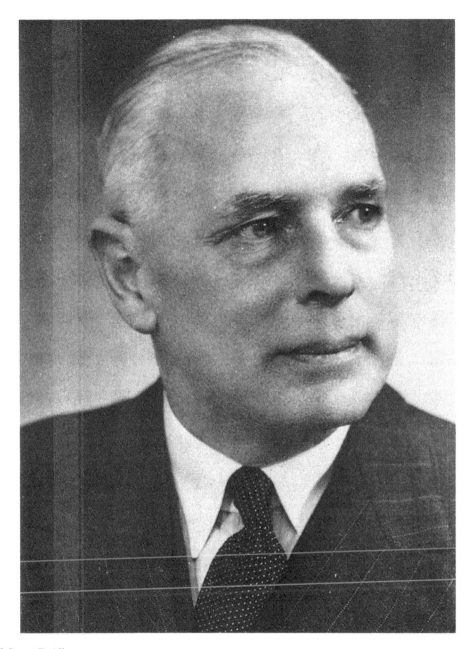

Figure 109 Stuart D.Allen

anidrosis supervened. However, this period was occasionally less, and in two instances the miliarial rash was still present on the patient's admission to hospital.

The onset is insidious. The patient first notices that exercise in the heat of the day, especially in bright sunshine, produces an unusual degree of exhaustion, as well as dyspnoea, palpitation, epigastric discomfort

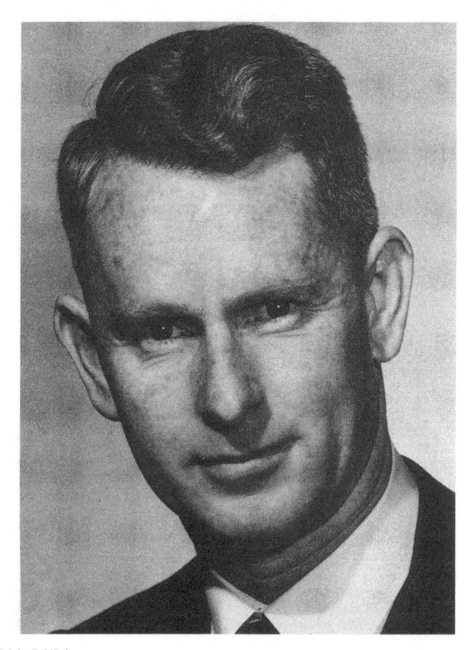

Figure 110 John P.O'Brien

and slight or severe frontal headache with giddiness. A hot, congested or tight prickling feeling in the skin may also be a symptom. At this stage he may notice that he is sweating less than usual; however, he often does not volunteer this information as he considers it unimportant. Previously sweating has been normal. In the humid atmosphere of the tropics profuse and continuous sweating occurs in normal subjects even on only slight exertion.

With rest, especially in a cool place, these symptoms pass off in from half to two hours, but once established, they are reproduced more readily and severely by less and less exertion, until extreme exhaustion or actual unconsciousness occurs when an attempt is made to carry out some relatively slight physical effort. In severe cases slight symptoms may be present in the hottest part of the day, even while the subject is resting.

When examined during or shortly after such an attack, the patient is extremely distressed and apprehensive. Respiration is increased in depth and rate, up to 46 per minute, the mouth temperature is elevated to between 100° and 102°F., while the pulse rate may be as high as 140 per minute.

Characteristic skin changes are present. On the forehead and face, sweating may be profuse. The palms and soles and perhaps the axillae are normally moist; but with these exceptions, the rest of the body is completely devoid of sweat and the skin is perfectly dry. Over the anterior and posterior aspects of the trunk and arms, but to a less degree over the forearms, the lower extremities and rarely the palms and soles, the skin appears much coarser than normal; on superficial examination, it looks like exaggerated "goose flesh." On close inspection, the affected skin is seen to be studded with innumerable greyish-white papule-like elevations, which, however, do not surround the hairs as in "goose flesh." The average size is remarkably constant at about 1 mm. in diameter. In one case larger lesions were present, obvious vesicles 3 mm. in diameter. There is no surrounding red areola. The intervening parts of the skin may be normal in colour or more often, a little paler than the same patient's resting skin. In other words, the flushing of the skin which is expected after exercise does not occur.

When one of the elevations is pricked with a needle, a minute drop of watery fluid may be obtained. The elevations are therefore caused by small vesicles, which are, however, a little deeper than the vesicles of dermatitis. Nor in any other way do the skin lesions resemble those of dermatitis.

The whole arm and fingers, and to a lesser extent the thighs, may be obviously swollen, with obliteration of the natural folds and creases.

To the touch the skin feels rough, tense and inelastic, and is extraordinarily hot and dry. It does not pit on pressure, and consequently the oedema observed is intracutaneous and not subcutaneous.

The axillary and inguinal lymph glands are in most cases moderately enlarged and tender, but not painful.

No significant changes are found in the nervous system, and there is no alteration in the blood pressure or composition of the urine, which is secreted in normal amounts.

With rest in a cool atmosphere, the temperature, pulse rate and respiration rate return to normal in from one to two hours, the skin regains a comparatively normal appearance and the patient again feels comfortable. The lymph glands, however, decrease in size more slowly, and some enlargement remains for a few days or longer, even though the patient rests.

It is extremely common to find soldiers who show isolated patches of the characteristic skin changes without general symptoms. The latter arise only when the change is widespread and sweat production seriously reduced. A mild degree of generalized clinical folliculitis is observed in a proportion of the severe cases. Ichthyoid desquamation has also been seen, especially on the legs.

Clinical Course. After a minimum period often to fourteen days, during which symptoms and signs readily recur on exertion, an increasing ability to undertake exercise with gradual re-establishment of

---

* Med. J. of Australia, 2:335, 1944.

sweating occurs. In all cases sweat production reappeared first on the trunk, whilst the upper and lower limbs regained this function irregularly and later.

Complications. The only complication seen was impetigo of the face when sweating had been most profuse and continuous. No instance of heat by hyperpyrexia complicating this disease was observed; though such a circumstance might reasonably be anticipated.

It is believed that the skin changes frequently lead on to dermatitis. The relationship is at present under investigation.

O'BRIEN'S GRANULOMA

Actinic Granuloma: An Annular Connective Tissue Disorder Affecting Sun- and Heat-damaged (Elastotic) Skin

The following account is based on information supplied by clinical colleagues and also on my own observations.

Actinic granuloma typically affects the exposed, weather-beaten skin of patients who are at least 30 and usually 40 years old or more. Favored sites are the neck, face, chest, and arms. A blond and freckled skin is a predisposing factor; in Australia, this implies that the person has either an Anglo-Saxon or more particularly a Celtic genetic background. Affecting male and female patients in about equal numbers, the disease begins insidiously as light amber, skin-colored, pink or dusky pink, single or grouped papules and progresses through a plaque stage to a complete or incomplete annulus of firm superficial dermal thickening. The border of the ring is smooth, pearly, only slightly raised, and measures between 0.2 and 0.5 cm in width. Scaliness is rarely observed. The ring expands exceedingly slowly and may become scalloped, while the center may return to a fairly normal appearance or else it may display slight or dubious atrophy. Depigmentation is variable; it is sometimes extreme and sometimes absent. There is no bright yellow (lipoidica) color, there is no telangiectasia, and the hairs are not destroyed. The largest ring found in this study measured 6.0 cm in diameter, while the number has varied from one to about ten. The latter figure is arbitrary, since some of the rings are compounded from smaller lesions. If single papules and nodules are counted, the tally may become innumerable.

Since they were asymptomatic, most patients allowed their lesions to progress to the ring stage before reporting to a physician. At times the skin as a whole displays so much actinic change, such as pigmentation, freckling, lentigo, macular depigmentation and elastosis, that the disease may be obscured and overlooked. Often the actinic elastosis is latent or *subrugose* and needs to be demonstrated by compressing the skin in its own plane, when the characteristic wrinkled, flaccid texture becomes obvious.

The duration of a single ring is months or years after which spontaneous remission may occur, leaving depigmentation or else very little aftermath. As resolution takes place, new areas may become involved, thus prolonging the condition. There is no anesthesia of the affected skin. No lesions have been found on the continuously covered parts of the body.

Although the typical disease is insidious and symptom-free, in a few instances it is more severe, with bright-red, itchy lesions. An episode of severe sunburn seems to precipitate these less common "acute" variants.

The general health of all patients has been normal, and diabetes has not been manifest.

Microscopical sections show that there is an infiltrate composed mainly of foreign-body giant cells, the cells being engaged in digesting and absorbing the abnormal elastotic fibers.

The disorder, which occurs on several continents, should probably be regarded as a phenomenon of repair within damaged connective tissue. The name *actinic granuloma* indicates its external or environmental origin and distinguishes it from other granulomas with which it is constantly being confused.

Actinic granuloma and granuloma annulare appear to be related. In *granuloma annulare,* a productive and resorptive process also occurs, but its nature remains obscure.

Actinic granuloma may be misdiagnosed as "atypical necrobiosis lipoidica" or as sarcoidosis.*

* Arch Dermatol *111:*460, 1975.

Johannes Fabry

Angiokeratoma Corporis Diffusum (Fabry's Disease)

JOHANNES FABRY was born in Germany in 1860. Following his M.D., he received training at the Royal Clinic for Skin and Venereal Diseases in Bonn from 1886 to 1889. His career of four decades was spent as Director of the Skin Clinic in Dortmund. In his youth he suffered the loss of a leg, but this was never to interfere with his joie de vivre, nor with his astonishing productivity (cf. Gianotti). His contributions covered the many facets of dermatology. He was especially concerned in the prevention and therapy of syphilis and cutaneous tuberculosis, so common at that time. He recognized tar as a carcinogen, and the ubiquitous nature of ringworm. His indefatigable energy transformed a clinic of but a few beds to one of 180 beds by 1925.

He was a charming teacher, always surrounded by eager post-graduate students. Recognizing the need for shared experiences he founded the Westphalian Dermatological Society. In recognition of his contributions and his moral way of life, the rank of Professor was conferred on him in 1919.

Although William Anderson, a surgeon at St. Thomas's Hospital in London, reported a case of angiokeratomas the same year as Fabry, history has denied him eponymous rights. To Fabry's credit he continued to report on this strange fatal disorder. June 29, 1930 saw the death of Fabry. Strangely, it was also the year of the death of his patient, as well as the publication of Fabry's final paper describing the autopsy findings on his patient.*

ANGIOKERATOMA CORPORIS DIFFUSUM

Ein Beitrag zur Kenntniss der Purpura haemorrhagicum nodularis (Purpura Papulosa Haemorrhagica Hebra)*

Emil Honke, 13 years old, from Langendreer. Both parents living. The father is 42 years old, a miner, always in good health, as is the mother. The paternal grandmother lived to the age of 64 and was always in good health. The grandfather had died of kidney disease at age 49. The maternal grandfather is alive and well at age 73, never having suffered a skin eruption. The maternal grandmother had died at age 63 of uterine cancer. On the father's side are skin eruptions, not identified. The mother of the patient has suffered for 7 years with polyarthritis deformans.

---

* Obit.: Dermatol. Wehnschr., *92*:319, 1931.

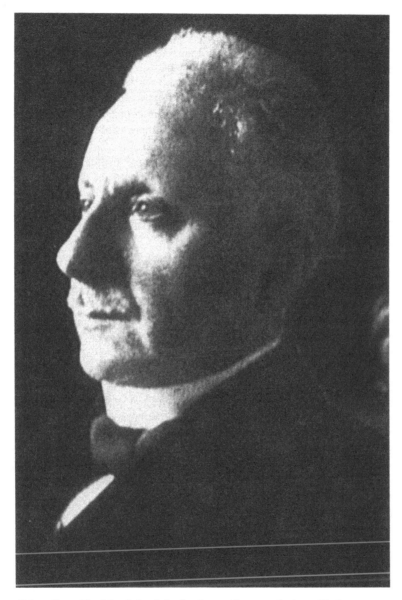

Figure 111 Johannes Fabry. From *The Man Behind the Syndrome*. Courtesy Springer-Verlag

The patient was always strong and healthy as a child, but had measles at age 5 without sequelae, and attends school regularly. There had been no discomfort, no pain, and no swelling in the skin noted by either the patient or parents during the 4 years preceding the appearance of small nodules in the left popliteal space. Then over the course of a year the eruption gradually spread over the posterior thigh and trunk. In the past year similar nodules were noted in the right popliteal space. The illness has given the patient relatively little discomfort, though the youth has become somewhat weaker in the past year. Attendance at school and learning suffered, as well as his appetite, and the patient became emaciated.

Physical Findings. The youngster is relatively strong. The mucous membranes are, however, anemic, his face is swollen, and the lips and the lids slightly edematous. Investigation of the inner abdominal and chest organs revealed no enlargement of the liver, spleen or heart and the heart sounds likewise were normal. In the left posterior region there are short sounds and in the apex expiratory wheezes. A similar finding is elicited on left anterior pulmonary apex. The urine is free of protein and sugar and in sedimented urine there is no evidence of microscopic casts or blood constituents. There is absolutely no evidence to support the diagnosis of central nervous system disease.

Blood studies were undertaken revealing a perfectly normal hemoglobin; the white cells were not increased in relation to the red cells. Finally, we observed the number of eosinophils was neither decreased nor increased.

When we examined the patient's body we found multiple indolent, tender, enlarged lymph nodes of the groin, nape of the neck, and in the throat. The skin color is pale and especially pigmented. The teeth are perfectly normal.

The body shows an exanthem, which is most striking on the chest, back, sacrum, and groin. The largest single lesions are in the popliteal areas, being more diffuse over the sternum and the back. Smaller clusters of excrescences appear over the whole body, i.e. they were on the entire anterior surface of the body, on the extensor surface of the upper and lower legs and on the entire periphery of the upper extremities. Inspection of the skin at sites where the exanthem is less prominent one sees, on paying closer attention, countless smaller and smaller puncta just as one observes the firmament on a starry night, one is struck by the larger constellations at first glance, only on prolonged observation to perceive numberless smaller and smaller stars.

So, for example, one sees a rather prominent eruption on the forearms, the extensor surface of the lower legs, and both sides of the knee. Likewise, there are rather large clusters in the umbilical region.

Essential next is the color of the exanthem. The larger nodules appear dark blue, going toward black. In the site where the exanthem is extending superficially, one can upon looking at a well-defined area think of a flat nevus vasculosus, so similar is the bluish-red color of the eruption. Small white scales are on the surface of the larger excrescences at isolated sites. We have already indicated the impressive papular nature of the eruption observed on direct observation of the lesions, and this impression is confirmed by running the palm over the affected sites and thereby obtaining evidence of the smaller and smallest changes in elevation of the normal skin surface. Stroking one's hand over the back and over the skin of the chest, one gets the typical feeling of a grater, which has been described by authors for lichen accuminatus and Darier's disease. The larger papular formations of the skin, as well as on the back and upper legs are conglomerate confluent papules.

As to the mucosa, careful inspection of the patient revealed papules in the mouth, on the cheeks, and near the corners of the mouth on both sides.

The patient came to the Skin Clinic of the city hospital for more days of careful examination and during that time could be observed for either the appearance of new papules or the fading of those already present. Also during those visits observations were made for mucosal bleeding or changes in his lungs, intestinal tract, or ever so little change in the kidney. The patient's skin changes were not associated with any complaints, itch, paresthesias, pain or discomfort, only some fatigue and weakness.

---

* Archiv. Dermatol. Syph., *43:*187, 1898.

Agostino Pasini and Luis E.Pierini

Atrophoderma of Pasini and Pierini

AGOSTINO PASINI (1875–1944). A graduate of Pavia University, he was a resident in the Department of Dermatology in Parma, headed by Mibelli. In 1905 he started his career in a Milanese Hospital, developing a small Unit of Clinical Research. Rapidly he became teacher of Dermosyphilology in the post-graduate courses and, soon after, he was the first Professor and Chairman of Dermatology at the University of Milan that was founded in 1924. Subsequently, he organized a large university hospital clinic with facilities for teaching and research and, in addition, he founded the first Library of Dermatology within the Department.

He was an invited lecturer to many national and international symposia and congresses. Author of 175 scientific papers on different fields of dermatology and venereology, he focused his interest on Pringle's diseases, on bromodermas (he was able to demonstrate the presence of bromides in the lesion) and, above all, on the well-known *"albo-papuloid bullous atrophic cutaneous dystrophy"* he described in 1927.

His studies in the fields of clinical and experimental syphilis, cutaneous mycosis and tuberculosis and the description of *"albo papuloid"* form of epidermolysis bullosa are also notable. Besides his remarkable clinical achievements, he was a man of broad culture, a sociologist, a famous teacher and Editor of the *Italian Journal of Dermatology and Syphilology*.* LUIS ENRIQUE PIERINI was born on July 3, 1899, in Montecassiano, a small town in the Commune of Macerata, Province of Ancona, Italy.

At the age of 3 months he moved with his parents and brothers to Argentina, and they established their residence in the town of Dolores, 200 Km from the city of Buenos Aires.

When he was 16 years old he began his studies of Medicine at the University of Buenos Aires, where he obtained his M.D. in 1923.

His first steps in Dermatology were accomplished under the guidance of Professor Maximiliano Aberastury, a pioneer in the fight against leprosy. Syphilis and leprosy were, at the time of Luis Pierini, the most frequent cause for hospitalization. He worked at the Infectious Diseases' "Francisco Muñiz" Hospital, where he described the Histamine test that allows the early diagnosis of leprosy, by demonstrating the absence of nerve conduction in the Lewis' triple response.

In 1929 he was appointed as Head of Service of Dermatology at the Pediatric Hospital of the Beneficence Society of Buenos Aires, where he had to deal with a tinea capitis epidemic of around 2,000 cases that he treated with thallium acetate instead of the X ray treatment that was the mainstay of the time.

---

* Personal communication, Professor Ruggero Caputo, Milan.

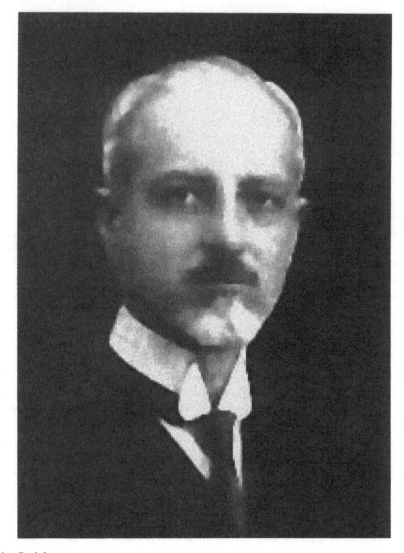

Figure 112 Agostino Pasini

Between 1943 and 1949 he was Head of the Department of Dermatology at the Italian Hospital, and after 1949 he was the Chairman and Professor of Dermatology at the "Guillermo Rawson" Hospital in Buenos Aires.

His career in the Faculty of Medicine of the University of Buenos Aires began under the guidance of Professor Pedro Baliña, and he rose to the highest position of Professor of the Graduate Chair of Dermatology in 1949.

He started an Annual Course of Dermatology that every November gathers dermatologists from all over the country and Latin America. This course has been continued by his successors until today, and it has been named "Curso de Perfeccionamiento Dermatológico Luis E Pierini" in his homage.

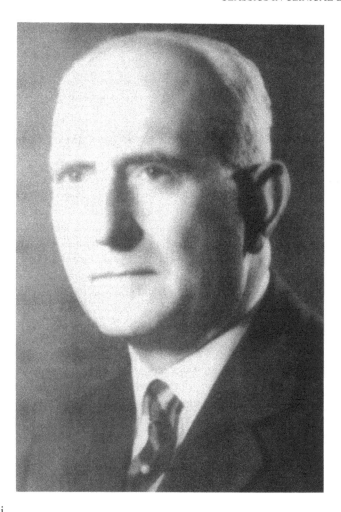

Figure 113 Luis E.Pierini

With a small group of pupils he founded a journal, *Archives Argentinos de Dermatología,* providing a site for the exchange of experiences between dermatologists of Argentina and Latin America.

Luis E.Pierini, "Don Luis" to his pupils, and "Gigio" to his relatives, was a simple man, extremely modest, not only fully dedicated to his profession but also with great interest for the arts. He loved literature, music and plastic art. He always said that he loved Dermatology because it presents a great canvas where different artists have expressed their impressions: the Renaissance represented by the balanced and well defined lesions of the pityriasis rosea, Impressionism expressed through the ill delineated cutis marmorata, and Surrealism seen in the factitial dermatoses.

He also liked to be remembered for his modest origins, and he dedicated much of his time to the care of the poor people. Probably because of this contact and his interest in all the matters dealing with the development of the humanity he became an expert in "the lunfardo" (the "slang" of Buenos Aires lower class), and was a full member of the Argentine Academy of Lunfardo.

He died in Buenos Aires, July 10, 1987, leaving an incomparable heritage, which includes his grand-nephew, Adrian-Martin Pierini, Secretary General of the 21 st World Congress of Dermatology to be held in Buenos Aires, October 1–5, 2007.*

ATROPHODERMA OF PASINI AND PIERINI

Atrofodermia Idiopatica Progressiva (Studio Clinico ed Istologico)[†]
Professor A.Pasini

Case Report. M.Rosa, a 21-year-old unmarried girl, a weaver from Lonate Pozzolo (Milan), seen on June 19, 1922.

The cutaneous eruption had first appeared about 4 years ago. The girl was recovering from influenza and broncho-pneumonia of the left side. The first lesions came out on the back between the scapulae and became evident with a slight feeling of warmth and tingling. Giving a look at that body site she saw a small round spot with a light blue cyanotic lesion, slightly depressed from the surrounding skin. There was no evidence of inflammation in the depressed lesion nor in the surrounding area. From then on the depression slowly enlarged in a continuous fashion with relapses and remissions from the upper part of the back to the lower part, to the sacral region, to the sternum, to the right shoulder and around the trunk, like a belt. The disease slowly progressed with subtle and asymptomatic progression, but with no inflammation or symptoms other than a slight sense of warmth, sometimes with itching and the appearance of a light blue color, and atrophic thinning of the skin.

Current Description of the Dermatosis. The eruption is actually composed of several large areas of cutaneous atrophy with thinning and depression of the skin without any change in firmness or appearance, other than a change in the color between cyanotic and light blue.

In the other parts of the skin the patient had a normal white coloring with no pigmentation, with a thick subcutaneous fat layer, good elasticity, but diminished sweat and sebaceous secretion. The pilosebaceous unit is normal with ordinary fine hair of brown color.

The responses to touch, temperature and pain are normal. There is an intense dermographism, which causes urticaria in the scratched area, with an erythematous border 3–4 mm all around. The reaction appears immediately after the scratching and lasts 10–15 minutes.

The normal appearance of the uninvolved skin results in an enhanced contrast with the areas of the skin that have become atrophic.

The involved areas have all the same appearance and with the exception of size and dimension; they are all monomorphic. They all appear depressed below the skin surface, with an abrupt border that defines the normal skin from the affected area without any sign of inflammation or dermo-epidermic infiltration, and without signs of visible erythema in the atrophic skin or on any part of the normal skin. In the atrophic areas there is a difference of 1–2 millimeters between the pathologic and normal skin.

The depressed skin is flat, smooth, and regular, with no change in keratinization and is in no part scarred. In the involved areas all the glandular ducts are present, even if they are less than in the normal skin and the skin ridges are also normal. Consistency and elastic properties are normal and if you pull the atrophic skin, it returns quickly to its location.

---

* Pierini, A.-M., Personal communication.

[†] Gior. Ital. Mal. Vener., *64:*785, 1923.

What you can see on the atrophic skin, other than some thinning, is a certain transparency of the skin that allows the observer to see some slight blood stasis without seeing any specific vessels. The atrophic patches have a diffuse light-blue color, similar to *"maculae ceruleae"* that allows one to see them clearly even from some distance.

The skin of the atrophic patches is also different from normal due to a slight tingling sensation and sometimes a sense of warmth, as compared to normal skin. The atrophic patches have normal sensitivity and there is no difference between the atrophic and normal areas regarding the dermographism reported above.

The normal skin changes into the atrophic with an abrupt edge, and in many places with an indentation with the outer borders, not very regular, sometimes sinuous, but never with dendritic aspect. The altered skin involves many body sites with large areas. The biggest atrophic area is on the back. From the infrascapular region the area goes down involving almost all the back, more on the right side and below the lumbar line the area divides itself in two parallel and lateral longitudinal patches that curve around the abdomen to join at the umbilicus.

Another large atrophic patch can be found at the sacral area with an irregular ellipsoid shape with a transverse diameter of 14 cm. A third large area almost round, with a diameter of 7 cm lies between the two areas described above the sacral area, to the right side of the back. Other large areas occupy the entire right deltoid region and the sternal region. Some smaller areas, all round or round-like, with the size of a pea to a coin are rare. Seven are on the trunk and nine over the arms, on the extensor and also the flexor side. The patches are not symmetric and are not in a distribution that is related to the nervous system.

Dermatoscopic Examination. Under dermatoscopic examination with an intense light a good distribution of superficial arterial vessels can be visualized on the normal skin that surrounds the atrophic areas with red vessels normally shaped with a linear distribution. In the atrophic areas the vessels are even more abundant, a little larger and dilated, with a tortuous distribution, almost cirsoid. This distribution is more pronounced over the papillary ridges, less pronounced in the interpapillary spaces.

Summary. After an intense investigation and a good clinical observation Pasini thinks he has found a pathogenic and perhaps also an etiologic relation between the cutaneous atrophy and the existence of clinically invisible microscopic inflammatory processes, with a specific inflammation only after an injection of tuberculin. The cutaneous atrophy is idiopathic only from a clinical point of view but is probably related to a chronic dermal inflammation. This is caused by a tuberculous process, virtually not apparent elsewhere in the body. Hence, these clinical features can be related to the tuberculids with a cutaneous atrophy secondary to that process.

ATROPHODERMA OF PASINI AND PIERINI

Atrofodermia Idiopatica Progressiva (Pasini)*
Luis E.Pierini and Donate Vivoli

Case Report. This is a 19-year-old woman with antecedent tuberculosis and signs of a chronic left pleuritis. Approximately 4 years ago there had been the appearance and enlargement of large areas of cutaneous atrophy, especially on the trunk, without any sign of clinically relevant inflammation or any other disease, and characterized by a marked decrease in skin thickness with a depression of the skin level from the surrounding skin and by a peculiar clear colour similar to the one caused by the *Pthirus pubis* (body louse). The atrophic skin retains its elasticity and softness and there is no tendency to sclerosis. The dermatoscopic examination reveals oedema of the capillaries and a serpiginous pattern of these same vessels in the atrophic areas. There are no neurologic alterations. Blood and urine tests are normal. A sympathic-hormonal test reveals a sympathomimetic tendency of possible suprarenal origin. The Wassermann and Sachs-Georgi tests are negative. The intradermal reaction to human tuberculin is positive, with fever during the time of the reaction in the skin surrounding the atrophic areas, with small intradermal inflammatory lesions visible through the normal epidermis. Transplants in guinea pigs are negative. Histologically, there is a reduction of the thickness of the reticular dermis in the atrophic areas but with no degeneration of the connective tissue and the collagen, and with perfect preservation of the elastic tissues. In all areas that appear thicker there is a decrease of reticular dermis. There is vasodilatation with a slight stasis in the deep blood vessels of the atrophic skin. There are small and isolated areas of infiltration in the reticular dermis consisting of small round mononuclear cells with no relation to known diseases. Microorganisms are absent.

Summary. Treatment consisting of the injection of extracts of the anterior lobe of the pituitary and the x-ray irradiation of the dorsal column slows the progression of new lesions as well as ameliorating those already present.

In our opinion, this unusual case appears to be similar to that described in 1926 by Pasini, and to which he gave the name *"atrofodermia idiopatica progressiva."*

---

* Gior. Ital. Derm., *77:*403, 1936.

Louis A. Brunsting

Pyoderma Gangrenosum

LOUIS ALBERT BRUNSTING was born in Grand Rapids, Michigan on July 7, 1900. He received his M.D. from the University of Michigan and his dermatologic training at the Mayo Graduate School of Medicine. He joined the staff of the Mayo Clinic in 1930 and remained associated with that institution for the next 35 years. By 1953 he was Chief of the Section of Dermatology, a position he held until his retirement in 1962. His remarkable clinical acumen manifested itself early. While still a resident, he observed and linked together five cases of chronic ulceration to create a "new" dermatologic entity, *pyoderma gangrenosum*. His creation, noted below, has stood the test of time.

Brunsting also made valuable contributions to our knowledge of scleroderma, lupus erythematosus, and porphyria. His name is associated as well with the localized form of bullous pemphigoid known as *"Brunsting-Perry disease,"* which he described in collaboration with his associate at Mayo, Harold O. Perry.

In 1965, Brunsting escaped from the frigidities of the North and set up a private practice in Tucson, Arizona. He retired in 1976 and moved to San Diego, California, where he died on October 8, 1980. We remember his crinkly smile and his taut comment, "You are not a leader, if no one follows you."*

PYODERMA GANGRENOSUM

Pyoderma (Echthyma) Gangrenosum*

The term "pyoderma" denotes a purulent infection of the skin due to pyogenic organisms, usually staphylococci. During the last two or three years we have observed a number of rare instances of extensive sloughing ulceration of the skin, similar in many respects to fulminating echthyma gangrenosum, but essentially a form of pyoderma in which the hemolytic streptococcus and staphylococcus were found repeatedly.

Besides the cutaneous lesions, each patient presented a serious infectious process of longstanding elsewhere in the body, which served to prepare the way for the ulcerations of the skin by producing marked constitutional debility. During the period of observation in each case throughout a series of exacerbations

---

* Crissey, J.T., et al: Historical Atlas of Dermatology and Dermatologists. Parthenon, 2002.

* Arch. Dermatol. Syphilol., *22*:655, 1930.

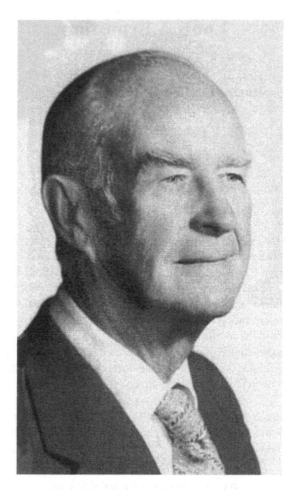

Figure 114 Louis A.Brunsting

and remission it appeared evident that there was a parallel relationship between the underlying debilitating disease and the cutaneous manifestations.

Of the five patients whose cases form the basis of this report, four had chronic ulcerative colitis, with recurrences dating back over a period of from two to nine years; the other had empyema of six months' duration following influenza. The latter patient died following an attempt to drain the empyema cavity. The others were under observation in the hospital for many months because of the ulcerations of the skin and the bowel, and afforded opportunity for ample study.

The bowel appeared to be the site of the major nidus of infection, control of which was essential to the successful management of the entire problem, including the ulcerating pyoderma. The activity of the cutaneous lesions at any one time depended on the particular state of the underlying disease.

During the most active stage of ulceration, the lesions of the skin presented an unusual appearance. They were single or multiple and sometimes involved the entire extent of the abdominal or thoracic wall. The borders of the ulcers were well defined because of their striking blue color, which clearly outlined the lesion as it extended peripherally in rough serpiginous configuration. The blue zone consisted of an edematous boggy strip from 5 to 8 mm wide in which there had been extensive undermining and necrosis of the subcutaneous tissue, the epidermis remaining as a thin, gray, translucent film extending over the crater of the lesion in a ragged, irregular fashion. On the advance of the undermining process, often at the rate of 1 to 2 cm in twenty-four hours, a zone of erythema extended as an areola into the area of normal skin.

The base was moist and covered with mucopurulent exudate of pus and tissue debris, which extended from the area of necrosis. Pressure on the border caused considerable gelatinous pus to ooze into the wound. Granulations were dependent on the stage of activity of the ulceration as a whole. During the acute phase they were digested away, when the advance was less active and the general condition of the patient improved, the granulations appeared in profusion.

Healing occurred by epithelial outgrowths from the periphery, with resulting thin, atrophic scarring, with some brownish pigmentation. After healing the scars maintained the serpiginous outline, making them practically indistinguishable in themselves from a syphilitic scar. In certain areas healing was delayed and small fistulous tracts remained, from which pus could be obtained on pressure. In such areas the epidermis and scar tissue would frequently assume a vegetative or verrucous character, similar to that seen in dermatitis vegetans.

Certain of the patients did not have elementary lesions. It was during a stage of acute exacerbation in one of the cases that the essential features in the production of the ulcers could be followed. The lesions appeared in crops as small, discrete pustules surrounded by an inflammatory areola. Within a few days the center of the pustule softened and the covering skin became blue and broke down. The lesion either underwent involution or extended peripherally to coalesce with others adjoining to form a larger, superficial ulcerative process, as described.

Friederich Wegener

Wegener's Granulomatosis

FRIEDERICH WEGENER, noted German pathologist, was born in Veral, Oldenburg 7 April 1907. Son of a well-known physician, he studied medicine in Munich and Kiel and graduated as M.D. in 1932. In 1935 he accepted a teaching position in Breslau and during this period published his minutely detailed classic 1939 report on "Wegener's granulomatosis." He himself never used that eponymic term, but the condition is so firmly associated with its describer that it appears to have no other official name. Case 2 from the report, shown below, displays the key elements associated with the disease.

Wegener served as a pathologist in the German army in World War II, and was taken prisoner by the British. He returned to civilian life and eventually became Professor at the Lübeck Medical Academy.

Wegener was a large man, big enough to be dubbed by colleagues "the Max Schmeling of German pathologists." He was a noted athlete and a life-long physical fitness enthusiast and Turn Verein booster. He participated in many sports and in 1931 became the German hammer-throwing champion. In retirement he enjoyed the affection of 17 grandchildren. Wegener suffered a severe stroke in May 1990 and died two months later.*

WEGENER'S GRANULOMATOSIS

Ueber eine eigenartige rhinogene Granulomatose mit besonderer Beteiligung des Arteiensystems und der Nieren*

Case 2. 36 year old housewife. Scarlet fever as a child. Questionable arthritis in 1926. Present illness began as a cold early in December 1935, accompanied at first by a mucoid secretion of pus and later by a dry nose. Staff examination in March 1936: inflammatory changes in the mucous membrane of the septum and both lower turbinates, perforation of the septum. The picture more or less resembled gummatous destruction. Wassermann reaction was negative. Biopsy showed non-specific granulation tissue. In mid-April, second day in the Ear Clinic: Patient in poor condition, fever, shaking chills. Admitted to the Medical Clinic. The interior of the nose was covered with malodorous crusts. Perforation of the septum, streaks of puss on the posterior part of the throat. A cough began, productive of mucoid pus.

---

* Dtsch. Med. Wochenschr., *116:*113, 1991

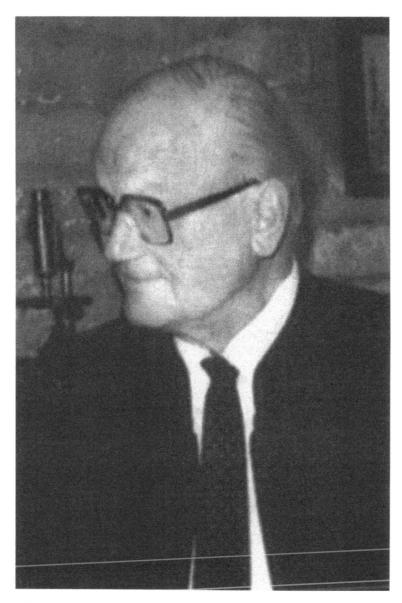

Figure 115 Friederich Wegener

Septic clinical picture: T. 38.5–39.8°. Agglutinations for typhus, paratyphus, dysentery, Flexner, Y., Bang and Weil negative. EKG showed myocardial damage. Anemia (2,840,000 erythrocytes, Hb 48%). Leucocytosis (16,200) Differential: Segmenteds 74%, lymphocytes 18%, eosinophils 5%, Basophils 1%. Sed Rate (Westergren) 44/90. Blood pressure R.R. 90/60. Besredka positive. Urine: positive for albumen. Sediment: erythrocytes, leucocytes, and isolated hyaline cylinders. Pain in the right kidney region. 23/IV Roentgenologic evidence of bronchopneumonia of the left lower lobe. Throat swab: Di negative. Sputum:

tbc negative; pneumostreptococci negative. On 8 V. *Staphylococcus aureus* and non-hemolytic streptococci. 15. V. more Gram-positive cocci along with leptothrix and streptothrix bacilli. 3.VI. Streptococci, pneumococci, and leptothrix.

Therapy: roentgen radiation of the left lower breast area. 30. V. Concentration test: Isosthenuria confirmed. From the beginning of June: profuse nasal secretions, cough, large amounts of malodorous sputum. One week before death a pustular skin eruption appeared. 15. VI. Patient expired."

Similarly, a skin eruption appeared in Case 3, a 33 year old housewife, shortly before death: "A hazel-nut size, elevated lesion, crusted and bleeding slightly, was present over the right parietal bone. Bluish colored blisters were present on the left cheek and on the left back. On pressure they exuded blackish colored blood."

Albert Sézary

Sézary's Syndrome (T-cell Erythroderma)

ALBERT SÉZARY (1880–1956) was born and raised in Algiers. A brilliant student, he pursued his medical studies in Paris, rose steadily through the standard hospital ranks to Professor agrégé in 1927, and served as Physician to l'Hôpital St. Louis from 1928 to 1945. He learned his dermatology on the service of Edouard Jeanselme, whom he succeeded. Sézary also had credentials in neurology, having served some two years as an interne under Joseph Jules Déjerine.

Author of more than 800 publications that are remarkably diverse in nature, Sézary was equally at home in the worlds of neurology, venereology, endocrinology, hematology, and dermatology. The latter two disciplines are combined harmoniously in his many studies on the malignant cutaneous reticuloses that resulted in the classic 1938 report on "Sézary's syndrome," noted below.

Throughout his life, Sézary maintained the traditions and friendships of his Algerian origins, and he did much to acquaint his French-born associates with the outstanding talents available among their colleagues to the South.*

On December 1, 1956, Sézary died in his beloved Paris.

SÉZARY'S SYNDROME

Erythrodermie avec Presence de Cellules Monstreuses dans le Derme et le Sang Circulant*

We are presenting today an unusual case of erythroderma characterized by the presence of giant cells in the dermis and circulating blood which, it seems, do not appear to belong to the blood line, but could, from their appearance, be considered as neoplastic.

P., 58 years of age, a factory guard, consulted us on November 25, 1937 for a generalized erythroderma that began in September 1937. The first symptom she noticed was itching, which began in July. This itching, which was severe enough to interfere with sleep was limited at first to the interscapular area.

Redness appeared in the same area around the 15th of September. This erythema spread slowly, encircling the waist first, then the shoulders and upper extremities, flanks, and abdomen. It spread next to

---

* Bull. Soc. Fr. Dermatol Syphilig., *66:*6, 1957.

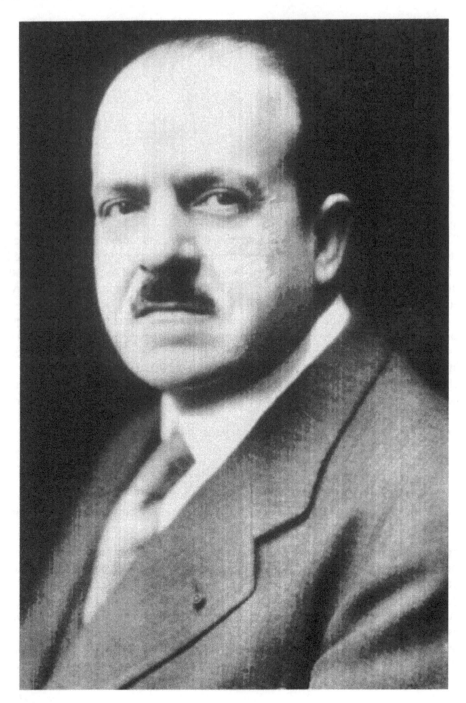

Figure 116 Albert Sézary

the lower extremities, and finally the face. As the erythema continued to extend little by little to involve the entire integument, the itching diminished and finally disappeared almost completely.

The erythroderma reached its final stage of development around November 13, some two months after it began; it was accompanied by neither fever nor any sort of illness. Since then the eruption has remained unchanged and, discouraged by its persistence, the patient decided November 25 to enter l'Hôpital St. Louis.

Her condition at that time was as follows. The patient is a rather obese woman, whose skin is bright red in color, truly boiled lobster-like. The hue is slightly violaceous in the folds, dependent parts, and distal areas of the extremities. The face and neck are uniformly red, the scalp a little less so. The color is also a little less intense on the shoulders, the deltoid and axillary areas, and on the palms and soles, which are, however, definitely involved.

On palpation, elevation of local temperature is clearly evident. The redness can be made to disappear with vitro-pression, but with difficulty.

In addition, a nearly generalized edema is evident. Infiltration is particularly evident in the face, where puffiness of the eyelids is striking, the abdominal wall, on which numerous stretch marks stand out clearly in relief, and finally, on the legs and the dorsum of the feet. For the most part, the edema is firm; it can, however, be made to pit on pressure over the anterior surface of the tibia.

There is little desquamation, but at the same time it cannot be said to be completely absent. In fact, a number of very small and fine, dry, white scales are evident on the face, anterior surface of the thighs and legs, and also on the epigastrium. Everywhere else they are absent, and to the touch the skin feels dry.

Superimposed on the erythematous background, a large number of small, punctiform, purpuric spots can be seen; they are more evident following vitro-pression. These miniscule petechiae, which appear following the application of pressure, are particularly numerous on the ankles and legs in an area extending above to garter level. They can also be found on the palms and soles.

This erythroderma appears to be directly attributable to the presence in the dermis of giant cells with a large nucleus, notched or bearing small rounded or angular extensions. The protoplasm of these cells is hyaline, scanty, and arranged in bands, or strips. The exact nature of these cells has not been determined. We have also found them in abundance in circulating blood.

* Bull. Soc. Fr. Dermatol. Syphiligr., *45*:254, 1938.

Masao Ota

Nevus Fusco-coeruleus Ophthalmomaxillaris, Oculodermal Melanocytosis (Nevus of Ota)

MASAO OTA was born in Ito-City, Shizuoka Prefecture, Japan on August 1, 1885. He grew up to be a unique individual with a distinguished career in two totally disparate fields, viz., dermatology and literature. His name at birth is known to every dermatologist worldwide, but it is under the pen name of *Mokutaro Kinoshita* that a wide Japanese readership knows him. It was his Kinoshita who wrote novels, poems, and essays, which in the lifetime aggregate were published in a complete series, comprising 25 volumes. He also wrote an *Atlas of 100 Herbals*.

To turn to his parallel career in dermatology, Ota received his M.D. in 1911 and then trained under the world renowned Professor Dohi at the University of Tokyo (then known as the Tokyo Imperial University). Dohi was the father of the specialty of dermatology in Japan and Ota was one of his brilliant students destined to ascend to the same chair as Dohi in 1937. Before that he was Professor of Dermatology at the South Manchurian Medical College (1918–1926), a research fellow at the Pasteur Institute in Paris (1921–24), Professor of Dermatology in Nagoya (1924–28), and later Sendai (1926–37).

Throughout all this he inspired and trained scores of students and residents. His special skills centered on the classification of fungi, recognized by France which awarded him their Legion of Honor Medal in 1941. In 1937 he had already written his classic description of what came to be known as the *Nevus of Ota*. It was only 15 years later that a Japanese colleague, Ito, received eponymic recognition for describing the same type of nevus localized to the shoulder.

Ota/Kinoshita died on October 15, 1945 in Tokyo, a victim of cancer of the stomach, but his name and writings live on in two worlds.*

NEVUS FUSCO-COERULEUS OPHTHALMOMAXILLARIS

The Relationship of the Common Japanese Nevus Fusco-Coeruleus Ophthalmomaxillaris to Eye Pigmentation*

Cases. Based on a study of 26 patients we can categorize into four types the congenital brownish-blue pigmentation of the orbital, periorbital and maxillary regions. As shown in the illustration Type la shows

---

* Kukita, A.Emeritus Chairman of Dermatology, Tokyo University, Personal Communication.

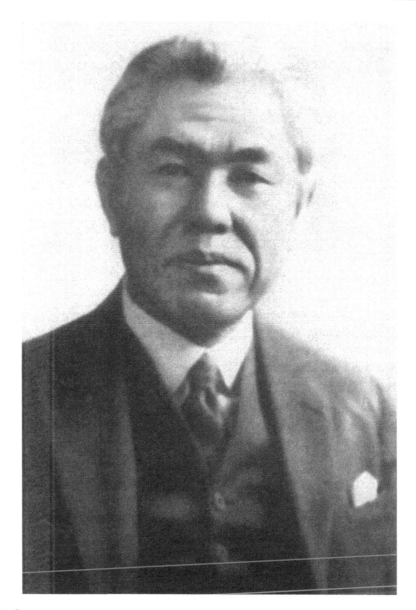

Figure 117 Masao Ota

mild pigmentation distributed in the periorbital area and was seen in 7 patients. Type Ib involves the cheek and was seen in 5 patients.

Type II, seen in 7 patients presents a medium degree of pigmentation and Type III shows a more extensive and intensive pigmentary change. Type IV shows bilateral pigmentation. IV is the rarest and was seen in only 3 patients.

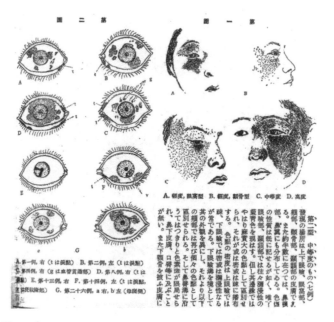

Figure 118 Ota's original illustration

Ocular melanosis was a common finding. The varied associated eyeball pigmentation patterning seen in these patients is shown in the illustration.

These pigmentary changes were seen at birth in 17 infants. The remaining 9 developed the discoloration later. There appears to be no hereditary cause. Only 2 female cousins presented with this nevus.

Malignant change was not observed in any instance.

---

* Tokyo Med. J., *63:*1243, 1939 (in Japanese).

S. William Becker

1.   Necrolytic Migratory Erythema (Glucagonoma Syndrome)

2.   Becker's Nevus (Melanosis and Hypertrichosis)

SAMUEL WILLIAM BECKER was born on July 11, 1894 in Benton Harbor, Michigan. As a boy his interest was in radio and electrical engineering, but following his father's wishes he earned an M.A. and M.D. from the University of Michigan in 1920. His dermatologic training was under John H.Stokes at the Mayo Clinic and Bruno Bloch in Zurich, Switzerland. He returned to be the first head of the Department of Dermatology at the University of Chicago, where he remained for 15 years. During this period he pioneered in instructing the public about the threat of syphilis with his 1937 book, *Ten Million Americans Have It*. By 1940 his classic textbook, *Modern Dermatology and Syphilology* had appeared. All this time he was instrumental in founding *The Society for Investigative Dermatology* and establishing the first dermatopathology laboratory in Chicago. He was a master teacher. No patient of his ever left without an awareness of the physiologic factors in psychosomatic disease. "Don't sweat the small stuff" could have been his mantra. No resident ever left without an appreciation of his imagery that seborrheic keratosis is the benign equivalent of basal cell carcinoma.

In 1942, he passed the torch of his chairmanship to Stephen Rothman while he pursued private practice. In 1955, his academic reincarnation took place in California as Chair in Dermatology at the Long Beach Veterans Administration Hospital. With the title of Professor at the University of Southern California he taught countless students and residents the arcane magic of his world of clinical care, library research and chess. An additional joy was seeing his son, Samuel, and his daughter, Bess, become accomplished dermatologists. He worked ceaselessly until only a few weeks before his death on August 15, 1964 from a coronary occlusion. His mind was never to wear out, only his heart.*

NECROLYTIC MIGRATORY ERYTHEMA (GLUCAGONOMA SYNDROME)

Cutaneous Manifestations of Internal Malignant Tumors*

Case 1. Mrs. C.F., a Polish housewife aged 45, was admitted to the University of Chicago clinics on Jan. 2, 1940 with a widespread symmetric eruption, which had started eight months previously. She had lost 17 pounds (7.7 Kg.) during this period and had noticed increasing weakness for several months. In May 1939 a

---

* Arch. Dermatol., *91*:97, 1965.

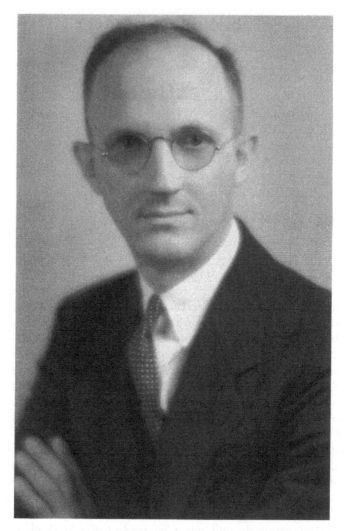

Figure 119 S.William Becker

pruritic erythematovesicular eruption with exudation appeared on the dorsa of the feet. Four exposures to roentgen rays and the application of numerous ointments gave only temporary relief. After one or two months, red scaly "spots that later turned brown" extended up the leg toward the groin. One month prior to admittance, similar lesions appeared on the sides of the chest and later in the anal crease, in the groins and about the vulva. A finely vesicular patchy eruption then appeared on the dorsa of the hands and fingers. All the lesions were so pruritic that at times they interfered with sleep.

Examination revealed symmetric diffuse erythema on the dorsa of the hands, fingers and feet with tiny vesicles and serous crusting. The dorsum of the right foot exhibited a punched-out ulcer, 0.75 to 1 cm in diameter, with a fairly clean granulating base and an elevated firm rolled border. The fingernails and toenails were distorted, with pitting, longitudinal striae and deposits of yellowish white grumous material beneath the nails.

Macular erythema with few large scales were present in widespread patchy distribution on the thighs and legs. Annular erythema with central clearing and small sanguineous crusts occurred below each patella. The groins, gluteal folds and vulva exhibited diffuse erythema, edema and serous crusting. Numerous scattered patches consisting of papules and macular lesions with some brownish crusts were present on the trunk. There was perioral perlèche. The tip and the lateral borders of the tongue were red, smooth and tender.

Monilia was demonstrated in the nail scrapings and later cultured in material from the lesions of perlèche and from those in the groin and on the tongue. Repeated cultures of material from the other cutaneous lesions and from those developing subsequently showed no organisms. The routine intracutaneous dermotrichophytin (Bischoff) test gave a strongly positive reaction.

During six weeks in the hospital, the dermatosis at first became more widespread with extension of the pruritic erythematous macular lesions over the trunk anteriorly and posteriorly. Many of these lesions then became purpuric and later large confluent patches showing superficial necrosis resulted. The necrotized epidermis formed a thin dark crust, which was cast off in a few days, and healing occurred with hyperpigmentation. These necrotic lesions resembled a superficial chemical burn in their appearance and course. Meanwhile an erythematous papulovesicular eruption appeared on the cheeks and across the bridge of the nose.

A biopsy specimen from an area of superficial necrosis on the abdomen showed the following picture. The pathologic changes were confined to the superficial portion of the section. The stratum corneum was thick, parakeratotic and acidophilic throughout. In one place it had been loosened by a collection of serum. The stratum mucosum was of about normal thickness and showed an increased number of mitotic figures in the basal portion. The papillae were edematous; the capillaries were dilated, and the endothelial cells were swollen. The vessels of the superficial cutis also showed endothelial swelling, perivascular edema and moderate perivascular infiltrate with round cells. The deeper portions of the section were essentially normal. A diagnosis of subacute dermatitis was made.

The following features were observed in a biopsy specimen from a crusted lesion on the chest. The stratum corneum was greatly thickened, parakeratotic and separated into several layers by collections of serum and remnants of what appeared to have been mononucleated cells. The stratum corneum had been separated from the stratum granulosum in some places by serum. The stratum granulosum was irregularly thickened and thinned and in some places showed liquefaction necrosis with practical disappearance. There was intercellular and intracellular edema, chiefly the former. There was an abnormally large number of mitotic figures in the basal portion. The papillae were edematous. The papillary and subpapillary layers of the cutis were involved in polymorphonuclear leukocytic infiltration. The blood vessels showed endothelial swelling and a perivascular round cell infiltrate. A diagnosis of acute and subacute exudative dermatitis was made.

Local treatment consisted of local applications, roentgen irradiation and ultraviolet irradiation; systemic medication consisted of iodides, ferrous sulfate and a high vitamin diet, reinforced by vitamin B complex and ascorbic acid. The anemia persisted (hemoglobin, 10 to 11 gm.) despite iron therapy and two transfusions. The white blood cell count was 6,000 to 8,400 at first and later 11,500, with 60 to 70 percent polymorphonuclear neutrophils and 0 to 3 percent eosinophils.

Although the skin cleared considerably, no general improvement was evident. However, the termination was rather sudden. During the hospital stay there developed an unusual tendency of the patient's blood to clot rapidly (clotting time on admission, two minutes and thirty seconds, and on February 7, thirty-four

---

* Arch. Dermatol. and Syphilol. *45*:1069, 1945.

seconds). Her left leg became swollen and dusky overnight, and the arteries, pulseless. Then the arteries of the right leg became pulseless. Acute thrombosis of the left iliac vein was diagnosed. Death ensued several hours later, on February 14, the picture being that of circulatory collapse and respiratory failure.

Postmortem examination revealed a neoplasm replacing the body and tail of the pancreas, with invasion of the adjacent lymph nodes and the left adrenal gland. Microscopic study suggested the islet cell type of pancreatic carcinoma.

Comment. The interpretation of case 1 is extremely difficult because of the complexity of the pathogenic factors (pancreatic neoplasm, metabolic changes, signs of deficiency disease and monilia infection) and because of the multiplicity of the cutaneous changes. These lesions do not correspond to those observed in other cases in which there were eruptions due to internal neoplasms. Although the two cardinal symptoms of such eruptions—intense pruritus and accentuated hyperpigmentation—were also present in our patient, the morphologic aspect and the course of the eruption seemed to be unique, not only in connection with internal neoplasms but also in general. Especially, the diffuse progressive epidermal necrosis with consecutive hyperpigmentation similar to a chemical burn seemed to be an entirely new manifestation, which up to the present time has not been described as occurring in moniliasis or in any dermatosis of internal origin.

Cutaneous changes due to pancreatic neoplasm have not been described as yet, and the peculiarity of the eruption may be due to the site of the tumor in the pancreas. It is probable that the disturbance in carbohydrate metabolism (mild borderline diabetes) was due to the neoplasm and that the monilial infection might have been a consequence of the metabolic disturbance. A further consequence of pancreatic insufficiency might have been deficiency symptoms. The following observations are from the autopsy report by Dr. Humphreys of the Department of Pathology:

"There is no direct evidence (diarrhea or fatty stools) pointing to an exocrine defect. However, it is not impossible that there was some digestive-absorptive defect. The character of lesions of the lip and tongue and of some of those on the skin, the atrophic gastritis and the slight metaplasia in the tongue, esophagus and pancreatic ducts all suggest deficiency disease. Also, the improvement in the cutaneous lesions while the patient was on the vitamin-reinforced diet should be noted. There is no doubt that moniliasis (superficial) was responsible for some of the lesions; however, it was probably secondary —superimposed on mild diabetes and/or a deficiency disease."

Thus, a comment on our first case seems to be impossible at present and we restrict ourselves to the recording of it. Only the observation of other cases of pancreatic tumor will decide whether the cutaneous changes in our case were primarily due to the neoplasm.

BECKER'S NEVUS

Concurrent Melanosis and Hypertrichosis in Distribution of Nevus Unius Lateris*

Case 1. G.B., a boy aged 17, had had alopecia areata at the age of 12, with recurrence of the disorder at 16. At the age of 11, after severe sunburn, a blotchy brown area developed over the right shoulder. Two years later, hair grew in the area. Since that time, the patient had been treated for nephrolithiasis, injury to the semilunar cartilage of the right knee and Bell's palsy.

---

* Arch. Dermatol. Syphilol., *60:*155, 1949.

Clinical Examination. There was patchy, light brown pigmentation over the right shoulder, extending from the midline down onto the arm. The central area was more diffuse, while the periphery showed islands of hyperpigmentation with their long axes in the lines of cleavage. The pigmentation appeared more pronounced about the follicles. In the pigmented plaques were numerous short, heavy, black hairs, their presence more pronounced near the center. There were no subjective symptoms. For this reason, and because the area was covered by the clothing, no treatment was attempted.

Microscopic Examination. Sections stained with hemalum, erythrosine and saffron revealed no alteration of the epidermis or dermis, except that there was increased pigment in the basal portion of the epidermis. Sections treated with a 2 percent solution of silver nitrate for two hours and fixed with a cold saturated solution of sodium thiosulfate for two minutes showed a large, heavily pigmented hair, with increased melanin in both the epidermis and the superficial dermis. Under high power, the basal cells were seen to contain large amounts of melanin, the pigment often filling the entire cell with the exception of the nuclear region. In some of the basal cells and in some of the more superficial cells, the melanin was localized in nuclear caps. Melanin granules were seen in decreasing numbers in the more superficial cells, even in the stratum corneum. It was difficult to identify melanoblasts, and no dendritic melanoblasts were apparent. The papillae and the superficial dermis contained melanin-laden chromatophores. No nevus cells were seen in either the epidermis or the dermis. The diagnosis was melanosis with hypertrichosis.

Comment. Since the terms "nevus" and "nevoid" have been used rather loosely, the disorder observed in the 2 patients could be called "acquired nevus pigmentosus et pilosus." In an effort to establish pathologic designations for various forms of nevi, such as those of the vascular variety, Becker and Obermayer stated, "Thus we suggest that the term nevus should be used only to designate nevus unius lateris and nevus pigmentosus." Nevus pigmentosus always contains nevus cells. They suggested confining the designation of nevus unius lateris to three types of disorder: (1) verrucous, (2) keratotic and (3) comedonicus. On this basis, the condition reported in this paper would not qualify for the diagnosis of nevus. For this reason, the designation "melanosis and hypertrichosis in distribution of nevus unius lateris" was employed. The preexisting sunburn in both instances is interesting and may have played a role in causing the disorder.

Clarence S. Livingood

Dhobie Dermatitis

CLARENCE S.LIVINGOOD was born on August 7, 1911 in a small town near Philadelphia. After graduating from nearby Ursinus College, he went on to obtain his M.D. and take a 2-year internship and a 3-year residency in Dermatology at the University of Pennsylvania. Working under the world famous syphilologist, John H. Stokes, he pursued his own research interests, developing a topical formulation still sold today as Pragmatar®.

World War II had broken out and Livingood volunteered for service in the Medical Corps in 1941, months before Pearl Harbor. The following year saw publication of his classic *Military Manual for Dermatology,* a straight and simple pictorial guide for the thousands of physicians entering the armed services with marginal knowledge of how to diagnose and treat the skin diseases they were seeing. Although written solely by Livingood, the manual was published with the name of the two ranking dermatologists in the Army and Navy (Pillsbury and Sulzberger) as the senior authors.

Army service in India, where he was Chief of Dermatology for a 2,000-bed hospital, led to his signal contributions on cutaneous diphtheria, dhobie mark dermatitis, and quinacrine dermatitis. By the time of his discharge in 1946, he was Chief Consultant in Dermatology for the U.S. Army.

Livingood's entire academic life was spent at Henry Ford Hospital in Detroit, follo wing brief stays at the University of Pennsylvania, Jefferson Medical School, and the University of Texas in Galveston. In each of these centers he received awards as an outstanding teacher. Always the consummate clinician, Livingood trained over a hundred dermatologists. Meanwhile, as Director of the American Board of Dermatology for nearly 20 years, he brought recognition and distinction to what was formerly a neglected, if not ignored, specialty.

In 1962 Livingood served as Secretary General for the XII International Congress of Dermatology held in Washington, DC. Here, as with the Board, his genius in the use of the telephone and in conducting committee meetings served the world of dermatology well.

But beyond all this he had another life—baseball. He was team physician, confidante, and father figure for the two-time World Championship Detroit Tigers for more than 20 years. He earned the respect, admiration, and love of all the players, managers and owners, even as he did in dermatology.

Working everyday to the very end of his 87 years of life, he died July 27, 1998 in Detroit.*

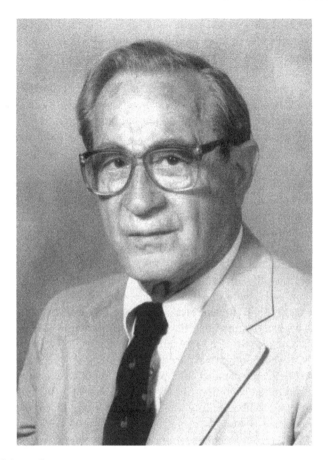

Figure 120 Clarence S.Livingood

DHOBIE DERMATITIS

Dhobie Mark Dermatitis[†]

When the personnel of the 20th General Hospital was first exposed to dhobie laundered clothes, soon after arrival in the C.B.I. theater, a small epidemic of patchy dermatitis made its appearance, which in all instances was distressing and in a few was temporarily incapacitating. The exact localization of the circumscribed patches of dermatitis on that part of the skin in contact with the dhobie mark and the course of the lesions made it quite obvious that this represented a contact dermatitis induced by the marking fluid which the native dhobies or washermen used in making their characteristic laundry marks.

   Clinical Data and Incidence. Of 55 officers exposed there were 11 cases; of 344 men exposed there were 41 cases. The manifestations were similar in all cases and the only variation was in the severity of involvement. Susceptible individuals invariably noted localized pruritus at the site of contact with the mark, sometimes within a few hours after the first exposure but more frequently after one or two exposures extending over a total period of time varying from eight to twenty-four hours. This was followed by localized lesions varying in severity from moderate erythema and edema to definite vesiculation, oozing and crusting. One or more of the following sites was always involved: nape of the neck and upper back, waist line (anterior, posterior or on one side), sides of the ankles, dorsal surface and sides of feet and lower one third of the legs. In every case the sites of the lesions correspond exactly with one or more of the dhobie marks on the recently laundered clothes worn by the individual. In more sensitive persons the dermatitis extended beyond these sites and in a few very sensitive ones a generalized "id" eruption occurred. The pruritus was intense in all cases and in some instances almost intolerable; it increased in severity as exposure to the mark was prolonged and in some cases recurred within thirty minutes after the marked clothes were worn. The itching disappeared and the lesions began to heal as soon as dhobie marked clothing was discarded. A few severe cases, however, required as long as two weeks for complete recovery. Recurrence of lesions was noted promptly if "marked" clothes were again worn.

The Dhobie Mark. The marking fluid used by dhobies throughout India is obtained from the nut of the ral or bella gutti tree, which is said to be common in this country. A straight pin is pushed through the hard capsule of the nut and enough dark brown or black fluid adheres to the pin to make possible the marking of clothes with small crosses, dots or lines in various combinations sufficient to identify the clothing. The marks are fairly permanent and with-stand repeated washings. Khaki shirts and cotton undershirts are usually marked inside the back of the collar, cotton shorts and khaki trousers inside the waistband and socks near the top or sides and occasionally above the heel. There is a common superstition among the natives of this country that the ral or bella gutti tree has strong "likes" and "dislikes" for certain individuals, expressing its dislikes by "poisoning" its enemies when they approach the tree. On close questioning of several intelligent natives, we have learned that the poisoning referred to is manifested by itching, edema, erythema and vesiculation on exposed parts. It would seem that the foliage of this tree causes an acute contact dermatitis when sensitive persons are exposed.

Patch Tests. Of previously affected persons, 80.5 percent were positive to patch tests (1 to 4 plus), which duplicated under standard controlled conditions the exposure to marking fluid. The remaining 19.5 percent were positive only when tested with marking fluid obtained from green nuts. Only 13.4 percent of previously exposed but unaffected persons were positive to patch test (1 plus) and in this group all of the reactions were minimal. Marking fluid obtained from green nuts caused a higher percentage of positive patch tests and more pronounced reaction than fluid obtained from older (dried) nuts.

Comment. It has been accepted as a fact that dhobie laundered clothes are responsible for the transmission of fungous infections, particularly tinea cruris. Physicians and laymen alike use the term "dhobie itch" and "tinea cruris" interchangeably, and some extend the use of the term to include epidermophytosis and tinea of the glabrous skin. The Suttons in their authoritative book define the term "dhobie itch" as follows:

"Dhobie itch (washerman's itch) is tropical epidermophytosis, the eczema marginatum of other climates. Owing to warmth and perspiration the symptoms are greatly exaggerated, and violent scratching and secondary pyogenic infection soon render the parts raw and inflamed, often with resultant impetigo, infectious eczematoid dermatitis and even furunculosis."

Strong similarly states:

"Tinea cruris: Under the name "dhobie itch" this fungous affection is probably better known to Europeans than any tropical skin disease. The name "dhobie" or "washerman's itch" has been given on

---

* Arch. Dermatol., *136:*1150, 2000.

† J.A.M.A., *123:*23, 1943.

account of associating it with the infection of the underclothing while being washed with the garments of those who have the affection. This view probably has some foundation but it has been difficult to verify it."

We believe that it is erroneous and misleading to use the term "dhobie itch" as a synonym for cutaneous fungous infections of any type.

Eugene M.Farber

Hypertensive Ulcer

EUGENE MARK FARBER was born in Buffalo, New York on July 24, 1917. He grew up in a family of books, brains, and brothers. Four of his brothers became doctors—one the internationally renowned Sidney Farber, the founder of the field of chemotherapy for cancer and also of eponymic fame: Farber's lipogranulomatosis. The fifth brother became a professor of philosophy. He left his home city to attend college at Oberlin in Ohio, where he excelled in basketball and track. Returning to the University of Buffalo for his M.D., he subsequently took a residency in dermatology at the Mayo Clinic in Rochester, Minnesota. There, he not only published on the previously unrecognized hypertensive ulcer, but also proved the effectiveness of the first antihistaminic, Benadryl®. By 1948 he had joined the faculty at Stanford Medical School in San Francisco. They provided him with only a 4×8 foot cubicle for his research, but it was in a matrix of unmatched intellectual stimuli. He dedicated his life to teaching, clinical care, and basic research, focusing on psoriasis in all its forms.

He trained 180 residents, wrote 225 papers, and centered his attention on ambulatory day-care and self-help workshops for psoriasis patients. Author of a popular book, *Conquering Psoriasis,* he lectured in 44 different countries and received awards and honorary membership in 26 foreign dermatologic societies. He established the first International Symposium on Psoriasis in 1971, which still meets every five years.

When he retired as Professor and Chairman of Dermatology at Stanford he had created a huge world-class center for clinical care and research out of the 32 square feet he had been given 38 years before. Not missing a step, Farber became President of a richly endowed Psoriasis Research Institute, which has provided research scholarships for physicians from more than a dozen countries. His enthusiasm for travel, Stanford sports, and his family remained undiminished until a brain tumor suddenly caused his death on November 10, 2000.*

HYPERTENSIVE ULCER

Ulcer of the Leg due to Arteriosclerosis and Ischemia, Occurring in the Presence of Hypertensive Disease (Hypertensive-Ischemic Ulcers): A Preliminary Report[†]

For several years we have observed a small group of patients who had painful ulcers of the legs, which were difficult to heal and did not fit into any of the usual clinical classifications of ulcers of the leg. The lesions did not have the appearance of typical stasis ulcers but were ischemic and similar to the ulcers that result from spastic or occlusive involvement of the smaller arteries, such as occurs in chronic pernio, livedo

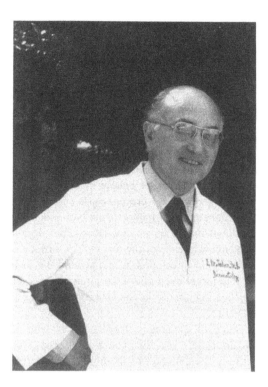

Figure 121 Eugene M.Farber

reticularis or senile changes in the skin. However, in this particular group of patients none had any of the commonly recognized conditions producing ischemic or stasis ulcers and no dermatitis was present. The usual diagnosis was ischemic ulcer of undetermined etiology.

After observation of several patients it was noted that, aside from the fact that they were all women with the same type of ulcer of the legs, they had one condition in common: namely, hypertensive disease of long duration and considerable sclerosis of the retinal arterioles of the chronic hypertensive type. It was postulated that changes similar to those in the retinal arterioles could also occur in the small arteries of the skin and subcutaneous tissues and could give rise to small areas of infarction of the skin. As the result of trauma, or for some unknown reason, the skin might break down and such an ischemic ulcer would form.

We are presenting this group of eleven cases as a possible new syndrome with the hope that additional observation and study will further clarify the cause and treatment of these lesions. Three representative cases will be reported in detail.

Our associate, Dr. Barker, has called our attention to a report by Martorel, which recently arrived in this country. He described a somewhat similar type of ulcer attributed to hypertension, which he had observed in four cases. His cases differed somewhat from ours in that the lesions were usually symmetrical and considerable pigmentation of the skin of the legs was associated.

---

* Arch. Dermatol., *137:*938, 2001.

† Proc. Staff. Mtgs. Mayo Clinic, *21:*377, 1946.

Description of a Typical Lesion. The ulcers often were located on the lateral surface of the ankle, although in four cases the lesion was on the lateral surface of the lower part of the leg, and in two low on the posterior surface of the leg. Lesions ranged in size from about 1 to 7 cm. in diameter. The ulcer usually had a purpuric base and in five cases a purpuric circle surrounded the ulcer. The ulcers were usually superficial and had a rather punched-out appearance. The base of the ulcer appeared to be ischemic and granulation was not extensive. Little serous or purulent exudates were present. The ulcers seemed to enlarge by a process of extension of the purpuric, hemorrhagic portion into the normal skin around the edges of the ulcer and by a subsequent breaking down of the skin. The ulcer was usually painful when fully developed.

Development and Course of Ulcer. The lesion may have been initiated as the result of slight local trauma, although the majority of our patients could remember no injury at the time of onset. Usually, the first abnormality that was observed was a painful red plaque in the skin, which, within a week or ten days, became blue and purpuric, or a plaque was not present but a small, flat area of bluish discoloration of a purpuric nature had appeared spontaneously. A hemorrhagic bleb would develop soon on the surface of the initial lesion and would break down into a superficial ulcer. The ulcer then gradually increased in size, usually by extension around the circumference of the lesion. The surface of the ulcer became sensitive and painful. In several cases sufficient pain developed in and around the lesion to prevent normal use of the extremity. The lesion often became larger even after a program of complete bed rest and local treatment of the ulcer was instituted. When healing finally began, it progressed slowly and from one to six months passed before the lesion healed entirely.

Pathology. Histopathologic study of specimens from the ulcers and of the adjacent skin in five cases revealed organic changes in the arterioles. The most common changes were an increase in the thickness of the arteriolar wall and a decrease in the diameter of the lumen. An increase in the number and size of the nuclei and hyaline degeneration in the media, intimal proliferation and periarteritis also were noted.

Differential Diagnosis From Various Ulcers Primarily Due To Peripheral Vascular Disease. *Stasis ulcers due to chronic venous insufficiency*—In none of our cases was there a history of thrombophlebitis. No evidence of significant varicose veins, or chronic venous insufficiency, such as hyperpigmentation of the skin of the stasis type, of indurated cellulitis or of dermatitis was found. The lesions were usually located in regions not commonly involved in chronic venous insufficiency; that is, on the lateral surface of the leg or ankle or the posterior surface of the leg. In contrast, the usual location of stasis ulcers is now on the medial surface of the leg.

Chronic pernio and livedo reticularis—The lesions in chronic pernio usually are multiple and appear in crops. In contrast, the lesions in our cases were only rarely multiple. The clinical picture typical of livedo reticularis was not present in any of our cases.

Senile ulcers of the skin—Occasionally in aged people, usually those in the eighth and ninth decades of life, ischemic appearing ulcers occur on the extremities. These ulcers are thought to be due to arteriosclerosis involving vessels supplying blood to the skin. Usually trauma is an important factor in initiating and aggravating such lesions. Only one of our patients was more than seventy years of age. The range of age in the group was from forty-three to seventy-three years.

Chronic occlusive arterial disease—It is unusual for localized gangrene or ischemic ulcers to occur around the ankle or in the leg in cases of thrombo-angiitis obliterans or arteriosclerosis obliterans. In these diseases ulcers and localized gangrene are most commonly located on the toes.

Tentative Criteria For Diagnosis. Tentative criteria for the diagnosis of hypertensive-ischemic ulcer of the leg should include (1) hypertension, (2) an ischemic appearing ulcer, (3) indolence of ulcer, (4) moderate to severe pain, (5) poor response to conventional treatment and (6) typical changes of the blood vessels in and near the lesion as indicated by biopsy. The following should be ruled out before the diagnosis is made: (1) significant chronic venous insufficiency, (2) occlusive arterial disease, (3) syphilis, (4) blood dyscrasia, (5) cutaneous sensitivity to drugs, frostbite, seasonal variations affecting the occurrence of the lesions, or serious local injury and (6) other disease on pathologic study of the lesion.

Sophie Spitz

Spitz Nevus (Benign Juvenile Melanoma)

SOPHIE SPITZ was born in Nashville, Tennessee on February 4, 1910. Her parents were Jewish immigrants from Germany and her father was a champion checker player. Sophie was an avid reader and played the violin until her brothers smashed the instrument. Her uncle, Dr. Herman Spitz, taught her clinical pathology in his private pathology laboratory in Nashville while she worked as a technician during her high school and college years. She received her B.A. and M.D. from Vanderbilt University. It was 1933, so as a woman she was barred from the surgical residency she desired.

Having served her rotating internship at the New York Infirmary for Women and Children, she elected to continue on as a resident in pathology. She remained on the staff for the next 20 years. She served concurrently as Attending Pathologist at the Memorial Hospital for Cancer and held the position of Assistant Professor of Pathology at Cornell Medical College.

During this period, Sophie was a strong advocate of the Papanicolaou test for cervical cancer, which many authorities ignored. Her wartime service was with the Army Institute of Pathology in Washington, DC. It was an assignment from Heaven, since her new love and husband, pathologist, Arthur Allen, had been inducted into the army and assigned to that same station. It was here in a whirlwind of productivity that she prepared study sets of tropical diseases for the army and almost all of the medical schools. Not only did she co-author with Colonel James Ash the invaluable text, *Pathology of Tropical Diseases,* but she also did signal work in neoplastic and orthopedic pathology.

After the war she returned to New York, spending much of her time doing autopsies and surgical pathology at Memorial Hospital. It was from this vantage point that she wrote the classic article on the non-fatal melanoma in childhood, *the Spitz nevus.* In off moments, she took most of the photomicrographs for both her husband's much-admired books, *The Skin* and *The Kidney.* Her skill as a pathologist was unrivaled as she took infinite pains to find and define the details. Despite all this, Sophie found time to enjoy the theater of New York, cruises around the world, and the hobbies of painting and photography.

Her life was cut short by colon cancer, the same malignancy as suffered by her father. At the age of 46 this mistress of all of pathology died on August 11, 1956.*

---

* Am. J.Clin. Pathol., *30:*553, 1958.

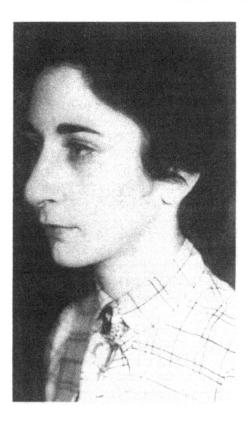

Figure 122 Sophie Spitz

SPITZ NEVUS

Melanoma of Childhood*

It has become apparent over a period of years that even when a histologic diagnosis of malignant melanoma has been made in children the clinical behavior rarely has been that of a malignant tumor. The disparity in behavior of the melanomas of adults and children, despite the histologic similarity of the lesions occurring in the different age groups, is obviously a matter of fundamental importance and the following questions immediately arise: Does the histologically malignant melanoma of children differ in any structural detail from that of adults? Can the clinical behavior of these lesions be predicted from their histologic structure? What, if any, are the factors known to influence the clinical behavior? Should the melanomas of children be treated any differently from the melanomas of adults?

    Material. The material for this study is comprised of 13 cases diagnosed histologically as juvenile melanoma during the past 13 years and occurring in children ranging in age from 18 months to 12 years. For purposes of comparison, a group of melanomas occurring in young adults of from 14 to 19 years of age also was reviewed. In addition, 50 consecutive cases of benign nevus occurring in children ranging in age from 1 month to 12 years were included in the comparative study. Blue nevi (Jadassohn) and Mongolian spots were not included in this study since they form a recognizable entity usually easily segregated from malignant melanomas both in histologic appearance and in their generally benign clinical behavior.

Clinical Features. In the group of childhood melanomas (juvenile melanomas) there were 5 males and 8 females. Three were less than 2 years of age; one was 3 years of age; one, 5 years old; and the remaining 8 patients ranged in age from 8 to 12 years. The clinical appearance was varied: 10 of the 13 patients had lesions under 1 cm. in diameter and only 3 lesions were between 1 and 3 cm. In a few, the lesions were described as being smooth with sharply delimited edges, but in the majority they were verrucous with irregular margins. All were elevated above the skin surface. The color was described as pink to red in 5, whereas 7 varied from brown to black. One lesion was said to have been subcutaneous. None was described as hairy.

The lesions had been noted for the duration of life in 6 cases but were said to have existed for from 6 weeks to 4 years in 7 cases. Three of the patients were presented for treatment within 1 year of the first appearance of the lesion. There was a history of gradual increase in size in all cases except one in which there was rapid growth for 6 weeks only.

Five of the lesions occurred on the face, one on the trunk, 2 on the upper extremity, and 5 on the lower extremity; only one of the latter category occurred on the sole. The parents of all these children stated that the lesions were in locations where they were frequently traumatized during the course of daily activities but none gave a history of frequent bleeding and none of the lesions was grossly ulcerated at the time of examination. Treatment consisted only of local surgical excision in all cases; in one case a group of obviously metastatic nodes was later removed from the groin.

All but one of the 13 children was alive and has shown no evidence of recurrence either locally or in drainage sites. They have been followed clinically for periods up to 13 years. Only 2, both female, have been followed for as short a time as 3 years and both of these have now passed their menarche. The remaining 10 have been seen regularly for from 5 to 13 years; 6 of these have passed the age of puberty.

One of the 13 cases had been clinically malignant and the child is dead. This one fatality occurred in a female child whose lesion was first noted at the age of 12 years; there had been no development of secondary sex characteristics and she had menstruated. This lesion occurred on the sole of the foot but was not described as involving the skin. After rapid growth over a period of 6 weeks, a soft white tumor, 2 cm. in diameter, was resected from the plantar fascia. One month after the initial excision there was a bulky local recurrence, thrombosis of the femoral vein, and metastasis to inguinal lymph nodes. Within 4 months the child was dead of generalized metastases.

Histologic Features. In general, it was concluded that differentiation histologically between the juvenile and adult melanomas could not be made with certainty in most cases. The one feature, found in almost one-half of cases of juvenile melanoma, that seemed to permit a histologic distinction from adult melanoma, was the presence of giant cells. In view of the survival of patients having this type of tumor, these have been regarded as an indication that the lesion is benign. This is so despite the fact that, except for the giant cells, such lesions have all the histologic criteria for the diagnosis of malignant melanoma.

Summary and Conclusions. Of 13 cases of juvenile melanoma in this series, only one (7.7 percent) has had a clinically malignant and fatal course despite the similarity of the juvenile lesions to the malignant melanoma of adults.

The juvenile melanoma may be distinguished histologically from adult melanoma in about one-half the cases by the presence of giant cells in the former, which seldom occur in the latter.

---

* Am. J.Pathol., *24:*591, 1948.

There is a precipitous rise in the capacity of melanomas to metastasize after puberty despite the histologic similarity to the usually non-metastasizing juvenile melanoma.

The possible influence of sex-linked hormonal activation of the growth capacity of melanomas at the age of puberty seems a logical conclusion.

Accordingly, since metastases from juvenile melanomas occur only rarely, conservative surgery, rather than the radical surgery usually indicated for adult melanomas, seems justified.

PART V

THE LAST 50 YEARS

Walter F.Lever

Bullous Pemphigoid

WALTER FREDERICK LEVER was born December 13, 1909 in Erfurt, Germany. Both he and his twin brother, Kurt, became dermatologists, following their father, Alexander Lever, Chief of Dermatology at the Municipal Hospital in Erfurt. After receiving his M.D. from the University of Leipzig in 1934, Lever moved to Boston in 1936 where he took a residency at Massachusetts General Hospital. This was followed by service at the Harvard Medical School where he sighted a new disease, *bullous pemphigoid*.

In 1961 he was appointed Professor of Dermatology and Chairman at Tufts University School of Medicine. His distinguished career focused on dermatopathology, culminating in 1949 with his classic *Histopathology of the Skin*. It was a beautifully written, lucid, didactic masterpiece, which went through seven editions and was translated into five languages. In 1965 he produced a classic monograph, *Pemphigus and Pemphigoid*.

Honorary membership in 16 foreign dermatological societies attests to his international status. He served as President of both the Society for Investigative Dermatology and the American Society of Dermatopathology. In 1989 he was awarded the Hebra Medal in Austria and in 1990 he received the Rothman Medal from the Society for Investigative Dermatology. He was awarded an honorary M.D. by both the University of Berlin and his own University of Leipzig.

In 1976 he retired, moving in 1984 to Tübingen, Germany, where in 1988 he and his wife, Gundula Schaumberg-Lever, wrote a color atlas of dermatopathology. Not only did he scale the heights of dermatology with several hundred papers, he also scaled the heights of many mountain peaks, including the Matterhorn in 1955.

He died on his 83rd birthday, December 13, 1992, in Germany, mourned by his students and colleagues around the world.*

BULLOUS PEMPHIGOID

Pemphigus[†]

Bullous pemphigoid (Pemphigus vulgaris chronicus, pemphigus vulgaris benignus,? Bullous dermatitis herpetiformis). This chronic, relatively benign and often self-limited bullous eruption does not belong in the pemphigus group because it does not show the histologic criterium of pemphigus, which is acantholysis. Clinical differentiation from malignant pemphigus vulgaris can be accomplished, as a rule, without

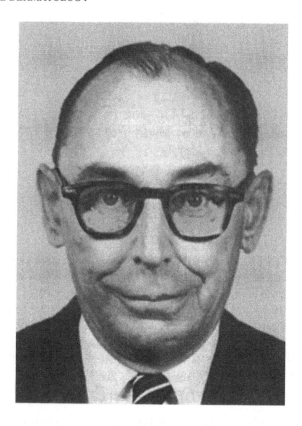

Figure 123 Walter F.Lever

difficulty; but differentiation from dermatitis herpetiformis may be very difficult. There is a tendency, especially among French, Belgian and some American authors, to regard this disease as a bullous type of dermatitis herpetiformis. This view is not without merit, and more will be said about it later.

Cutaneous Lesions. The cutaneous lesions consist of tense bullae. Only when part of the fluid they contain drains out or is reabsorbed do they become flaccid. The bullae may attain considerable size and often have an irregular outline. They do not break as easily as they do in pemphigus vulgaris malignus. When they break the resulting denuded areas usually do not increase in size materially; rather they show a good tendency to heal. Thus, bullae predominate the clinical picture throughout the course of the disease and the denuded areas rarely are large. Although the distribution of the bullae may be haphazard over the entire skin surface, the groins, axillae and flexor surfaces of the forearms often show the largest number of lesions. The bullae usually arise on normal appearing skin but they may arise on erythematous patches, which are present in most cases, in addition to the bullae. These erythematous patches are somewhat edematous and tend to show a serpiginous outline with an active border and central clearing. These erythematous patches greatly resemble those seen in erythema multiforme and may suggest that diagnosis.

---

* J.Am. Acad. Dermatol., *30:*141, 1994.

† Medicine, *32:*1, 1953.

Occasionally, the bullae are arranged in groups as in dermatitis herpetiformis. The amount of itching varies. It may be absent; but in most patients it is present and sometimes it is severe.

Mucous Membranes. The oral mucosa often is free from lesions. When lesions are present they usually are small in size and few in number.

Course. The disease is chronic and may last from a few months to several years. There are remissions and exacerbations and occasionally after months or even years of quiescence, there may be a recurrence. In most instances, however, such a recurrence is less severe than the first attack. The general health, except in old patients, is not greatly impaired, although the discomfort caused by the presence of innumerable bullae and erosions may be great. The prognosis as to life is good except in the old age group where general debility is liable to cause death.

Bullous pemphigoid occurs predominantly in older adults but also not infrequently in young children.

Own Patients. Forty-four patients with bullous pemphigoid were admitted to the Massachusetts General Hospital between 1937 and early 1952.

Eleven patients, namely 10 adults and 1 child, received treatment with corticotropin or cortisone. All have responded well.

Max Jessner

Jessner's Lymphocytic Infiltrate

MAX JESSNER was born in Stolp, Pomerania on November 2, 1887.

His father, Samuel Jessner, was a prominent Docent in Dermatology at the University of Königsberg. Thus, it was not surprising that Max trained in this field with Albert Neisser in Breslau. Soon his career and practice were entwined with the heroic figure of Josef Jadassohn at the Breslau University Clinic. By 1921 he had already reached eponymic fame by describing focal dermal hypoplasia. This entity was virtually unrecognized by English-speaking dermatologists until Goltz's report in 1962. Jadassohn retired in 1931 and Jessner succeeded him as Professor and Head.

With the rise of Hitler, Jessner's position was in jeopardy because of his Jewish heritage. By 1933 he had already lost one of his distinguished staff members, Rudolf Mayer, who went on to head the Ciba Research Unit in the U.S. where he developed one of the first antihistamines, pyribenzamine. By the following year Jessner was relieved of his teaching post and he left for Switzerland to collaborate on the classic *Jadassohn Handbook*. In 1941 he emigrated to New York City to join the staff at New York University, enriching research, practice and teaching at this great center.

Jessner's contributions ranged far beyond superb teaching and patient care. He was a major force in introducing Thorium X as one of the first radioactive isotopes for medical use. He was author of numerous papers on the immunology of mycotic infections and he stressed the role of iodide sensitivity in dermatitis herpetiformis. Not only was he an investigator of the ravages of syphilis on the heart and blood vessels, but he also organized forces for the control of all venereal disease.

Jessner retired from the New York University in 1971 moving back to Switzerland where he died in August, 1978 at the age of 91.*

JESSNER'S LYMPHOCYTIC INFILTRATE

Lymphocytic Infiltration of the Skin*

Discussion. Dr. Kanof and I presented a group of cases, the nature of which I began to recognize about 10 years ago. We summarize the clinical picture, course, diagnosis, and histology as follows: The lesions are flat, discoid, more or less elevated, pinkish to reddish brown, starting as small papules, expanding

---

* Hautarzt, *8:*478, 1957.

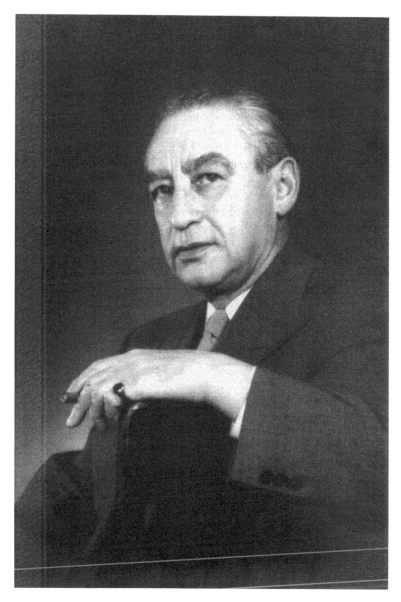

Figure 124 Max Jessner

peripherally, sometimes clearing in the center, sometimes showing a circinate arrangement. The surface is smooth, occasionally uneven. There is no follicular hyperkeratosis. The consistency is firm. There may be only one, a few, or numerous lesions. They persist for weeks or months or longer, disappear without sequelae, and may recur in the same or other areas and cause practically no subjective symptoms. The face is obviously the area of predilection, but other parts of the body may or may not be affected. These cases must be distinguished particularly from cases of chronic discoid lupus erythematosus, under which label they are invariably described; also from sarcoid tuberoserpiginous syphilid, and drug eruption.

There are no enlarged lymph nodes. The blood cell count shows only an occasional relative lymphocytosis. The bone marrow smear reveals no abnormalities.

Histologically, the findings are rather constant. The epidermis may be stretched but is otherwise uninvolved. There may be edema in the subpapillary region in fresh lesions; older ones show none. Distributed through the cutis are rather sharply circumscribed lymphocytic infiltrations, sometimes extending to the subcutaneous fat, frequently, but not always, around vessels and/or appendages. The infiltrates consist of lymphocytes, mostly small ones, and usually a few histiocytes and plasma cells. The infiltrates are often enmeshed in a fine reticulum. There are no eosinophiles, no germinal centers or germinal center-like formations.

The evaluation of therapy in a condition so prone to spontaneous remission is extremely difficult, but speedy resolution has been noted following the administration of penicillin, bismuth, arsenic, sulfapyridine, quinacrine dihydrochloride, paraaminosalicylic acid, x-ray therapy, and Staphylococcus ambotoxoid.

We reviewed the pertinent European and American literature to separate this group from (a) the "true lymphocytomas" as described in 1935 by Stephan Epstein, from the Breslau University Hospital, and more recently by Loveman and Fliegelman and Mopper and Rogin; (b) the "reticuloses" of the French literature, named by Werner Jadassohn, and (c) the Spiegler-Fendt sarcoid and lymphoblastoma.

---

* Arch. Dermatol. Syphilol., *68:*447, 1953.

Ferdinando Gianotti and Agostino Crosti

Gianotti-Crosti Syndrome (Papular Acrodermatitis of Childhood)

FERDINANDO GIANOTTI was born in 1920 in Corsico, a little town near Milan, Italy. Coming from a very poor family he started to work in a tannery once he had finished grade school. An accident at work led to the loss of his left forearm. In compensation his employer supported his return to school where he proved to be an outstanding student, graduating from medical school with high honors in 1947. He chose dermatology because of its great opportunities for discovery.

He trained in the great Department of Dermatology in Milan, which the famed Agostino Pasini had founded in 1924, and now headed by Professor Crosti. A rapid rise to professorship in 1956 was followed by his becoming Director of the Institute of Dermatology and thus the successor to his colleague, Crosti.

Gianotti loved taking care of children. "They do not speak and moreover the smile of a cured child is of inestimable value." With a phenomenal memory and a genius for close observation, he was able to enrich the dermatologic literature with more than 200 publications ranging from genodermatoses to histiocyte and mastocyte syndromes. Included were his classic papers on papular acrodermatitis of children and benign cephalic histiocytosis, the latter written with the dermatologist to succeed him, Ruggero Caputo.

Away from children, Gianotti was an introvert, reserved and taciturn, who taught his disciples not to rely on him for a diagnosis, but closely observe, to read widely and to inquire by thinking.

Gianotti died in 1984 leaving a rich heritage, including the very first department of pediatric dermatology, which he founded in 1953 and a million smiles from the children of Milan.*

AGOSTINO CROSTI was born in Milan, Italy on February 16, 1896. He received his indoctrination into dermato-venereology from the master clinician, Agostino Pasini. It was here in Milan that he doubtless saw the atrophoderma his professor was first to describe. By 1929 he was called to head the University of Perugia Skin Clinic, which he transformed into a major center in the subsequent 10 years.

In 1939 he moved to the University of Palermo. There, despite the obstacles of the war and the occupational forces, he again molded another major dermatologic center. Not surprisingly, in 1947 he was invited to the Chair back in Milan, a position he held for the next 20 years. Here he established a center for the treatment of sexually transmitted diseases.

Crosti's productivity was phenomenal, 170 personal papers and an additional 500 with collaborators. Highlights were his studies on the factors determining the localization of skin disease, the role of sulfonamides in therapy, the multiplicity of serum antibodies in syphilis and especially his definitive 1956

---

* Caputo, R.: "Ferdinando Gianotti," Communication à la Société française d'Histoire de la Dermatologie, le 4 décembre 1998. Available at: http://www.bium.univ-paris5fr/sfhd/ecrits/ gianno.htm. Accessed February 27, 2003.

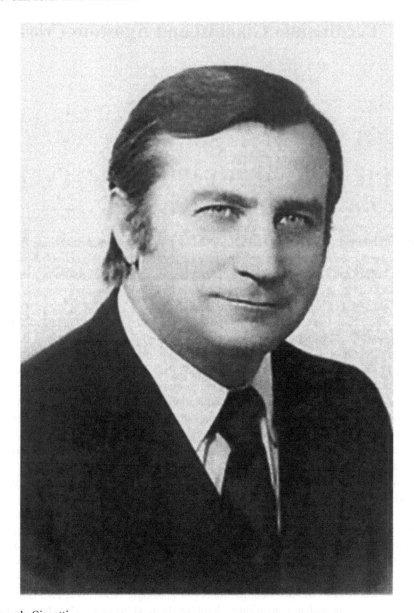

Figure 125 Ferdinando Gianotti

paper on the pathogenic role of the hepatitis virus in papular acrodermatitis of childhood. This disease had been first described the year before by Gianotti, one of his faculty members.

Crosti served as President of the Italian Society of Dermatology and Venereology and in 1961 he was appointed President of the Faculty of Medicine at his beloved University of Milan. Numerous foreign dermatologic societies prided themselves on having him as an honorary member.

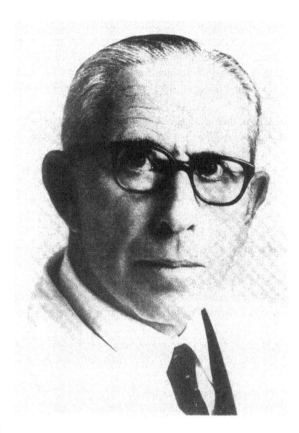

Figure 126 Agostino Crosti

His residents found him strict and fair, reserved and dignified. He was the Maestro of Italian Dermatology, whose disciples filled many of the Chairs in the universities. After his retirement in 1966 he continued to advise and assist his associates, even as he became an avid student of the arts and literature.

His powerful inspiration and his peerless influence on our specialty have been enormous. He died in Milan in 1988 at the age of 92, a revered and beloved patriarch of 20th century dermatology.*

PAPULAR ACRODERMATITIS OF CHILDHOOD

Rilievi di una Particolare Casistica Tossinfettiva Caratterizzata da Eruzione Eritemato-Infiltrativa Desquamativa a Focolai Lenticolari, a sede Elettiva Actoesposta[†]

Case 1. G.Giuseppi, age 3. The skin from the shoulders to the fingers and from the superior iliac crest to the buttocks and on to the inguinal region and down to the toes is involved with a disseminate, erythematous, barely infiltrated eruption, at times purpuric, showing branny scaling, with elements equal in size to lentils, distinct one from another and, for the most part, at follicular orifices, to a great degree appearing on the extensor surfaces and confluent only around the elbows and knees. The superficial palms and soles are covered with erythematous macules. The remaining skin and mucosa are completely free of these lesions.

The singular element of about 2 mm in diameter is a dull red brownish, without prominent margins, barely infiltrated with a small branny scale desquamation. On diascopy only a hazel-colored spot remains.

The inguinal lymph nodes are palpable pea-sized firm bodies, distinct from the surrounding skin. Pruritus is uncommon.

Laboratory studies were negative, including the Wassermann and an intradermal tuberculin test.

Course. After a few days following the visit to the clinic the erythema and infiltration began to fade retreating at 8 days to only brownish, scaling macules. The desquamation continued another week, but with subsequent auxiliary therapy with ointment the dermatitis resolved completely.

Summary. The author reports three cases of a dermatitis observed in children between 3 and 8 years of age, presenting a dense aero-situated eruption of erythematous, circular, more or less papular and partially purpuric elements, about 2–3 mm large, isolated from one another, mainly in follicular position. This eruption begins, without prodromes of any kind, on the legs, extends within the next two or three days to the buttocks, the upper limbs, face and neck, undergoing no further modification of its localization for the whole duration of the illness, which lasts about 25–45 days. The skin of the trunk was never involved.

In the course of the evolution, all elements were covered simultaneously with branny scales, adhering at their core, which came off when the dermatitis resolved. No itching was noticed.

The subcutaneous lymph nodes involved in the inflammatory process became enlarged and returned to normal only after recovery.

The liver may be enlarged, but there was no splenomegaly. A slight rise in body temperature accompanies the course of the dermatitis. Two of the cases presented a feverish follicular or herpetic tonsillitis.

The general condition of the little patients was good; only one of them complained of slight asthenia during the leukopenic period. Prognosis was good in all of them.

Laboratory data showed a modest anaemia, normal leucocytosis or leukopenia, a varying degree (3–20) of monocytoid and lymphocytoid histiocytes in the peripheral blood, together with some mitotic cells and rare Türck's cells. The sedimentation rate was normal.

Serum electrophoresis showed a modest increase of the alpha and gamma globulins. The Paul-Bunnel-Davidsohn test was slightly positive (1:64) in one case. Cold agglutinins were present in low concentrations (1:32) in another one.

Histologically there was a capillaritis and perivascular infiltration of mono-histocytic cells in the papular and upper dermal layers. In the latter, monohistiocytes were to be found in small, not well circumscribed, extravascular masses.

The pattern described is considered to be the expression of an infective reticulo-endotheliosis, probably of viral origin.

The development of a feverish illness (herpetic or follicular tonsillitis, subcutaneous lymphopathy, presence of circulating histiocytes similar to those observed by the author in the reported cases in children hospitalized in the same room as one of the aforementioned little patients, confirms the probable infective origin of this dermatitis.

---

* Puccinelli, V.: In Memoria, Prof. Agostino Crosti 1896–1988. Giorn. Ital. Dermatol. Venereol., July–August, 1989.

† G.Ital. Derm. Sif., *96*:678, 1955.

Ian Bruce Sneddon

1. *Sneddon's Syndrome*

2. *Sneddon-Wilkinson Disease*

I.B.SNEDDON was born in Sheffield on March 6, 1915 and lived there for most of his life. His father, William, was a Scottish general practitioner who died when Ian was still a schoolboy. After graduating from the University of Sheffield he became House Physician and lost his heart to dermatology. The onset of the Second World War called him up for naval service in the Pacific. It was sailing in dinghies in Sydney Harbor that grew into a lifetime passion, a highly prized yacht master certificate and sailing his 10-tonner to and from France. Fly-fishing and painting rounded out his extra-dermatological talents.

On return to Sheffield in 1946 he continued his dermatologic pursuit, becoming a consultant. His genius for enthusiastic teaching resulted in his appointment as Clinical Dean. In that position he instituted a system of tutorial instruction for medical students.

His sharp analysis of unusual skin syndromes led to over a hundred articles and a small influential textbook, *Practical Dermatology,* which enjoyed four editions. A witty and fluent speaker he gave numerous lectures all over the world. He was President of the British Association of Dermatology at its 50th Anniversary in 1970. Awarded the coveted CBE in 1974 he never retired, but in 1968 a coronary thrombosis induced him to relinquish his clinical deanship. With an admirable work ethic he continued his private practice and writing clinical classics until the very end. He died while consulting on October 10, 1987 at the age of 72.*

SNEDDON'S SYNDROME

Cerebro-Vascular Lesions and Livedo Reticularis[†]

The physical sign livedo reticularis is caused by capillary stasis in areas of skin furthest from the cutaneous arteriolar supply. In the type known as cutis marmorata, due to the effect of cold on normal blood vessels, the network of bluish discoloration is continuous but transient, as it disappears when the skin is warmed.

A broken livedo, which is present even in warm surroundings, denotes more permanent damage to skin arterioles. Though originally described in syphilis and tuberculosis, in recent years it has been increasingly

---

* Br. J.Dermatol., *118:*721, 1988.

† Br. J.Dermatol., *77:*80, 1965.

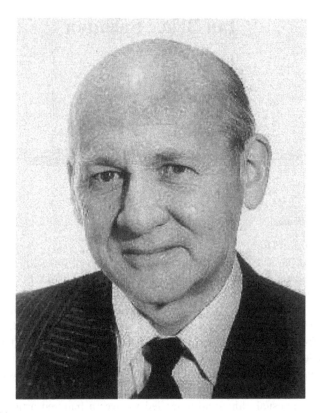

Figure 127 Ian Bruce Sneddon

recognized as a skin manifestation of polyarteritis nodosa but it is then usually accompanied by nodules. Lyell and Church (1954) drew attention to this and suggested that in the majority of cases of polyarteritis where livedo was found, the skin was the main target organ and there was little involvement of other systems. More recently, reticular livedo has been described in disseminated lupus erythematosus (Golden, 1963) and essential thrombocythaemia (Champion and Rook, 1963), superficial thromboses and, of course, a high platelet count.

My interest in livedo was aroused when I was asked to see the first of the following patients.

Case Reports. Case 1—A coal miner aged 42 in 1957, whilst at work at the coal face, suddenly became unable to speak and developed weakness of his right arm. There was no unconsciousness or headache.

He was admitted to a neurological unit where his blood pressure was found on admission to be 180/110 mm. of mercury and he had the signs of a partial right hemiplegia. Investigations, including a left carotid angiogram, C.S.F. protein, cells and W.R., were negative and the only constant positive findings were a diastolic blood pressure of 110, a trace of albumin in the urine and a widespread reticular livedo on the arms, forearms, buttocks, thighs and legs. It should be mentioned here that the possible significance of this skin lesion was not appreciated until after the second case had been seen on the neurological unit. Some months after this incident I was asked to see him and on the basis of the very gross, irregular but constant livedo suggested a diagnosis of polyarteritis nodosa. This diagnosis was supported when he was demonstrated at a North of England Dermatological Society meeting in 1958. However, after several months the neurological signs cleared and a skin biopsy specimen did not show histological evidence of polyarteritis nodosa.

For the subsequent history of this patient I am indebted to Dr. J.Caley, Physician at Mansfield Hospital, where the patient was admitted in March, 1962, five years after the first incident. On this occasion he had a sudden onset of weakness of the right arm and leg and difficulty in speaking, but no unconsciousness. Examination showed a partial right hemiplegia associated on this occasion with more severe hypertension (B.P. 200/140) and hypertensive fundal changes of Grade 3 type. No evidence of polyarteritis was found on muscle biopsy and all other investigations, including renal function, were substantially normal, as before. Again, he made a good recovery with hypotensive drugs and is alive though unfit for work.

Within a few months another patient with similar findings was seen.

Case 2—A girl aged 20 who in November 1957 was referred to the neurological department because of a sudden attack of weakness of the right arm and leg and difficulty in micturition. A left carotid angiogram revealed a partial blockage of the middle cerebral artery.

A month after the onset a purplish mottling of the forearms, arms, legs and thighs was noted and I was asked to see her. There was a broken irregular livedo, typical of that seen in polyarteritis nodosa. The hemiplegia spontaneously improved without treatment. She remained well with a blood pressure of 150/100 until August 1962 five years after the original incident, when she was re-admitted because of a dizzy attack in which her right hand became numb and weak and she developed aphasia. On this occasion the reticular livedo was more obvious than ever, particularly over the abdomen. The right hemiparesis had returned and she had a right foot drop. A repeat carotid angiogram again showed a partial branch occlusion of the left middle cerebral artery. An E.E.G. revealed changes, presumably of vascular origin. She recovered with physiotherapy and when seen in November 1963 her livedo persisted but the neurological signs had disappeared and she had no hypertension.

In the last five years four other women have been seen in Sheffield with the full-blown syndrome of livedo, cerebrovascular lesions and moderate but benign type of hypertension.

Summary. Extensive livedo reticularis has been observed in one man and five women who have suffered from a series of cerebrovascular lesions. The neurological disabilities have included aphasia, homonymous hemianopia and hemiplegia but have been remarkable for the degree of recovery that has occurred. It is presumed that the livedo which has been found in only one patient without neurological lesions is related to the cerebrovascular incidents. Investigations have failed to show any evidence of polyarteritis nodosa, disseminated lupus erythematosus and thrombocythaemia and an arteritis of unrecognized type is suggested as the etiology.

Darrell Sheldon Wilkinson

Subcornial Pustular Dermatosis (Sneddon-Wilkinson Disease)

D.S.WILKINSON was born in Gillingham, Kent, England on August 7, 1919. After graduating from Epsom College, he went on to medical school at St. Thomas Hospital. Following wartime service in the Royal Navy (1942–1946) he returned to St. Thomas for dermatologic training under the legendary G.B.Dowling. By 1949 he was named Consultant in Dermatology in the small county of Buckinghamshire. To paraphrase Shakespeare, it proved to be *"a dukedom large enough."* It was the dukedom that gave him a global view of dermatoses, unlike the fragmented, transitory experience of those in the great urban teaching centers of the world. In Aylesworth, England, he could study the long-term course of disease in a controlled population of 250,000. It was here in a regional, non-teaching hospital that he set up specialized clinics in contact, occupational, and environmental dermatoses, as well as venereology. His dukedom permitted him to detect and eliminate the worldwide problem of photosensitization due to soaps containing tetrachlorosalicylanilide. His patients permitted him to recognize toxic reactions never suspected in short-term testing, for example, necrotizing balanitis due to a newly formulated quaternium ammonium antiseptic. In his dukedom he described such entities as forefoot dermatitis, perioral dermatitis, equestrian chilblains, occupational sensitization to wood, and the glucagonoma syndrome.

By 1968 his clinical acumen led to his co-editorship of Rook's encyclopedic text, which he nurtured through four editions. He became President of the British Association of Dermatology, and was recipient of many other honors, including the *Sir Archibald Gray Gold Medal*. It was he who conceived and initiated the Dermatology Training Center in Tanzania and who has spent a life in cross-fertilization of the English and French dermatologic cultures.

In 1983 he retired as consultant and entered private practice, with music, reading and cooking filling the interstices.

Wilkinson gave the Prosser White Oration in 1984, in which he presented a charming Greek mythical story embracing his philosophy and his wonderful adventures in his dukedom of dermatology.*

SNEDDON-WILKINSON DISEASE

Subcorneal Pustular Dermatosis[†]

From time to time patients are shown at dermatological meetings who have unusual chronic blistering eruptions not readily recognized as belonging either to the dermatitis herpetiformis or to the pemphigus

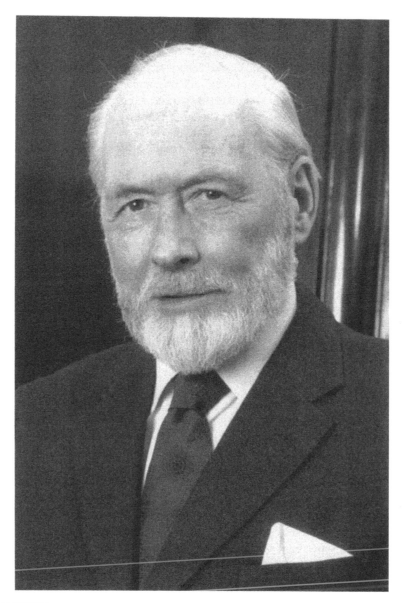

Figure 128 Darrell S.Wilkinson

group. Discussion on these cases is often long, and the diagnoses offered are tentative, dermatitis herpetiformis and impetigo herpetiformis being the most usual.

Case Reports. Case 2—A housewife aged 65 had suffered for six years from a recurrent blistering eruption on the abdomen and thighs. Severe outbreaks lasted two to three weeks and then subsided; she was rarely without a few lesions. Acute outbreaks were ushered in by severe itching. During the previous year, treatment with sulphapyridine had not influenced the eruption. In addition she was subject to occasional attacks of asthma and both her sister and niece suffered from hay fever.

Examination revealed numerous gyrate and annular erythematous and blistering lesions. Where they were subsiding a leafy scale could be seen, and in the center of other lesions crusts gave an appearance of circinate impetigo. Pigmentation was present on the abdomen and in the lumbar region at the site of healed lesions. No abnormal physical signs were found in other systems.

Investigations—Histology showed a subcorneal aggregation of polymorphonuclear leucocytes with no evidence of acantholytic change in the underlying epidermal cells.

Blood count: WBC 8,000. Differential count—no eosinophilia. Culture from vesicles was sterile and no organisms were seen on a Gram-stained film. Treatment with dapsone 50 mg. b.d. was followed by rapid resolution of the eruption within seven days. The treatment was stopped after some weeks and no recurrence has occurred up to the present.

Comment. The main feature of these cases is the onset in middle life of a recurrent vesicopustular eruption that runs a harmless but protracted course over a number of years.

The axillae, groins, abdomen and flexor aspects of the proximal parts of the limbs have been particularly affected. The hands, feet, face and mucous membranes have been entirely spared. The individual lesions consist either of a pustule from the start, or of a vesicle which rapidly becomes a pustule, flaccid, turbid and often oval rather than circular; there is a faint and short-lived erythematous flare surrounding it at the beginning. Within a few days the pustule ruptures, leaving a scale or crust. Pustules tend to collect to form little groups of annular or gyrate shape with an actively spreading edge, incomplete and irregular, in which are seen pustules, crusts and in places leafy dry scales about to fall off. After healing, either a reddish stain or sometimes a more definite brown pigmentation is left. There is no atrophy.

This configuration spreads outwards in an irregular arc from the folds of the breasts, armpits and groins on to the adjoining areas of the body. In successive attacks the same area of skin may be completely involved and further spread may occur at the periphery, or isolated groups of pustules may form within the now pigmented area and die away before they have spread very far. The eruption has phases of alternate quiescence and activity lasting a few weeks, though in some cases the skin has been almost continuously affected by successive waves of pustules overlapping each other. On the other hand, the eruption may subside completely after an attack and a spontaneous remission occur, lasting several months.

The constant histological feature of every case has been a subcorneal blister filled with polymorphonuclear leucocytes. No change in the epidermal cells such as acantholysis, has been seen and usually edema was absent in the epidermis, though spongiosis was observed in one case. Polymorphonuclear leucocytes were sometimes also found in the upper corium and here there seems to have been an increase of eosinophils in some cases. Some, but by no means all, of the blisters have communicated with hair follicles.

Local or systemic treatment with antibiotics has not influenced the eruption. It will be seen that diamino-diphenyl sulphone ("dapsone") was successful in 3 and partly successful in another one of the 5 cases in which it was used, and appears therefore to be the most effective remedy.

Summary. Six cases of a chronic vesicopustular eruption, which affects mainly middle-aged women, are described.

The pustular nature of the eruption that histologically shows a subcorneal blister filled with polymorphonuclear leucocytes has been a feature of all the cases. Diamino-diphenyl-sulphone (dapsone)

---

* Clin. Exp. Dermatol., *11:*1, 1984.

† Br. J.Dermatol., *68:*385, 1956.

was successful in controlling the eruption in 4 of the 6 cases. It is suggested that the eruption is distinct from dermatitis herpetiformis, though similar in the grouping of its lesions, its protracted course and its response to remedies.

Until its position as a separate entity or otherwise has been established, we suggest the descriptive name of "subcorneal pustular dermatosis".

Alan Lyell

Toxic Epidermal Necrolysis (Lyell's Syndrome)

ALAN LYELL, well-known Scottish dermatologist was born in India on November 4, 1917. He received his medical degree from Cambridge University in 1942. He served as a medical officer in the British Army and was wounded in the Normandy invasion of 1944. Following the war he received his dermatologic training at Addenbrooke's Hospital in Cambridge, later joined G.H.Percival at the Edinburgh Royal Infirmary, and in 1962 was appointed in charge of the Skin Department of the Glasgow Royal Infirmary. He remained with that institution until his retirement in 1980.

Lyell's dermatologic interests are many. He has published valuable studies on warts, cutaneous bacteriology, self-induced dermatoses, and delusions of parasitosis. His best known production, noted below, is his 1956 classic description of toxic epidermal necrolysis (TEN). The relationship of TEN to erythema multiforme and the staphylococcus scalded skin syndrome continues to generate controversy, but whatever the taxonomic truth turns out to be, the vivid picture of the skin changes painted by Lyell has enabled clinicians everywhere to recognize the condition when they see it.

Although retired more than 20 years, Lyell keeps a watchful eye on the dermatologic literature. He believes that the name TEN, which he created, should be abandoned, along with "Stevens-Johnson syndrome" and erythema multiforme bullosum, and that all should be united under the name "exanthematic necrolysis."*

TOXIC EPIDERMAL NECROLYSIS

Toxic Epidermal Necrolysis: An Eruption Resembling Scalding of the Skin*

The purpose of this paper is to describe the course of events in four cases of a toxic eruption, which closely resembles scalding in its clinical appearance and in the sensations to which it gives rise in the patient. It is probable that this type of reaction is not uncommon and that it has been classified as a toxic eruption, toxic erythema with blistering, or something similar. But the features of the reaction are so definite and they concern the epidermis so intimately—to the exclusion of the dermis—that I believe it to be useful and important to recognize this sequence of events as a distinct syndrome in which some circulating toxin specifically damages the epidermis and results in its necrosis.

---

* Personal communication.

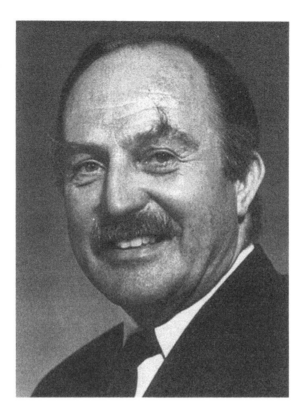

Figure 129 Alan Lyell

Case 1. Eight years ago a woman aged 34 came to Dr. C.Whittle's clinic in Cambridge with a history that she had suffered from five attacks of a blistering eruption which was always preceded by pain in the right loin. She looked perfectly well but assured us that she now had the pain and that the blisters could be expected within a matter of hours. She did not seem agitated by the prospect, but we admitted her to the ward for observation, and there straightaway developed a blotchy erythema, mostly on the thighs and buttocks. The skin was tender and she felt ill with fever.

The next day the red skin began to loosen and could be pulled and pushed about with the finger into creases and wrinkles, having separated so extensively that it had an extraordinary mobility, though it would rupture if it was pulled too hard. Apart from this spontaneous epidermolysis neighboring areas which were still apparently normal could be loosened by the finger in what amounted to a caricature of the Nikolsky test. The formation of blisters was an incident in the process and depended upon the collection of fluid in the potential space beneath the loosened layer. The blisters that did form were flaccid, the fluid within them was distributed in levels according to the force of gravity, and the extent of the blister could always be enlarged by the application of external pressure. Soon the loose skin peeled off in shreds and exposed a dark red, raw surface, very tender, and liable to bleed if touched. It was later evident that the force of the toxemia had spent itself within the first few days for she soon began to feel better, the temperature abated, and no

---

* Br. J.Dermatol., *68:*355, 1956.

new lesion appeared. But it took some weeks for the skin to heal, which it did without scarring. After the initial toxemia had subsided the severity of the skin condition contrasted with the untroubled demeanor of the patient; her serenity proved justifiable in the event.

It seems, then, that these four cases are clinically comparable since in all of them large areas of skin have loosened. The loosening has been preceded by erythema and tenderness, and has been followed by peeling, so that a dark red, excessively tender surface has been revealed which has healed rapidly without scar formation. In three of the cases fluid collected beneath the loose skin and formed flaccid blisters. The clinical resemblance to scalding was close, both in the appearance of the lesions and in the sensations of the patient, but it is not complete in that there was no shock or exudation such as one sees after a scald. There is no doubt that Case 4 with her 80% involvement of the skin would never have survived a scald of such extent. Nevertheless the analogy with a scald is appropriate, for it is evident that in scalding, as in this syndrome, the damage all occurs at the beginning of the illness and the subsequent events are the logical result of the damage and are proportional to its severity. As a corollary to this one can predict complete recovery of the skin provided that the toxemia does not irreparably damage such organs as the lungs and kidneys, and provided that the patient can be nursed through the early stages of healing. This is a situation in which skilled nursing is of paramount importance and there is no doubt that the last patient owes her life to the nurses of the City Hospital, Aberdeen, as well as to her own courage and endurance. The nursing was made easier by the turning frame, which I can certainly recommend for ill patients who have extensive raw surfaces, particularly if, as in this case, postural drainage of the chest is a necessity. The prodromal symptoms, which these patients suffered, were presumably the result of toxemia. As regards the nature of the toxin, a drug, butazolidin, was suspected in Case 4, but in the other cases no cause could be found. In Case I a subsequent attack occurred and suspicion was eventually directed towards drugs because of a severe, but different, reaction which followed the exhibition of Dover's powder with aspirin. Case 3 died with pyaemia and nephritis; perhaps the toxin, which damaged the skin, damaged the kidneys also, and the infection was secondary.

It is essential to stress that the pathogenesis of this syndrome is epidermal necrosis, in distinction to reactions such as erythema multiforme, dermatitis herpetiformis, and pemphigoid, which depend upon dermal inflammatory changes. In these latter diseases the blisters have a different character which is consistent with their mode of formation by fluid which, exuding from dermal vessels, collects beneath and raises the epidermis. They are therefore tense, and they break rather than spread when pressed upon. Blisters are almost incidental to the syndrome under discussion. Fluid fills the cleft which has been opened up by epidermolysis, and since the amount of fluid is small in relation to the potential space the blisters are flaccid, can be spread readily by external pressure, and often display fluid levels.

Conclusion. I have tried to describe a clinical syndrome, which resembles scalding both objectively and subjectively, brought about by necrosis of the epidermis, which results from toxemia. The toxemia, which is short-lived, produces the prodromal symptoms. If the patient survives the initial toxemia, and if he can be nursed through the subsequent complications, he can look forward to a complete recovery; but should the toxemia be repeated at any time the skin will be liable to react in the same way as before.

Such a very definite syndrome as this is should have a name to distinguish it from other toxic erythemas and bullous eruptions, and I suggest that it might be called "Toxic epidermal necrolysis." The word necrolysis avoids the ambiguity of epidermolysis and the picture of ulceration and gangrene, which is conjured up by necrosis. It avoids any reference to blistering, which is not an essential part of the process and is therefore better omitted.

Walter B.Shelley

1. *Larva Currens*

2. *Cold Erythema*

3. *Aquagenic Urticaria*

4. *Autoimmune Progesterone Sensitivity Dermatitis*

5. *Piezogenic Pedal Papules*

6. *Pincer Nails*

7. *Mid-dermal Elastolysis Wrinkles*

8. *Adrenergic Urticaria*

9. *Non-pigmenting Fixed Drug Eruption*

10. *Autoimmune Estrogen Dermatitis*

11. *Abacus Nodule*

12. *IgE Bullous Disease*

13. *Aquadynia*

WALTER BROWN SHELLEY was born in St. Paul, Minnesota February 6, 1917. He earned an M.D. and Ph.D. in Physiology at the University of Minnesota 1937–1943. After several years of conducting research on heat stress at the Armored Medical Research Laboratory at Fort Knox, KY, he took his residency at the University of Pennsylvania. Following a year with Walter C.Lobitz at Dartmouth Medical School he returned to Penn, joining Donald M.Pillsbury in practice. The next 30 years saw him dividing his time equally between clinical research and private practice. The practice yielded more than a dozen new dermatologic entities and the research half of this life saw him with his associates demonstrating the role of sweat retention in Fox-Fordyce disease, as well as in miliaria. Studies on pruritus with Robert P.Arthur led to the isolation of mucunain, the proteolytic enzyme responsible for the effect of itch powder. Another first was the histologic demonstration of unmyelinated C fibers in the epidermis, which conduct the itch sensation.

Hyperhidrosis studies with Harry J.Hurley led to the development of anhydrous aluminum chloride antiperspirants, the introduction of botulinum toxin therapy for palmar hyperhidrosis, and the surgical

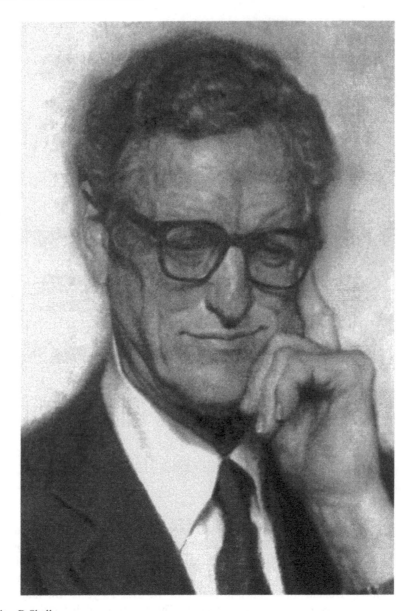

Figure 130 Walter B.Shelley

treatment of axillary hyperhidrosis. They were the first to study pure apocrine sweat and to show that axillary odor resulted from bacterial contamination.

Immunological research was a fourth area of investigation. With Lennart Juhlin he developed the basophil test, which miniaturized anaphylaxis onto a glass slide. He further developed the fibrin star test for the detection of endotoxin hypersensitivity. With Hurley he discovered a new class of allergic reactions, the allergic granuloma typified by the zirconium deodorant granuloma. Further, Juhlin and Shelley were the first to demonstrate that the Langerhans cell is a phagocyte engulfing antigens that enter the epidermis. They coined the term, *reticulo-epithelial system,* to emphasize this unique function. A more recent observation centers on the contractility of the stratum granulosum, of significance in the pathogenesis of wrinkles.

He named *aquagenic pruritus,* but his most significant coinage was the word, *keratinocyte,* which he introduced in 1956. Before that time the epidermis was viewed as four distinct layers with no name for the mother cell.

In 1980, he left Penn to marry E.Dorinda Loeffel, the only woman dermatologist at that time to hold a departmental chair. Now settled at the Medical College of Ohio in Toledo they have continued to research and write together. Their most recent contribution has been *Advanced Dermatologic Therapy II* and *Shelley's 77 Skins.* Both Shelleys have retired, immersed in their library of 30,000 books and a small farm boasting over 100 birds and animals.*

LARVA CURRENS

Larva Currens: A Distinctive Variant of Cutaneous Larva Migrans due to Strongyloides Stercoralis[†]

Report of a Case. The patient, a white 46 year old housewife, developed a pruritic erythematous urticarial lesion of the medial aspect of the left midthigh on April 15, 1957. The eruption progressed from time to time in an irregular serpiginous linear fashion. Systemic chloramphenicol (Chloromycetin) and erythromycin therapy for 10 days was without effect. Admitted to the hospital on April 28, she was considered to have a possible cellulitis, lymphangitis, or thrombophlebitis. On the left thigh she presented tender erythematous serpentine cords, which showed periodic urticarial extensions. She had marked enlargement of the left inguinal nodes.

We were called in consultation on May 3, at which time the entire left thigh was encircled by a wide, rapidly extending band of urticaria. It was actually possible to see advancement of the lesion within a matter of 10 minutes. After a period of hours the lesion would cease moving, only to resume movement at an unpredictable time the following day. The urticaria subsided slowly, leaving a distinct brownish track consisting of a brownish, slightly infiltrated line. The patient presented only one track, all of her lesions being traceable as one continuous line.

On May 8 an intradermal injection of crystalline lyophilized trypsin (1 ml. of a concentration of 10^{-3} in isotonic saline solution) was made at the most advanced point of the lesion. This single injection was curative, since no further extension of the skin lesion developed.

Comment. The clinical result with trypsin delighted us, but we continued to puzzle over the strange clinical pattern we had seen. We had seen a "racing larva" move inches in hours, and we had seen a giant urticarial band develop. We had previously seen patients with fine linear slow-moving larva migrans, but here was a different problem.

We despaired of any precise elucidation of the type of larva migrans in our patient until we read the masterful review article of Beaver.

---

* Int. J.Dermatol., *39:*710, 2000.

† Arch. Dermatol., *78:*186, 1958.

Beaver made it apparent that we most likely had been observing and treating a case of *Strongyloides stercoralis* larval infection.

All of the reported clinical cases of creeping eruption proven to be due to *S. stercoralis* larvae have had the following unique clinical features: (1) involvement of perianal area, due to autoinfection from larvae coming out with the fecal matter; (2) an extraordinary band of urticaria associated with the presence of the larva in the skin; (3) a burrow advancing with almost unbelievable speed, as much as four inches an hour.

We have proposed a name, larva currens (Latin: racing larva), to indicate the nature and uniqueness of this specific form of larva migrans. An alternate descriptive term, strongyloidiasis cutis, fails to indicate the major clinical feature of rapidity of larva movement.

COLD ERYTHEMA

Cold Erythema: A New Hypersensitivity Syndrome*

Report of a Case. The patient was a 5-year-old boy with a history of lifelong hypersensitivity to cold. The parents reported that ever since the first month of life the child had screamed and turned red whenever exposed to a cool environment. The pain and erythema were limited to the areas of chilled skin. As the child matured and was given cool liquids to drink, it was found that this invariably was followed by emesis. Furthermore, bowel training appeared to induce the pain and local erythema reaction. In the words of his mother, "After the age of 4 months, having a B.M. regularly caused a terrible spasm. His legs were so stiff they couldn't be straightened out, and he was in such severe pain, he couldn't be touched." The muscle spasm would gradually subside, but the child would scream continuously for up to an hour during which time his legs and lower trunk remained vividly red.

During the past year the patient has gradually overcome the problem of constipation and now has normal, regular bowel movements. The cold sensitivity, however, has persisted and has resulted in very serious restriction of the child's social and physical activity during cool weather. Indeed, in the summer even swimming is not possible. All cool beverages and foods are completely avoided, as well as contact with cool objects. The child's fear of anything cold has been overwhelming, and he guards against contact with ice as one would guard against contact with an open flame.

His parents described a generalized muscular spasm occurring after intense cold (e.g., ice) or cooling of a large area. The child collapses to the floor screaming and with all extremities flexed in rigid, tonic spasm. He has never lost consciousness during one of these attacks. No urticarial element has been noted by the parents, but rather they describe sudden reddening of the exposed areas, which persists for 30 to 60 minutes.

Physical examination and routine laboratory studies were normal, as were specialized studies on serum and urine. The ice test produced pain and erythema without urticaria and was blocked by previous infiltration with procaine hydrochloride. Intradermal injections of histamine and bradykinin produced typical reactions; serotonin produced marked erythema without a wheal. Injected plasma from cold-incubated, autologous blood also resulted in marked erythema. Passive transfer tests were negative. Therapeutic trial with several classes of compounds offered only slight relief. It is felt that this cold sensitivity may be mediated by local serotonin release.

---

* J.A.M.A., *180:*639, 1962.

AQUAGENIC URTICARIA

Aquagenic Urticaria: Contact Sensitivity Reaction to Water*

Report of Cases. Case 1—In July, 1963 a 15-year-old girl first noted the sudden onset of hives 30 minutes after water skiing. The lesions appeared as punctate wheals over her upper arms, upper back, anterior chest, abdomen, and flanks. Each wheal was surrounded by a large area of erythema, and the associated pruritus was severe.

Since her initial attack, urticaria has developed regularly in these same areas whenever she takes a bath or shower, swims, exercises, or perspires heavily. However, the hives have not been precipitated by psychological stress. Initially, she notes pruritus and blotchy erythema five to eight minutes after immersion in water. This is followed in three to five minutes by the appearance of small follicular hives, which persist 30 to 90 minutes, depending on the duration of water exposure. Longer exposure also greatly increases the number of lesions that develop. She notes no relationship of water temperature to the process. Following an urticarial attack, there is a relative to absolute refractory period of several hours.

Antihistaminic therapy (chlorpheniramine maleate) has successfully controlled the attacks, and at no time have systemic symptoms been experienced.

A towel wet with 0.9% sodium chloride solution and placed on the patient's back for ten minutes induced 50 small urticarial lesions. The same procedure using 5% sodium chloride solution induced more marked urticaria (20 more lesions which were larger than with 0.9% sodium chloride solution). Many lesions were induced by a towel wet with tap water on the back for ten minutes. A towel wet with tap water, placed on the back with a water-repellent polyethylene film (Saran Wrap) interposed for 15 minutes failed to produce hives. No hives were induced by a towel wet with absolute alcohol or one soaked in mineral oil.

Comment. Our 3 patients presented the classic features of "cholinergic urticaria". Such urticaria is readily distinguished from ordinary hives, cold urticaria, or dermographism by the patterning and by the critical challenge.

Interestingly, stress, tension, and pain did not initiate hives in our patients. This is understandable when it is realized that such stimuli did not produce any gross sweating and hence could not serve as a trigger factor. Sweating from exercise did prove to be an adequate stimulus. Here again, the surface "water" was the stimulus for hives.

The mechanism whereby water on the surface of the skin initiates hives and itching is not clear, but the follicular localization suggests that some toxic substance is formed by water acting on the sebum or sebaceous gland. This substance in passing through the pilosebaceous unit exerts a degranulating effect on the local mast cells. The released histamine produces pruritus, a pinhead-sized hive, and the flare.

AUTOIMMUNE PROGESTERONE SENSITIVITY DERMATITIS

Autoimmune Progesterone Dermatitis: Cure by Oophorectomy*

Report of a Case. A 27-year-old woman was referred to us in June, 1963 for evaluation of an extremely pruritic, grouped, vesicular eruption of five years' duration. The onset was in June, 1958, one week after delivery of her second child. Interpreted as a photosensitivity, the eruption cleared slowly over a period of

---

* J.A.M.A., *189:*895, 1964.

months only to recur explosively in November, 1960, after the birth of her third child. With but rare, short-lived remissions, this eruption has persisted. Dermatologic consultation coupled with biopsies had led to conflicting diagnoses ranging from dermatitis herpetiformis to a neurogenic disorder. Sulfapyridine, systemic steroids, griseofulvin, antihistaminics, sedation, as well as a score of topical agents had been without remarkable effect. The most striking feature of the history was the fact that the eruption usually became much more severe just prior to her menses. Her general medical history was noncontributory except for the removal of an ovarian cyst in 1959. Her menstrual cycle had been normal at all times. Menorrhagia or metrorrhagia had never been noted.

Physically she presented flaccid bullae in arciform patterning on her back and shins. These were on an erythematous base. Crusts, hyperpigmentation, and depigmented excoriation scars were much in evidence over the entire back and arms, as well as her anterior legs. General physical examination disclosed no gross abnormalities.

Our initial clinical impression brought forth the following differential list: dermatitis herpetiformis, lupus erythematosus, bullous lichen planus, drug eruption, dermatitis factitia, trichophytid, porphyria cutanea tarda, and erythema multiforme.

Hormonal challenges showed an oral dose of 1 mg Estradiol, 16 mg triamcinolone, 50 mg methyl testosterone, and 20 mg chlordiazepoxide hydrochloride (Librium) to have no effect. Administration of progesterone, 20 mg, resulted in a flare with new vesicles. Significant clinical improvement was demonstrated with intravenous administration of 25 units of corticotropin (ACTH).

Following discharge from the hospital, a progesterone desensitization program was initiated. Daily oral dosage of progesterone was 0.1 mg, with daily increments of 0.1 mg. Within ten days the dermatitis had become much more severe with many new lesions on the back, buttocks, upper anterior chest and mouth.

Ovulation was suppressed with estinyl estradiol in an oral dosage of 0.05 mg three times a day. This was followed by dramatic clearing. Within three days after stopping estinyl to permit menstruation, the eruption reappeared suddenly; it persisted until the estinyl was resumed.

After six months, estrogen therapy was discontinued. A bilateral oophorectomy and total hysterectomy was then done. The ovaries were grossly normal and histopathological study revealed normal tissue.

Within ten days the patient experienced a dramatic and complete remission of her dermatitis. She has had no pruritus or vesiculobullous lesions in the subsequent three months. Only residual postinflammatory pigmentation remains.

Comment. We have hence elected to label the findings in this patient as autoimmune progesterone dermatitis. It could be induced by progesterone or progesterone-like compounds, and presumably was triggered premenstrually by the elevated progesterone levels normally developing at this time. Hence, the endogenous progesterone triggering has been viewed as a form of autoimmune reaction.

PIEZOGENIC PEDAL PAPULES

Painful Feet due to Herniation of Fat*

Report of a Case. Tired, painful feet developed in a 20-year-old student after one week of summer employment as a railroad trackman.

At rest the foot appeared normal, but immediately on standing or applying pressure on the heel, firm papules developed along the medial aspect of the lower heel. Their induction by pressure was so characteristic that we have described these papules as "piezogenic." Numbering about a dozen on each foot, they could be made to appear and disappear as often as desired by simply regulating the pressure applications. Significantly, application of a blood pressure cuff at supra-systolic pressure (200 mmHg) failed to prevent their appearance, nor did intrasystolic pressure held at 150 mmHg produce them when the patient was prone.

The extrusions were soft and became painful with the passage of time. Relief was achieved only by avoiding long periods of standing.

Comment. The papules on the heels of this patient were viewed as true dermatoceles, i.e., the herniations of fatty subcutaneous tissue into connective tissue defects in the fascial layer we consider the dermis. The extrusion of fat with its vasculature and associated nerves could be presumed to lead in time to anoxic pain and hence explain the initial complaint of "painful feet on standing." Such pressure-induced pseudopapules are unique in our experience, but can be viewed as yet another example of skin changes due to physical forces.

PINCER NAILS

Pincer Nail Syndrome[†]

Report of Cases. Case 3. A 60-year-old white woman was seen in the Dermatology Clinic of the Hospital of the University of Pennsylvania, November 1966 for a problem of pain and swelling about the distal interphalangeal joints of her fingers accompanied by excessive transverse curvature of her nails. She stated that the condition began in 1961 when she noted the onset of her swelling and pain in the distal finger joints with a gradual exacerbation over the years. In 1965 she received a nine-month course of griseofulvin 250 mg four times a day without benefit. She denied the use of nail hardeners.

Physical examination showed swelling and deformity of the distal phalangeal joints of all fingers except thumbs. There was also a marked transverse curvature of all the fingernails. The left middle fingernail showed the greatest involvement to the point that the two lateral sides of the nail virtually met to form a tunnel. This finger also showed a marked loss of pulp. All toenails were thickened and curved in a similar fashion. Examination of toe and fingernails was negative for fungal elements. X-ray examination of the hands showed loss of tufts of the terminal phalanges of the third left finger and osteoarthritis of distal interphalangeal joints with hypertrophic spurring and narrowing of the distal joint space. No evidence of rheumatoid arthritis was noted. Serum latex fixation study for rheumatoid factor was negative.

The nail of the left middle finger was removed due to the associated pain occurring from the dystrophy of the nail. Postoperatively, the patient experienced relief of pain. Culture of the nail plate on Sabouraud's medium did not produce any growth.

Comment. Although excess transverse curvature of the nail has been recently described by Samman, we feel that the examples reported by us deserve a special name since they produce a pathologic degree of pinching of the underlying soft tissue, often to the point of disabling pain. The chronic constrictive forces of

---

* J.A.M.A., *205:*308, 1968.

† Arch. Surg., *96:*321, 1968.

the distorted nail plate may produce not only pain, but also loss of pulp tissue and resorption of bone as reflected in the radiologic patterns seen by us. The pathogenesis of this abnormality is obscure.

MID-DERMAL ELASTOLYSIS WRINKLES

Wrinkles due to Idiopathic Loss of Mid-dermal Elastic Tissue*

Case Report. A 42-year-old white woman had noted for 2 years widespread areas of crinkling of her skin, which gave it an inappropriate aged appearance. It was most evident on the antecubital fossae, the arms and trunk. Although large plaques were involved, areas of skin with normal appearance were evident. The affected skin was asymptomatic, normal in colour, and did not show atrophy or macules of herniation. Tension on the skin would completely obliterate the fine wrinkling.

Past history revealed that seven years prior to the present problem the patient had had recurrent unexplained urticarial lesions for more than a year. Actually, the initial wrinkling of the skin of the waist was first noted after an urticarial attack. The patient has endometriosis for which she has received contraceptive therapy (Norlestrin) for 10 years. Otherwise, her health has been excellent. There was no history of atopy. The parents, as well as her brothers and sisters, are in good health and show no signs of premature aging of the skin.

A general physical examination, complete blood count, urinalysis, thyroid studies and an SMA 12 screen showed no abnormalities. Histological study of 1–5 cm excisional biopsies of affected and normal skin from the right flank was made. The involved area showed thickening of the papillary dermis, some thinning of the rete and vacuolation of the basal cell zone. The small vessels of the superficial dermis were prominent, but there was no cellular infiltrate. The elastic tissue stain showed a remarkable and total absence of elastic fibre throughout the mid-dermis, except for a few fibres passing along the vascular structures.

Discussion. The large areas of fine wrinkled skin, which appeared in this woman at the age of 40, were unique in our experience. The process was not an anetoderma in the classical sense of a macule of atrophy. No atrophy of the dermal connective tissue was evident. Nor was it a form of striae distensae; no scarring was evident, only the fine crinkled surface. It was not acrodermatitis chronica atrophicans, since there was no inflammatory change, nodules, sclerotic change, or predilection for the extremities. Only wrinkles were seen, which left lichen sclerosis et atrophicus as well as poikiloderma vasculare atrophicans out of the differential diagnosis. The wrinkles were fine and superficial, not the pendulous folds of acquired cutis laxa.

No less unique than the anachronistic clinical appearance of our patient was the histological finding of complete absence of elastic fibres from the mid-dermal zone of connective tissue. The skin was otherwise microscopically normal. There was no inflammatory infiltrate nor was there a change in or recognizable absence of collagen. The elastic fibres present in the papillary dermis, as well as those in the deep dermis, were normal and showed no clumping or degenerative change.

The specific disappearance of elastic tissue would seem unquestionably to be the significant cause of the superficial fine wrinkling this patient developed at age 40. The absence of elastic tissue, whether it be in post acne scars (Dick et al., 1976) or in a wide variety of elastoses (Jarrett, 1974), regularly leads to wrinkling, since elastic tissue is the major element responsible for maintenance of a taut firm skin (Ross & Bornstein, 1971; Montagna & Parakkal, 1974). It is the unparalleled ability of elastic tissue to return rapidly to original size after being stretched to virtually twice its length, which gives skin its close fit!

---

* Br. J.Dermatol., *97*:441, 1977.

The selective disappearance of a specific band of elastic fibres remains unexplained. The loss of fibres was not from aging, since degenerative elastic change was not observed histologically. Nor did sunlight or actinic damage play a role. The key areas of involvement were not in exposed sites. One can postulate an immune elastolysis involving a sensitivity to elastin-bound progestational steroids, which she took for many years. One can think of specific destruction of elastin by the elastase known to exist in granulocytes (Janoff, 1970) and macrophages (Werb & Gordon, 1975), which participate in inflammatory processes. However, for neither of these hypotheses could we summon supportive evidence.

In conclusion, our patient demonstrates the need for a continuing awareness of the heterogeneity of wrinkles. Her wrinkles proved to have the fascination of a specific, histologically identifiable entity.

ADRENERGIC URTICARIA

Adrenergic Urticaria: A New Form of Stress-Induced Hives*

Case Reports and Results. Case 1—Five weeks after being in a serious truck accident a 28-year-old white male truck driver began having attacks of hives, which have recurred for 1 year. Face and jaw injuries had necessitated a three-day admission to hospital, but investigations including computed tomographic scanning of the skull had revealed no other ill-effects. A subsequent fear of driving led to a diagnosis, through psychological testing, of post-traumatic stress disorder.

The skin lesions had a half-life of about an hour and varied from 4–5 mm red macules to 1–3 mm papules with or without a 5–10 mm blanched halo. No lesions showed the erythematous flare seen in cholinergic urticaria. In severe attacks he experienced dyspnea and very large urticarial wheals. The hives appeared within 10–15 minutes after emotional stress—such as the fear invariably induced by the sight of his truck. Tension and coffee or chocolate intake also precipitated hives. Hydroxyzine 50 mg and diphenhydramine 50 mg both provided relief during attacks. He had a history of allergies to penicillin and lincomycin. Vitiligo was present on his hands, the onset of which he associated with the accident.

Our studies over six months revealed normal blood count and blood chemistries, serum IgE 210 U/ml (normal <60 U/ml), acetylcholine receptors normal, and no cryoglobulins. Plasma histamine, dopamine, and serotonin were normal before and during attacks. Total catecholamines increased from a baseline average of 379 pg/ml during hive-free periods to 838 pg/ml during an attack (normal 140–730 pg/ml). Noradrenaline similarly increased from 366 to 738 (normal 120–680 pg/ml) and adrenaline from <10 to 50 pg/ml (normal <60 pg/ml) during attacks.

A skin biopsy specimen of a hive showed only oedema and a sparse non-specific inflammatory infiltrate. Electron microscopy of his normal skin and three of the hives showed degranulation of the mast cells in the hives.

On intradermal skin testing a small red papule in a halo of blanched skin was induced by noradrenaline (3–10 ng in 0.02 ml saline). A similar response was seen with adrenaline in a dose of about 15 ng; larger amounts gave intense constriction, no hive. Injections of histamine, serotonin, and acetylcholine gave normal responses as did injection of noradrenaline and adrenaline intradermally in 7 normal subjects.

Therapy with the beta-adrenoreceptor-blocker propranolol (20 mg three times daily) has prevented nearly all hives over the past four months. When propranolol was discontinued for 72 h, the hives reappeared and a trial of an alternative beta-blocker, atenolol, was not successful.

---

* Lancet, 2:1031, 1985.

Discussion. Cholinergic urticaria is the only form of urticaria known to have a neural basis. Triggered by stress, heat, or emotion, it has a distinctive, readily recognizable appearance, e.g., a small papule in the center of a large bright red flare of axon-mediated vasodilation. It represents a unique response to acetylcholine released by the autonomic nerves and can, in many patients, be specifically replicated by an intradermal injection of acetylcholine (0.02 ml of a dilution of 10^{-3} to 10^{-5}).

This report describes a new distinctive form of urticaria, also stress-related, but due to a unique response to nor adrenaline. It can be readily distinguished from cholinergic urticaria since the primary urticarial papule is surrounded by a halo of blanched vasoconstricted skin. We have named these halo hives "adrenergic" urticaria, to distinguish them from and at the same time relate them to the congener, cholinergic urticaria. We suspect that this type of hive was previously lumped together with the cholinergic hive, since they have in common a tiny urticarial papule and similar precipitating factors of autonomic origin.

Adrenergic urticaria can and should be distinguished from cholinergic urticaria by its distinctive clinical appearance, by the halo hive induced with noradrenaline skin testing, and by a negative acetylcholine skin test. Patients currently classified as having "cholinergic urticaria" despite a negative acetylcholine skin test should be retested with noradrenaline, as well as with other neurotransmitters such as dopamine since other forms of "autonomic urticaria" may exist. The specificity of noradrenaline is noteworthy, and extremely dilute solutions (0.02 ml of 0.5×10^{-6}) must be used to avoid excessive vasoconstriction.

NON-PIGMENTING FIXED DRUG ERUPTION

Non-pigmenting Fixed Drug Eruption as a Distinctive Reaction Pattern: Examples Caused by Sensitivity to Pseudoephedrine Hydrochloride and Tetrahydrozoline*

Case Report. Case 1—A 7-year-old girl presented for emergency evaluation of large, erythematous plaques of the cheeks, axillae, groin, and buttocks of 4 hours duration. The lesions were bright red and slightly tender. The child felt sick, and there was associated joint tenderness and swelling. She had complained of malaise the previous night and had slept poorly. The only medication given had been 1 teaspoonful of Night-Time cold formula (anti-histamine with pain reliever, cough suppressant, and decongestant). There was no evidence of pharyngitis or otitis media.

The patient had been in excellent health, and there was no history of exposure to infectious disease. Her parents and 3-year-old brother were well.

Remarkably, the patient had had two identical attacks with skin lesions localized to the same sites. The first attack, 2 years previously, followed a cough and runny nose and required 3 days of hospitalization. A diagnosis of toxic erythema was made, and treatment was limited to acetaminophen and diphenhydramine. Within 3 days the eruption faded without residua. The second attack, 10 months before the present one, had been identical and had cleared after office treatment with diphenhydramine elixir and an intra-muscular injection of 20 mg of methylprednisolone acetate (Depo-Medrol).

A 5-day tapered course of prednisone (40, 40, 20, 10, 10 mg) led to resolution of the current lesions, followed by marked scaling of the involved sites. After 3 weeks the skin was normal. A diagnosis of nonpigmenting fixed drug eruption was made.

---

* J.Am. Acad. Dermatol., _17:_403, 1987.

The patient was then challenged orally with 1 ml of Night Time Cold Formula. Within 6 hours the same erythematous eruption appeared at exactly the same sites as her three former attacks. The erythema spontaneously remitted within 2 days. An oral challenge with 3 mg of d-pseudoephedrine (one third of the dose in a teaspoonful of Night Time Cold Formula) was also followed, 5 hours later, by the appearance of tender red plaques in all the previously affected sites, as well as swelling and pain in her hips and knee joints, so that walking became difficult. The inflammatory skin and joint changes involuted spontaneously within a week without residual pigmentation. Subsequent separate challenges with the other four components of Night Time Cold Formula (i.e., acetaminophen, doxylamine succinate, dextromethorphan hydrobromide, and tartrazine) showed negative results. A skin biopsy of the right hip 24 hours after the pseudoephedrine challenge showed a normal epidermis, edema of the papillary dermis, and occasional neutrophils and eosinophils in the upper portion of the reticular dermis, particularly around the blood vessels. The absence of epidermal change was interpreted by the pathologist as precluding the diagnosis of a fixed drug eruption.

In the subsequent year, the patient has avoided all pseudoephedrine-containing medications and has had no further attacks.

Discussion. For us, the nonpigmenting fixed drug eruption has become a recognizable clinical entity. All three patients whose cases are presented here had remarkably similar symmetrical erythematous plaques that had recurred at the same sites, particularly the groin areas. The margins of the plaques showed fine punctate erythematous macules. These lesions were identical to those caused by the d-pseudoephedrine isomer of ephedrine in the two patients carefully studied by Brownstein.

We became convinced that our first patient's skin lesions were truly a fixed drug eruption after seeing and photographing skin lesions on three separate occasions after drug ingestion. We suspect that similar recurrent eruptions occurring months to years apart go unrecognized as appearing at identical sites.

In this patient, specific symmetrical areas of the skin were sensitized and responsive to pseudoephedrine, which caused a "fixed" eruption. However, in contrast to the pigmenting fixed drug eruption, the lesions were symmetrical and not followed by pigmentation. Presumably, the dermis, rather than the epidermis, was the primary site of the drug sensitivity response. Without epidermal melanocyte incontinence, ready recognition of the "fixed" nature of the response becomes difficult. An eruption is "fixed" if it repeatedly recurs in a previously affected (hypersensitive) area of skin or mucous membrane; duration and pigmentation are inconsequential. Only by serial photography or careful cartographic drawings can the fixed nature of the eruption be documented and appreciated. Otherwise, most physicians pay little heed to the patient's statement, "It's back in the same places."

Recognition of the nonpigmenting dermal type of fixed drug eruption as an entity will come with improved documentation of the localization of recurring lesions. We should direct our attention and our patient's attention to all medications used or taken in the 24-hour period preceding any attack. Challenges can then be performed safely with small doses of suspected medications and their ingredients.

AUTOIMMUNE ESTROGEN DERMATITIS

Estrogen Dermatitis*

Case Reports. Case 1—A 34-year-old woman was first seen in January 1986 because of a papulovesicular facial eruption that she had had 13 years. It began after a serum sickness reaction to gamma globulin. Her facial eruption persisted despite numerous types of treatment. In July 1983 a biopsy specimen revealed an inflammatory cell infiltrate of eosinophils and lymphocytes with marked focal edema and erosion of the epidermis, consistent with granuloma faciale. In June 1984 another biopsy specimen showed allergic vasculitis, with focal necrosis of the epidermis, fibrin deposition, an intense inflammatory infiltrate of eosinophils and neutrophils around vessels in the papillary dermis, and a lymphocytic infiltrate in the reticular dermis extending into the fat.

Examination revealed patchy erythema, edema, and vesicles on the face with secondary impetiginization. After controlling the secondary infection and having the patient keep a diary, it was evident that her lesions worsened and new ones appeared premenstrually. The diagnosis then became autoimmune progesterone dermatitis. She was treated with injections of triamcinolone acetonide suspension at 3- to 6-week intervals and later with terfenadine and chlorpheniramine. This was continued for 4 years, at which time astemizole was substituted. Vesicles and papules reappeared whenever the antihistamines were stopped.

In November 1989 duplicate intradermal skin tests on the arm and thigh were done; medroxyprogesterone (Depo-Provera 0.1 ml, 1 mg/ml) was negative at 20 minutes and 2 days; estrone (Theeline Aqueous 0.1 ml, 1 mg/ml) was negative at 20 minutes, but within 3 hours became urticarial. By 5 hours her face showed blotchy erythema and within 12 hours vesicles and papules appeared on her face. The estrone skin test sites remained indurated and edematous for more than 24 hours, and the facial eruption persisted for 3 days. We diagnosed "estrogen dermatitis."

She was then given the estrogen antagonist tamoxifen (10 mg twice daily) during the second half of the menstrual cycle, with marked improvement. Her follicular phase serum estrogen and progesterone levels were normal. For the next 3 years she remained free of lesions while taking terfenadine (60 mg twice daily) and tamoxifen (10 mg twice daily) for 4 days premenstrually. At her last visit she had not taken tamoxifen for 3 months and has had no recurrence of her eruption.

In October 1993 she was tested with the 15 hormones listed in (Table 1). All yielded negative results. At that time a luteal phase serum hormone panel also gave normal findings.

Discussion. The disorder demonstrated in our seven patients and first recognized by Zondek and Bromberg a half century ago is considered to be "autoimmune estrogen dermatitis." It refers to patients who have a positive estrogen skin test or a positive oral challenge to estrogens. We believe that this term is inappropriate for diseases in which immune modulation by estrogens occurs rather than direct sensitivity to estrone. We also recognize that the criteria for inclusion of this disease within the strict immunologic definition of autoimmunity have not yet been met.

The hallmark of estrogen dermatitis is the cyclic premenstrual flare. This may be difficult to discern in a chronic dermatosis, which to the patient is "always worse." Some patients experience the problem only menstrually. Sometimes a patient will volunteer in a routine history that "it always gets worse before my period." Dismissing the patient's observations may lead to missing the diagnosis.

The clinical picture is varied. Sometimes it presents as pruritus, either generalized or localized, as in pruritus vulvae and pruritus ani. In others the reactive pattern is urticaria, unremitting and daily, but always peaking premenstrually. One of our patients had inflammatory vesicles and papules, largely limited to the face and neck. A second patient had inflammatory papules on the neck, upper trunk, and arms. This localization may reflect estrogen receptor density, which is highest in the skin in the face and surrounding areas.

Intradermal tests are necessary to establish the diagnosis. It is essential that intradermal test material be injected subepidernally to raise a superficial bleb and minimize rapid lymphatic removal. We recommend 0. 1 ml of a 1:1,000 dilution (1 mg/ml) be injected with a tuberculin syringe with a 27-gauge needle. Ideally,

* J.Am. Acad. Dermatol., *32*:25, 1995.

sterile aqueous suspensions of pure estrone and other hormones should be used, but preliminary testing can be done by diluting Theelin (aqueous estrone) to half strength with sterile saline solution. Persistence of a papule for more than 24 hours is considered a positive test. Even more convincing is the reactivation of the test site during future premenstrual periods, as the skin test site acts as a mini-fixed drug eruption. In urticaria the positive test is an immediate urticarial wheal that fades in hours.

Oral challenge may also be done with ethinyl estradiol, but a positive result supports only an estrogen-aggravated dermatitis. To show sensitization, a superficial injection is required. Injections of progesterone (10^{-3} aqueous suspension) are routinely given to rule out autoimmune progesterone dermatitis.

A specific treatment is the antiestrogen tamoxifen (10 mg one to three times a day for 10 to 14 days before each period). Tamoxifen interferes with the clinical expression of estrogen sensitivity, possibly via its competitive binding of the estrogen receptors.

ABACUS NODULE

Photovignette: The Abacus Nodule (Mobile Encapsulated Lipoma)*

For the past six months this 76-year-old man had been intrigued by a small, painless, non-inflammatory mass in the skin of his left forearm. It simply would not hold still and moved up and down along his forearm. Measuring about 1 cm in size it had a territorial range of about 15 cm. We could move it like an abacus bead in a linear path to any desired spot. At surgery, the mass proved to be a firm yellow ball of fatty tissue 0.8 cm in diameter. Histologic study showed a discrete nodule of fat tissue surrounded by hyalinized collagen containing punctate spindle cells and blood vessels. The center portion was hyalinized suggesting some degeneration. We suspect the nodule derived its mobility and nutrition from a thin umbilical string of connective tissue.

Healing was uneventful but the patient wistfully misses his little worry bead.

IGE BULLOUS DISEASE

IgE Bullous Disease[†]

Case 1. A 69-year-old woman developed numerous pruritic blisters behind her ears in April 1991, five months prior to our examination. The blisters gradually became more generalized, with the largest ones being concentrated over the left anterior thigh. In September 1989 she fractured her left femur, requiring hip surgery with a dynamic chondylar screw, a buttress plate with allografting, and an osteogenic bone growth stimulator battery. Otherwise, she was in relatively good health. Tense bullae on erythematous urticarial bases, 0.5–3.0 cm in size, were noted on her face, neck, upper trunk, back, and left thigh, each filled with clear or slightly haemorrhagic fluid. Nikolsky's sign was negative. Ruptured bullae left mildly inflamed crusted erosions. Mucous membranes were not affected.

Routine laboratory investigations, including the eosinophil count, were normal, as were the serum antinuclear antibody (ANA), BMZ antibody, intercellular antibody titres, and serum immunoglobulin IgG,

---

* J.Geriatric. Dermatol., *3*:A6, 1995.

† Clin. Exp. Dermatol., *22*:82, 1997.

IgM, and IgA concentrations. Her serum IgE concentration, however, was markedly elevated at 1250 U/ml (normal <88 U/ml).

Skin biopsy revealed a subepidermal bulla containing numerous eosinophils and rare neutrophils, while in the upper dermis there was a dense perivascular infiltrate composed of eosinophils, lymphocytes and occasional mast cells. Immunofluorescent staining for IgA, IgG, IgM, C3, fibrinogen, and albumin, performed on several occasions, was negative in lesional, perilesional and uninvolved tissue from various sites.

In May 1994, further skin biopsy showed identical results, as did further routine immunofluorescent studies. However, special immunofluorescent staining for IgE revealed numerous IgE-positive cells inside a bulla and in the upper dermis. However, no deposition was seen along the basement membrane or in non-lesional skin, while indirect immunofluorescence failed to demonstrate circulating anti-skin IgE antibodies.

Improvement again occurred when the patient was given cefadroxil monohydrate (500 mg, twice a day), although new lesions still continued to appear, particularly on the left thigh overlying the subcutaneous battery ('EBI OsteoGen' Long bone SN 511540; EBI Medical Systems, Parsippany, NJ) installed to stimulate bone healing. Hypersensitivity to the battery was thus suspected, but patch tests to the battery materials (titanium, platinum and silicone) were negative, while subsequent patch tests with the T.R.U.E. Test® (Kabi Pharmacia Service A/S, Hillerod, Denmark) and standard patch tests to 24 allergenic compounds were negative as well.

Intradermal tests with various metallic salts (0.1% solutions of potassium dichromate, cobalt sulphate, gold chloride, titanium lactate, nickel sulphate and copper sulphate) were also negative.

In October 1994, the battery was surgically removed, the tissue surrounding the battery being found to contain adipose tissue with dense fibrosis and chronic inflammation, all staining negative for bacteria and fungi. This removal was followed by rapid clearing within days of the skin lesions, while during the next twenty months, only occasional small bullae have continued to appear on the left hip, neck and face. The serum IgE level has also decreased (422 U/mL (11/1994); 390 U/mL (12/1994); 360 U/mL (02/1995); 320 U/mL (07/1995); 257 U/mL (08/1995)).

Discussion. Our two cases are unique in having IgE as the only immunoglobulin present in their skin lesions, although the finding of IgE in the lesions of bullous pemphigoid is not new, IgE having been seen as linear deposits along the BMZ and on inflammatory cells in bullae in up to 70% patients with the disease. In all cases, however, IgG or C3 were also present in the lesions or in perilesional skin.

We, therefore, speculate that microbial antigens from the orthopaedic device (patient one) and the necrotic leg ulcers (patient two) triggered IgE production, and that binding of IgE antibodies to target cells in the skin, mainly eosinophils, may have induced the bullous lesions. In fact, eosinophils are believed to be directly responsible for blister formation in bullous pemphigoid, exerting cytotoxic effects through their specific granule proteins, including in particular MPB, and since eosinophils participate in IgE-mediated antigen presentation, very low concentrations of allergen could cause continuous activation of the immune system with increased IgE production. Thus, the presumptive triggering infections were surgically removed in our patients, their serum IgE levels gradually declined.

We now suspect that 'IgE bullous disease' is a subset of the bullous dermatoses clinically similar to bullous pemphigoid, in which routine immunofluorescent stains are negative, and for this reason we suggest that routine direct immunofluorescence staining technique be expanded to also include the detection of IgE antibodies.

AQUADYNIA

Aquadynia: Noradrenergic Pain Induced by Bathing and Responsive to Clonidine*

Case Reports. Case 1—An 82-year-old woman had severe generalized burning pain after every bath. For more than 6 years, it had not responded to bicarbonate baths or to hydroxyzine and other antihistamines. Her pain began within minutes after she got out of the bath and lasted 45 minutes. It was so severe that she limited her bathing to once a week. The pain did not occur while she was in the water. Although remaining in the bath for a prolonged period lessened subsequent symptoms, she had not been able to desensitize herself by repeated baths at short intervals. Treatment with propranolol (60 mg/day) provided some relief, but the pain intensity and duration continued to increase, with some attacks lasting more than an hour.

Her past history included a hysterectomy, tonsillectomy, and cholecystectomy. She did not smoke or drink. Her medications included hydrochlorothiazide plus triamterene daily for 10 years and atenolol for 2 years. A complete blood cell count, chemistry profile, urinalysis, sedimentation rate, antinuclear antibody test, rapid plasma reagin test, and rheumatoid factor test were normal. Results of her skin examination were normal and dermographism was absent. Findings of a general physical and neurologic examination were normal. Two skin biopsy specimens were normal, including the mast cell count.

After 2 years her hemoglobin had risen to 19.0 gm with a hematocrit of 57.6 and a red blood cell count of 6.82. Polycythemia was diagnosed, although her platelet count was normal and there was no splenomegaly. Her blood cell count returned to normal after phlebotomies (500 ml/week×4), but this had no effect on the pain after bathing. She then told us that a sister had polycythemia vera with associated aquagenic pruritus, but no pain.

In January 1994, studies showed elevated serum epinephrine, norepinephrine, and catecholamine levels during her attacks of pain. Accordingly, clonidine 0.1 mg twice a day was prescribed: it gave complete relief of pain. She has taken clonidine daily for 3 years, and bathes regularly without symptoms.

Discussion. Severe burning pain in the skin that follows brief contact with water and lasts 15 to 45 minutes without observable skin changes is rare. Previously included with aquagenic pruritus, the pain seems severe enough to deserve a separate diagnosis, aquadynia.

We found no psychosomatic explanation or evidence of feigned symptoms. Xerosis from over-bathing was not a factor. It was not an inflammatory skin disease, as in erythromelalgia, nor was it drug-induced or caused by iron deficiency. There was no evidence of Fabry's disease, hyperesthesia, or allodynia. Our first patient had polycythemia, sometimes associated with aquagenic pruritus, but elimination of the polycythemia did not affect her aquadynia.

The pathogenesis of the pain appears to involve sympathetic nerves that can mediate pain, but we have no explanation of the mechanism. Studies on reflex sympathetic dystrophy (causalgia) have shown that sympatholytic intervention can abolish pain and hyperalgesia. The application or injection of norepinephrine in an area of causalgia can induce intense pain. Significantly, the topical application of clonidine, an alpha-2 adrenergic agonist, eliminates hyperalgesia to mechanical and cold stimuli in causalgia.

We propose that the pain of aquadynia may in some patients be of noradrenergic origin because systemic clonidine and propranolol were effective treatments in our patients. Propranolol, a beta-adrenergic blocking agent, was less effective than clonidine, an adrenergic inhibitor. The persistence of pain for up to an hour

---

* J.Am. Acad. Dermatol., 38:357, 1998.

may correlate with the time to deplete norepinephrine granules from nerve endings. Aquagenic pruritus probably has a similar noradrenergic origin, because we have successfully treated four patients with clonidine.

William Bennett Bean

Blue Rubber-Bleb Nevus Syndrome (Bean's Syndrome)

WILLIAM BENNETT BEAN was born on November 9, 1909 in Manila, Philippines. His father was an anatomist and physical anthropologist studying Philippine tribesmen at the time. After the family returned to the US, Bean's life through college and medical school centered on the campus of the University of Virginia where his father became Head of the Anatomy Department. William's scholastic achievements were legendary, with his grades higher than ever seen in the history of that university.

After graduation in 1935 he interned at Johns-Hopkins and was a resident at Harvard and the University of Cincinnati. There, with others, he demonstrated that nicotinic acid was the key missing nutrient in alcoholic pellagrins. Next came 4 years of study of heat stress in tanks at the Armored Medical Research Laboratory at Fort Knox, KY. Shortly after the war he was appointed Head of the Department of Internal Medicine at the University of Iowa where he brought his staff enthusiasm, culture and skills in reading and writing. He graced medical literature with 527 published papers, 693 book reviews and gave 980 formal talks.

In 1969 he resigned his headship of the Department of Medicine and later moved to be the Director of the Institute of Humanities in Medicine at Galveston, Texas. By 1980 he returned to Iowa as a beloved Professor Emeritus, still full of roguish wit and infinite wisdom.

His paper of 35 years of monthly recording of the growth of his fingernails, as well as his monograph on vascular spiders, endeared him to dermatologists.

William Bennett Bean died at his home March 1, 1989 after a long struggle with colon cancer.*

BEAN'S SYNDROME

Blue Rubber-Bleb Nevi of the Skin and Gastrointestinal Tract[†]

There is a characteristic variety of bluish nevus of the skin found in association with angiomas of the gastrointestinal tract which cause serious bleeding. The larger angiomas have some of the feel and look of rubber nipples, are compressible and refill fairly promptly from their rumpled compressed state. I have called them rubber-bleb nevi, though they vary in size, shape and number. This lesion has been described by surgeons but has not been emphasized in writings of internists and gastroenterologists. In association with Dr. Robert Tidrick I have observed a child with this condition and there are records from *Surgical Pathology* of others. In Albuquerque with Dr. Lyle Carr I saw another patient, a Latin American girl, with dark brown

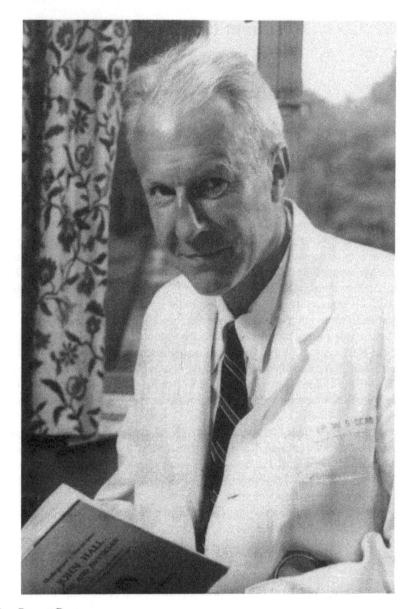

Figure 131 William Bennett Bean

skin who had bled from the bowel, was anemic, and had the characteristic lesions of the skin. At the same time sections of the resected specimen from another patient were inspected.

While much less common than hereditary hemorrhagic telangiectasia, the syndrome of erectile bluish nevi of the skin and angiomatosis of the gut associated with enteric bleeding is definite. It should be known better.

Case Report. In March 1944, a three month old boy was admitted to the Pediatric Service because his mother discovered a swelling of the medial aspect of the right knee. It had been present at birth. There was no restriction of motion or pain on movement and no therapy was tried. He was next seen in the spring of 1949 with the same complaint and the soft, nontender mass, which prevented full extension of the leg at the knee. Numerous solitary telangiectases on the trunk, the extremities, and the soles of the feet and soft, bilateral nontender masses in the parotid regions were found. An operation was done to remove the large hemangioma, which extended into the knee joint. He was seen twice in 1950, having had no recurrence of the lesion. Motion at the joint was normal. In the spring of 1951 he was admitted for persistent anemia and given iron and transfusions. There had been the passage of some bloody stools. Hemangiomas were noted on sigmoidoscopic examination. X-rays of the upper and lower parts of the alimentary canal revealed no obvious abnormality. The hemoglobin, despite transfusions and the use of iron, ranged between 3.5 and 10 gm. per 100 ml. In May 1951 a resection of part of the small bowel was performed. Though there was some occult blood in the stool after operation, the hemoglobin returned to normal but has fallen at times, usually responding to iron therapy. At intervals there is probably bleeding but there has been no gross hemorrhage. He has done well most of the time but has been given two transfusions. Once in 1956 he had a convulsion involving the left arm and leg. An electroencephalogram revealed a few focal spikes in the right temporal region. On his last visit, he was asymptomatic, there were no new findings, and the hemoglobin was 11.5 gm.

In the syndrome exemplified by these few cases we have a spectrum of angiomatous lesions distributed widely throughout the body. I emphasize the fact that in a rare case angiomas of the gut can be inferred with assurance from their presence in the skin. In number, size and location, the vascular lesions may range from the trivial single lesion of the skin or gut to the disastrous destructive angiomatosis when the lesion is almost everywhere. The family history is negative. There is no sign of lesion in the parents or siblings of our patient.

The bluish nevi of the skin seen in this syndrome may occur in three main forms. One is the large disfiguring cavernous angioma, which may replace vital structures, or growing to large size, obstruct the airway, alimentary canal, or some other important tubular structure. Another variety is the blood sac, looking like a blue rubber nipple covered with a milk white tissue of thin skin. These can be emptied of much or all of their contained blood. From the irregular mussed and rumpled state they resume their distended state by the gradual influx of blood. The third major variety of lesion is the irregular blue mark, sometimes with punctate blackish spots, merging with the adjacent normal skin in a series of color gradations through pale blue to white. Such lesions are elevated above the skin surface only if they are large. The small ones may or may not blanch on pressure. There is rarely complete fading perhaps because of the complex tangle of coiled vascular spaces, which trap blood when the structure is compressed.

---

* Trans. Assoc. Am. Physicians., *103:*LXXX vii, 1990.

† Bean, W.B.: Vascular Spiders and Related Lesions of the Skin. Charles C.Thomas, Springfield, IL; pp 178, 1958.

Earl W.Netherton

Netherton's Syndrome

EARL WELDON NETHERTON was born in Gallatin, Missouri on April 7, 1893. After a boyhood in Gallatin he graduated from the University of Missouri and went on to receive his M.D. in 1917 from Washington University in St. Louis. Following a residency in Dermatology at Barnard Skin and Cancer Hospital in St. Louis and service in the U.S. Army, he joined the Cleveland Clinic, establishing and nurturing their outstanding Department of Dermatology. A splendid teacher and astute clinician, he published numerous incisive clinical papers on a variety of subjects ranging from beryllium granulomas to vaccine therapy. But, it was his story of the child with bamboo hair that gave him eponymic recognition.

After retirement from the Clinic in 1958, he joined his dermatologist son, Thomas, in private practice. He died November 2, 1967.*

NETHERTON'S SYNDROME

A Unique Case of Trichorrhexis Nodosa—"Bamboo hairs"[†]

Report of a Case. A girl, aged 4 years, was admitted to The Cleveland Clinic on November 22, 1949, because the hair on the scalp had failed to grow to normal length (there had been no area of baldness), and a pruritic eruption had been present since birth. The mother stated that at birth the patient's entire cutaneous surface was extremely red and that for several weeks thereafter there was a generalized exfoliative dermatitis emitting a foul odor. The erythroderma gradually disappeared, leaving a persistent papular squamous eruption disseminated over the trunk and the extremities. Partial remission of this eruption occurred during each summer season, although it had never disappeared entirely.

At the age of 2 years, the patient had had vaccinia. Since infancy she had had frequent attacks of upper respiratory infection. The mother stated that the child was "frequently restless, irritable, and difficult to feed because of her preference for liquid foods."

There was no familial history of hay fever, asthma, or eczema. Two siblings, aged 8 and 2 years, were normal.

---

* Szymanski, F.J.: Centenial History of the American Dermatological Association 1876–1976.

[†] Arch. Dermatol., *78*:483, 1958.

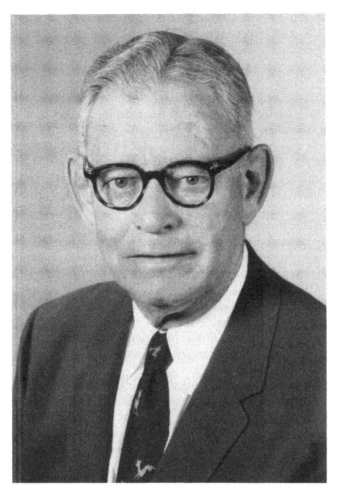

Figure 132 Earl W.Netherton

Physical examination disclosed that the patient was thin and poorly nourished. The skin was abnormally dry, and there were poorly demarcated areas of pink scaly dermatitis on the forehead and neck. There was excessive seborrheic scaling on the scalp, but there were no follicular keratosis pilaris-like papules on the scalp. Patches of subacute erythematous scaly dermatitis, which resembled chapping, were scattered over the trunk and extremities, as well as groups of small discrete acuminate pink follicular papules. Some of these papules had apical keratotic spines. Pruritus was paroxysmal and was said to be usually more severe during the night. The teeth and nails were normal. The lymph nodes of the neck, axillae, and inguinal regions were palpable. The spleen and liver were not enlarged.

The hair on the scalp was dry and fragile and lacked the luster and beauty commonly seen in the hair of young girls. Hairs on the occiput and sides of the scalp were no longer than 3 or 4 cm and developed transverse fractures so easily that it was difficult to remove them from the follicles by traction. Casual inspection did not reveal nodes involving the hairs of the scalp.

Microscopic examination of hairs from the scalp and the eyebrows revealed a unique type of nodosity or jointed swelling of the hair shafts. Apparently the jointedness accounted for the easy fracturing of the hair shaft and its failure to grow to a normal length. Some eyelashes and downy hairs from the arms showed small nodes, but they were not the well-developed jointed swellings of the type seen in the hairs from the scalp.

A biopsy specimen from the scalp unfortunately was not obtained. However, tissue from an erythematous plaque on the patient's back was removed. Sections from this biopsy specimen revealed surprisingly few significant histopathologic changes.

Almost seven years after the initial examination, in September, 1956, I had the privilege of examining the patient again in her home city. The hair on the scalp was dry, without normal luster, and fragile. The hair on the sides and posterior surfaces of the scalp had failed to grow to normal length. Hairs removed from the scalp showed the same unique type of joint-like nodose swelling of the shaft, which was observed at the first examination in 1949.

Laboratory Studies. Hairs from the scalp were mounted in balsam for study of the morphologic details of the hair shafts. The nodose swellings showed great variation in size. The earliest indication of abnormality comprised a narrow indentation of the cortex of the hair, forming a shallow sulcus, which appeared to surround the shaft. This change was sparse or frequent, occurring at irregular intervals and throughout the length of the hair. One hair showed early indentation of the atrophic portion of the shaft, immediately distal to the orifice of its follicle. As the abnormality had progressed, swellings of the shaft had developed, the sulcus had enlarged, and, on the proximal portion of the hair shaft, a concavity had formed into which fitted the adjacent enlargement of the distal portion of the hair. These combined changes had resulted in the formation of a pseudojointed nodose swelling that, as previously stated, closely resembled the appearance of the joints of a bamboo pole.

Changes observed in the large nodes suggest that there had been an invagination or intussusception of portions of the hair shaft. Cultures of hairs planted on Sabouraud's medium did not show growth of a pathogenic fungus.

Comment. The most familiar diseases in which fragility and nodose swellings of the hair shaft are prominent characteristics are trichorrhexis nodosa and monilethrix. Nodose swellings that resemble those seen in trichorrhexis nodosa have been observed in pili torti. Nodular concretions of infectious origin surrounding the hair shafts in piedra nostros and lepothrix differ greatly in appearance from those seen in trichorrhexis nodosa and monilethrix. Formerly, the concept was widely accepted that abnormal changes involving the hair shaft in trichorrhexis nodosa are of infectious origin. This concept now has been largely discarded, and the present consensus is that the longitudinal splintering of the shaft and the formation of nodes, which resemble the interlocking of two small brushes at sites of fracture of the hair shaft, probably are the sequelae of too-frequent shampooing and excessive dryness of the hair. Some chemicals commonly applied to the hair may be important etiologic factors.

Pili torti and monilethrix are examples of ectodermal defects. Monilethrix usually is hereditary and is characterized by numerous small discrete papules, similar to those of keratosis pilaris, on the scalp, and sparse growth of short fragile beaded hair. The nodose swellings are uniform in size and shape and are located at regular intervals throughout the entire length of the hair. There is a notable constriction of the hair shaft between the nodes. Abnormal dentition and other manifestations of the ectodermal defect may be present. Twisting of the hair around its long axis occurs in some of the beaded hairs. However, this change is minor and does not approach the degree of rotation seen in pili torti. Danforth has pointed out that normal hair tends to be ribbon-like and frequently is rotated to some degree around the long axis. He believed that this feature of normal hair had been neglected by previous observers.

In regard to this case, Drs. M.F.Engman, Lee McCarthy, Herman Pinkus, Richard Weiss, Harold Cole, Fred Weidman, and others, were unanimous in stating that never had they seen similar nodosa swellings of the hair shaft.

Harold O.Perry

Reticular Erythematous Mucinosis (REM Syndrome)

HAROLD OTTO PERRY was born in Rochester, Minnesota on November 18, 1921, and received his B.S. from the University of Minnesota in 1944 and his M.D. in 1947. After an internship at the Naval Hospital in Oakland, California, his dermatologic training was at the Mayo Clinic under Paul O'Leary. He joined the faculty at the Mayo Clinic in 1952 and continued to practice and teach there until his retirement in 1989. Although throughout his career Perry was concerned with the whole of dermatology, the wealth of material at Mayo provided him with ample opportunity to identify and study in depth the rarer entities in the dermatologic catalogue. His work on pyoderma gangrenosum has done much to clarify and identify the ramifications of that mysterious entity, and he has made valuable contributions to our knowledge of bullous diseases, pilomatrixoma, drug eruptions, cutaneous signs of internal disease, and the treatment of psoriasis. His keen clinical eye is evident in his 1960 classic account, excerpted below, of the condition now known as *reticular erythematous mucinosis*.

President of four national dermatologic societies in the U.S., honorary member of many international and national societies, he received the Gold Medal of the American Academy of Dermatology in 1998 for his visionary leadership. A consummate clinician and gentleman, he is admired and loved by his students all over the world.*

REM SYNDROME

Plaque-Like Form of Cutaneous Mucinosis*

That mucin may be deposited in the skin independent of any apparent associated endocrinopathy is now a well-established fact. Initially, generalized myxedema in association with hypothyroidism was considered the only situation in which this occurred. Subsequently, nodules and large plaques of mucin were found, particularly in the pretibial area, in association with patients who had, or had been treated for, hyperthyroidism.

As the problem of localized pretibial myxedema was further studied, it was appreciated that patches of localized myxedema could occur in the absence of any thyroid dysfunction; cutaneous deposits of mucin were found in the skin widespread over the body, and in this group of patients a normal endocrine function

---

* Who's Who in America, 2003.

* Arch. Dermatol. *82:*980, 1960.

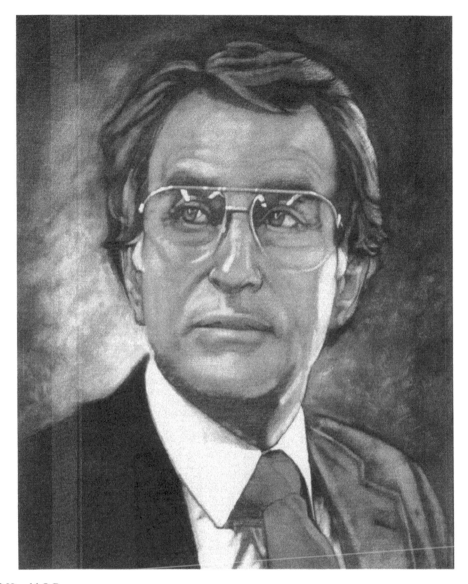

Figure 133 Harold O.Perry

so far has been the rule. The term "lichen myxedematosus" (papular mucinosis, lichen fibromucinoidosus) has been employed to classify this latter group clinically.

The deposits of mucin in cutaneous mucinosis, referred to in the past as lichen myxedematosus, occur in various morphologic forms. Montgomery and Underwood have outlined these forms as (1) generalized lichenoid papular, (2) discrete papular, (3) localized or generalized lichenoid plaques, and (4) urticarial and nodular forms. We have had the opportunity of studying three patients, two women and one man, each in the middle decades of life, each presenting symmetrically disposed, essentially asymptomatic eruptions of closely set, somewhat urticarial papules on the anterior and posterior aspects of the upper part of the trunk, and each displaying histologically the deposition of mucin in the upper corium. It would seem on the basis of the peculiar truncal involvement in these three patients that still another type of cutaneous mucinosis may be seen and that this may be an additional subgrouping of lichen myxedematosus (papular mucinosis). Because the histopathologic features of the three cases were so very similar, the results of skin biopsies will be discussed together, after the case reports.

Summary. Three patients are reported who have had persistent erythematous plaques on the anterior and posterior aspects of the thorax that histologically fulfill the criteria for the diagnosis of lichen myxedematosus. The plaques, composed of closely set erythematous, somewhat urticarial papules, have persisted essentially unchanged for periods up to eight years after obtaining their present size soon after onset, have been asymptomatic except for some pruritus, and have been unassociated with systemic disease. These three patients seem to form another subgroup among those forms of cutaneous mucinosis classified as lichen myxedematosus (papular mucinosis); however, it is probably best to continue to classify them under this term, which is in general usage at this time, and adequately separates these lesions from those of generalized myxedema and localized pretibial myxedema.

Albert M. Kligman

Telogen Effluvium

ALBERT MONTGOMERY KLIGMAN was born March 17, 1916 in Philadelphia and has remained there as an indigenous treasure to this day. He received his Bachelor's Degree at Pennsylvania State University where he was Captain of their Olympic-qualifying gymnastic team. After a Ph.D. in Botany and authoring the only monograph on the care and feeding of mushrooms, he received his M.D. and took his residency in dermatology, all at the University of Pennsylvania. There he has spent all of his life, lifted to full professorship by a phenomenal 1,700 papers and 5 textbooks. He became an international institution, training over 600 fellows in dermatology from all over the world. His zest for research and for living infects all who have ever encountered him in his lab, in the lecture hall, or in his writings. His great love is teaching. He has a flair for clothing his thoughts in regal phrase. At the blackboard he converts chalk into the gold of wisdom.

His research has included a ladder of investigations, centered on study of volunteers in the local prisons of Philadelphia. He brought them hope and they brought him knowledge. Not surprisingly, his knowledge of botany led to his early investigations of tinea capitis and the PAS stain for detecting fungal hyphae. He proceeded to explore contact dermatitis, developing predictive screening for compounds, as well as desensitization for poison ivy. At the very top of the ladder are his discoveries of retinoic acid for the topical treatment of acne and photo-aging.

Kligman coined the word, *cosmeceuticals* and minted many a product in this very field. His royalties have enabled him to be one of dermatology's greatest philanthropists.

His hobbies express his exuberance for life. Everything he does can be described only in superlatives. His gymnastic athleticism evolved into ballet dancing, figure skating, skiing, and golfing. He has, indeed, leaped into the air, ballooning as well as flying his private plane; all this, while he remains a cosmonaut exploring the outer reaches of the universe of dermatology.

In summation, it is *Albert the Great* who has changed the face of man…and the mind of dermatology.*

TELOGEN EFFLUVIUM

Pathologic Dynamics of Human Hair Loss. I. Telogen Effluvium[†]

Specific Formulation. The thesis is simplicity itself. Whatever the cause of hair loss, the follicle tends to behave in a similar way. To etiologic diversity it reacts with stereotyped singularity. The follicle traumatized sufficiently to lose its hair, regardless of the nature of the insult, is precipitated into catagen and

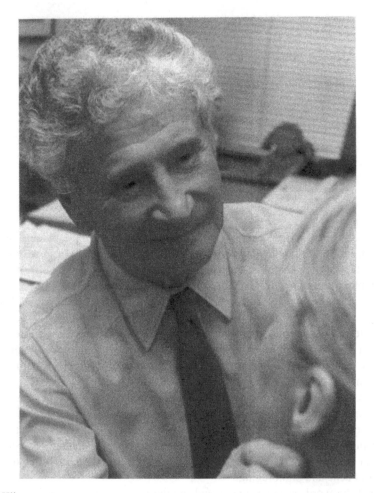

Figure 134 Albert M.Kligman

transforms into a resting stage, which mimics telogen. Ignoring teleological undertones, the strategy of the harassed follicle is to protect itself by regressing to an inactive embryonal stage. In so doing, it utilizes a built-in model, namely, the pattern of catagen, which is its accustomed means of involution at the end of anagen. We thus have before us another example of one of the paramount axioms of pathology. The normal contains the seed of the abnormal; the normal and the pathologic reciprocally illuminate each other.

Only temporary reversible hair loss is being considered; excluded are situations in which the matrix or papilla is totally destroyed with no potential for regrowth left.

There is some variation in the degree to which the traumatized follicle succeeds in following its built-in tendency to enact the terminal events of its normal life cycle. Theoretically, the ideal would be formation of a telogen follicle, which in no way differed from the normal. This is the biologically perfect defense and, indeed, is achieved after certain systemic stresses unaccompanied by cutaneous inflammation. The defluvium consists entirely in the loss of normal club hairs and in no sense can the follicle be considered "diseased." The dynamic event is merely a premature termination of anagen. The ceremony of catagen is impeccably performed. Excessive loss of club hairs will be termed *telogen effluvium*[‡].

The excessive shedding of normal club hairs from normal telogen follicles is brought about by a variety of stresses. The stress identifies the clinical species of the genus viz., postfebrile, postpartum, psychogenic, systemic, etc. Recognition of such a phenomenon is by no means new, but its characteristics have not been crisply defined nor dynamics suitably exposed. To my knowledge only gross observations have been made and these are of the sketchiest kind. Previous terms are *symptomatic alopecia* and more classically, but vaguely, *defluvium capillorum*.

Telogen Counting—It is diagnostically important to be able to determine the proportion of resting hairs. This can be done with an epilating forceps, making sure to remove *all* the hairs in the sampled site to avoid the skewness, which might result from not removing the more firmly inserted anagen hairs. Some experience is required to avoid breaking the hairs; these should be pulled parallel to their angle of insertion. Van Scott's, et al. technique of epilating a cluster of about 50 hairs with a surgical needle-holder is quite useful. Before extraction, the hairs should be cut short. For ease of counting they may be floated on a film of water in a scored petri dish. A modest magnification (10X to 20X) is helpful.

As a practical working figure, counts higher than 25% are diagnostic of telogen effluvium; above 20% is presumptively abnormal.

Postfebrile Telogen Effluvium. Hair loss after febrile illness is the best known of the classical varieties of telogen effluvium. Nowadays physicians have little opportunity to observe devastating febrile illness. Our medical forebears, however, had a plethora of experience and were well acquainted with the hair loss following typhoid fever, scarlet fever, pneumonia, etc.

Observations: Four cases of postfebrile alopecia have been studied: pertussis (1), lobar pneumonia (2), and influenza (1). All 4 were mentally defective children, inadequately treated and in relatively poor health. Each case was biopsied at the height of the shedding, which began after 3 to 4 months. Only club hairs were shed. Hair loss seemed to develop suddenly and to continue copiously for 3 to 4 weeks. The telogen counts were respectively 34%, 39%, 46%, and 53%. Regeneration was quite well under way within 6 weeks after excessive shedding stopped. A clinical degree of alopecia manifested as diffuse thinning became apparent in each case. There were no histologic abnormalities. An increased number of perfectly normal telogen follicles were seen.

Postpartum Telogen Effluvium. Folklore and "old wives' tales" give a better account of hair loss after childbirth than is to be found in the annals of medicine. Obstetricians know it is commonplace, and laymen accept it as one of the minor nuisances of childbirth. Nevertheless, a peculiar deep silence prevails in the medical literature.

Observations: Thirty-five subjects were observed with varying degrees of excessive shedding. Only a few were seen more than twice. Eight of the more severe cases were biopsied. The shedding generally began about 2 to 4 months after parturition. The loss was diffuse throughout the scalp. In the usual case, shedding continued for 2 to 5 months, but may be considerably longer, up to one year and even more, if one can place credence in the patients' recitations. Eventually, restitution is complete unless some other process intervenes. The patient who subsequently develops female-patterned baldness (akin to male-patterned

---

[*] J.Soc. Cosmetic Chemists, *17:*502, 1966.

[†] Arch. Dermatol., *83:*175, 1961.

[‡] I have deliberately chosen the word *effluvium* rather than *defluvium* because the former does not carry the connotation of sudden conspicuous hair loss of the latter.

baldness) may connect, falsely, the onset of the irreversible balding process with an episode of postpartum shedding.

The telogen counts in 21 subjects ranged from 20% to 55% with a mean of 32%. The clinical appearance of 32 of the 35 subjects was not appreciably changed; there was no obvious loss of hair, although many thought their hair was "thinned out."

Psychogenic Telogen Effluvium. There are no convenient Koch's postulates to prove emotional etiology.

Observations: Five cases have been studied in detail, including scalp biopsy. Another 11 were observed in which the circumstantial evidence for an emotional etiology seemed substantial.

The circumstances of one really spectacular, though decidedly unusual, case will be presented, which dissolved my own doubts concerning a psychogenic type of telogen effluvium. A prisoner under my close surveillance was implicated in a murder and had stood trial on 3 occasions, each time escaping the death penalty on a legal technicality. His uncertain status in this world had continued for a period of about 3 years. The fourth trial resulted in a conviction of murder in the first degree. About a month later he presented transverse depressions (Beau's lines) in the proximal portions of all his fingernails. The distal segments were duly shed in about another 10 weeks. He was showered with scales from an extraordinary amount of simple dandruff. He began to complain of hair loss approximately 10 weeks after sentencing, but this was put down to imagination since there was no obvious change in his appearance. He saved every single hair fanatically, but since there was no indication of baldness, I remained indifferent to the bundles of hair he offered in evidence. I was not at the time sensitive to the dynamics of telogen effluvium; besides, prison experience instills skepticism much beyond that required for the prosecution of research. My obtuseness was finally pierced, when about 14 weeks after sentencing, thinning was obvious to everyone. Biopsy was done then. He had been shedding excessively for about 3 weeks before developing a manifest alopecia. The man was definitely a scientific bookkeeper, having saved the daily harvest for 3 weeks during the height of the shedding. The average daily loss during the height of the shedding was 1,100 hairs ranging from 600 to 1,500! All were club hairs. There were no histologic changes except for an increased number of telogen follicles. On 2 occasions the telogen counts were 41% and 54%. Substantial restitution was in progress within about 8 weeks after shedding had subsided. This case was unique in that there was a phasic wave-like loss of hair resulting in clinical alopecia. The reader interested in macabre details will perhaps rejoice that this highly observant colleague was subsequently pardoned and set free *after* complete hair regrowth.

Chronic Systemic Illness. Observations: Telogen counts were made on 28 hospitalized patients with a variety of debilitating chronic illnesses, viz., terminal carcinoma, ulcerative colitis, leukemia, tuberculosis, malnutrition, etc. Only 6 had counts above 25%; the range was 26% to 64%.

Telogen Effluvium of the New Born. Observations: Eight infants whose mothers sought professional advice because of marked alopecia were examined.

The shedding begins any time immediately after birth up to 4 months of age. It may occur as a wave leading to almost complete alopecia or, more commonly, in a gradual form, which may be scarcely perceptible. Whether sharp or blurred, there is evidently a total replacement of the first terminal pelage completed before the first 6 months of life.

The Daily Rate of Hair Loss—Since increased shedding is the primary feature of telogen effluvium, will not counting of the hairs lost daily provide a more direct and reliable diagnostic procedure than telogen counting or clinical evaluation of alopecia?

The duration of anagen is derived by dividing the final length in millimeters by the daily growth rate. Pinkus holds that the longevity is 2 to 6 years with an average of about 3 years (1,000 days). The fact that there is singular agreement on this figure reflects less on its probable accuracy than trust in authority.

Thirty healthy white women between the ages of 19 and 50 saved for each of 3 to 5 consecutive days the hairs obtained by one daily routine combing and brushing. They did not wash during this time or do anything else, which might cause incidental hair loss. Every hair was counted as a club hair, though some were doubtlessly broken anagen hairs. The average for the group, 47.

Shedding During Telogen Effluvium—The number of hairs shed daily during an episode of telogen effluvium gives an idea of the diagnostic usefulness of the normal values. Eleven adults with telogen effluvium brushed and combed their hair in routine fashion once daily for 3 to 5 days with an average daily loss between 121 and 646.

General Summation. Telogen effluvium signifies the loss of normal club hairs from normal resting follicles, which have performed the ritual of involution, catagen, in the prescribed fashion. Inflammatory signs or other histologic abnormalities are necessarily minor or absent or else the follicle could not conclude its growing phase in the normal way. Telogen effluvium is obviously a nonspecific reaction pattern provoked by a host of different stimuli —a syndrome, not a disease. It has only the barest qualifications as a pathologic state in that it merely represents a shortening of the follicle's life expectation, a premature death, as it were.

John Thorne Crissey

Calcaneal Petechiae (Black Heel, Talon Noir)

JOHN THORNE CRISSEY was born in Tonawanda, NY on July 19, 1924. He received his M.D. from the University of Buffalo School of Medicine in 1946. He specialized in Dermatology at the University of Pennsylvania under Donald Pillsbury. He returned to Buffalo in 1952, joined Earl D.Osborne in practice, and took over the didactic training of dermatologic residents in the University program. In 1964 he joined the faculty of the University of Southern California Medical School, where he continues to teach with distinction. In 1991 he became full Professor of Dermatology.

Author of seven books and numerous scientific papers, Crissey has maintained a continuing interest in fungal diseases, dermatologic entomology, and related fields. In 1952, along with Gerbert Rebell and John Laskas, he demonstrated for the first time that trichomycosis axillaris is not mycotic, but is caused instead by corynebacteria. He called the species isolated in his studies *Corynebacterium tennis*. In 1961 he published the classic account of calcaneal petechiae, given below. The condition is commonly called *"black heel,"* or *"talon noir."* In 1985 he received the Gougerot Prize for his work.

Crissey also has an abiding interest in music. He studied composition with Aaron Copland, has composed for many different combinations, and plays the piano, organ, and flute.*

BLACK HEEL

Calcaneal Petechiae*

In the past 2 years we have observed 16 cases of a highly characteristic traumatic petechial eruption of the heels. It is interesting as a stigma peculiar to basketball players, and although it is of no real significance in itself, it has been mistaken by the untrained eye for plantar verrucae, and even for malignant melanoma.

Clinical Picture. The eruption is usually bilateral and roughly symmetrical. It is sharply limited to the posterior and lateral surfaces of that convex part of the heel between the insertion of the tendo calcaneus and the portion of the fat pad, which rests upon the ground. The lesions are discrete and confluent, deep-red, deep-seated petechiae, sometimes randomly distributed within the area, but usually aggregated into groups. In mild cases only 3 or 4 lesions may be present, but in severe examples a continuous magenta-colored band

---

* Pittelkow, R.B.: History of the American Dermatological Association, 1994.

* Arch. Dermatol., *83:*501, 1961.

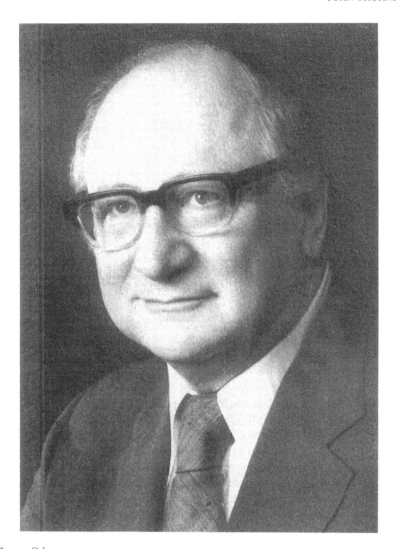

Figure 135 John Thorne Crissey

may extend completely around the heel. Callosities and the diffuse thickening of the stratum corneum common on this part of the heel may blur the sharpness of the lesions.

The eruption is asymptomatic, and was the presenting complaint in only 4 of the cases. One was referred to us as a possible malignant melanoma and 3 as plantar warts. The remaining 12 were discovered incidentally in examination of the feet for other dermatologic complaints. All examples appeared in basketball players during basketball season. The lesions began in the early weeks of play and persisted until 4 or 5 weeks after the final game. From a survey conducted among 12 area coaches we believe the condition is very common among basket-ball players, and that the 16 cases reported here could easily be raised to any number. One coach was certain he had seen similar lesions on the heels of trackmen and football players, but so far we have discovered none.

Robert W.Goltz

Focal Dermal Hypoplasia Syndrome (Goltz Syndrome)

ROBERT WILLIAM GOLTZ was born in St. Paul, Minnesota on September 21, 1923. After receiving his B.S. and M.D. at the University of Minnesota, he was permitted a nine-month residency under Henry Michelson before entering the Army. Here, he served for 2 years as the only dermatologist for the entire Pacific Theater. He returned to Minneapolis to complete his residency and to enter private practice in 1950. His research in dermatopathology, which was accomplished in evenings and weekends was so outstanding that it led to his appointment in 1964 as Chairman of Dermatology at the University of Colorado. He pioneered in demonstrating that cutis laxa and reticulohistiocytosis are the cutaneous signs of a widespread systemic pathologic process.

With Gorlin he was the first to describe the basal cell nevus syndrome with its telltale cysts of the jaw. This was followed by seminal observations on the graft-versus-host reactions, an entirely new arena of dermatology, the heritage of advances in surgical transplantation. By 1971 he was invited to become the first full-time Chair back at the University of Minnesota. There he remained for 14 productive years. His energies spread in all directions and forms. He was responsible for crafting the special American Board Certification in Dermatopathology, as well as in Immunopathology. He trained over 100 dermatologists, 11 of whom became heads of dermatologic programs. He has served as Advisor to the Surgeon General of the Air Force, as well as President of seven national dermatologic societies.

In 1985, unwilling to even consider retirement, he accepted a professorship at the University of California at San Diego where he continues in the youth of his eighties to garner the admiration and love of students, residents, and physicians alike. His career continues as an inspiration to all of dermatology.*

GOLTZ SYNDROME

Focal Dermal Hypoplasia*

Case Presentations. Case 1—She was born at term in 1958 after an uneventful pregnancy. At birth her general condition was good, but she had a generalized scaling and erosive dermatosis. This was most severe on the extremities, especially the flexor aspects. After systemic and topical antibiotic therapy the condition improved, and by the ninth postnatal day her skin had assumed its present appearance.

---

* Who's Who in America, 2003.

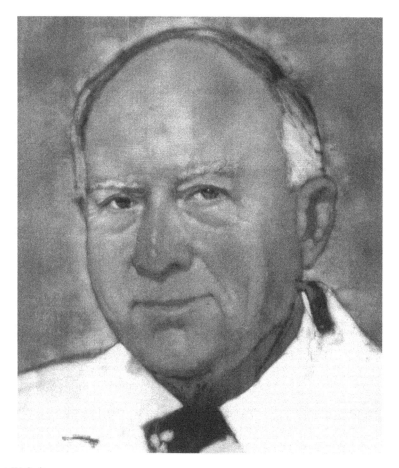

Figure 136 Robert W.Goltz

Examination now shows irregular circumscribed areas in which the skin is thinned and its surface depressed. These areas are brownish-red and considerably darker than the nearby normal skin. On the scalp they measure 2 to 3 cm. in diameter, and the hair growth is sparse. Similar plaques are present on the chin, chest, and extremities. On the trunk and extremities some of the depressed areas are small and lighter than the normal skin, and are arranged in linear groupings, particularly on the arms. Here they are accompanied by varying degrees of atrophy of the subcutaneous structures as well, most markedly illustrated by depression of the hypothenar eminence of the right hand. Most remarkable skin lesions appear in a group in the region of the right cubital fossa where there are a number of soft yellow baggy herniations of subcutaneous fat covered only by the thinnest of integuments. These excrescences measure up to 2 cm. in diameter. We know of no other cutaneous lesions with which they could be confused.

Histopathology. One of the most remarkable features of these specimens was that even when the corium had been almost completely replaced by fat cells and existed only as a thin band beneath the epidermis and around pilosebaceous follicles, the epithelial structures appear to be entirely normal.

Comments. It is apparent that the type of hypoplasia of the dermis in which we are here interested is only one of a number of malformations of the ectoderm and mesoderm, which affect these patients to a varying degree. These malformations include central nervous system and optical defects, anomalies of the heart, osseous defects such as absence of digits, and syndactylism, a number of dental abnormalities, as well as a number of less well-defined abnormalities such as shortness of stature and slightness of build. In addition to the fine texture and fragility of the skin, cutaneous defects include nail deformities, papilloma formation, and possibly congenital absence of large areas of skin.

In regard to differential diagnosis, several conditions come into consideration. Perhaps the most closely related are the various linear lesions seen in the syndrome described by Thomson as congenital poikiloderma. Congenital poikiloderma does not show the hypoplasia of the collagen which we are emphasizing, but rather is characterized by atrophy of the epidermis, disappearance of the papillae, hydropic degeneration of the basal layer, and remarkable dyskeratosis of the epidermal cells, followed in many cases by the appearance of outright carcinomas. The histologic changes are therefore quite different from that in focal dermal hypoplasia, in which the principal change is in the corium, while the epidermis and appendages remain unaffected.

Heredity—It will be noted that all 5 of the reported children with this defect have been female and that similar defects in their ancestors and relatives have been found only in females. It is also true that there is a high incidence of miscarriages in these families, and it is postulated that the defect is neither sex-linked nor limited in occurrence to females, but rather is incompatible with survival of life in male fetuses beyond early months of gestation.

---

* Arch. Dermatol., *86:*708, 1962.

Peter Samman

Yellow Nail Syndrome

PETER DERRICK SAMMAN was born in 1914 in the beautiful Indian hill station of Darjeeling. After his father retired in 1914 as Commissioner in the Indian Civil Service, the family of seven children moved to the Isle of Man. Peter was educated at King Williams College. He had begun his clinical training in Medicine at King's College Hospital when World War II broke out. As a volunteer in the Royal Air Force he rose to the rank of Squadron Leader. After discharge he went on to get his MRCP in 1946. Further training in dermatology at King's and a stint at Bristol led to his appointment to the staff of St. John's Hospital where he remained for his academic lifetime, with his private practice being conducted at his home. His research skills were honed by a sabbatical at the University of Pennsylvania in 1958.

His life was dedicated to clinical investigation centered on diseases of the nails and on cutaneous lymphomas. His book, *The Nails in Disease,* enjoyed the popularity of five editions. His superb clinical acumen allowed him to distinguish chronic superficial dermatitis from the serious mimic, mycosis fungoides. He kept meticulous records, which led to seminal papers on the reticuloses.

Soon patients from all over the UK came to him for care and comfort. He was shy and self-effacing, but in his quiet way he was more beloved than some of his flamboyant peers. And everyone knew he was never late to his clinics or meetings.

He wrote *A History of St. John's Hospital for Diseases of the Skin 1963–1988,* as well as three sections for *Rook's Textbook.* His work on lymphomas earned him the prestigious Parkes-Weber Medal in 1976 from the Royal College of Physicians.

Gardening was his joy and chrysanthemums his special delight. He derived equal pleasure from world travel and cheering at cricket matches.

The last period of his life was blighted by Parkinson's Disease, but he had had a most productive career as Consulting Physician to the Skin Department at Westminster Hospital, Physician to St. John's Hospital for Diseases of the Skin and Dean of the Institute of Dermatology. He died December 1, 1992.*

YELLOW NAIL SYNDROME

The "Yellow Nail" Syndrome[†]

The present report is based on 13 cases. In addition to the nail changes most of the patients complain of ankle oedema. The oedema may, however, not appear until some years after the nails have become abnormal. The age at onset of symptoms has varied between 22 and 65 years. One patient had oedema of

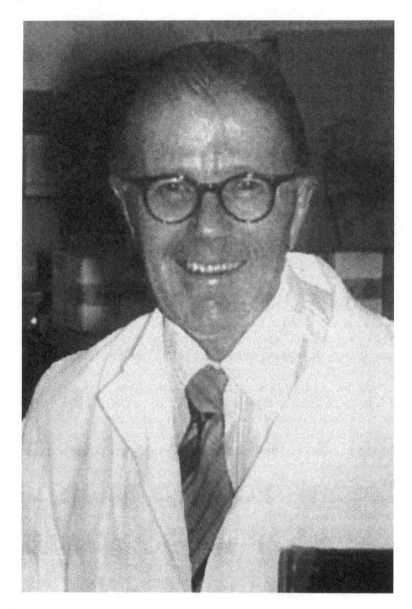

Figure 137 Peter Samman

the face and no ankle oedema. It is proposed here to show that this oedema is due to abnormalities of the lymphatic vessels in some cases and it seems probable that it is so in most.

The nail changes are characteristic and can immediately be recognized. The patient will often state that the nails seem to have stopped growing before the appearance becomes altered. Measurements have shown that the nails, in fact, continue to grow, but very slowly. In most cases watched for a period long enough for accurate measurements to be made, the rate of growth of the fingernails has been less than 0.2 mm per week compared with the normal 0.5 to 1.2 mm per week. The nails usually remain smooth, they are excessively curved from side to side so that the lateral edges are less covered by the surrounding soft tissue than is normal and the cuticles are deficient. The colour change usually affects the whole nail plate but sometimes the proximal third or half of the nail is of normal colour. The colour is usually pale yellow but it may be slightly greenish and occasionally the edges of the nails are rather darker than the remainder. The colour change may be present in both finger- and toenails, and in toenails which, are not otherwise diseased, the yellow colour is often more obvious than in the fingernails. The reason for the colour is not known but it does not appear to be due to infection with *Candida* or *Pseudomonas pyocyanea*. Onycholysis (separation of the nail from its bed) may affect one or more fingernails and the separation may extend so far towards the matrix that the nail is shed. The nail is later replaced but only very slowly. Some of the partially separated nails show a distinct hump. Occasionally the nails will show cross-ridging owing to variations in the rate of growth from time to time.

Oedema is the other feature of the syndrome. Several of the patients have had unexplained ankle oedema for a number of years, but often the nail changes occur before the oedema becomes obvious. The patient may not complain of the oedema but readily admits to it when questioned. The oedema usually affects the ankles and not infrequently is a good deal worse on one side than the other.

Six of the thirteen patients had abnormal lymphatics. Four other cases had oedema of the ankles and it is likely that they too had anomalous lymphatics.

The appearances of the nail are probably dependent on the slow rate of growth, but is this in its turn due to the impaired lymph drainage? The late onset of oedema in patients with defective lymphatics is readily explained on the assumption that the lymphatics are able to manage satisfactorily until some extra stress such as infection or hypostasis is placed upon them.

Summary. A new syndrome is described consisting of slow growing nails, which have a characteristic appearance, and oedema, usually affecting the ankles, probably due to defective lymph drainage.

---

* Obituary, Br. J.Dermatol., *128:*699, 1993.

† Br, J.Dermatol., *76:*153, 1964.

R.D.Sweet

Acute Febrile Neutrophilic Dermatosis (Sweet's Syndrome)

ROBERT DOUGLAS SWEET was born in Weybridge, Surrey, England on December 26, 1917. He attended school in New Zealand, at Wanganui. He received his medical education at Cambridge and was awarded his M.D. in 1943. This was followed by two years of service as an R.A.F. Squadron Leader. His dermatologic tutelage was at St. Thomas Hospital in London.

Entering practice in 1950 as consultant for the Plymouth group of hospitals he enjoyed a full and varied practice until retirement in 1982. His inquiring mind searched out the rare and unusual forms of skin disease. Many of his writings received wide approval, including one on acidental X-ray burns and another on the treatment of basal cell carcinoma by curettage. But, it was the paper in 1962 on the disease bearing his name that led to his fellowship in the Royal College of Physicians, as well as to worldwide recognition and many lectureships. He served for a year as consultant in charge of the Skin Department at the University of West Indies, Jamaica.

His administrative skills were greatly appreciated, as he served as Chief of Staff at Plymouth Hospital. A man with a wonderful smile, an engaging personality, and a great sense of humor, he was a joy to his staff and patients.

In retirement Sweet focused his attention on his moorland farming and promotion of conservation. His true love was horse riding and he was an enthusiastic member and subsequently Chairman of the Spooners and West Dartmoor Hunt. He died on September 28, 2001 and his funeral service ended with a triumphant horn sounding his final call to the Hunt.*

SWEET'S SYNDROME

Acute Febrile Neutrophilic Dermatosis[†]

In the course of the last fifteen years I have encountered eight patients who have had what seems to be a distinctive and fairly severe illness. It is accompanied by a skin eruption which, although presumably reactive in nature and somewhat resembling erythema multiforme in appearance and duration, is I believe clinically and histologically distinctive. The four cardinal features are fever, neutrophil polymorphonuclear

---

* H.M.Leather, courtesy D.S.Wilkinson, Personal communication.

[†] Br. J.Dermatol., *76:*348, 1964.

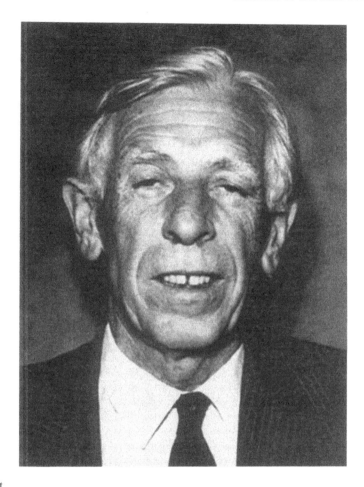

Figure 138 R.D.Sweet

leucocytosis of the blood, raised painful plaques on the limbs, face and neck, and histologically a dense dermal infiltration with mature neutrophil polymorphs. No evidence of infection is to be found. Response to corticosteroid drugs is rapid and complete.

The object of this paper is to draw a composite picture of the condition and behaviour of these patients and to describe briefly their variations. I hope that thereby others who have seen similar cases may at least have the intellectual satisfaction of being able to classify them, even though they will remain as ignorant as ever about their essential nature.

Clinical Picture. All eight patients have been women between the ages of 32 and 55. One or more erythematous patches about 1 cm in diameter appeared asymmetrically on the forearms, face or neck and in the course of the next week became larger, more numerous and widespread, darkened, raised in a plateau and progressively more and more painful. During the first week the patient felt unwell, took to her bed and was found to be febrile, the temperature usually swinging between 100° and 102°F. Fresh lesions continued to appear for two to three weeks and older ones became confluent. There was considerable variation in size from about 0.5 cm to 4 cm in diameter. The surface of larger lesions invariably became raised, usually abruptly, and was often mamillated, sometimes giving the illusion of a multilocular blister. Occasionally, small pustules formed under this raised irregular surface and in one case formed the salient clinical features. Some of these pustules burst and healed without scarring. In the other cases the surface of the lesions did not break down.

The active phase of the illness lasted between one and two months in three of the four patients in which it was not terminated artificially with steroids. Improvement was then rapid with an abrupt fall of temperature and cessation of tenderness. The lesions flattened and disappeared apart from some residual staining within a further three weeks, though in the fourth case they persisted in all for over six months. There was no scarring.

Apart from the fever and the rash, general physical examination revealed no abnormalities. Regional lymph glands were not enlarged. Several patients had transient albuminuria. In five of the six who were examined there was a neutrophil polymorphonuclear leucocytosis in excess of 12,000 cells per cu mm during the second and third weeks. In two, a blood count was not carried out in the first month and in the remaining patient, suffering from an influenzal bronchopneumonia at the time, there was a leucopenia. Except in the latter case, no abnormality was seen in chest x-rays. L.E. cells were not found. The W.R. was negative. The E.S.R. was moderately raised. Pustules, when present, were sterile and attempts to grow organisms from biopsy sections have been unsuccessful. In short, all efforts to unearth infection in these patients with fever and leucocytosis have been unsuccessful.

André Bazex

1.   Acrokeratosis Paraneoplastica (Bazex Syndrome)

2.   Follicular Atrophoderma and Basal Cell Carcinoma Syndrome (Bazex Atrophoderma)

ANDRÉ BAZEX was born on February 14, 1911 in Montestruc Sur Gers, France. André grew up in Auch as the son of the local physician who died when André was 14. Determined to follow in his father's footsteps he went to Toulouse for medical training and specialization in Dermatology under famed Professor, André Nanta.

By 1941 he was Director of the Venereological Department. His distinguished career continued with his appointment in 1954 as Chairman and Professor of Dermatology at the University of Toulouse. His numerous publications included the description of unique cutaneous changes resulting from underlying cancer, as well as a distinctive inherited atrophy of the hair follicles. These are referred to as *Bazex Syndrome* and *Bazex Atrophoderma,* respectively. He went on to become President of the Societé Francaise de Dermatologie and to honorary membership in many foreign dermatologic societies.

Curiosity was his passion and his remarkable histopathologic and clinical skills made for exciting Grand Rounds. His fellow professors in internal medicine, anatomy, and biochemistry considered themselves privileged to join him in the search for knowledge of skin disease. Students came from all over Europe to his clinic in Toulouse, inspired by this modest, reserved, hard-working leader. And, his many honors and medals attested to his scientific productivity.

In 1980 Bazex retired, enjoying philosophic discussion groups, as well as intensive study of World War II. His death on October 18, 1988 left dermatology a treasured heritage: a distinguished Professor of Dermatology, his son, Jacques Bazex.*

BAZEX SYNDROME

Syndrome Para-Neoplasique Á Type D'hyperkeratose Des Extrémitiés: Guerison après le traitement de l'epithélioma larynge*

Mr. C…Jean-Marie, 60-years-old was referred to us by his doctor January 13 for hyperkeratotic lesions of the extremities of fairly recent onset. To be frank, the patient has a low I.Q. and it is difficult to obtain an exact history. The lesions are polymorphic: plantar keratoderma appearing on the dorsum of the toes, on the

---

* Wallach and Tilles: Dermatology in France, p 675, 2002.

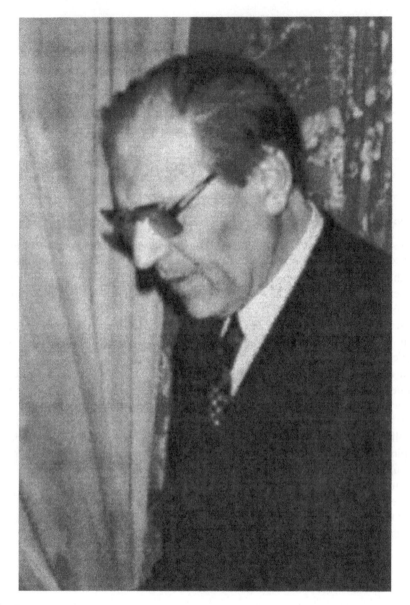

Figure 139 André Bazex

palms, and on the back of the fingers, dry follicular parakeratosis of the nose, ichthyotic changes on the face and ears, and pseudo-tinea amiantacea of the scalp. This ensemble brings to mind pityriasis rubra pilaris, a localized ichthyosiform process or a seborrheic dermatitis.

Physical examination of the patient reveals the presence of submaxillary and jugular adenopathy, which permits us to discern the existence of a neoplasm in the buccal-laryngeal, pharyngeal area that only hoarseness would have led us to suspect. It proved to be a very advanced epithelioma, possibly only responsive to palliative cobalt therapy, preceded by local injections of endoxan and methotrexate in the superior thyroid artery.

From the initiation of this treatment and parallel improvement of the epithelioma, the keratotic lesions cleared and presently the hands and face are entirely cured.

This case, therefore, meets the necessary criteria to be considered as a paraneoplastic dermatosis as delineated by the Bureau and H.O.Curth of the XI Congress of the Association of French Dermatologists. In effect, we note in the case of this patient, the almost simultaneous onset of the dermatosis and the neoplasm, as well as the parallel evolution of the dermatosis and the neoplastic lesion. We can even speak here of it being a marker dermatosis.

This report can be compared with, but is not identical to: 1) The palmar-plantar keratoses associated with epitheliomas of the upper esophagus reported by Howel-Evans (palmar and plantar tylosis); 2) The ichthyosiform changes accompanying palmar-plantar hyperkeratosis (reported by Glasebrook).

BAZEX ATROPHODERMA

Atrophodermie Folliculaire, Proliferations Baso-cellulaires et Hypotrichose[†]

We are describing under this term a new dystrophic complex of dominant inheritance observed in 6 members of the same family. This genodermatosis is similar to both the observations of Miescher and H.O.Curth (follicular atrophoderma, pseudo-pelade, congenital chondrodystrophy) and the observations of Caubet (follicular atrophoderma, milia, sebaceous cysts and, trichorrhexis nodosa). All these types of genodermatoses have an essential common element: follicular atrophoderma, a term created by Miescher to designate a particular atrophic change in the skin, expressed as small cupolaform depressions centered at the follicular orifice.

Our Observations. The three major clinical symptoms: 1) Hypotrichosis —It is congenital. It involves not only the scalp and the hirsute areas (eyebrows, chin, pubes and axillae), but also the entire integument, arms, legs, trunk where hair is sparse and sometimes replaced by a fuzz which is equally sparse; 2) Follicular atrophoderma—It manifests itself as small punctate depressions centered on the pilosebaceous orifices, funnel shaped, which in reality appears to be simply an exaggeration of the normal follicular infundibulum. This abnormality is particularly evident on the hands and feet; the majority of these depressions are empty, in others we can see with a loupe a fine fuzz, a few others have in their center a thin hair. It seems that the skin has always had this appearance and there was no preceding eruption in childhood; 3) The basal cell elements are essentially found on the face: some are small nodular skin-colored or whitish formations, some are milia sized, others are comparable to sebaceous adenomas, predominantly around the eyes, near the upper and lower eyelids; others are more voluminous, the size of a big pea, with heterogeneous pigmentation. Finally, the most striking are the degenerative elements on the lips, forehead or eyelids. These elements exhibit rapid growth and a crusted but non-ulcerative appearance. Some pigmented macules are found on the forearms and the dorsae of the hands. The nevoid elements appeared only at puberty and the degenerative change around the age of 16 or 17.

The other less important abnormalities contributing to this syndrome include hypohidrosis; we can even note anhidrosis of the face, as is the case in patients who can't recall ever having drops of sweat on their

---

* Bull. Soc. Fr. Dermatol. Syphil., *72*:82, 1965.

† Ann. Derm. Syph., *93*:241, 1966.

forehead even in extreme heat or during heavy labor. On the rest of the body sweating occurs but is less profuse than in a normal subjects.

Three biopsies of the degenerative tumors show the appearance of basal cell epitheliomas with trabecular differentiation and nuclear mitotic abnormalities. A fourth biopsy done on less advanced lesions gives the appearance of a basal cell nevus.

Case 1—An 8-year-old child of Asiatic descent whose parents were born in Poland. Immediately after birth the mother notes a large part of the scalp and body are covered with red crusts, some are small and thin; others are confluent and form large adherent plaques.

The mother is told at Day Care that it is eczema. After a few weeks the crusts fall. The skin of the body becomes normal though there are some dilated pores. The scalp shows areas of hair loss. On examination there are more lesions on the right than on the left side of the body. They are found on the chest, right arm and forearm, on the back of the right hand, the knee and tibial surface, and the right thigh. The left arm and left knee are also afflicted. The involved areas form plaques or bands, more or less circumscribed, exhibiting small funnel-like depressions the size of a pinhead, without fuzz in the follicular orifices. The depressions form a regular vermicular aspect. Most of the scalp is covered with normal hair but on the frontal area there are atrophic sites and multiple bald spots.

At their periphery we find crusts attached to the base of each hair. There are no follicles in the atrophic sites.

Ervin Epstein

Acanthoma Fissuratum

ERVIN EPSTEIN was born May 17, 1909 in Vallejo, California. When he was a teenager his family moved to San Francisco where he attended college and medical school at the University of California. Following a residency in Dermatology in Los Angeles, he entered a lifetime of private practice in Oakland, California, interrupted in 1942–1945 for service in the U.S. Army. His commitment to teaching led to Associate Professorships at Stanford and the University of California.

His productivity resulted in over 240 papers and nearly a dozen books. His fame also rests squarely on his success in bringing forth the specialty of skin surgery. He achieved this in no small part, his classic text, *Skin Surgery,* which spawned six great editions. Equally significant was his impact on the clinical practice of dermatology as a co-editor and later Editor of the *Schoch Monthly Newsletter* for over 25 years.

He retired from practice in 1989, but never from writing. His was a career that epitomized the best in patient care, teaching prowess, and in ferreting out the secrets of the skin. He did all of this with wisdom, wit and will.

Ervin Epstein died on January 22, 2002, leaving Dermatology the richer for his presence, but also leaving his legacy of a distinguished dermatologic son, Ervin Epstein, Jr.*

ACANTHOMA FISSURATUM

Granuloma Fissuratum of the Ears*

Report of Cases. Case 1—Mrs. M.F., a 49-year-old white woman, consulted me on March 4, 1963 because of a growth at the superior pole of her left postauricular area. The growth had been present for three months. It had not been growing during the past two months or more. On examination she presented a firm smooth neoplasm. The central portion was depressed in a furrow but was not ulcerated. The two wings were folded over the furrow. The lesion tended to be smooth and somewhat pearly so that a clinical diagnosis of basal-cell epithelioma was entertained. The growth was removed by electrodesiccation and curettage under local anesthesia. The tumor separated easily from the underlying skin.

---

* J.Am. Acad. Dermatol, *15:*1319, 1986.

* Arch. Dermatol., *91:*621, 1965.

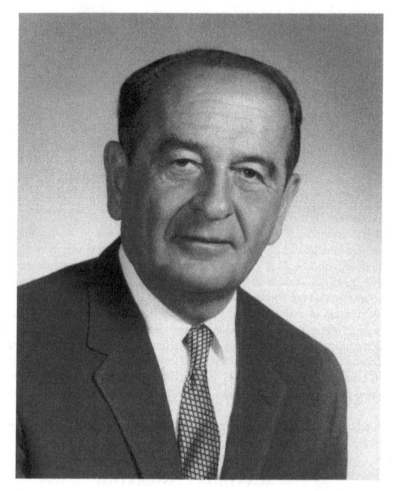

Figure 140 Ervin Epstein

Histopathologic examination failed to confirm the clinical impression. There was a moderate amount of hyperkeratosis with parakeratotic changes. The epidermis was markedly acanthotic, the pegs being elongated and broadened. Both intracellular and extracellular edema was present. The basal-cell layer was intact. Edema of the corium was noted, especially superficially. A mild round-cell and elongated fibroblastic cell infiltration was intermixed and scattered through the dermis. There was no predilection to form cellular masses around vessels or appendages.

Further questioning elicited the information that the patient wore glasses that "did not fit right over the left ear." It seemed to rub in this area. This had been bothering Mrs. F. for about four months. The earpieces were made of clear plastic surrounding a metal wire. Rubber guards were recommended for use around the plastic. There has been no recurrence to date.

Comments. It is strange that one can practice dermatology for 35 years, see a "new condition," and then encounter a second example on the following day. Yet, this is what transpired in this instance. No further lesions of this type have been seen since.

Marvin Chernosky

Disseminated Superficial Actinic Porokeratosis (DSAP)

MARVIN ERNEST CHERNOSKY was born in Austin, Texas on March 29, 1926. He grew up in Austin, and following a 3-year Army service he received his B.A. degree in Biology from the University of Texas in 1948. He was granted the M.D. by Tulane University in 1952. His residency at Charity Hospital in New Orleans was in surgery followed by dermatology. He entered practice in Houston, Texas with an appointment at Baylor University, rising to the rank of Clinical Associate Professor. In 1972 he was named Chairman and Clinical Professor at the University of Texas Medical School, at Houston, a position he held until 1982. He has held numerous hospital staff appointments and continued in practice until 1998 when he retired.

Author of 130 papers, he has received many honors and served as President of the Society of Dermatologic Surgery as well as Vice-President of the American Academy of Dermatology. His academic life has been devoted to serving the needs of innumerable medical societies. His love of surgery, his skill at patient care, and his enthusiasm for teaching led to him being the only dermatologist ever to receive the Herman Hospital Distinguished Physician Award, a prestigious citation given to only 66 doctors in its 72 year history.

Chernosky, now retired, continues to contribute to his beloved Texas community, when he isn't out hunting.

DISSEMINATED SUPERFICIAL ACTINIC POROKERATOSIS

Porokeratosis: Report of Twelve Patients with Multiple Superficial Lesions*

Porokeratosis is a chronic, progressive, morphologically distinct disorder of the skin first described in 1893 by Mibelli and by Respighi.

Descriptions and illustrations in most textbooks, as well as references in the literature, indicate that the lesions of porokeratosis are quite distinct and easy to identify. While this may often be true, in the patient with systematized, multiple, bilateral, superficial lesions of porokeratosis, the lesions are usually very faint, their borders not rising high above the skin level. They can easily be overlooked or confused with several other types of lesions.

---

* Southern Med. J., *59*:289, 1966.

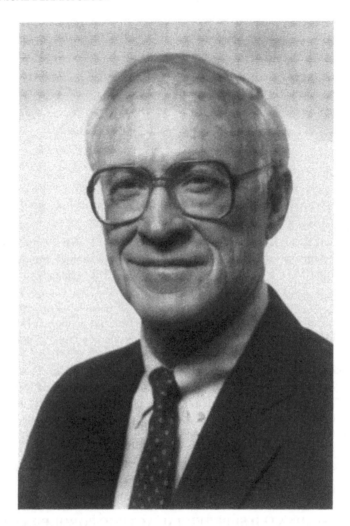

Figure 141 Marvin Chernosky

This report concerns 12 patients with multiple superficial lesions of porokeratosis.

The primary lesion noted in this condition is a very small (1 to 3 mm.) keratotic papule that sometimes is follicular in location. These tiny papules are frequently brownish or brownish-red, and sometimes a few telangiectatic vessels can be seen in them. They may have a depression in their summit resembling a minute volcano. The lesions tend to enlarge centrifugally and flatten out, usually leaving a somewhat atrophic area surrounded by a slightly raised keratotic ridge.

The central area may remain pigmented or erythematous and frequently it is separated from the lesion's peripheral edge by a hypopigmented area. Sometimes the central area loses the pigmentation and erythema and appears hypopigmented, or the same color as the surrounding skin. The center of some lesions may continue to have keratotic papules with delling and the keratotic material may remain adherent or the scaling may become loose and micaceous. Hairs in the central areas are usually missing and the surface feels dry. The lesion slowly enlarges by centrifugal spread of the keratotic ridge sometimes attaining a round or oval shape, though more frequently being irregularly circinate. In the multiple superficial type of porokeratosis lesions this ridge is only slightly elevated on the skin surface.

The greatest number of lesions occurred in the areas exposed most to sunlight. Women had more lesions on their legs than did men.

Histopathology. In each case the typical cornoid lamella was observed, a thickened column of keratin containing dark parakeratotic-like granules in a groove or thinned area of the stratum malpighii. The granular layer is absent in this area and usually one can see signs of disturbed maturation of the cells. The adjacent epidermis may be acanthotic and in the dermis a banal round cell infiltrate and capillary dilatation are usually present.

Treatment. In 5 patients cryotherapy, in the form of liquid nitrogen to individual lesions sufficient to produce bullous formation, was carried out. Observations 2 to 5 months later revealed that the treated lesions had remained smooth, with no evidence of a raised keratotic ridge. However, 3 of the 5 patients still show hyperpigmentation in the areas.

Discussion. Again, let me emphasize that these minimal, superficial lesions may easily be overlooked. For example, I observed one patient for another dermatologic complaint intermittently for several months before I first noticed the many lesions of porokeratosis on her extremities. I believe the frequent use of emollients, soap and water, particularly with a washcloth, tend to remove the keratotic material from the lesions and make them less noticeable.

The differential diagnosis must include actinic keratosis, xerosis, psoriasis, lentigines, lichen scler osus et atrophicus, lichen planus, pityriasis rubra pilaris, keratosis pilaris, verruca plana and acrokeratosis verruciformis.

It is possible that this condition is more prevalent in this geographic area where greater exposure to intense sunlight is common.

Amir H.Mehregan

Reactive Perforating Collagenosis

AMIR HOSSEIN MEHREGAN was born on June 12, 1931 in Tehran, Iran. After graduating from the University of Tehran School of Medicine he sought training in dermatology in the United States. He began his training in dermatology at the Skin and Cancer Hospital of Philadelphia. After two years in Philadelphia he sought additional training at the University of Wisconsin School of Medicine Hospital in Madison under Sture Johnson. During this time he was introduced to Frederic E. Mohs who provided many surgical dermatopathology specimens for Mehregan to review. During an O'Leary Meeting at the Mayo Clinic he met Hermann Pinkus and arranged for a dermatopathology fellowship in Detroit, Michigan from July, 1959 through August, 1961. After he completed training he accepted a position in Shiraz, Iran; however, in 1962 he returned to Detroit to join Pinkus at the Wayne State University School of Medicine. In 1964 he left to join the University of Alberta School of Medicine in Edmonton, Alberta, but returned to Detroit a year later. At that time, Mehregan joined Pinkus in his dermatopathology practice in Monroe, Michigan. Over the next 35 years he transformed this small part-time venture from a laboratory preparing 10 to 20 specimens a day to a regional dermatopathology laboratory reviewing 300 to 400 specimens daily.

In 1969 Mehregan and Pinkus published the first edition of *A Guide to Dermatohistopathology*. After the death of Pinkus in 1985 the 4th through 6th editions were renamed, *Pinkus' Guide to Dermatohistopathology* in honor of Mehregan's former partner.

Mehregan was president of the American Society of Dermatopathology 1981–1982. In 1984 he and Martin Brownstein became editors of the Journal of Cutaneous Pathology, prior to the transition of the journal to the American Society of Dermatopathology.

During his career, Mehregan had an interest in adnexal neoplasms. He wrote many articles, including observations of the tumor of the follicular infundibulum, epidermotropic eccrine carcinoma, generalized follicular hamartoma, pilar sheath acanthoma, pigmented follicular cyst, and basaloid follicular hamartoma. He also had an interest in perforating disorders of the skin, including reactive perforating collagenosis described in 1967 with Schwartz and Livingood, and perforating folliculitis described in 1968. In 1971 he and Jules Altman described another new entity, inflammatory linear verrucous epidermal nevus (ILVEN).

Amir Mehregan had a lifelong love of Persian archeology and history. He was also an avid fisherman. He was diagnosed with a glioblastoma multiforme, grade IV, in May, 2000 and died on September 28, 2000 in Monroe, Michigan.*

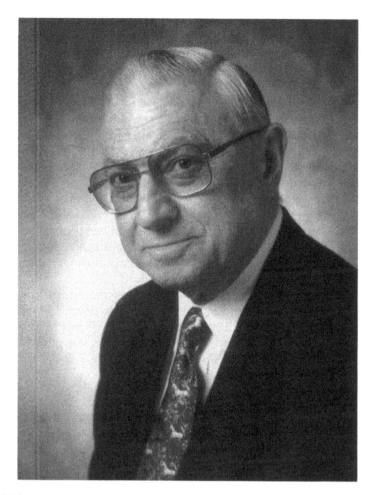

Figure 142 Amir H.Mehregan

REACTIVE PERFORATING COLLAGENOSIS

Reactive Perforating Collagenosis[†]

Report of a Case. The skin eruption appeared at the age of 9 months and consisted of numerous discrete papules located mainly over the extremities. As new papules continued to develop, the older lesions regressed and disappeared completely.

This patient has been followed for two years and is now 8½ years old and in good general health. Her present skin eruption consists of numerous discrete papules involving mainly the dorsa of the hands, forearms, elbows, and knees. Some papules are arranged in a linear fashion, suggesting a Koebner phenomenon. The earliest lesion is a pinhead-sized skin-colored papule. As it becomes older it increases in size and develops a small central area of umbilication containing keratinous material. Eventually, this central umbo becomes wider, and the keratotic plug becomes larger and assumes a dark brown color. The central plug has a tough leathery consistency. It is adherent and not easily removed without bleeding. The lesion reaches a maximum size of 5 to 6 mm in approximately three to four weeks; this is followed by a stage of regression in which the individual papules flatten out. The central umbo becomes shallow and the keratinous plug wears off. In a six- to eight-week period, the lesion disappears completely, leaving a small area of temporary hypopigmentation.

Comments. The life history of a lesion may be reconstructed as follows. In response to injury, certain changes take place in the connective tissue of the papillary layer of the corium. The epidermis becomes slightly edematous and the granular layer disappears, leading to parakeratosis. The epidermis eventually becomes atrophic, and multiple small areas of disruption occur within the suprapapillary areas. From the partially exposed tips of papillae, a mixture of necrobiotic connective tissue, degenerating inflammatory cells, and some normal appearing collagen bundles are extruded. This extruded material is mixed with parakeratotic keratin to form an adherent leathery mass, which fills a cup-shaped area of epidermal depression. As this process progresses with more necrobiotic material being extruded, the central plug becomes larger, and the crater becomes deeper. Somewhat later, perhaps because the supply of necrobiotic material in the corium is exhausted, there is regression and then cessation of the pathologic process followed by the reparative phase. Eventually, the epidermis resumes its normal structure, the central area of umbilication becomes shallow, and the leathery plug wears off.

In connection with our case we reviewed a case reported in the French literature by Laugier and Woringer under the title of "Collagenome perforant verruciforme." The case concerns an 18-year-old boy who received multiple lacerations on his forearm. The lacerations were due to broken glass and required sutures. After six weeks, papular lesions appeared at both sides of a linear scar on his forearm and within a somewhat irregular scarred area close to the antecubital region. The lesions consisted of individual or grouped skin-colored papules with slightly crusted centers. The histologic examination revealed the formation of transepidermal perforating canals resembling those seen in elastosis perforans serpiginosa. Through these canals, some necrobiotic collagenous tissue was being extruded to the surface. The corium showed areas of marked basophilic degeneration with some increase in PAS-positive material. In addition, there was also a granulomatous inflammatory infiltrate. There was no evidence of double refractile foreign-body material in the corium. The authors concluded that the injury to the skin produced certain histochemical changes in the connective tissue, and made it irritant and foreign to the surrounding tissue, thus provoking this peculiar chain of reactions. However, the possibility of irritation by a nonrefractile foreign material could not be completely excluded. The eruption appeared only in one attack.

The basic pattern of reaction presented in the case reported by Laugier and Woringer bears some similarity to that of elastosis perforans serpiginosa and to the reaction we have described for our case. However, the differences are quite obvious. In their case, the eruption followed an injury severe enough to cause definite pathologic changes in the entire thickness of the skin. The types of skin lesions were quite different, and the eruption occurred only in one period.

---

* Ackerman, A.B. Intl. J.Dermatol., *42:*29, 2003.

† Arch. Dermatol., *96:*277, 1967.

Tomisaku Kawasaki

Kawasaki Disease (Muco-cutaneous Lymph Node Syndrome)

TOMISAKU KAWASAKI was born in Tokyo on February 7, 1925. He received his M.D., and took his internship and residency in pediatrics, all at the Medical College in Chiba, Japan from 1943–1950. He then joined the Department of Pediatrics of the Japanese Red Cross Central Hospital where he did his studies on 50 infants and young children who had an unknown febrile illness, lymphadenopathy, and swollen hands and feet followed by desquamation. It became known as Kawasaki Disease, which, to date, has been seen in over 30,000 young patients.

The serious prognosis of these skin changes has evolved with recognition that the changes reflect an underlying medium-sized vessel vasculitis, which may involve the coronary arteries, with a fatal outcome.

Kawasaki has devoted his life to the study of his disease, heading national Kawasaki disease research committees for over two decades. In 1988 he was honored to be the Chairman of the 3rd International Kawasaki Disease Symposium. He served as Director of the Department of Pediatrics of the Japanese Red Cross Medical Center until 1990. At that time he became Director of the Kawasaki Disease Research Center, where he continues to serve today.

Not surprisingly, numerous honors and prizes have been showered on him. His careful, meticulous observations of all aspects of his sick little patients make him an international hero. No one knows more about Kawasaki Disease than Kawasaki. He has truly earned his eponym, which crosses the mind of any physician examining a febrile child with swollen glands and swollen hands.*

KAWASAKI DISEASE

Febrile Oculo-oro-cutaneo-acrodesquamatous Syndrome with or without Acute Non-Suppurative Cervical Lymphadenitis in Infancy and Childhood: Clinical Observations of 50 Cases*

In our series of 50 patients admitted to the Pediatric Department of the Japanese Red Cross Central Hospital in Tokyo from January of 1961 to November of 1966, the main clinical features were as follows:

---

* Kukita, A.: Emeritus Chairman of Dermatology, Tokyo University; Personal communication.

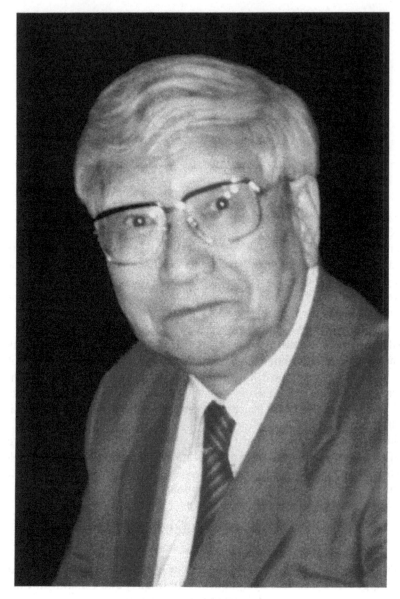

Figure 143 Tomisaku Kawasaki

1. All patients (50 cases) had a temperature of 38°C and higher, and its duration was at least 6 days in spite of antibiotic therapy.
2. In 49 (98%) of 50 cases bilateral injection of bulbal conjunctivae was seen. Pseudomembrane formation or corneal complications were not seen.

3. Forty-three cases (86%) in our series had skin eruptions. The lesions were basically erythematous, appeared over the whole body, especially on the palms and soles, characterized by an absence of vesicular or bullous lesions.

4. Forty-eight (96%) of the 50 cases showed dried, injected, eroded and fissured lips, sometimes with bleeding and crust formation. Mucous membranes of the mouth showed diffuse injection without any vesicular or aphthous lesions. Sometimes strawberry-tongue was present.

5. Thirty-three (66%) of the 50 cases had acute non-suppurative cervical lymphadenitis, which showed from thumb tip to hen's-egg and larger in size.

6. Angioneurotic edema of the hands and feet was seen in 22 cases (44%) in infants and small children.

7. Acrodesquamation from the junction of the nail and skin on fingers and toes was seen in 49 cases (98%). It began at almost the second week of illness. This desquamation was limited to hands and feet, and never seen on other parts of the body.

8. The age range was from 2-months-old to 9-years and 1-month. Over half of the patients (27 cases (54%)) were under 2 years of age.

9. This syndrome showed natural curability, no residual formation, no recurrence, and no contagious tendency among siblings.

From the clinical findings mentioned above, this syndrome seemed to be a new clinical entity.

* Arerugi (Jap. J.Allergy), *16:*178, 1967 (In Japanese).

Thomas B. Fitzpatrick

The Ash Leaf Macule of Tuberous Sclerosis

THOMAS BERNARD FITZPATRICK was born in Madison, Wisconsin on December 19, 1919, an early Christmas present to his family and to all of Dermatology. After his undergraduate studies at the University of Wisconsin he went on to get his M.D. at Harvard. He then collaborated with Aaron Lerner at the Army Chemical Center in Maryland where they were the first to demonstrate that tyrosinase is in human skin and that it converted tyrosine into melanin. This was followed by a residency in dermatology at the Mayo Clinic, where he also earned a Ph.D. He again joined Lerner who was now at the University of Michigan. The following year he was invited to head the Department of Dermatology at the University of Oregon. In 1958 on a sabbatical at Oxford in England he first isolated and named the melanosome. His triumphant return was to Harvard in 1959 as Department Head and Professor. There his passion with pigment led to the classic description of early melanoma. This recognition with Wallace Clark of its unique variegated color pattern and irregular border resulted in detection and excision of melanomas before fatal metastatic spread had occurred.

In the next decade he introduced photochemotherapy (PUVA) for the treatment of vitiligo and psoriasis. He had already developed an effective sunscreen with para-amino benzoic acid and was a leader in recognizing the role of sunlight in melanocyte carcinogenesis.

Meanwhile, his Department grew to 14 full-time dermatologists and 14 residents. Of the 138 he trained, 24 became full professors or department heads. Thirty-five fellows came from Japan, followed by a $90 million dollar grant from the Japanese cosmetic firm, Shiseido.

His influence continued to spread throughout the medical world with his monumental multi-authored text, *Dermatology in General Medicine.* Appearing first in 1971, we now eagerly await its sixth edition.

Always alert to the need for funding research he was the founding father of the Dermatology Foundation in the early 1960s. Now it is a major source of support for young investigators.

Recipient of numerous awards and medals, honorary fellowships, and President of the Society for Investigative Dermatology, the International Pigment Cell Society and the Association of Professors of Dermatology, Fitzpatrick resigned as Chairman in 1987. But there was no let-up in his productivity. He actively studied vitiligo, as well as the use of digital imaging of the life of nevi. Always a serious musicologist he specialized in Johannes Brahams. He continued to publish every single day a thought-provoking quotation from the arts, sciences and literature. This appeared every day from April, 1984 in the *Boston Globe,* which has a readership of 400,000. It is evident that Fitzpatrick had a profound effect not only on the skin but also on the mind of man. Thomas B.Fitzpatrick died Saturday, August 16th 2003.*

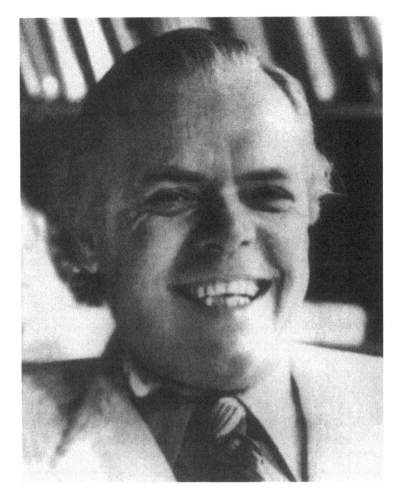

Figure 144 Thomas B.Fitzpatrick

THE ASH LEAF MACULE OF TUBEROUS SCLEROSIS

White Leaf-Shaped Macules: Earliest Visible Sign of Tuberous Sclerosis[†]

In the general physical examination every physician should be keenly aware of the clues on the skin that might lead to the discovery of diseases in other organs. The dermatologist should assume the prime role in the characterization of these "marker" lesions by a careful and clear description of the clinical morphology and the light-microscopic and electron-microscopic changes.

We wish to call attention to distinctive leaf-shaped white macules that appear to be the first harbinger of a serious dominant trait that causes mental retardation and convulsions, namely, tuberous sclerosis.

A 21-month-old Caucasian infant had a history of mental retardation and a convulsive disorder. This infant represented a sad situation for her parents and a diagnostic problem for the pediatrician and neurologist who were desperately seeking the etiology of the mental retardation and convulsions. The infant had six easily overlooked white macules. Because she was so young, there were none of the usual typical signs of tuberous sclerosis, such as the characteristic facial lesions or periungual fibromas. On the basis of the white spots, a diagnosis of tuberous sclerosis was suggested. The skull roentgenogram taken subsequently showed intracranial calcification of the left temporal area, and the electroencephalogram was abnormal. The white spots were thus the "marker" lesions that prompted studies that led to a diagnosis of this inheritable disease, made early enough to warn parents about the possibility of having other mentally retarded infants.

Hence, in infants with seizures and mental retardation, the presence of a few isolated white macules may be the earliest visible clue to tuberous sclerosis, inasmuch as the other important skin sign of this disease, adenoma sebaceum, does not appear until two to six years after birth.

This study is based on 31 patients whose ages range from 4 months to 36 years, all of whom have proved tuberous sclerosis. Ten of the infants in this series had white macules as the only visible manifestation of tuberous sclerosis. The white macules can persist into adult life, as may be seen in a 35-year-old patient with tuberous sclerosis and facial lesions.

The lesions may be distributed all over the body as irregularly scattered, isolated white macules, varying in number from 4 to more than 100. The macules are usually larger than 1 cm in diameter and are characteristically dull white, in contrast to vitiligo spots, which are pure white. On comparison of the white macules of tuberous sclerosis with those of vitiligo under visible or Wood's light, it is apparent that there is only a partial decrease of pigment in the macules of tuberous sclerosis.

A special feature of the white macule is its configuration, which may be oval or, in botanical terms, lance-ovate (tapering at one end and round at the other), which is most characteristic; this is the shape of the leaflet from the mountain-ash tree.

We are able to discriminate between the white macules of tuberous sclerosis and those of vitiligo with light-microscopic and electron-microscopic studies of these lesions.

We believe that, if infants have the typical white macules at birth, it is probable that tuberous sclerosis is present. If the combination of white macules and seizures is present, however, it then becomes highly probable that tuberous sclerosis is present. Therefore, it seems necessary to screen all newborns with Wood's light for the detection of these typical and easily overlooked white macules associated with tuberous sclerosis. In addition, all patients with seizures, regardless of age, should be examined for these white macules that may be the only visible sign of the disease.

As a result of these observations, it would be desirable to reword the familiar triad of epiloia. A more meaningful version, especially for the important early diagnosis, would be convulsions, mental retardation, and white macules.

---

* J.Invest Dermatol., *80:* suppl. 3s, 1983.

† Arch. Dermatol., *98:*1, 1968.

Lawrence M. Solomon

Epidermal Nevus Syndrome: Solomon's Syndrome

LAWRENCE MARVIN SOLOMON was born in Montreal, Quebec June 1, 1931. After graduating from McGill University he went on to receive an M.D. from the University of Geneva, Switzerland in 1959. Following a residency in medicine in Montreal he trained in dermatology at the University of Pennsylvania in Philadelphia. Joining the staff at the University of Illinois in Chicago, he rose to professorship and Head of the Department of Dermatology. His specialty is pediatric diseases of the skin. Together with Nancy B.Esterly he founded the Journal of Pediatric Dermatology, first published in 1983, and they remain the co-Editors 20 years later. In addition to his pioneer studies on nevi, he has written over 100 articles and eight books on subjects ranging from teaching by clinical simulation to the specialty of adolescent dermatology. He has held numerous visiting professorships around the world and served as President of the International Society of Pediatric Dermatology 1979–1983.

He retired from the University of Illinois in 2001 and now has a Chicago-based private practice limited to children. He has a lifelong addiction to mystery stories and possesses an enviable collection of rare books of this vintage.*

SOLOMON'S SYNDROME

The Epidermal Nevus Syndrome*

Since 1950, 15 patients have been seen at the Research and Education Hospital of the University of Illinois with a diagnosis of "epidermal nevus," "nevus unius lateris," "nevus verrucous;" or "acanthosis nigricans." Thirteen of these 15 patients agreed to return to the clinic for investigation and reevaluation, and a diagnosis was established by clinical and histological criteria. One of these reexamined patients had lichen planus (also associated with structural abnormality of the jaw). Of the remaining 12 patients (six males and six females), seven had lesions most consistent with a diagnosis of nevus unius lateris clinically and historically, two with bilateral epidermal nevi and three with ichthyosis hystrix or congenital benign acanthosis nigricans. Among the associated cutaneous lesions there were cavernous hemangiomas (cases 4 and 7), café au lait spots, melanocytic nevi, and webbing of the fingers (case 7). Neurological deficiencies were found in

---

* Pittelkow, R.B.: History of the American Dermatological Association, 1994.

* Arch. Dermatol., 97:273 1968

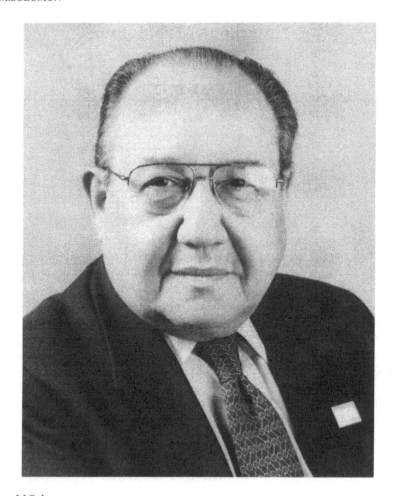

Figure 145 Lawrence M.Solomon

five of the 12 patients. The disorders were partial hemiparesis on the side of the lesion (cases 7, 8), epilepsy (cases 5, 1), mental retardation (case 8), and neural deafness (case 10).

The bony abnormalities associated with the epidermal nevi presented are widespread and involve not only leg length inequality but also deformities of the spine, hip, ankle, hands, and teeth (cases 1, 2, and 5 to 12). There seems to be no specific localization for the abnormality in the affected bones, and it was not possible to classify abnormalities under Rubin's classification. Three of the patients had mild deformities, three had moderate deformities, and four had severely disabling anomalies of the skeletal system. Membranous bones and enchondral bones were both affected. It was not possible to discern whether some of the static skeletal abnormalities were secondary to an underlying neurological deficit present in some of our patients or whether both the neurological and skeletal abnormalities were both due to a vascular accident which had occurred at some time in the past.

Whereas the cutaneous lesion is often the presenting complaint when a patient enters the physician's office, the associated bone pathology may have far more detrimental effects to the patient's well being than the cosmetic appearance of the skin lesion. Scoliosis may lead to grotesque deformity (cases 7 and 8). Untreated, the coxa valga subluxans could lead to an early form of osteoarthritis of the involved hip.

From the evidence presented, as well as that found in the literature, it seems reasonable to conclude that the incidence of bony and CNS abnormalities, which are found in association with extensive epidermal nevi are much higher than that expected in a normal population. Although certain anomalies, such as mild scoliosis and spina bifida, are relatively common, the incidence in the general population does not approach the 83% incidence of vertebral column disease found in our series. Furthermore, an abnormally high incidence (33%) of CNS disease was also found in our patients. It should be pointed out that our 12 patients with epidermal nevi were not randomly selected. They represent that group of patients who were willing to return to the hospital for reevaluation and therefore represent a degree of selection. Two patients in our series who were free of associated abnormalities had small (less than 10 cm long) isolated nevi. It would appear, therefore, that the larger the nevus, the more likely the association with other anomalies. The ensemble of findings suggests that extensive epidermal nevi form part of a syndrome including bony abnormalities and CNS disease.

We believe that nevus unius lateris, ichthyosis hystrix, bilateral linear epidermal nevi, and some instances of benign congenital acanthosis nigricans may be grouped under the name of epidermal nevi.

Summary. Nevus unius lateris, bilateral linear epidermal nevi, and ichthyosis hystrix may all be considered clinical variants of epidermal nevi. They were found in ten of 12 patients examined to be accompanied by congenital skeletal disorders. Five of these patients also had central nervous system (CNS) disease and two had other uncommon abnormalities, including a conjunctival fibroma and hepatosplenomegaly. The high frequency of associated abnormalities of bone and CNS in this study as well as the frequent reports of such findings in the literature strongly suggests the possibility that extensive epidermal nevi form part of a syndrome, including skeletal and CNS abnormalities. The presence of extensive epidermal nevi should be considered an indication for careful history and examination of the entire patient.

Ralph Grover

Transient Acantholytic Dermatosis (Grover's Disease)

RALPH WIER GROVER was born in Jersey City, NJ on December 26, 1920. He grew up on Long Island, where he remains to this day. With a degree from Harvard College, he went on to receive his M.D. from the Columbia College of Physicians and Surgeons. Two years at a Veterans' Hospital in Arkansas crystallized his interest in dermatology. He returned to New York to train at Skin and Cancer Hospital, as well as Presbyterian Hospital. Always a Long Islander at heart he opened a private office just outside New York City in the small suburban town of Floral Park, NY. There he practiced for 37 years until his retirement in 1988.

His love of pathology was not only clinical, but also histologic. He saw patients not only with his eye, but also under the microscope that was always at his elbow. Cytology intrigued him so that few patients escaped his nick of their skin for a smear. And so he came to recognize the acantholytic disease that bears his name. He notes with etymologic precision that he has seen over 500 cases of Grover disease, but only one case of Grover's disease, his own case.

Grover is a man of intense intellectual activity. He has studied seven languages ranging through Italian to savor Dante in the original, Swahili to enhance his visit to East Africa, and Russian to know the culture of Peter the Great. In retirement he spends long hours studying Beethoven's piano sonatas. A one-time scuba diver student of the ocean fauna and ham radio operator, he now is intent on studying the world of birds. It all began with his *"Watch Duck,"* a pet Peking, who for many years rode guard in the back seat of his car.[*]

GROVER'S DISEASE

Transient Acantholytic Dermatosis[†]

During the past five years I have observed six patients with unusual papulovesicular dermatoses which showed microscopic alterations suggestive of either Darier's disease (keratosis follicularis) or Hailey-Hailey's disease (familial benign chronic pemphigus), but which seemed clearly separable from these two diseases on clinical grounds.

---

[*] The Suffolk Times, November 14, 2002.

[†] Arch. Dermatol., *101:*426, 1970.

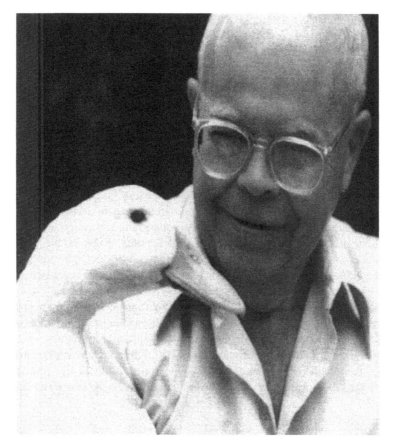

Figure 146 Ralph Grover

Case 2—A 62-year-old white lawyer was referred for consultation on May 11, 1965 because of a skin disease of two months' duration. The first lesions had appeared on his sternal area during the last week of a one-month vacation in Florida and had gradually spread widely on his trunk.

When first examined he had numerous isolated and irregularly aggregated, edematous, erythematous papules and vesiculopapules scattered about his trunk. The lesions were limited to those areas of his trunk, which he had exposed to the sunlight and were most prominent in his sternal area. They ended abruptly at his belt line and spared his axillae. His head, extremities, and the portion of his trunk below his belt line were not involved. A cytologic preparation revealed acantholytic cells and the histologic changes were interpreted as suggestive of Hailey-Hailey's disease.

Within the next two weeks the lesions of his trunk had begun to fade, but fresh spots continued to develop in a centrifugal manner on those areas of his extremities that had been exposed to sunlight. In the following six weeks the entire eruption gradually disappeared. At a recent examination, four years later, the previously involved areas appeared normal and he stated that he had not had any recurrence of the disease.

Comment. Each patient experienced an eruption of relatively acute onset with discrete, pruritic, edematous papular or papulovesicular elementary lesions. Some of the papules were crusted and occasionally small, tense blisters appeared at their summits. There was a tendency to form confluent groups of nummular or herpetiform aspect in the areas of maximal involvement.

In five of the six patients the disease began on the trunk. In both of the female patients it began on the back; in three of the male patients it began on the anterior aspect of the chest. The site of onset was not determined on one of the men, but the upper portion of his back was involved.

The disease appeared to run a self-limited course in each case, and its ultimate extent and duration seem significantly correlated with age. The two patients under the age of 50 had distinctly localized involvement, which lasted less than one month. The one patient in his 50's had moderate dissemination limited to the anterior aspect of his trunk, and his disease lasted approximately two months.

Microscopic findings—Acantholysis with vesicle formation was the principal finding and it should be emphasized that the demonstration of acantholytic cells in cytologic preparations done as a routine office procedure gave the preliminary evidence of the histologic nature of the disease in each case.

Clinical differential diagnosis—these patients did not appear to have any of the three generally recognized primary acantholytic diseases. The histologic suggestions of Hailey-Hailey's disease or Darier's disease, in particular, are not supported by the clinical features. None of the patients had the clinical hallmarks of familial benign chronic pemphigus, such as a tendency for the individual lesions to involve intertriginous areas and to spread centrifugally, or a tendency to chronic recurrence. In Darier's disease an onset so late in life would be most unusual, since it starts before the 40th year in 93% of cases, and less than 2% begin after the 60th year. Further, keratosis follicularis is a chronic and relentlessly progressive affliction in which a rapid onset, followed by healing within a few weeks or months, would be exceptional. The benign course of the disease is not compatible with common pemphigus and its variants.

The term "transient acantholytic dermatosis" seems a useful descriptive term for this group of patients. It indicates the basic pathologic change and, at the same time, indicates the principal point of clinical differentiation from the other forms of primary acantholytic disease—the characteristic of transiency.

Shigeo Ofuji

1.   Eosinophilic Pustular Folliculitis (Ofuji's Disease)

2.   Papuloerythroderma of Ofuji

SHIGEO OFUJI was born in Tokyo, Japan on September 9, 1917. He received his M.D. at the Kyoto University School of Medicine in 1941 and he also holds a Ph.D. For 30 years he served on the staff of the Department of Dermatology at Kyoto University, rising to Professorship and Chairmanship in 1962. By 1973 he was named Dean of their School of Medicine. As Emeritus Professor he later served for over 10 years as Director of Kansai Denryoku Hospital. Author of numerous papers, 48 in English, he is widely recognized for having identified a new form of folliculitis, as well as a unique erythroderma.

In his retirement, Professor Ofuji continues his hobby of sculpting images of Buddha and playing a fierce game of Go.*

OFUJI'S DISEASE

Eosinophilic Pustular Folliculitis[†]

Case Reports. Case 3—A 25-year-old Japanese engineer visited the Kyoto University Hospital on December 23, 1968. He first noticed a pruritic erythematous pea-sized skin lesion on the left eyebrow region. After a standstill for 2 months, the lesion gradually increased in size, taking an annular configuration and developing small pustules at its periphery. In the middle of December it involved the left half of the face. At the same time similar lesions appeared on the right cheek and submental region. Scattered papulopustules also developed on the back and extensor aspects of the upper extremities.

Laboratory findings. The blood count on the first visit revealed WBC 11,500 with a differential count of 43% neutrophils, 23% eosinophils, 3% monocytes and 31% lymphocytes. During the following 6 months the WBC ranged from 7,700 to 10,800 and the eosinophils from 12 to 45%.

Histological findings. In the hair follicle a vesicle was noted extending from the subcorneal portion of follicular ostium to the sebaceous gland. The wall of the vesicle consisted of a few layers of flattened cells of the outer root sheath. The vesicle was filled with numerous eosinophils and a small number of epithelial cells and mononuclear cells. At the follicular ostium the hair canal was preserved, including the hair, but

---

* Personal communication.

[†] Acta. Dermatovener (Stockholm), *50:*195, 1970.

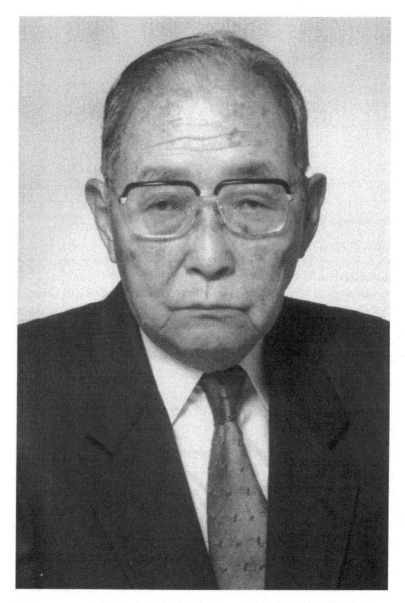

Figure 147 Shigeo Ofuji

serial sections of this specimen showed that the hair canal in the other portions was destroyed and the hair was floating in the vesicle.

Clinical course and treatment. During the following 3 weeks the skin lesions on the face enlarged and coalesced each other to involve almost the entire face. The papulopustules on the arms and back increased in number and formed many patches 5 to 10 cm in diameter, which developed papulopustules at their periphery, and pigmentation and some scales at their central areas. Thereafter, the skin lesions gradually faded and at the end of February, 1969, there were no skin lesions except for pigmented patches. However, exacerbations with a duration of about one month occurred twice after a remission period of 2 to 3 weeks.

Application of 0.12% betamethasone 17-valerate ointment was effective to some degree.

Discussion. The main feature of these three cases was the repeated development of crops of pruritic follicular sterile papulopustules in fairly well-defined areas. The skin lesions extended peripherally, i.e., fresh lesions appeared at the periphery as old ones faded in the center. When the plaques reached a certain size, they subsided leaving pigmentation. Subsequently, new lesions developed mostly in the pigmented areas and followed a similar course. The duration, interval and extent of these exacerbations varied. Although wide areas of the body surface were affected in the severest stage, the hands, feet and mucous membranes were always spared, and there were few systemic symptoms.

Because of the peculiar clinical, histologic and laboratory findings and of the characteristic clinical course, these cases are diagnostically distinct from pyoderma, dermatophytosis, syphilis pustulosa, impetigo herpetiformis, psoriasis pustulosa, acrodermatitis continua and dermatitis herpetiformis Duhring.

The diagnosis of contact dermatitis or drug eruptions was excluded by observations of the clinical course of the diseases. Eczematous dermatitis of unknown etiology occasionally occurs in follicular arrangement. The seborrheic skin observed in the patients, predilection sites, follicular papules with scales or crusts, and well-defined patch formation made us consider the possibility of seborrheic dermatitis. Follicular papules are seen frequently in atopic dermatitis and two of the four patients had atopic family history. However, pustules filled mostly with eosinophils are quite unusual findings in these three dermatoses. Pustules of erythema toxicum neonatorum resemble histologically those of the present cases in their pustule formation, filled mostly with eosinophils in the outer root sheath, but the clinical appearance of the two diseases is quite different.

Thus, these four cases seem to represent some entity with clinical and histologic features that do not correspond, to our knowledge, with any of the known dermatoses, including subcorneal pustular dermatosis. We, therefore, propose the name of eosinophilic pustular follliculitis to denote this disease.

Seborrheic facial skin and a present or past history of acne vulgaris were present in all four cases. The sites of predilection of the skin lesions were the face, chest, back and extensor surfaces of the upper arms. These facts suggest that sebaceous gland activity may have some relationship to the development of the skin lesions. However, clinical, histologic and laboratory findings did not clarify any etiological factors.

PAPULOERYTHRODERMA OF OFUJI

Papuloerythroderma*

Case Reports. Case 1—A 57-year-old company clerk visited Kyoto University Hospital on June 1, 1978. He had noticed pruritic papules scattered over the abdomen 3 months earlier. These papules had spread extensively over the entire surface of his body, increased in number, and became confluent.

Clinical findings—The skin of the trunk was almost entirely diffusely brownish-red, but the axillae, inguinal regions and the big furrows on the abdomen were spared with a fairly clear border. On the chest this diffuse lesion was composed of an assembly of slightly elevated, small macules 3–6 mm in diameter, quasi-square, quasi-rectangular, or irregular in shape. Each macule was bordered by the linear skin of normal color. On the back this pattern was not seen so clearly, but rather uniform, brownish-red discoloration was observed. On the upper extremities skin lesions were seen except in the cubital fossae and their surroundings. The extensor surfaces showed diffuse lesions similar to those of the trunk, while the flexor surfaces showed papules scattered, assembled, or confluent. The papules were 2–4 mm in diameter, brownish-red, clearly bordered, dome-shaped, smooth-surfaced, glossy, and solid. The skin lesions of lower extremities were nearly identical to those of the upper ones. In the neighborhood of the diffuse lesions, it was clear how papules assembled became confluent and formed the diffuse lesions. The palms and soles revealed marked hyperkeratosis with fissures. Both papules and diffuse lesions showed little scaling. The face and scalp were not involved. In the axillae and inguinal regions several indolent nonadhesive lymph nodes were palpable to the size of a little fingertip. Though moderate itching was complained of, it did not seem to be so intense as in exfoliative dermatitis or atopic dermatitis.

Laboratory findings—The blood count revealed a WBC of 8,100 with a differential count of 52% neutrophils, 22% eosinophils, 1.5% basophils, 6% monocytes and 18.5% lymphocytes. Serum IgE was below 500 IU/dl. Stools were free of ova and parasites.

Histological findings—A solid papule on the left forearm was biopsied. The main change was the relatively dense infiltration of lymphocytes and histiocytes mixed with a fair number of eosinophils in the upper and mid-dermis, chiefly around the blood vessels. PAS and alcian blue staining did not reveal any further findings.

Course and treatment—He was treated at our clinic while he continued to work. With the application of corticosteroid ointment and internal anti-histamine medication, the skin lesions improved gradually but very slowly. By August, 1979, about 1 year after the initial visit, the papules had become flatter, and the erythroderma-like lesions decreased in redness, becoming dark brown in tone. The blood eosinophilia returned to normal levels. By August, 1980, the skin lesions had nearly disappeared and, in March, 1982, he was completely normal.

Comment. Exfoliative dermatitis or erythroderma may follow eczema, psoriasis, lichen ruber, pityriasis rubra pilaris, pemphigus foliaceus, etc., and may also appear as skin manifestations of leukemia, mycosis fungoides, Sézary's syndrome, sarcoidosis and adverse drug reactions, but, in addition, is idiopathic in many cases, appearing mainly in older males. The initial rashes in our cases, solid papules, differ from the rashes of aforesaid skin diseases microscopically and microscopically, and are not observed in idiopathic exfoliative dermatitis.

It is characteristic in the macroscopic picture of these cases that the face, as well as the axillae, inguinal regions, big furrows on the abdomen, cubital and popliteal fossae are not involved, together with the presence of solid papules.

Clinical, histological and laboratory findings did not clarify any etiological factors and the name 'papuloerythroderma' is provisionally proposed.

---

* Dermatologica, *169*:125, 1984.

George C.Wells

Eosinophilic Cellulitis (Wells' Syndrome)

GEORGE CRICHTON WELLS was one of nine children of the distinguished Bedford Brewery Family of England. Born in 1917 he grew up excelling at rugby, swimming, high board diving, and rowing. Indeed, his collegiate eight won the Henley Cup in 1935. He qualified at St. Thomas Hospital and from 1942–1946 was with the Second Parachute Brigade of the Royal Army Marine Corps on their ambulance and surgical team. He saw action in North Africa, Greece, Italy and France.

After the war, Wells returned to St. Thomas Hospital to work with the celebrated Geoffrey Barrow Dowling. He left in 1951 for 3 years of research with Stephen Rothman at the University of Chicago. Back at St. Thomas he taught innumerable registrars, helped found the Dowling Club, and gave the Parkes-Weber Lecture in 1961. Then, in 1971, he described eosinophilic cellulitis with its distinctive flame figures.

His entire career was exemplified by an excellence in clinical teaching and research. He retired in 1979 and spent the next 20 years at his beautiful home in Sibton in Suffolk. There he had a textbook English garden, where he specialized in growing lilies.

Wells died in January, 1999.*

EOSINOPHILIC CELLULITIS (WELLS' SYNDROME)

Recurrent Granulomatous Dermatitis with Eosinophilia*

The four patients recorded here illustrate a changing symptom complex with a phase of the disease characterized by episodes of acute 'eosinophilic cellulitis' followed by 'granulomatous dermatitis' with its distinctive histopathology.

Case Reports. Case 1—*History*—This male clerk was first seen at St. Thomas' Hospital in 1958 when his age was 42, and when he had been getting periodic cutaneous swellings for about three years.

His eruptions start with an area of redness and swelling with irritation. Over one or two days the oedematous swellings spread outward and might cover the whole extent of a limb. The lesions are usually single, but may on occasion be multiple. The swellings show a distinct rosy or violaceous border. A brawny, bluish oedema persists for three or four weeks and slowly regresses, leaving the appearance of atrophy with slate grey pigmentation, which slowly fades over a month or two.

---

* Am. J.Dermatopathol., *24*:164, 2002.

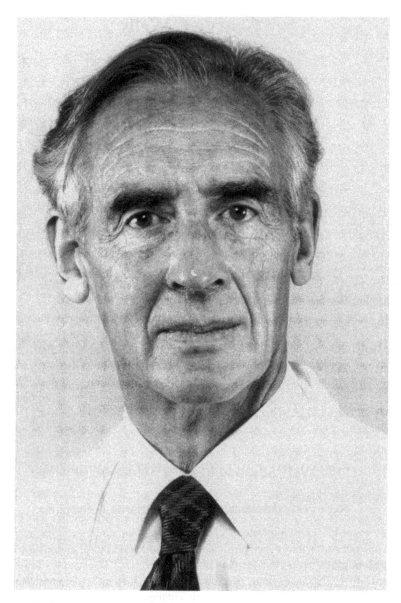

Figure 148 George C.Wells

Over the past three years there have been some very severe episodes of spreading oedema, resembling acute infective cellulitis, when bullae, some of them haemorrhagic, have appeared in parts of the plaques. There have been no constitutional symptoms with these attacks and he has had no fever. While lesions in the acute stage resemble cellulitis, during their gradual resolution they may look like morphoea.

Investigations—WBCs 9,200, neutrophils 46%, eosinophils 30, lymphos 15, monos 9, platelets 205.000.

Histology—In all cases the dermis was widely infiltrated with eosinophils and pale histiocytes and giant cells. Here and there in the dermis were striking foci of eosinophil debris adherent to connective tissue bundles with phagocytic cells ringed around.

Clinical Features. Our four patients had the characteristic severe swellings over a period of some years, before and after which there were undiagnostic cutaneous symptoms.

Eosinophilic cellulitis—An itching or burning sensation with redness and oedema of the skin appears suddenly and spreads rapidly over two or three days, sometimes with blistering. The 'cellulitis' covers the greater part of a limb or an area such as one shoulder. As it spreads the redness fades from the centre thus accentuating the margins of the lesion. Severe swellings may be quite painful for a few days.

Granulomatous dermatitis—The 'cellulitis' gradually resolves from the centre, which remains oedematous and slate-coloured for several weeks, while the border is rosy or violaceous. Further fading gives the impression of atrophy with a resemblance to morphoea. Eventually the skin recovers completely.

All patients have eosinophilia of the blood and marrow during active phases of the disease. One of our patients (Case 1) has had no other sign of disease, while our last patient (Case IV) had severe general symptoms including fever, asthma and arthralgia. The two others (Cases II and III) required corticosteroids for control of the more severe cutaneous swellings. In spite of these severe symptoms the three surviving patients have recovered and have been free from major attacks of granulomatous dermatitis for several years.

Histopathology. *Acute stage (eosinophilic cellulitis)*—Biopsy made within a few days of onset of the swelling shows massive infiltration of the dermis with oedema and eosinophils. Leucocytes (predominantly eosinophils) are massed in and around small venules and may be seen in transit through their walls. Apart from these vessel walls appearing oedematous and indistinct, no specific features of vasculitis are to be seen. Where blisters occur they are subepidermal and crowded with eosinophils.

Sub-acute stage (granulomatous dermatitis)—Biopsies taken one to three weeks from the onset of swelling show infiltration between the connective tissue bundles of eosinophils and large pale histiocytes. This granulomatous infiltrate causes some displacement of the fibres which is most apparent with elastic tissue stains. Besides this diffuse dermal infiltrate there are the sharply focal 'flame figures' characteristic of this condition.

The "flame figures"—These very striking aggregates are scattered in the mid or deeper dermis and show no relation to blood vessels. In a low power field one might see one, several or none. The central core is part of a collagen bundle and this is coated with eosinophilic debris. The eosinophilic flame-like mass is in turn surrounded by a palisade of large histiocytes and giant cells. In the extracellular debris can be identified loose cytoplasmic granules from disrupted eosinophils as well as Feulgen-positive nuclear material. The surrounding histiocytes and giant cells appear to be phagocytic for the eosinophil debris and some eosinophil granules are to be seen in their cytoplasm. The multinuclear giant cells are of foreign body type.

Summary. This is a study of the clinical features of four patients in the light of particular cutaneous histopathology. The characteristic eruption is periodic, tending to recur every few months, usually without systemic symptoms. The acute stage of *eosinophilic cellulitis* develops over a few days. Painful red oedema may cover a whole limb. Histologically, there is oedema and dermal infiltration with eosinophils.

The resolving stage of *granulomatous dermatitis* lasts about six weeks with brawny, slate coloured

---

* Trans. St. Johns Hospital, *57*:46, 1971.

oedema. Histologically, the dermis is infiltrated with eosinophils and histiocytes. Foci of phagocytosis of eosinophilic debris produce the characteristic flame figures.

A possible relationship to allergic granulomatosis of Churg and Strauss is discussed.

Peyton E. Weary

1.   Weary's Syndrome

2.   Cowden's Syndrome

PEYTON EDWIN WEARY was born in Evanston, Illinois on January 10, 1930. After attending Princeton University he received his M.D. at the University of Virginia where he has remained all of his life. It has been a life dedicated to the care of patients and to the care of his specialty of Dermatology. From 1972 to 1975 he served as Chairman of the Council of the National Program for Dermatology, helping to restructure the American Academy of Dermatology (A.A.D.). From 1975 to 1982 he chaired the A.A.D. Council on Governmental Liaison. No one in America has influenced governmental health policy in the field of skin disease more than Peyton Weary.

All of this led to skin diseases being recognized by the National Institutes of Health in their formation of a major institute, viz. The Institute of Arthritis, Musculoskeletal and Skin Diseases. This has had a significant impact on awareness and on funding for a field that garners less than 2% of the specialists in the US.

Throughout all of this, Weary has served as Chairman of his school's department of dermatology for 17 years. His small group is a crown jewel among training centers. But, above all, his total dedication to society has meant better health and better medical care for each of us in this nation, whether it be direct access to the right doctor, the right drug, or the right environment.*

WEARY'S SYNDROME

Hereditary Sclerosing Poikiloderma: Report of Two Families with an Unusual and Distinctive Genodermatosis*

A new widespread poikilodermatous and sclerotic disorder has been observed in seven members of two unrelated Negro families and is presented as yet another heritable disorder of connective tissue. By virtue of its inheritance pattern in one family, the disorder is thought to be inherited as a dominant trait and, thus, it is clearly different from poikiloderma congenitale (Rothmund-Thomson syndrome), which is transmitted as a recessive trait. We have been unable to find any description of a similar disorder in the literature, although

---

* Who's Who in America, 2003.

---

* Arch. Dermatol., *100:*413, 1969.

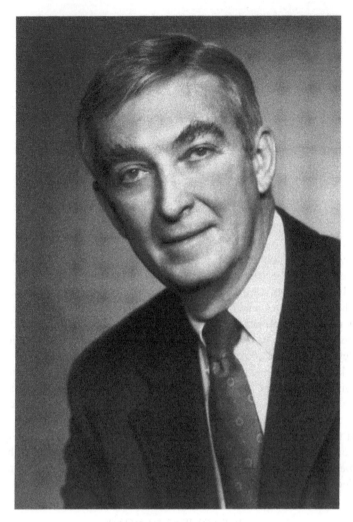

Figure 149 Peyton E. Weary

several other reported disorders may perhaps represent formes fruste of the picture encountered in our patients.

Summary of the Cutaneous Abnormalities in Affected Members of Family No. 1. In all affected members there was extensive mottled pigmentation, which was absent at birth, became apparent usually before the fourth year of life, and gradually increased in severity and extent with the passage of time. The most extensively affected members exhibited mottled pigmentation of all areas of skin except the upper chest (with the exception of the eyelids, which were involved with the scalp and ears). The lower legs were less severely affected than were other involved sites. The mottled appearance arose from irregular macular spots of hyperpigmentation, hypopigmentation, and depigmentation of varying size, up to about 1 cm in diameter, intermingled in a random fashion so as to totally confound any attempt to determine the normal skin color. In many of the regions no obvious atrophy or telangiectasia was visible so these regions cannot be said to be truly poikilodermatous. In other regions, however, such as the elbows and knees, obvious atrophy and telangiectasia was evident clinically providing justification for considering the process basically poikilodermatous rather than simply dyschromic. It was the impression of all observers that in those areas in which obvious atrophy was not present sweat gland function, thermoregulatory ability, sensory capability, and appendageal population density were probably unaltered.

The skin of the flexural regions of the axillae, antecubital fossae and, to a lesser extent, the popliteal fossae, in addition to accentuation of the mottling, exhibited a more unique cutaneous alteration in the form of reticulated and occasionally linear hyperkeratotic and sclerotic bands. These firm cord-like structures were 1 to 2 mm in width and elevated 1 to 2 mm above the surface of the skin.

The long axis of the majority of these hyperkeratotic bands was oriented perpendicular to the flexural creases. Because of a slight irregularity in width of the bands throughout the length, some appeared faintly beaded creating a slight resemblance to lesions of lichen rubra moniliformis. These sclerotic bands were thought to increase in number with the passage of time, since there was only one small area of such involvement in the left axillary vault of the youngest patient.

The extensor surfaces of the elbows, knees, knuckles, and interphalangeal joints exhibited the most intense poikiloderma with obvious atrophy and telangiectasia, but no sclerotic change was present in these regions. It was the skin of the palms, and to a lesser extent the soles, which most clearly demonstrated the diffuse sclerotic change with surface irregularity, which prompted us to liken the texture and appearance to shiny, scotch-grained leather. This firm, tense, shiny skin extended onto the medial and lateral aspects but it was not present on the dorsal aspects of the digits. In this way, the disorder differed greatly from scleroderma since there was no stretching of skin over the joints, no alteration of skin lines, and no impairment of the ability to fully flex the fingers.

COWDEN'S SYNDROME

Multiple Hamartoma Syndrome (Cowden's Disease)*

Summary of Cutaneous and Mucosal Lesions. The mucocutaneous lesions of our five cases are thought to be sufficiently distinctive as to represent the principal feature, which will more readily permit recognition of this uncommon and confusing disorder. The following is a synopsis of the mucocutaneous lesions that are encountered. It should be understood that while all patients exhibit mucocutaneous lesions, there is some degree of variability in the degree to which each type of lesion is encountered.

Cutaneous lesions—Lichenoid papules—Flat-topped papules that vary in size from less than a millimeter to 4 mm in diameter are the most common type of cutaneous lesion encountered. These lesions are of normal skin color and are not covered with scale. Many of these lesions contain a visible central pore or dell in which a small rough keratotic plug may be embedded. These flat-topped lesions tend to coalesce in some areas where they are found in profusion, but each lesion tends to retain its individual outline, giving to the surface a fine cobblestone or aggregated stone appearance. The pinnae and adjacent skin are the sites at which these lichenoid lesions are most apt to be found in profusion, but they also occur on the sides of the neck and in a centrofacial distribution with a tendency to cluster about the orifices of the eyes, nose and mouth. Although they are located over the glabella in all cases, they tend to diminish in number on the upper portion of the forehead. The lichenoid papules are not found on the trunk or elsewhere on the body. These lesions bear a rather striking similarity clinically to the cutaneous lesions of Darier's disease; however, as will be further described, the microscopic appearance shows them to be entirely unlike lesions of Darier's disease.

Papillomatous lesions—All patients exhibit to a more variable degree papillomatous and filiform verrucoid lesions, which also exhibit a tendency to cluster about orifices of the ears, eyes, nose and mouth.

Hyperkeratotic flat-topped papules—Lesions similar in appearance clinically to acrokeratosis verruciformis or flat warts are found on the dorsa of the hands and wrists but not on the dorsa of the feet.

Translucent keratoses—These lesions of the palms, soles and sides of the hands and feet, and palmar and plantar surfaces of the digits are seen in all patients. These lesions clinically resemble keratosis punctata palmaris et plantaris or arsenical keratoses.

Multiple lipomas—Some lipomas of large size or unusual distribution, are thought to be a feature of this disorder.

Cutaneous angiomas—These have been found in three of the cases, and in one, the angioma ultimately produced severe disability.

Mucosal lesions—Papular gingival and palatal lesions—Scattered over the surface of the gingivae and, to a lesser extent, the palates of all patients are small papular lesions, somewhat whiter than the surrounding gingival surface. These vary in size from 1 to 3 mm in diameter, and while they exhibit some tendency to coalesce, they retain a portion of their original outline, giving to the surface a faint cobblestone appearance.

Papillomatous lesions—Papillomatous and verrucoid lesions may be found in some of the patients on the buccal mucosa, faucial areas, and oropharynx. These same papillomatous lesions may extend into the region of the larynx, as in Case 3, interfering with phonation and requiring periodic removal. Also, the papillomatous tissue of the faucial region probably accounts for repeated tonsillectomies having been performed on Case 3.

Pebbly scrotal tongue—The tongue of cases 1, 2 and 4 exhibited a most unusual appearance. The surface was studded with hundreds of round, pearly papules, giving the surface a pebbly appearance. In addition, a degree of fissuring is present like that seen in scrotal tongue. The overall effect is that of a pebbly scrotal tongue.

Comment. *Summary of previous report*—To date, only one case of this disorder has been recorded in the literature, although it is entirely conceivable that other cases have been reported in series dealing with one or more of the facets of the overall syndrome. The one reported case, the family name was Cowden, was that of a 20-year-old girl with a remarkable hodgepodge of anomalies, of which the following were conceived by the authors to possibly represent a new symptom complex: adenoid facies with sharp beaked nose; hypoplasia of the mandible and maxilla; a high-arched palate; hypoplasia of the soft palate and uvula; microstomia; papillomatosis of the lips and oral pharynx; scrotal tongue; and multiple thyroid adenomas. Also included were bilateral virginal hypertrophy of the breasts with advanced fibrocystic disease and early malignant degeneration; pectus excavatum; scoliosis; probably cystic lesions of the head of one femur; and nonspecific dysrhythmic electroencephalographic abnormalities of the central nervous system associated with a course intention tremor. The patient exhibited cutaneous and mucosal findings, which were only described in a cursory fashion as multiple hyperkeratotic papillomata over the surface of the lips, most marked on the lower lip. The alveolar ridges and palate were covered with hyperkeratotic papules similar to those on the lips. There were numerous verrucae simplex on the dorsa of both hands and a linear area of hyperpigmentation was present over the vertebral spines from T6 to L2.

---

* Arch. Dermatol., *106:*682, 1972.

Rona M.MacKie

Juvenile Plantar Dermatosis

RONA MCLEOD MACKIE was born in Dundee, Scotland on May 22, 1946. After receiving her medical education at the University of Glasgow, she rose through the ranks to become Professor and Head of the Department of Dermatology. This was a singular honor, since she was the first woman ever to chair any department in the history of Glasgow University. Under her guidance, the Department gained international prominence, attracting postgraduate students from around the world.

Her reputation grew out of her dedication to the problems of malignant melanoma, lymphomas and atopic dermatitis. Author of over 400 research papers, sole author of a textbook of dermatology, now in its 4th edition, and editor of the *British Journal of Dermatology* (1984–1988), she has had influence far beyond being the first to christen juvenile plantar dermatosis.

A glance at her curriculum vitae shows a coruscating cascade of academic degrees and international honorary fellowships, memberships, gold medals, and presidencies. And England is proud, having given her the coveted CBE—Commander of the Order of the British Empire. She is truly the *"Queen of Dermatology"*. And her husband is the Nobel Laureate, James Black.

In the year 2000 she vacated her Chair of 28 years to become a Leuverhulme Senior Research Fellow in the study of environmental and genetic interactions leading to malignant melanoma.*

JUVENILE PLANTAR DERMATOSIS

Juvenile Plantar Dermatosis: A New Entity?*

Summary. 102 children with dermatitis, predominantly affecting the weight-bearing areas of the feet, are described. Despite a clinical appearance suggestive of an allergic contact dermatitis, only thirteen children had positive patch tests to any substance in the European battery, or to constituents of their own footwear.

Introduction. In the course of routine patch testing and paediatric dermatological practice, a group of children with a persistent dermatitis of the feet came to our notice. This group consisted mainly of primary school-aged children. The presenting complaint was scaling, fissuring and an itching or burning sensation of the weight-bearing areas of the feet. A search of the literature revealed reports of two rather similar

---

* The Medical Directory, 1990.

* Clin. Exp. Dermatol., *1:*253, 1976.

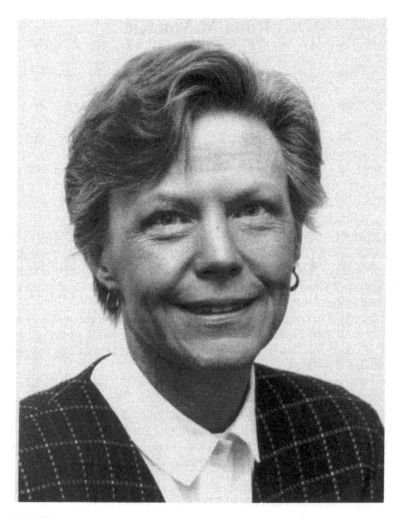

Figure 150 Rona M.MacKie

conditions; Moller in 1972 described a condition to which he gave the name "atopic winter feet", and Schultz and Zachariae, also in 1972, described a condition called "recurrent juvenile eczema of hands and feet". However, a study of our group of patients revealed firstly that atopy was not closely associated with this condition, and secondly that in no case studied was hand eczema an associated condition. We, therefore, carried out a study of these children in an attempt to explain this condition.

The patients. Fifty-five boys and forty-seven girls have been studied, with an age range of 2–14 years. All had lesions on the soles of the feet, which had been considered by the clinician concerned to be suggestive of contact dermatitis, and they had, therefore, been referred for routine patch testing. Erythema, scaling and fissuring of the ball of the foot and frequently of the under surface of the toes, was a constant feature. Involvement of the heels and insteps was less frequent, and no lesions were observed in the interdigital clefts or on the dorsa of the feet.

Duration of lesions—The majority had had lesions present for between 6 months and 2 years at the time of presentation, and once present the lesions tended to fluctuate in severity. The majority noted no clear-cut association between severity of the lesions and summer or winter weather, but seven children noted a clear deterioration of the condition during the winter months (December to March), whereas nine others found the summer months (June to September) the period when their lesions were most troublesome.

Relationship of the condition to sports or footwear—The majority of patients found that the condition of their feet deteriorated considerably after a period of vigorous physical activity; joining a football team or training for school sports were both mentioned by parents as being occasions on which rapid deterioration was noted. Five children (4 boys and 1 girl) noted increased discomfort and irritation after attending swimming baths. Six children reported increased discomfort after wearing Wellington boots, but other than this there was no clear-cut association between the condition and the use of rubber, leather or composition-soled shoes. Nearly all the children in the study habitually wore nylon socks and found little benefit in changing to wool or nylon-wool mixture socks. Cotton socks are becoming increasingly difficult to obtain, but the majority of children who changed to cotton socks found some improvement in their condition.

Mycology—Routine mycological examination was carried out in all patients with negative results in all cases.

Discussion. This group of children have a fairly chronic and, at times, painful and disabling condition. The majority gave a history of onset shortly after starting formal education at the age of 5 years. Only three children in the whole series presented prior to school entry, and two of those had atopic dermatitis. The natural history of the condition once present is of exacerbations and remissions with no complete clearance of lesions for a period of 2–3 years, after which time spontaneous resolution of the condition would appear to take place. Intermittent use of weak topical non-fluorinated steroids appears to be the most beneficial therapy in the majority of cases. Several children reported deterioration of the condition after using tar or dithranol preparations.

The children with positive patch tests to shoe materials had footwear free of the appropriate allergens supplied, but despite this the condition continued to be troublesome, indicating that allergic contact sensitivity was not a major causative factor.

We would suggest that a suitable name for this disorder is *juvenile plantar dermatosis*. It is at present a fairly common disorder among children attending paediatric dermatology clinics in the West of Scotland. Whether it is a new entity or one just recently recognized is a matter for speculation, but it seems surprising that if not a new entity, it was not recorded by dermatologists 30 and 40 years ago whose recognition of clinical conditions was generally so accurate.

A likely aetiological factor would seem to be the increasing use of synthetic materials for children's socks as in the past decade the use of natural fibre such as cotton or wool has become much less common, and the substitution of nylon almost universal.

Thomas J. Lawley

Pruritic Urticarial Papules and Plaques of Pregnancy (PUPPP)

THOMAS JOSEPH LAWLEY was born in Buffalo, NY on January 16, 1947. Growing up in Buffalo he remained there for his B.S. from Canisius College and his M.D. and internship from SUNY at Buffalo.

His dermatologic training was split between Yale, SUNY and the National Institutes of Health. From 1977 to 1988 he spent his time as a clinical research investigator at the NIH. He was then appointed Professor and Chairman of Dermatology at Emory University in Atlanta. In 1996 he became Dean of the medical school where he now wrestles with the problems of academic leadership, financial spreadsheets, and the internecine warfare of his departments. Yet, all this does not keep him from a regular weekly schedule of dermatologic research in the clinic and laboratory.

His productivity at the NIH and at Emory has been phenomenal. Beginning with studies on that remarkable drug, dapsone, his research has centered on the immunologic factors in disease. He has focused on the pathogenic role of immune complexes, the process of cell adhesion, as well as the functions of the endothelial cell itself. Since his seminal paper on PUPPP, he has continued to study the varied skin diseases seen in pregnancy.

Lawley has graced the staff of 32 universities as Visiting Professor, as well as writing nearly 50 chapters in a variety of textbooks and producing over a hundred original research papers. Overriding all this is the counsel and wisdom he has brought to the countless committees, review panels, editorial boards, directorships and councils on which he has served.*

PRURITIC URTICARIAL PAPULES AND PLAQUES OF PREGNANCY (PUPPP)

Pruritic Urticarial Papules and Plaques of Pregnancy*

Report of Cases. Case 1. A 26-year-old woman (gravida 1, para 0) in the 38th week of her first pregnancy noted the onset of an intensely itchy eruption on her abdomen that progressed within days to cover much of her thighs and buttocks, with less involvement of her arms and legs. The lesions were preponderantly urticarial plaques, but many small (1 to 2 mm) erythematous papules that showed blanching at their peripheries were also present. There was no evidence of excoriation. The patient had no prior history of skin

---

* Pittelkow, R.B.: History of the American Dermatological Association, 1994.

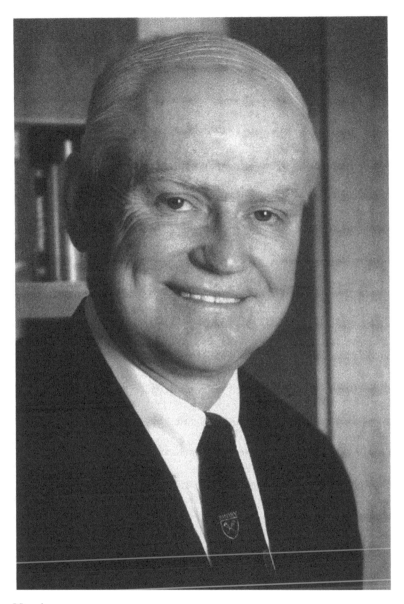

Figure 151 Thomas J.Lawley

disease and was taking no medications or vitamins. A complete blood cell count (CBC) and serum SGOT, SGPT, lactic dehydrogenase (LDH), alkaline phosphatase, bilirubin, and human chorionic gonadotrophin levels were within normal limits. A skin biopsy specimen showed a superficial perivascular and interstitial inflammatory cell infiltrate composed of lymphocytes, histiocytes, and a few eosinophils. The overlying epidermis was normal. Direct immunofluorescence of normal and lesional skin for IgG, IgA, IgM, IgE, and C3 was negative. The patient's symptoms abated somewhat with treatment with a fluorinated topical corticosteroid gel. Two days later she was delivered of a healthy girl, and within seven days thereafter the eruption abated.

Comment. Our seven cases closely resemble one another in terms of the clinical setting, symptoms, and morphological characteristics of the lesions. The eruption began in each patient in the third trimester of pregnancy. It started on the abdomen in all patients and frequently spread to involve the thighs. The buttocks and arms were also affected in some patients. Truncal lesions were rarely seen above the midthorax, and the face was never affected. The lesions consisted of erythematous urticarial plaques and small (1 to 2 mm) papules that were often surrounded by a narrow, pale halo. In most patients the plaques and papules were of such great number that the fate (e.g., time course and prodrome) of individual lesions could not be accurately determined. Six of the patients complained of pruritus sufficiently severe to keep them awake at night. Despite complaints of marked itching, excoriated lesions were extraordinarily infrequent.

The eruption in these patients differs considerably from almost all of the other previously described pruritic dermatoses of pregnancy. Herpes gestationis can be ruled out by its clinical and histopathologic features and by the absence of IgG or C3 deposits at the basement membrane zone of perilesional skin. The hallmark of prurigo gravidarum (intrahepatic cholestasis of pregnancy) is itching and clinical jaundice associated with notable aberration of liver function tests, although in mild cases jaundice may not be apparent. None of our patients demonstrated these findings. Papular dermatitis of pregnancy, as described by Spangler, et al., differs from the eruption in our patients because it consists exclusively of excoriated papules, has no major areas of predilection (the face is often involved), occurs any time from the first to the ninth month of pregnancy, and is characterized by elevated urine chorionic gonadotrophin levels. The morphological characteristics and distribution of lesions of prurigo gestationis of Besnier also differ considerably from those in our patients. They are excoriated papules without urticarial features. In addition, the lesions in prurigo gestationis are characteristically confined to the extensor surfaces of the extremities and rarely involve the trunk. Impetigo herpetiformis is a pustular eruption that is similar to, if not identical with, pustular psoriasis. None of our patients had pustules, and the histopathology of impetigo herpetiformis is different from that in our cases. Serious systemic toxic effects, which are common in impetigo herpetiformis, did not occur in our patients.

Details of individual cases, histopathology, and laboratory data are lacking in the description of the toxemic rash of pregnancy by Bourne. Despite this, the eruption in our patients is somewhat similar to that in the toxemic rash of pregnancy. Both are very pruritic and occur in the third trimester. Both begin on the abdomen and may subsequently involve the thighs, buttocks, and arms. Areas of sparing are also similar. Urticarial lesions occurred in only some of Bourne's cases, whereas this was a constant feature in ours. Crusting of lesions frequently occurred in Bourne's cases, but was uncommon in our patients.

Pruritic urticarial papules and plaques of pregnancy may be the most common of the pruritic diseases of pregnancy. The absence of previous reports is probably due to several factors. The eruption occurs late in pregnancy and usually remits shortly after delivery, so that most patients may never consult a dermatologist. Many patients respond well to topical therapy with corticosteroids and are probably seen no more than once. Moreover, the obscure nature of the pruritic gestational dermatoses tends to encourage lumping of these patients into the nonspecific category of "pruritus of pregnancy." Some cases are probably misdiagnosed as drug eruptions or are categorized as unusual cases of erythema multiforme. Finally, individual dermatologists may not see enough cases to arouse their suspicions to the similar clinical and histopathologic findings in this entity.

---

* J.A.M.A., *241:*1696, 1979.

Steven Kossard and Richard K. Winkelmann

Necrobiotic Xanthogranuloma

STEVEN KOSSARD was born in Shanghai on February 9, 1944. His career has centered on Sydney, Australia where he attended college and received his medical education and earned a Ph.D. at Sydney University in 1973 for his research on melanoma. After a year in dermatology at St. Vincent's Hospital he finished his residency at Mayo Clinic in 1979. As a dermatopathology fellow working with Winkelmann, he published this landmark paper on a unique necrotizing xanthogranuloma.

Currently, he is Associate Professor of Dermatology at the University of New South Wales and Chairman at St. Vincent's Hospital in Sydney. He heads the Dermatopathology Department of the Skin and Cancer Foundation Australia. To date, he has published 120 papers, which include studies on eruptive infundibulomas and postmenopausal frontal fibrosing alopecia.

His hobbies are photography, painting and his garden.*

RICHARD KNISELY WINKELMANN was born in Akron, Ohio on July 12, 1924. His student days make up a checkerboard of schools: University of Akron, Michigan State, Michigan, and Marquette where he received his M.D. in 1948. Subsequently, he was a research fellow with the Atomic Energy Commission and the Department of Anatomy at Washington University, as well as at the Medical College of Alabama. He had his fellowship in Dermatology at the Mayo Clinic, receiving a Ph.D. in that field from the University of Minnesota. Joining the Mayo Clinic staff in 1956, he has remained there for a most productive career, which led to his Professorship and Chair.

He also attained the rank of Associate Professor of Anatomy in the Mayo Graduate School of Medicine. In 1990 he moved to the Mayo Clinic/Scottsdale in Arizona, where he retired in 1994. Since 1998 he has been Research Professor of Plant Biology at Arizona State University, where he is an avid student of algae and diatoms in the St. Croix River back in Minnesota.

Winkelmann has introduced innumerable fellows to his excitement and his work ethic in clinical research. With them he has published over 775 papers ranging from esoteric histopathology to the therapeutic use of chlorambucil and intravenous immunoglobulin.

As a founding father of the American Society of Dermatopathologists, he went on to be its President. He has served as Editor or member of the editorial board of eight journals. Some twenty foreign dermatologic societies have given him honorary membership. He has graced the research faculty of the Institute of Dermatology in London for extended periods, studying urticaria.

---

* Personal communication.

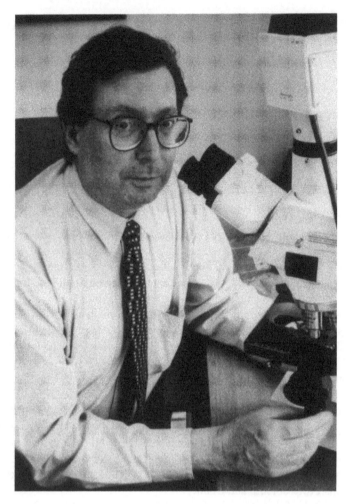

Figure 152 Steven Kossard

Winkelmann has spent a lifetime traveling through dermatology in cross section. And what he has told us of his adventures has been thrilling for all of us who seek to understand and treat skin disease.*

NECROBIOTIC XANTHOGRANULOMA

Necrobiotic Xanthogranuloma with Paraproteinemia[†]

We wish to describe eight patients in whom unusual multiple, inflammatory, ulcerative, and atrophic nodules and plaques with a xanthomatous quality developed in conjunction with paraproteinemia. Multiple skin biopsy specimens showed a mixture of xanthogranuloma with zones of necrobiosis. We believe that the clinical and histopathologic findings differ from those of normolipemic generalized plane xanthoma or other necrobiotic granulomas previously documented. In three patients, bone marrow changes were interpreted as showing either myeloma or B cell lymphoma.

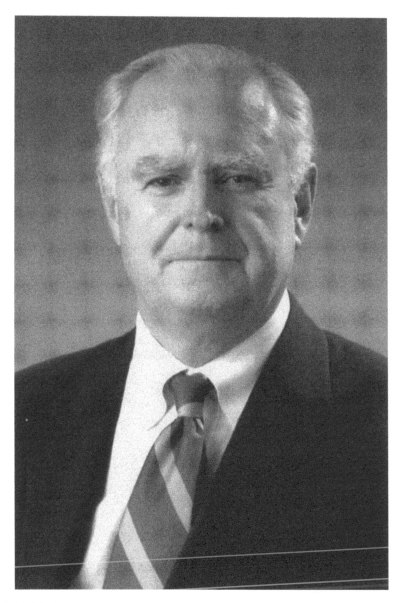

Figure 153 Richard K. Winkelmann

Case Report. A 51-year-old woman was referred for evaluation of cutaneous granulomas, which had developed during a 7-year period. The initial lesion was an asymptomatic, subcutaneous nodule over the left hip, and this was followed by similar lesions over the abdomen, buttock, arm, and face. The periorbital lesions were disfiguring and had ulcerated. The patient was well and had no symptoms of anorexia, nausea, night sweats, or bone pain. Previous skin biopsy specimens had been variously interpreted as showing changes consistent with granuloma annulare, palisading granulomatous dermatitis and panniculitis, or

Rothmann-Makai panniculitis. For the 5-year period before being seen at the Mayo Clinic, she had leukopenia, with counts as low as 1,900/mm^3. A bone marrow study performed at another institution was nondiagnostic. In December 1978, a monoclonal protein band was found on serum electrophoresis. Previous therapy included the use of intralesional and topical corticosteroids, low-dose methotrexate, azathioprine, and saturated solution of potassium iodide. The lesions decreased in size when potassium iodide was used.

Physical examination showed disfiguring ulcerated xanthomatous nodules in the periorbital area, with associated epidermal atrophy and telangiectasia. There were multiple subcutaneous nodules, which were flesh-colored or violaceous, located particularly over the back. Indurated plaques and papules were scattered over the trunk, buttocks, and hips. There was no adenopathy or hepatosplenomegaly.

The serum protein electrophoresis showed an elevated γ-globulin level of 2.42 gm/dl (normal, 0.5 to 1.6), with a monoclonal spike. Immunoelectrophoresis of serum showed this to be an IgGλ protein.

Histopathologic Findings. A consistent pattern of xanthogranulomatous disease was found in all sixteen specimens. Xanthogranuloma may be defined as an inflammatory, histiocytic, and foam cell lesion.

Comment. The principal differential diagnosis for this lesion is necrobiosis lipoidica diabeticorum. Clinical similarities to necrobiosis lipoidica were noted, particularly in Cases 2 and 6, in which lesions developed over the pretibial areas. In contrast to necrobiosis lipoidica, none of the patients had frank diabetes mellitus or lesions confined to the pretibial surfaces.

Various cytotoxic agents were used to treat four of our patients, with clinical evidence of improvement in skin lesions. Because of the slowly progressive nature of the condition and the frequent presence of leukopenia, low-dose alkylating agents appear to be preferable. Necrobiotic xanthogranuloma with paraproteinemia represents an important rare biologic phenomenon that can be recognized clinically and histologically and should be separated from other syndromes of generalized plane xanthomas and necrobiotic granulomas.

* Pittelkow, R.B.: History of the American Dermatological Association, 1994.

† J.Am. Acad Dermatol., *3:*257, 1980.

Grant J. Anhalt

Paraneoplastic Pemphigus

GRANT JAMES ANHALT was born in Shaunavon, Saskatchewan, Canada on December 14, 1952. His father was a dermatologist in Winnipeg and on the teaching staff until his retirement in 1992. Grant took his under-graduate work, his M.D., internship, and a year of internal medicine all at the University of Winnipeg. This was followed by 5 years of training in his father's field at the University of Michigan. He then moved to Johns Hopkins University where by 1996 he had risen to the rank of full Professor of Dermatology and Pathology. He currently serves as Vice Chairman of the Department.

His ascent was propelled by the publication of over 260 papers in the field of the immunopathology and therapy of pemphigus.

His work has attracted international acclaim and some 26 post-doctoral fellows from around the world. He has been the invited speaker for innumerable named lectureships, workshops, courses, and national and international meetings. Few can match his zeal and skill in modern basic molecular pathology.

His hobbies outside the game of pemphigus antigens are tennis, golf and numismatics.*

PARANEOPLASTIC PEMPHIGUS

An Autoimmune Mucocutaneous Disease Associated with Neoplasia*

Case Report (Index case). In early 1987 a 62-year-old man was given a diagnosis of malignant follicular large-cell lymphoma. The tumor initially responded to therapy with cyclophosphamide, doxorubicin (Adriamycin), vincristine, bleomycin, and intravenous and intrathecal methotrexate. In January 1988 a pruritic urticarial skin eruption developed; it was assumed to be an allergic reaction to diltiazem, but it did not resolve after discontinuation of the drug. In May 1988 the lymphoma recurred and was treated with chlorambucil and prednisone, but both the lymphadenopathy and the skin eruption responded only partially. A skin biopsy showed focal acantholysis, with granular complement deposition at the epidermal basement-membrane zone and weak deposition of IgG within the intercellular substance of the epidermis. Indirect immunofluorescence testing of the patient's serum on sections of monkey esophagus showed the presence of pemphigus-like anti-bodies at a titer of 1:80. Treatment with azathioprine (100 mg/day) and prednisone (60

---

* Pittekow, R.B.: History of the American Dermatological Association, 1994.

* N.Engl. J.Med., *323*:1729, 1990.

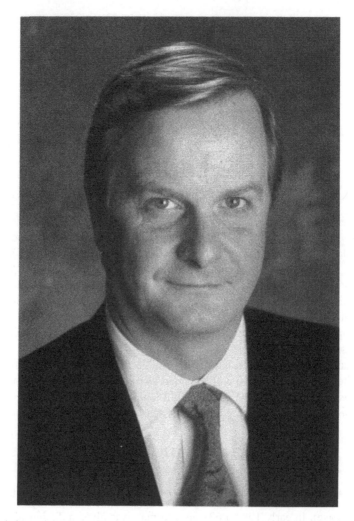

Figure 154 Grant J.Anhalt

mg/day) was started, but the skin eruption worsened. Numerous confluent vesicles and erosions of the conjunctivas, oropharynx, and esophagus developed, accompanied by severe dysphagia, malaise, myalgia, and fatigue and numerous erosions on the trunk and extremities. Staphylococcal sepsis developed, and the patient was admitted to a burn-care unit with a presumed diagnosis of toxic epidermal necrolysis.

On the 11th hospital day, new pruritic vesiculobullous lesions developed on the trunk and extremities and new oral and conjunctival erosions appeared. Biopsy of a skin lesion revealed an acantholytic intraepidermal blister consistent with pemphigus vulgaris. The epithelium adjacent to the blister showed vacuolar-interface change and necrosis of individual keratinocytes. Circulating pemphigus-like antibodies were present at a titer of 1:2560.

The lymphoma was considered to be incurable. The patient was discharged home, where he had recurrent episodes of pneumonia and died in December 1988.

Discussion. Paraneoplastic pemphigus is clinically distinct from pemphigus vulgaris and pemphigus foliaceus. Painful, persistent, and treatment-resistant erosions of the oral mucosa, vermilion borders of the lips, and conjunctivas were common to all cases. The initial skin lesions were polymorphous, often presenting as a pruritic papulosquamous eruption with subsequent blistering. The occurrence of blisters of the palms and soles suggested a diagnosis of erythema multiforme in three of our five patients, raising the interesting possibility that previously reported cases of erythema multiforme associated with underlying tumors may have in fact been unrecognized cases of paraneoplastic pemphigus. The clinical polymorphism is reflected by histologic variability. The combination of acantholysis with interface dermatitis or with keratinocyte necrosis within a single biopsy specimen seems characteristic of paraneoplastic pemphigus.

The autoantibodies of paraneoplastic pemphigus differ from those of pemphigus vulgaris and pemphigus foliaceus in their antigenic specificity, as demonstrated by immunofluorescence testing and by immunoprecipitation. The antibodies in our five patients had broad tissue specificity, reacting with all epithelia, and immunoprecipitated a characteristic complex of four high-molecular-weight antigens. The broad specificity may be due to binding of the autoantibodies to desmoplakin I, a protein that is common to the cytoplasmic plaque of desmosomes in all epithelia and that has regions of marked homology with the 230-kd antigen of bullous pemphigoid. At present, we employ indirect immunofluorescence testing of rodent bladder as a convenient and cost-effective method of screening for this syndrome, since bladder epithelium has numerous desmosomes, but the antigens of pemphigus vulgaris and pemphigus foliaceus are not expressed in this tissue.

Index

Abacus nodule, 548
Acanthoma fissuratum, 589
Acanthosis nigricans, 239
Acaro-dermatitis urticarioides, 360
Achor, 9
Acne keloidalis nuchae, 166
Acne vulgaris, 55
Acrodermatitis continua, 202, 288
Acrodermatitis infantile lichenoid, 518
Acrokeratosis paraneoplastica, 583
Actinic granuloma, 460
Acute febrile mucocutaneous lymph node syndrome
   (Kawasaki disease), 601
Acute febrile neutrophilic dermatosis, 581
Addison, T., 84
Adenoma sebaceum, 227
Adrenergic urticaria, 543
Alibert, J.L., 29
Allen, S.D., 455
Anetoderma, 234
Angeiomata, eruptive, 122
Angiokeratoma, 259
Angiokeratoma corporis diffusum, 464
Angiokeratoma of the scrotum, 272
Angioma serpiginosum, 187, 360
Angioneurotic edema, 180
Anhalt, Grant J., 641
Aquadynia, 550
Aquagenic urticaria, 537
Arsenical keratosis, 186
Ash leaf macule of tuberous sclerosis, 604
Athrepsie, 115
Atopic dermatitis, 245
Atrophia maculosa cutis, 335
Atrophic glossitis, 67
Atrophoderma of Pasini and Pierini, 470
Autoimmune estrogen dermatitis, 546

Autoimmune progesterone sensitivity dermatitis, 538

Bateman, T., 4, 18
Bazex, André, 583
Bazex atrophoderma, 585
Bazex syndrome, 585
Bazin, E., 80
Bean, William Bennett, 552
Bean's syndrome, 554
Becker, S.William, 488
Becker's nevus, 492
Behçet, H., 444
Behçet's disease, 444
Besnier, E., 243
Benign juvenile melanoma, 502
Black heel, 570
Bleb, 8
Bloch, B., 420
Bloch-Sulzberger, 436
Blue rubber-bleb nevus syndrome, 554
Blum, P., 412
Boeck, C., 294
Botryomycose humaine, 280
Bowen, J.T., 373
Bowen's disease, 375
Breisky, A., 190
Brocq, J.L., 85, 256, 303
Brooke, H.G., 247
Brunsting, Louis A., 474
Bulla, 8
Bullous pemphigoid, 510
Burchardt, M., 78
Bury, J., 205
Buschke, A., 324
Busse-Buschke's disease, 324

Calcaneal petechiae, 570

Cancroides, 34
Castellani, A., 410
Cazenave, A., 60
Cerion, 9
Cheilitis exfoliativa, 52
Cheilitis glandularis, 130
Chernosky, Marvin E., 591
Chondrodermatitis nodularis chronica helicis, 390
Chromoblastomycosis, 387
Chronic atypical epithelial proliferation, 375
Cold erythema, 536
Colloid milium, 195
Congenital ichthyosiform erythroderma, 312
Contagious pustular dermatitis, 434
Cowden's syndrome, 626
Crissey, John T., 569
Crosti, A., 515
Curth, H., 324
Curth, W., 324
Cutaneous diphtheria, 44
Cutis laxa, 319
Cutis verticis gyrata, 338

Darier, J., 393
Darier's disease, 395
Dartre pustuleuse disseminee, 55
Dartre pustuleuse miliaire, 55
Dartre rongeante, 31
Dermatitis exfoliativa, 122
Dermatitis gangrenosa infantum, 200
Dermatitis herpetiformis, 150
Dermatitis papillaris capillitii, 166
Dermatitis repens, 202
Dermatolysis, 38
Dermatomyositis, 196
Dermatose hétéromorphe, 38
Dermatosis papillomatosa capillitii, 166
Dermatosis papulosa nigra, 411
Devergie, A., 73
Dhobie dermatitis, 496
Dieulafoy, 42
Disseminated superficial actinic porokeratosis (DSAP), 592
Duhring, L., 145
Dysidrosis, 136

Ecthyma, 51
Eczema, 21, 329
Eczema impetigenodes, 21

Eczema marginatum, 214
Eczema rubrum, 23
Edema neonatorum, 115
Ehlers-Danlos syndrome, 319
Ehlers, E., 317
Engman, M.F., 328
Eosinophilic cellulitis, 621
Eosinophilic pustular folliculitis, 614
Epidermal nevus syndrome, 607
Epidermolysis bullosa, 177
Epithelioma adenoides cysticum, 249
Epstein, Ervin, 588
Erysipeloid, 192
Erythema annulare, 101
Erythema annulare centrifugum, 399
Erythema contagiosum, 332
Erythema diffusum, 101
Erythema elevatum diutinum, 204
Erythema exudativum multiforme, 101
Erythema figurata perstans, 356
Erythema fugax, 101
Erythema gyratum, 101
Erythema gyratum perstans, 231
Erythema induratum, 82
Erythema infectiosum, 332
Erythema iris, 101
Erythema laeve, 101
Erythema marginatum, 101
Erythema multiforme, 101
Erythema nodosurn, 15, 101
Erythema papulatum, 101
Erythema tuberculatum, 101
Erythema urticans, 101
Erythèma centrifuge, 64
Erythrasma, 79
Erythrodermia desquamativa, 351
Erythrodermies pityriasiques en plaques, 316
Erythroplasia, 367
Escherich, T., 331
Estrogen dermatitis, 546
Exanthema, 8
Exfoliative dermatitis, 108, 122
Exudative discoid and lichenoid chronic dermatosis, 439

Fabry, Johannes, 462
Fabry's disease, 464
Familial benign chronic pemphigus, 448
Farber, Eugene M., 498
Favus, 9

Fitzpatrick, Thomas B., 602
Focal dermal hypoplasia syndrome, 574
Fogo salvagem, 451
Folliculitis decalvans, 218
Fordyce, J.A., 270
Fox, T.C., 229
Fox-Fordyce disease, 323
Fox, G.H., 321
Fox, T., 132
Framboesia non syphilitica capillitii, 166
Furfura, 8

Garbe, W., 436
Gianotti-Crosti syndrome, 518
Gianotti, F., 515
Gibert, C., 92
Glucagonoma syndrome, 490
Goldscheider, A., 176
Goltz, Robert W., 572
Goltz syndrome, 574
Gougerot, H., 412
Grain itch, 360
Granuloma annulare, 208
Granulosis rubra nasi, 336
Grocer's itch, 21
Grover, Ralph W., 610
Grover's disease, 611

Hailey, H.E., 446
Hailey, W.H., 446
Hallopeau, H., 285
Hardaway, W.A., 172
Hereditary edema of the legs, 252
Hereditary hemorrhagic telangiectasia, 277
Herpes circinatus, 104
Herpes iris, 104
Hidrocystoma, 267
Hutchinson, J., 181, 205
Hutchinson's triad, 181
Hydroa aestivale, 183
Hydroa vacciniforme, 83
Hypertensive ulcer, 499

Icthyose noire cornée, 223
Ichthyosis, 13, 222
IgE bullous disease, 548
Impetigo contagiosa, 134
Impetigo herpetiformis, 112, 157
Incontinentia pigmenti, 422

Infectious eczematoid dermatitis, 329

Jacobi, E., 343
Jadassohn, J., 333
Jessner's lymphocytic infiltrate, 514
Jessner, Max, 512
Juvenile plantar dermatosis, 629

Kaposi, M., 164
Kaposi's varicelliform eruption, 170
Kawasaki's disease, 601
Kawasaki, Tomisaku, 599
Keloid, 34
Keloid of Alibert, 90
Keloid true, 90
Kératose pilaire blanche, 307
Kératose pilaire rouge, 307
Keratosis blennorrhagica, 255
Keratosis follicularis, 222, 398
Keratosis pilaris, 307
Kligman, Albert M., 563
Kossard, Steven, 636
Kraurosis vulvae, 191

Lane, C.G., 387
Larva currens, 535
Lawley, Thomas J., 632
Leiner, C., 351
Leiner's disease, 351
Lepra alphoides, 12
Lepra nigricans, 12
Lepra vulgaris, 10
Leucoderma acquisitum centrifugum, 386
Lever, Walter F., 509
Lichen annularis, 209
Lichen annulatus serpiginosus, 213
Lichen circumscriptus, 312
Lichen nitidus, 349
Lichen plan atrophique, 288
Lichen planus, 118
Lichen sclerosus et atrophicus, 287
Lichen scrofulosorum, 105
Lichen simplex chronique, 311
Lichen urticatus, 21, 183
Lichen variegatus, 315
Lingua nigra, 53
Lipschuetz, B., 379
Little, G., 181, 395
Livingood, Clarence S., 494

Localized elastolysis, 234
Lupus erythematosus, 64, 426
Lupus vulgaris, 31
Lyell, Alan, 529
Lyell syndrome, 530
Lymphocytic infiltration of the skin, 514

MacKie, Rona M., 628
MacKee, G., 270
Macula, 8
Macular atrophy, 335
Majocchi, D., 281
Mal de Meleda, 46
Malum perforans pedis, 71
McDonagh, J.E., 369
Mehregan, Amir H., 595
Melanoma, benign juvenile, 502
Melanosis and hypertrichosis, 490
Mibelli, V., 258
Mid-dermal elastolysis wrinkles, 541
Miliaria rubra, 458
Milroy, W.F., 251
Moeller-Barlow disease, 67
Moeller's glossitis, 67
Moeller, J.O.L., 67
Molluscum, 19
Molluscum contagiosum, 19
Monilethrix, 163
Morphea, 90
Multiple benign tumor-like new growths, 234
Multiple idiopathic hemorrhagic sarcoma, 167
Mycosis fungoides, 36
Myxadenitis labialis, 130

Necrobiosis lipoidica diabeticorum, 432
Necrobiotic xanthogranuloma, 639
Necrolytic migratory erythema, 490
Nélaton, A., 69
Netherton, Earl W., 556
Netherton's syndrome, 556
Nettleship, E., 127
Neumann, I., 158
Nevrodermites, 310
Neurodermatitis circumscripta, 310
Neurotic excoriations, 124
Neutrophilic dermatosis, 581
Nevoxantho-endothelioma, 369
Nevus araneus, 122
Nevus fusco-coeruleus ophthalmomaxillaris, 487

Nevus of Ota, 487
Nigrities, 53
Non-pigmenting fixed drug eruption, 544
Nummular eczema, 75

O'Brien, J.P., 455
O'Brien's granuloma, 460
Oculodermal melanocytosis, 485
Ofuji's disease, 614
Ofuji's papuloerythroderma, 614
Ofuji, Shigeo, 614
Orf, 434
Ota, Masao, 485

Pachyonychia congenita, 340
Paget, J., 138
Paget's disease, 140
Papula, 8
Papular acrodermatitis of childhood, 518
Papular urticaria, 21
Papuloerythroderma of Ofuji, 617
Papulo-vesicular aero-located syndrome, 518
Parakeratosis variegata, 315
Paraneoplastic pemphigus, 642
Parapsoriasis, 314
Parapsoriasis en gouttes, 315
Parapsoriasis en plaques, 315
Parapsoriasis lichenoides, 315
Parchment skin, 168
Parkes-Weber, F., 406
Parrot, J., 114
Pasini, Agostino, 466
Pautrier, 305
Peculiar progressive pigmentary disease, 359
Pediculoides ventricosus, 362
Pemphigus, 15, 426, 448, 451
Pemphigus erythematodes, 426
Pemphigus foliaceus, 61, 451
Pemphigus, paraneoplastic, 642
Pemphigus vegetans, 160
Periadenitis mucosa necrotica recurrens, 384
Pernet, G., 417
Perry, Harold O., 560
Peterkin, G.A.Grant, 434
Phialophora verrucosa, 387
Phlyzacium, 9
Pian fongoïde, 36
Pierini, Luigi E., 466
Piezogenic pedal papules, 540

Pigmented purpuric lichenoid dermatitis, 415
Pincer nails, 540
Pinkus, F., 347
Pityriasis, 52, 75, 93, 108
Pityriasis labrum, 52
Pityriasis pilaris, 75
Pityriasis rosea, 93
Pityriasis rubra, 108
Pityriasis rubra pilaris, 75
Plantar dermatosis, juvenile, 629
Plumbe, S., 54
Poikilodermia vascularis atrophicans, 343
Pollitzer, S., 237
Polymyositis, 196
Pompholyx diutinus, 15
Poncet, A., 279
Porokeratosis, 261
Porrigo, 57, 134
Pregnancy, PUPPP, 634
Pringle, J.J., 225
Progesterone dermatitis, 538
Prurigo, 106
Prurigo agria s. ferox, 107
Prurigo diathésique, 245
Prurigo of Hebra, 183, 245
Prurigo hiemalis, 147
Prurigo nodularis, 173
Pruritic urticarial papules and plaques of pregnancy
    (PUPPP), 634
Pseudo-colloid of the lips, 273
Pseudo-paralysis of Parrot, 114
Pseudopelade, 306
Pseudo-xanthoma elasticum, 397
Psoriasis, 9
Psorospermose folliculaire végétante, 395
Psydracium, 9
PUPPP, 634
Pusey,W.A., 321, 354
Purpura angioslereux prurigineux, 415
Purpura annularis telangiectodes, 283
Pustule, 9
Pyoderma gangrenosum, 475
Pyogenic granuloma, 280

Queyrat, L., 365
Quincke, H.I., 179
Quinquaud, C., 217

Radcliffe-Crocker, H., 198

Rash, 8
Rayer, P.F., 4, 49
Reactive perforating collagenosis, 597
Relapsing non-suppurative nodular panniculitis, 408
REM syndrome, 561
Rendu, H., 276
Rendu-Osler-Weber's disease, 276, 406
Reticular erythematous mucinosis, 561
Rhinoscleroma, 110
Riehl, G., 402
Riehl's melanosis, 404
Roberts, L., 210
Robinson, A.R., 266
Rosenbach, J.F., 192
Rosenthal, F., 54

Samman, Peter D., 576
Sarcoidosis, 296
Scab, 8
Scale, 8
Schamberg, J.F., 357
Schamberg's disease, 359
Schenck, B.R., 292
Schweninger, E., 233
Scleredema adultorum, 326
Sclerema neonatorum, 27
Sclérose atrophique, 346
Scrofulides érythémateuses, 82
Scurf, 8
Seborrheic dermatitis, 212
Seborrhoeal eczema, 212
Senear, F.E., 423
Sézary, Albert, 481
Sézary syndrome, 483
Shelley, Walter B., 533
Skin-bound, 27
Smith, W.G., 162
Sneddon, Bruce Ian, 521
Sneddon syndrome, 522
Sneddon-Wilkinson disease, 525
Solid edema, 185
Solomon, Lawrence, M., 606
Spitz nevus, 504
Spitz, Sophie, 502
Sporotrichosis, 292
Squama, 8
Stigma, 8
Stokes, J.H., 430
Strophulus pruriginosus, 183

Stulli, L., 46
Sturge-Weber-Kalischer's disease, 406
Subcornial pustular dermatosis, 527
Sulzberger, M.B., 436
Summer prurigo, 183
Sutton, R.L., 382
Sutton's nevus, 386
Sweet, R.D., 580
Sweet's syndrome, 581
Sycosis barbae, 24
Sycosis menti, 24
Symmetric erythema of the soles, 417
Symmetrical lividities of the soles, 417
Syphilid, 31

Talon noir, 570
Telangiectasia macularis eruptiva perstans, 406
Telogen effluvium, 565
Tinea capitis, 57
Toxic epidermal necrolysis, 530
Transient acantholytic dermatosis, 611
Trichoepithelioma, 249
Triple symptom complex, 444
Tropical anidrosis, 458
Tropical anidrotic asthenia, 458
Trousseau, A., 42
Tubercle, 8
Tuberculosis verrucosa cutis, 402
Tuberous sclerosis, 604

Ulcus vulvae acutum, 379
Underwood, M., 26
Unna, P.G., 210
Urbach, E., 430
Urticaria pigmentosa, 127
Usher, B., 423

Van Harlingen, A., 147
Verruca necrogenica, 95
Vesicle, 8
Vesicula, 8
Vidal, E., 254
Vieira, J.P., 451
Vitiligoidea, 86
Von Hebra, F., 99
Von Volkmann, R., 129

Wagner, E.L., 194
Walker, N., 329

Weary, Peyton E., 623
Weary's syndrome, 624
Weber-Christian's disease, 406
Weber-Cockayne syndrome, 406
Weber-Klippel syndrome, 406
Wegener, F., 478
Wegener's granulomatosis, 480
Wells, George C., 619
Wells' syndrome, 621
Wende, G., 354
Wheal, 8
White, J.C., 220
Wilkinson, Darrell S., 525
Wilks, S., 94
Willan, R., 3, 18
Wilson, E., 116
Winkelmann, Richard K., 636
Winkler, M., 390

Xanthogranuloma, necrobiotic, 639
Xanthoma, 86
Xeroderma pigmentosum, 168

Yellow nail syndrome, 578

T - #0052 - 101024 - C14 - 235/191/31 [33] - CB - 9781842142073 - Gloss Lamination